Sports Medicine

Sports Medicine

Edited by **Pablo De Souza**

Callisto Reference
New York

Published by Callisto Reference,
106 Park Avenue, Suite 200,
New York, NY 10016, USA
www.callistoreference.com

Sports Medicine
Edited by Pablo De Souza

International Standard Book Number: 978-1-63239-698-3 (Hardback)

Printed in China.

Contents

Preface

Every book is a source of knowledge and this one is no exception. The idea that led to the conceptualization of this book was the fact that the world is advancing rapidly; which makes it crucial to document the progress in every field. I am aware that a lot of data is already available, yet, there is a lot more to learn. Hence, I accepted the responsibility of editing this book and contributing my knowledge to the community.

This book provides comprehensive insights into the field of sports medicine. Sports medicine is a part of medical science that deals with treating and preventing injuries incurred while playing sports and the general physical fitness of the player. Every team or individual sports person has his or her own sport medicine specialist. These doctors treat injuries like ankle sprains, joint dislocations, tendonitis and osteoarthritis, etc. This field is rapidly progressing and therefore, this book has been complied in such a manner that it provides the readers with all the latest theories and advanced application in this area. It includes contributions of experts and scientists to help readers understand the subject better. Those with an eye for detail will find this text a highly beneficial source of knowledge.

While editing this book, I had multiple visions for it. Then I finally narrowed down to make every chapter a sole standing text explaining a particular topic, so that they can be used independently. However, the umbrella subject sinews them into a common theme. This makes the book a unique platform of knowledge.

I would like to give the major credit of this book to the experts from every corner of the world, who took the time to share their expertise with us. Also, I owe the completion of this book to the never-ending support of my family, who supported me throughout the project.

Editor

1

Measuring Dyspnea and Perceived Exertion in Healthy Adults and with Respiratory Disease: New Pictorial Scales

Paolo T. Pianosi[1*], Zhen Zhang[2], Paul Hernandez[4] and Marianne Huebner[3]

Abstract

Background: Dyspnea or perceived exertion during exercise is most commonly measured using Borg or visual analog scales, created for use in adults. In contrast, pictorial scales have been promoted for children due to skepticism concerning applicability of the said scales in pediatrics. We sought to validate our newly created, pictorial Dalhousie Dyspnea and Perceived Exertion Scales in adult populations and compare ratings with the Borg scale.

Methods: Dyspnea and perceived exertion ratings obtained with both modified Borg CR-10 and Dalhousie scales during maximal cycle exercise were compared in 24 healthy adults and 17 with various pulmonary disorders. Scale ratings for perceived exertion were plotted against work while ratings for dyspnea were plotted against ventilation using previously developed alternative models to simple power law. Goodness of fit was determined by lowest root-mean-square error or by corrected Akaike information criterion.

Results: Pictorial ratings of dyspnea and perceived exertion measured by both scale ratings rose as expected with increasing exercise intensity, and individual trajectories obtained by either scale were virtually superimposable in 90 % of subjects. In general, the lowest root-mean-square error or corrected Akaike information criterion was found with models which incorporated a time delay, defined as the fraction of maximum work or ventilation at which point a clear increase in ratings above resting level was reported.

Conclusions: The Dalhousie Dyspnea and Exertion Scales offer an equally good alternative to the Borg scale for measuring dyspnea and perceived exertion in adults.

Key Points

1. Dalhousie Dyspnea and Perceived Exertion Scales offer an alternative to Borg CR-10 scale in adults and were preferred by half our healthy subjects.
2. Most healthy subjects appear to have a lag or delay below which they report minimal changes in dyspnea or perceived exertion during incremental exercise, whereas most pulmonary patients do not, particularly for dyspnea.
3. Quadratic-delay model display improved fitting of observed trajectories of dyspnea perceived exertion during incremental, maximal exercise over simple power function.

* Correspondence: pianosi.paolo@mayo.edu
[1]Department of Pediatric and Adolescent Medicine, Mayo Clinic, 200 First St. SW, Rochester, MN 55905, USA
Full list of author information is available at the end of the article

Background

Dyspnea is defined as a subjective experience of breathing discomfort that consists of qualitatively distinct sensations that vary in intensity [1]. Several scales have been employed to measure task-specific dyspnea: the most commonly employed is the Borg scale and modifications thereof [2–4]; another is a visual analog scale (VAS) [5–7]. Both VAS and Borg scales were developed and studied in adults, and the Borg scale specifically was originally conceived to rate the distinct but related sensation of perceived exertion. It has undergone a few iterations from its original description but remains the principal tool for quantitating these sensations during exercise. Borg scale ratings for dyspnea and leg effort conform to a stimulus–perceptual sensation relationship defined by [8] the following: $S = kI^a$, where S is the magnitude of the particular sensation of interest (e.g., dyspnea), I the stimulus intensity, k a constant, and a the exponent, which lies somewhere between 1 and 2 in adults [2, 9].

We recently described mathematical modeling and perceived exertion ratings during incremental exercise to voluntary exhaustion in children and adolescents using the Borg scale [10]. We created an alternative scale for use in children and adolescents, Dalhousie pictorial scales [11], to measure dyspnea and perceived exertion during work requiring leg exercise such as cycling or running. We reported that the Dalhousie scales accurately track dyspnea and perceived exertion during a maximal exercise test in a pediatric population of individuals with and without respiratory disease [12]. Most recently, we demonstrated excellent correlations between ratings of dyspnea and ventilation, or perceived exertion and work intensity, during incremental exercise in children and adolescents [13]. We now report validation studies for our Dalhousie Dyspnea and Perceived Exertion Scales in adults, both healthy and with pulmonary disease, via three steps: (1) comparison with the current "gold standard," i.e., Borg scale (concurrent validity); (2) Dalhousie pictorial ratings of dyspnea should rise with increasing ventilation and of perceived exertion should rise with increasing work (content validity); and (3) determination that rating trajectories conformed to a power function (internal validity). We studied adult subjects in order to open the door for potential use in adults with language or comprehension obstacles that could impair ability to dyspnea and perceived exertion using scales employing written and numeric cues.

Methods

Participants

Healthy adult subjects were recruited from hospital personnel or their friends at the IWK Health Centre in Halifax, Canada. Adult pulmonary patients underwent progressive exercise testing prior to beginning pulmonary rehabilitation at the Queen Elizabeth II Health Centre in Halifax, Canada. The Research Ethics Board of the IWK Health Centre approved this study, and subjects signed informed consent. All procedures were conducted in accordance with the Helsinki declaration of 1975.

Procedures

Healthy adult subjects performed a maximal exercise test with step increments of either, 50, 100, or 150 kpm/min depending on a subject's size and age on an electrically braked Collins ergometer. Increments were chosen to achieve test duration of 8–12 min, until voluntary, symptom-limited exhaustion (maximum work capacity, Wmax). Ventilation and gas exchange were measured on the same apparatus (CPX Plus, WE Collins, Braintree MA, USA). Adults with pulmonary disease performed incremental, symptom-limited exercise tests on a cardiopulmonary test system (Vmax Series 229, SensorMedics Corporation, Yorba Linda, CA) on an electronically braked cycle ergometer (Lode Corival 400, Groningen, Holland). The initial exercise work rate was set at unloaded pedaling and was increased using a ramp protocol at a rate of 100 or 150 kpm/min, depending upon the subjects' self-reported functional exercise capacity. Tests were considered maximal in as much as subjects were encouraged to pedal to voluntary exhaustion or until the physician stopped the test for safety reasons.

Symptom Measurement

Each scale was mounted in front of the participant. The Dalhousie Dyspnea and Perceived Exertion Scales consist of a sequence of seven pictures depicting three dyspnea contructs: chest tightness, throat closure, and breathing effort, plus an additional pictorial scale to depict leg exertion/fatigue (Fig. 1). The research assistant gave participants an explanation of the pictorial scales at the outset as follows:

> The purpose of this test is to see how your breathing feels and how your legs feel during exercise. There is no right or wrong answer. The pictures in front of you show how your breathing might feel, from no difficulty at all, to the most difficulty you can imagine. You might feel this difficulty breathing in your chest or in your throat. Another scale simply asks you to tell us how hard it is to breathe – from nothing at all, to the hardest breathing imaginable. With the final set of pictures, tell us how your legs feel – from nothing at all, to the hardest imaginable. We will ask you the same using this other scale (pointing to the Borg CR-10).

Ratings using the pictorial scales at rest and during exercise were prompted by the questions:

> "How does your breathing feel?" or "How do your legs feel?"

While ratings using the Borg scale were prompted by the questions:

> "How hard is your breathing?" or "How tired are your legs?"

Ratings were recorded at each workload during the final 15–20 s of each work rate in the exercise tests on healthy controls but at rest and *every other* minute

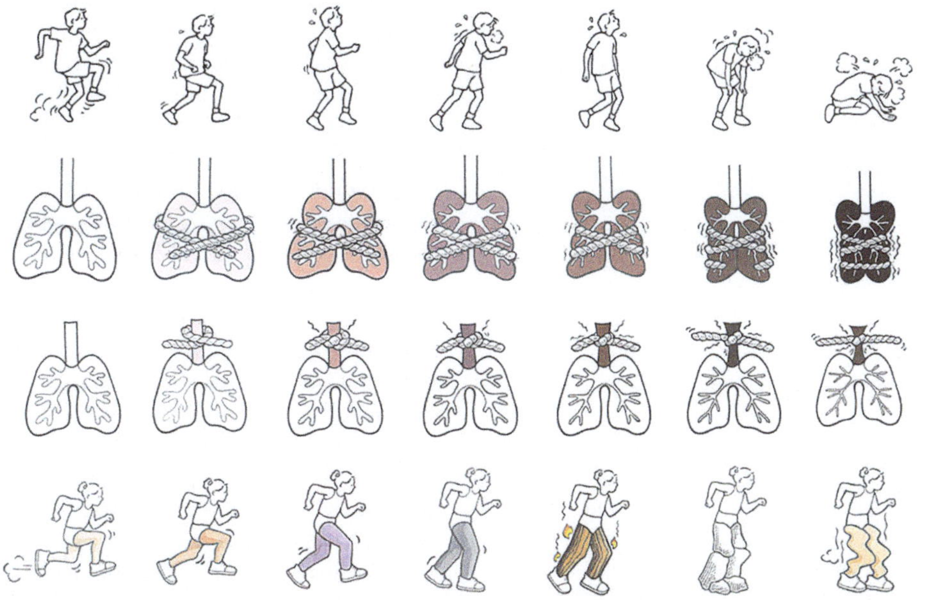

Fig. 1 Dalhousie Dyspnea and Perceived Exertion Scales. Each scale depicts specific construct with severity increasing from left to right. The top row depicts breathing effort; the second set of pictures depict the construct of chest constriction or tightness; the third row throat narrowing; whereas the bottom row depicts the perceived exertion scale (for predominantly leg exercise)

(alternating with blood pressure measurements) in pulmonary patients.

Analysis

Baseline characteristics were summarized as mean ± SD or median (interquartile range [IQR]). We report and compare perceived exertion using the Borg CR-10 and Dalhousie pictorial (leg fatigue) ratings, as well as dyspnea ratings using the Borg CR-10 and Dalhousie pictorial (breathing effort) scales for simplicity. Concurrent validation was done with the premise that Borg's scale is the gold standard. Dalhousie and Borg ratings were evaluated using canonical plots that compare actual ratings of one scale to the average ratings of the other scale at the same workload. Similar curves would indicate that ratings on one scale map well to the other scale. Internal validity was assessed by plotting dyspnea and perceived exertion ratings during increasing exercise intensity from measurements obtained using both Dalhousie and Borg scales and computing the mathematical stimulus–response relationship to determine the psychophysical function. For each individual subject, four models were defined with a delay or with a power term used to estimate a best fit mathematical model of leg fatigue or exertion vs work, and dyspnea—specifically, the breathing effort sub-scale—vs exercise ventilation (content validation). A delay was defined as %Wmax at which point a clear increase in ratings of leg symptom occurred or percentage of maximal ventilation at which dyspnea rating rose above resting level. A quadratic-delay model is defined as follows:

$$\mathrm{S} = a + b_1(I\text{–}d)^+ + b_2\left((I\text{–}d)^+\right)^2$$

where a is an adjustment factor, b_1 and b_2 coefficients of the linear and quadratic term, respectively, and d denotes the delay. The coefficients of these models were estimated with a quasi-Newton algorithm. We calculated root-mean-square error (RMSE) and the Akaike information criterion (AIC) for model assessment, where the preferred model is the one with the lowest RMSE or AIC. These analyses were performed using R version 3.1.0: R Core Team (2014) (R Foundation for Statistical Computing, Vienna, Austria).

Results

Anthropometric, spirometric, and maximal exercise data on all subjects are shown in Table 1. Diagnoses in pulmonary patients were as follows: chronic obstructive pulmonary disease (COPD) 8, asthma 3, lung cancer 2, interstitial respiratory disease 2, pulmonary embolism 1, and bronchiectasis 1. Unfortunately, sub-maximal gas exchange data on five (Fig. 2) pulmonary subjects were lost due to computer malfunction (COPD 3, ILD 1, bronchiectasis 1). Adults with respiratory disease were older than healthy controls ($p < .025$). There was a 50:50 split among subjects when asked about scale preference following the test.

Table 1 Subject characteristics and maximal exercise data (means ± SD)

	Healthy controls	Pulmonary patients
M:F	15:9	12:5
Age (years)	37 ± 16	54 ± 15
Height (cm)	173.5 ± 10	171.6 ± 7
Weight (kg)	70.3 ± 13.5	91.6 ± 24.3
FVC (L)	5.33 ± 1.24	3.23 ± 0.64
FEV_1 (L)	4.37 ± 0.94	2.09 ± 0.74
FEV_1/FVC	0·82 ± 0·04	0·64 ± 0·16
$\dot{V}O_2$ (%predicted)[a]	105 ± 15	69 ± 13
$\dot{V}O_2$ ($L \cdot min^{-1}$)	2.72 ± 1.01	1.53 ± 0.31
$\dot{V}_E$ ($L \cdot min^{-1}$)	113 ± 34	53 ± 10
$\dot{V}_E/35 \cdot FEV_1$	0·88 ± 0·28[a]	0·79 ± 0·24
Pulse (%predicted)	100 ± 6	80 ± 10

FVC forced vital capacity (L), *FEV_1* forced expired volume in first second (L), *$\dot{V}O_2$* oxygen uptake, *$\dot{V}_E$* ventilation

[a]peak $\dot{V}O_2$ = 0.046 (Ht) -0.021 (age) -0.62 (sex) -4.31 L/min peak pulse = 202 -0.72 (age), *after* [33]

Results of model fitting these data are shown in Table 2. Inclusion of a delay term improved model fit [10]. Overall, a quadratic model with a delay term offered the best fit of any power function ($exp = 2$) from the data obtained based on lowest RMSE or AIC criteria. Median and quartiles of parameters for the quadratic-delay model are shown in Table 3. Curves for each individual subjects showing dyspnea rating using each scale vs ventilation and perceived exertion vs work are shown in Fig. 2. Ratings obtained with the throat and chest sub-scales of the pictorial scales mirrored those obtained using the perceived effort of breathing scale and are not shown. Two features differentiated pulmonary patients from healthy controls. There was clearly a steeper trajectory for dyspnea vs ventilation and for perceived exertion vs workload (parameter b_1 in Table 3) for pulmonary patients than for healthy controls, regardless of which scale used; and there was a shorter delay between exercise onset and initial change from resting value (parameter d in Table 3) notwithstanding that healthy adults had more ratings (workloads) during

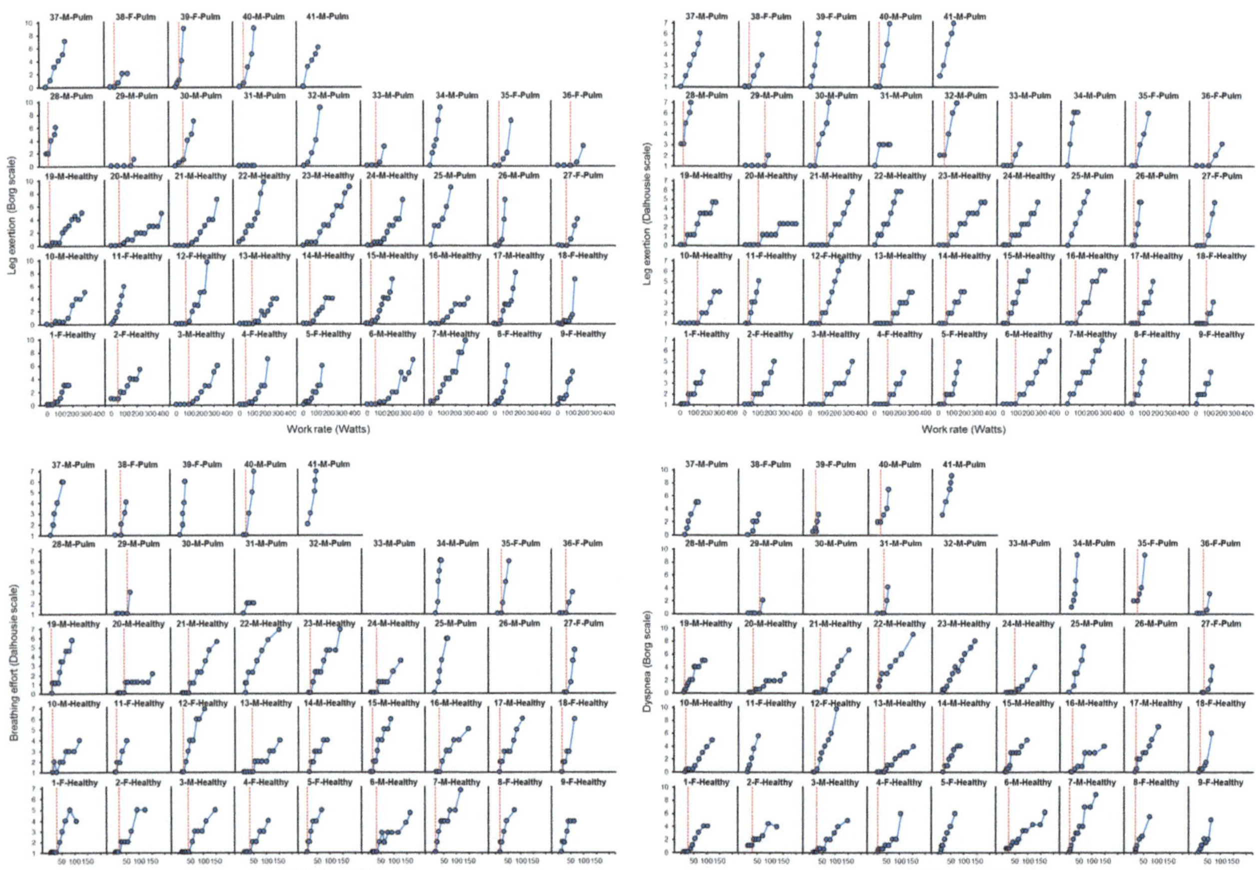

Fig. 2 Line plots of dyspnea ratings obtained with breathing effort sub-scale of the Dalhousie scales and Borg dyspnea rating for each individual subject, plotted vs ventilation; and of perceived leg exertion obtained by Dalhousie and Borg scales vs work. *Dashed red vertical lines* indicate delay ("d" term in Table 3). One can see a general upward trend during incremental exercise but with marked inter-individual variability irrespective of diagnosis

Table 2 Summary of model fitting

	Model	RMSE	AIC
Dalhousie legs vs W	Power	0.292	6.977
	Delay	0.245	−12.669
	Delay-power	0.247	6.454
	Delay-quadratic	0.196	−9.87
Borg leg fatigue vs W	Power	0.481	16.375
	Delay	0.418	−2.159
	Delay-power	0.395	15.809
	Delay-quadratic	0.344	−3.064
Dalhousie breathing effort vs $\dot{V}_E$	Power	0.337	11.145
	Delay	0.324	3.976
	Delay-power	0.264	8.805
	Delay-quadratic	0.237	−2.157
Borg dyspnea vs $\dot{V}_E$	Power	0.433	12.926
	Delay	0.352	−0.231
	Delay-power	0.295	9.901
	Delay-quadratic	0.269	−2.77

exercise. The variation in the delay terms was large among individual subjects across all scales, but the largest differences were observed in Borg exertion ratings between healthy adults and patients with pulmonary disease: for Borg leg exertion scale vs %Wmax, the median delay was 64 % [IQR 42–100] vs 24 % [IQR 0–60] of their respective Wmax (Table 3). Canonical plots in Fig. 3 demonstrate that ratings by respective scales mirrored each other very well at light to moderate exercise then diverged slightly at peak exercise, as there was slightly more variability when ratings obtained by both scales during heavy exercise were compared. In spite of the fact that Dalhousie ratings ranged from 1 to 7, while the Borg ratings ranged from 0 to 10, ratings clearly differed at peak exercise in only two subjects: nos. 1 and 13 for dyspnea or nos. 14 and 16 for perceived leg exertion.

Discussion

We demonstrated that dyspnea and perceived leg exertion ratings obtained using the Borg CR-10 scale closely tracked analogous ratings obtained using our Dalhousie scales in adult, rising more steeply in patients with pulmonary disease than in healthy controls but exponentially in both groups during incremental exercise. The coherence between measurements and similar trajectories obtained with either scale as exercise intensity grew implies that the Dalhousie pictorial scales can be used in adult populations with equal confidence and are arguably superior to the Borg scale in adults who have difficulty understanding the latter, e.g., patient 31.

We created the Dalhousie scales primarily as a tool to measure degree of dyspnea including the overall sense of breathing effort or discomfort and secondly perceived exertion with specific focus on the legs—the principal muscle groups involved in most ergometry systems. In his thesis, Borg stated the concept of overall perceived exertion could be regarded as a gestalt made up of perceptions from several important cues [3]. He later

Table 3 Estimated model parameters for quadratic-delay model

	Model parameters	Healthy	Pulmonary dis.
Dalhousie legs vs %Wmax	*a*	1 (1.0, 1.05)	1 (1, 1.05)
	*b*1	0.02 (0.02, 0.02)	0.05 (0.03, 0.08)
	*b*2	0 (0, 0)	0 (0, 0)
	d	40.7 (27.7, 81.1)	26.7 (5.7, 41.5)
Borg leg fatigue vs %Wmax	*a*	0.18 (0.02, 0.36)	0.19 (0, 0.25)
	*b*1	0.02 (0.02, 0.03)	0.04 (0, 0.06)
	*b*2	0 (0, 0)	0 (0, 0)
	d	63.9 (41.6, 105)	24 (0, 60.4)
Dalhousie breathing effort vs %max $\dot{V}_E$	*a*	1 (1, 1.15)	1 (1, 1.01)
	*b*1	0.06 (0.04, 0.11)	0.15 (0.08, 0.22)
	*b*2	0 (0, 0)	0 (0, 0)
	d	17.7 (14.9, 24.5)	23.7 (15.9, 29.8)
Borg dyspnea vs %max $\dot{V}_E$	*a*	0.03 (0, 0.21)	0.02 (0, 1.68)
	*b*1	0.07 (0.04, 0.11)	0.11 (0, 0.22)
	*b*2	0 (0, 0)	0 (0, 0.01)
	d	20.2 (16.4, 30.0)	24.7 (15.9, 41.9)

Shown as median (1st, 3rd quartiles) for ratings perceived exertion and dyspnea, using Borg CR-10 scale or using Dalhousie scales. Model: $S = a + b_1(I - d)^+ + b_2((I - d)^+)^2$

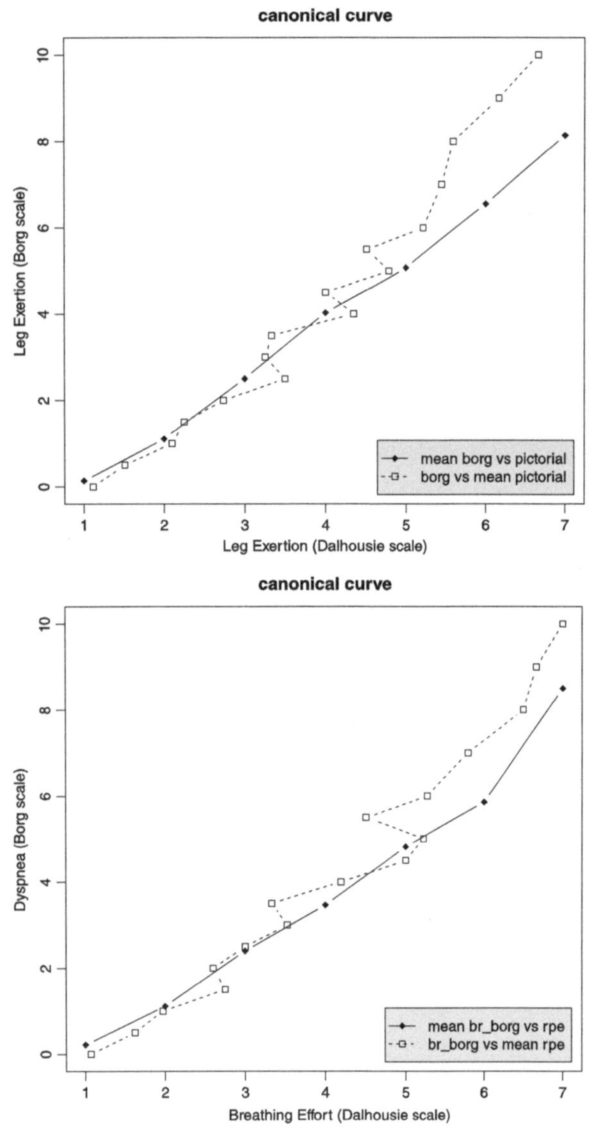

Fig. 3 Canonical plots comparing ratings made by each scale. For example, when Borg perceived exertion rating was 10, Dalhousie leg fatigue ratings averaged just under 7 (*dashed line*). Alternately, when subjects rated leg fatigue with the sixth picture on the Dalhousie scales, averaged Borg rating fell between 6 and 7 (*solid line*). Similarly, when Borg dyspnea rating was 10, Dalhousie leg fatigue ratings averaged 7. Alternately, when subjects rated dyspnea at the fifth picture of the Dalhousie scales, averaged Borg rating was approximately 5

developed a category (C) scale with ratio (R) properties by adding numbers along his line at specific distances and adding descriptive adjectives to this non-linear numeric scale [4]. We submit that our pictures serve as the equivalent of, or replace, the descriptive categories for subjects who cannot grasp these sometimes-subtle, quantitative semantics. We further speculate that they embody the "qualitatively distinct sensations" [1] and the gestalt made up of perceptions from several important cues [3]. The larger variability in ratings obtained by the two scales seen during heavy exercise in canonical plots could simply be due to the additional gradations of sensation available on a CR-10 scale, but these extras matter little if a subject cannot distinguish "very strong" (7) from "extremely strong" (10). Killian argued that the Borg CR-10 scale adheres to principles of an absolute scale with ratio properties [14]. The Dalhousie Dyspnea and Perceived Exertions Scales function at least as interval scales with perceptual anchors ("from nothing at all, to the hardest breathing imaginable"), and our findings confirm their ratio properties as well. The novel finding of this study was that ratings of dyspnea and leg exertion derived from either Borg or Dalhousie pictorial scale conformed better to a trajectory that includes a delay term than to the expected simple power function.

Borg found it necessary to include one and sometimes two extra basic constants in his original equation (for the absolute threshold, or describing basic "noise") [3, 4]. Borg and Kaijser ignored this delay term (eqtn.1 in their paper) [2], whereas Killian et al. noted thresholds in relative power output below which leg effort and dyspnea did not change appreciably from resting level [9]. This delay amounted to somewhere between 20 and 65 % (longest with Borg CR-10) of healthy subjects' Wmax and accounts for some of the variability in dyspnea and perceived exertion ratings. It was markedly different between our healthy subjects and those with respiratory disease (Table 3) but we did not seek matched controls for purposes of this study since our aims were to compare scales, not healthy controls vs patients. In general, trajectories rose quite steeply in pulmonary patients from the outset, markedly different than growth function(s) in healthy controls. A model that accounts for variable delays *and* variability in rate of rise will be intuitively superior to a simple power function. The delay model that includes a linear and a quadratic term had the lowest RMSE and AIC, though coefficients for the quadratic terms were small. While ratio scales in general function well empirically, alternative modeling of the sensory–perceptual function, specifically incorporating a delay term, can reduce inter-subject variability in ratings.

Dyspnea is a complex sensation that relies on mechanical, chemical, and cortical inputs and incorporates numerous sensations, with a common theme of an imbalance or inappropriateness between neural output to, and mechanical output from, the respiratory pump [15–18]. Clearly, one becomes more aware of one's breathing and the effort it requires as exercise becomes progressively harder or prolonged, but it does not become unpleasant or perceived as dyspnea so long as afferent signals from the respiratory apparatus remain in harmony with the efferent drive to the muscle(s) of breathing. This balance becomes upset by dynamic hyperinflation with exercise onset in patients with COPD or asthma in order to compensate for flow limitation [19–21] by low lung compliance coupled with flow limitation in ILD [22], whereas increased neural drive rather than mechanical ventilatory displacement appears to play a greater role in obesity [23]. Chemical stimuli arising from blood-gas abnormalities, particularly hypercapnia, both magnify and alter perceived dyspnea (and consequent affective response) [24], a common scenario in patients with respiratory disease. Patients with different disease processes tend to describe their sensation of dyspnea with typical descriptors [25–28]. Our pediatric focus group interviews during scale development differentiated the separate and distinguishable concepts of shortness of breath from increased breathing effort, prompting creation of the "breathing effort" sub-scale [2, 11]. There is now general agreement based on descriptor studies that perceptions of "work and effort," "air hunger or unsatisfied breaths," and "chest tightness" are separable qualities of dyspnea, and recent work suggests they are likely distinct [29]. In our study, all sub-scale (breathing effort, throat, or chest) ratings rose more or less in unison. We instructed subjects at the outset that their difficulty breathing might be perceived in the chest or throat, but we did not instruct them to choose one sensation or location over the other. "Descriptor" literature was a contemporaneous phenomenon during our scale development (1998) and work that elucidated mechanisms explaining separate but distinguishable types of dyspnea was only beginning when we conducted exercise tests. We demonstrated that dyspnea rose more steeply and to a greater extent in adults with pulmonary disease using our pictorial scales having receiving generic instructions. Future studies in this population can examine whether rephrasing instructions to patients prompts them to select one scale over another to describe their sensory-perceptual experience. For example, it seems intuitive that an asthmatic experiencing bronchoconstriction may select the chest constriction scale, but will a COPD patient be drawn toward the throat narrowing scale to convey a sense of or unsatisfied inhalation (a common descriptor offered by adolescents with exercise-induced glottic obstruction) while both gravitate toward the breathing effort scale to describe exercise hyperpnea?

This issue may pose a limitation on applicability of the Dalhousie dyspnea and perceived exertion scales. One could argue that only the breathing effort and perceived leg exertion pictorial scales are all that are required, although one hopes that localization of the site of perceived difficulty might permit separation of patients with different disorders. No patients with cardiac disease were tested in our study, and utility of the Dalhousie scale in this population cannot be presumed. The pathophysiologic bases of dyspnea and perceived exertion scale in this population are arguably more complex [29, 30]. On the other hand, recent studies have considered the multidimensional aspect of dyspnea [30] that comprises three major aspects: a sensory-perceptual domain and a symptom impact both in physical and affective terms. Sensory-perceptual dimension includes ratings of dyspnea intensity and its quality, i.e., "what breathing feels like." One might argue that there will be less precision differentiating perceived intensity levels denoted by solely by pictures without accompanying numbers. The pictorial nature of the Dalhousie scales implies de facto they are imbued with qualitative as well as quantitative information. It has been recently recognized that dyspnea, like pain, is a complex symptom with both sensory and affective domains, the latter thought to be processed in central limbic neural structures. Functional MRI has shown regions in the CNS where unpleasantness of perceived dyspnea is received, perceived, and processed [31, 32]. Furthermore, even verbal cues in the absence of any breathing load can evoke affective responses, which themselves are influenced by fatigue, anxiety, and somatic hypervigilance [32]. It is not unreasonable to presume that visual cues could do likewise, although we have no data for or against this notion. The Dalhousie pictorial scales were developed to quantify and discriminate qualitative aspects of the sensory perception of effort and difficulty associated with breathing in health and disease. Although the ratings are modulated by affective state in individual subjects, the pictorial scales were not developed to specifically assess the affective domain of dyspnea; further research would be necessary to develop pictorial scales to quantify the affective dimension of dyspnea. Finally, the perceived exertion scale is predicated on large-muscle, leg exercise—either treadmill or cycle ergometry. Arm cranking exercise is seldom performed in children (unless paraplegic), and thus, we convened no focus group to create the analogous arm-scale for this modality. Such would have to be created de novo if one wished to study perceived exertion with arm exercise. Such multiplicity of scales may render the entire pictorial concept unwieldy, but we believe this limitation will be more than compensated by the richness of information they yield.

Conclusions

We conclude the Dalhousie Dyspnea and Perceived Exertion Scales yield comparable results to the Borg CR-10 scale in measuring dyspnea and perceived leg exertion during bicycle exercise in healthy adults and in adults with pulmonary disease. We already demonstrated feasibility and reproducibility of using the Dalhousie scales in a population of Italian children running on a treadmill in the hope that the pictorial nature of the scales would obviate need for verbal descriptors that might limit scale comprehension in subjects with limited literacy or understanding [13]. By the same reasoning, the Dalhousie scales can now be employed in exercise testing of adults in whom a clinician might have similar concerns. Our modeling to the stimulus–perceptual function suggests additional advantages of the Dalhousie Dyspnea and Perceived Exertion Scales. Specifically, efficacy of measures aimed at reducing exertional dyspnea can now be gaged either by reduction in dyspnea at the same absolute work, lengthening of the delay before dyspnea rises above resting level, or alteration in trajectory of dyspnea during progressive exercise, after an intervention.

Competing interests
Paolo Pianosi, Paul Hernandez, Zhen Zhang, and Marianne Huebner each declare no conflict of interest.

Authors' contributions
PP created scales and conducted tests in healthy adults. PH conducted tests in adults with pulmonary disease. MH and ZZ conducted statistical analyses and generated plots. All authors read and approved the final manuscript.

Acknowledgements
Funded by Lung Association of Nova Scotia grant. Funding agency played no other role in conducting research or preparing manuscript. Authors express gratitude to, and acknowledge contributions of, Dr. Patrick McGrath who was instrumental in creation of the Dalhousie Dyspnea and Perceived Exertion Scales.

Author details
[1]Department of Pediatric and Adolescent Medicine, Mayo Clinic, 200 First St. SW, Rochester, MN 55905, USA. [2]Department of Statistics, University of Chicago, Eckhart 7 #5. 5734 S. University Avenue, Chicago, IL 60637, USA. [3]Department of Statistics and Probability, Michigan State University, 619 Red Cedar Rd, Rm C422 Wells Hall, East Lansing, MI 48824, USA. [4]Department of Medicine, Queen Elizabeth II Health Sciences Centre and Dalhousie University, 1796 Summer Street Halifax, Halifax B3H 4G2 NS, Canada.

References

1. American Thoracic Society. Dyspnea: mechanisms, assessment, and management: a consensus statement. Am J Respir Crit Care Med. 1999;159:321–40.
2. Borg E, Kaijser L. A comparison between three rating scales for perceived exertion and two different work tests. Scand J Med Sci Sports. 2006;16:57–69.
3. Borg G. Physical performance and perceived exertion. Studia Psychologica et Paedagogica (Series altera, Investigationes XI). Lund: Gleerup; 1962.
4. Borg GAV. A category scale with ratio properties for intermodal and interindividual comparisons. In: Geissler H-G, Petzold P, editors. Psychophysical Judgement and the Process of Perception. Berlin: VEB Deutscher Verlag der Wissenschaften; 1982. p. 25–34.
5. Adams L, Chronos N, Lane R, Guz A. The measurement of breathlessness induced in normal participants: validity of two scaling techniques. Clin Sci. 1985;69:7–16.
6. Harty HR, Heywood P, Adams L. (1993). Comparison between continuous and discrete measurements of breathlessness during exercise in normal participants using a visual analogue scale. Clin Sci. 1993;85:229–36.
7. Wilson RC, Jones PW. A comparison of the visual analogue scale and modified Borg scale for the measurement of dyspnea during exercise. Clin Sci. 1989;76:277–82.
8. Stevens SS. On the theory of scales of measurement. Science. 1946;103: 677–81.
9. Killian KJ, Summers E, Jones NL, Campbell EJM. Dyspnea and leg effort during incremental cycle ergometry. Am Rev Resp Dis. 1992;145:1339–45.
10. Huebner M, Zhang Z, McGrath PJ, Therneau T, Pianosi PT. Determination of the psychophysical function for Borg ratings of leg exertion during maximal cycle ergometer exercise in children and adolescents. BMC Medical Research Methodology [Internet]. 2014;14:4. http://www.biomedcentral.com/1471-2288/14/4. doi:10.1186/1471-2288-14-4.
11. McGrath PJ, Pianosi P, Unruh AM, Smith CP. Dalhousie Dyspnea Scales: construct and content validity of pictorial scales for measuring dyspnea. BMC Pediatr. 2014;5:33. doi:10.1186/1471-2431-5-33. Available from http://www.biomedcentral.com/1471-2431/5/33.
12. Pianosi PT, Huebner M, Zhang Z, McGrath PJ. Dalhousie dyspnea and perceived exertion scales: psychophysical properties in children and adolescents. Respir Physiol Neurobiol. 2014;199:34–40. doi:10.1016/j.resp.2014.04.003.
13. Pianosi PT, Huebner M, Zhang Z, Turchetta A, McGrath PJ. Dalhousie pictorial scales measuring dyspnea and perceived exertion during exercise in children and adolescents. Ann Am Thorac Soc. 2015;12:718–26. doi:10.1513/AnnalsATS.201410-477OC.
14. Killian KJ. Measurements of dyspnea during bronchoconstriction. Eur Respir J. 1999;13:943–6.
15. Mahler DA, O'Donnell DE. Recent Advances in dyspnea. CHEST. 2015;147:232–41.
16. Hudson AL, Laveneziana P. Do we "drive" dyspnoea? Eur Respir J. 2015;45:301–4.
17. Parshall MB, Schwartzstein RM, Adams L, Banzett RB, Manning HL, Bourbeau J, et al. An Official American Thoracic Society Statement: update on the mechanisms, assessment, and management of dyspnea. Am J Resp Crit Care Med. 2012;185:435–45.
18. Manning HL, Schwartzstein RM. Pathophysiology of dyspnea. New Engl J Med. 1995;333:1547–53.
19. O'Donnell DE, Webb KA. Exertional breathlessness in patients with chronic airflow limitation. Am Rev Respir Dis. 1993;148:1351–7.
20. Banzett RB, Dempsey JA, O'Donnell DE, Wamboldt MZ. Symptom perception and respiratory sensation in asthma. Am J Respir Crit Care Med. 2000;162:1178–82.
21. Binks AP, Moosavi SH, Banzett RB, Schwartzstein RM. "Tightness" sensation of asthma does not arise from work of breathing. Am J Respir Crit Care Med. 2002;165:78–82.
22. Marciniuk DD, Sridhar G, Clemens RE, Zintel TA, Gallagher CG. Lung volumes and expiratory flow limitation during exercise in interstitial lung disease. J Appl Physiol. 1994;77:963–73.
23. O'Donnell DE, Ciavaglia CE, Neder JA. When obesity and chronic obstructive pulmonary disease collide. Physiological and clinical consequences. Ann Am Thorac Soc. 2014;11:635–44.
24. Banzett RB, Pedersen SH, Schwartzstein RM, Lansing RW. The affective dimension of laboratory dyspnea: air hunger is more unpleasant than work/effort. Am J Respir Crit Care Med. 2008;177:1384–90.
25. Elliot MW, Adams L, Cockcroft A, MaCrae KD, Murphy K, Guz A. Language of breathlessness: use of verbal descriptors by patients with cardiorespiratory disease. Am Rev Resp Dis. 1991;144:826–32.
26. Harver A, Mahler DA, Schwartzstein RM, Baird JC. Descriptors of breathlessness in healthy individuals. CHEST. 2000;118:679–90.
27. Mahler DA, Harver A, Lentine T, Scott JA, Beck K, Schwartzstein RM. Descriptors of breathlessness in cardiorespiratory diseases. Am J Resp Crit Care Med. 1996;154:1357–63.
28. Simon PM, Schwartzstein RM, Weiss JW, Lahive K. Distinguishable sensations of breathlessness induced in normal nolunteers. Am Rev Respir Dis. 1989;140:1021–7.
29. Scano G, Innocenti-Bruni G, Stendardi L. Do obstructive and restrictive lung diseases share common underlying mechanisms of breathlessness? Respir Med. 2010;104:925–33.
30. Lansing RW, Gracely RH, Banzett RB. The multiple dimensions of dyspnea: review and hypotheses. Respir Physiol Neurobiol. 2009;167:53–60.
31. von Leupoldt A, Sommer T, Kegat S, Baumann HJ, Klose H, Dahme B, et al. The unpleasantness of perceived dyspnea is processed in the anterior insula and amygdala. Am J Respir Crit Care Med. 2008;177:1026–32.
32. Herigstad M, Hayen A, Evans E, Hardinge FM, Davies RJ, Wiech K, et al. Dyspnea-related cues engage the prefrontal cortex: evidence from functional brain imaging in COPD. CHEST. 2015;148:953–61.
33. Jones NL, Makrides L, Hitchcock C, Chypchar T, McCartney N. Normal Standards for an Incremental Progressive Cycle Ergometer Test 1–3. Am Rev of Respira Dis. 1985;131(5):700–708.

2

The efficacy of exercise in preventing injury in adult male football: a systematic review of randomised controlled trials

Tom Porter* and Alison Rushton

Abstract

Background: Injury prevention measures might reduce the impact of injury on footballers and football clubs. Increasing research has evaluated the use of exercise for injury prevention. However, research has focused on adolescent females. No high-quality systematic reviews have evaluated the efficacy of all forms of exercise on preventing injury in adult male football.

Objective: Our objective was to conduct a systematic review to evaluate the efficacy of exercise in preventing injury in adult male football.

Data sources: Comprehensive searches of electronic databases CINAHL (Cumulative Index to Nursing and Allied Health Literature), MEDLINE, Embase, AMED (The Allied and Complementary Medicine Database), the Cochrane Central Register of Controlled Trials, PEDro (The Physiotherapy Evidence Database), SPORTDiscus™, the National Research Register, Current Controlled Trials website (York), and http://www.ClinicalTrials.gov were conducted using predefined search terms to identify relevant studies published up to 1 March 2013. Screening of references, searches of grey literature, and hand searches of relevant journals were also employed.

Study selection: Included studies were randomized controlled trials using injury incidence as an outcome measure to evaluate the efficacy of an exercise intervention on uninjured male footballers aged 16 years and over. Articles not written in English were excluded.

Data extraction: Two researchers independently searched data sources, screened studies for eligibility, evaluated risk of bias, and extracted data using predefined criteria.

Study appraisal and synthesis methods: Risk of bias of included trials was assessed using the Cochrane Collaboration's tool for assessing risk of bias. There was insufficient trial comparability (outcome measures, interventions, injury type) for meta-analysis, and a qualitative analysis was performed.

Results: Eight trials ($n = 3{,}355$) from five countries met the inclusion criteria. All trials were assessed as having a high risk of bias. Two trials reported statistically significant reductions in hamstring injuries with eccentric exercise, and two reported statistically significant reductions in recurrent ankle sprains with proprioceptive exercise. Four trials showed no statistically significant difference in injury incidence with exercise interventions targeting a range of injuries.

Limitations: Notable limitations of included trials included poor reporting and limited blinding. A high risk of bias and insufficient comparability across trials prevented quantitative data synthesis.
(Continued on next page)

* Correspondence: tomporter_@hotmail.com
School of Sport, Exercise and Rehabilitation Sciences, College of Life and Environmental Sciences, University of Birmingham, Edgbaston, Birmingham B15 2TT, UK

(Continued from previous page)

Conclusions: Limitations in the context of study quality and heterogeneity resulted in an inability to reach a clear conclusion regarding efficacy of exercise for injury prevention in adult male football. Future low risk of bias, properly powered, and comprehensively reported trials are warranted to evaluate the efficacy of exercise on injury prevention. The use of eccentric hamstring exercise for hamstring injury prevention and proprioceptive training for recurrent ankle sprain prevention might be a good focus for future trials, as existing trials with a high risk of bias suggest an effect.

Key points

- The use of eccentric hamstring exercise may be efficacious in hamstring injury prevention.
- Proprioceptive training may be efficacious in recurrent ankle sprain prevention.
- A lack of high-quality randomised controlled trials of injury prevention in the adult male football population is contradictory to the number of publications on injury epidemiology and risk factors in this population.

Introduction

Rationale

Football (soccer) has been described as the world's most popular sport, with over 265 million registered players [1]. Injury is a major factor influencing player availability up to the highest level of the sport [2,3]. Top European clubs have a mean of 14% of a squad unavailable due to injury at any one time, with players experiencing a mean of two injuries a season [4,5]. This could have a significant impact on team performance and results [6], which in turn could have financial implications for clubs [7,8].

The impact of injury on footballers can be multifaceted. Injuries can result in a detraining effect, with loss of physiological adaptations and fitness, and may become psychological burdens for players [9,10]. Some injuries also have long-term implications, such as the risk of developing early-onset osteoarthritis [11]. This implies that injury prevention measures may benefit player well-being as well as enhancing a team's chance of success. Some clubs include exercises aimed at preventing injuries in their training [12].

There has recently been an increase in research evaluating the use of exercise to reduce the risk of injury to athletes. A number of studies demonstrate that neuromuscular training programs may reduce the risk of injury to females, particularly during adolescence [13-16]. A systematic literature review evaluating the prevention of non-contact anterior cruciate ligament (ACL) injuries with neuromuscular training in female athletes reported a prophylactic effect on injury incidence in all of the five included trials [17]. Interestingly, a meta-analysis evaluating the influence of exercise intervention on the risk of ACL injury in a range of sports included trials with participants of both genders and concluded that injury prevention exercises that include a proprioceptive neuromuscular training component may be more effective in males, reporting a risk reduction of 52% in females and 85% in males [18]. This meta-analysis included eight trials; only one trial (a non-randomized controlled trial evaluating the efficacy of proprioceptive exercise on ACL injury incidence in male footballers) included male participants [19]. The absence of randomization in this trial introduced a risk of selection bias [20], and the predominantly female cohorts evaluated in the review limit extrapolation of the findings to males.

Two systematic reviews evaluate the use of exercise for injury prevention specific to football. Both review the efficacy of interventions on players of all ages and either gender. Kirkendall and Dvorak [21] included trials evaluating any exercise-based intervention and concluded that both specific and generic exercise interventions are effective in preventing injuries. The review used these findings to inform the development of an exercise warm-up program. However, the validity of the findings is limited, as the review had several methodological limitations [22]. Notably, the literature search was inadequately reported, narrow search terms were used, only one database was searched, there were no clear eligibility criteria for study selection, and the risk of bias of included trials was not assessed [22,23]. These limitations limit confidence in the review findings.

The more recent review by van Beijsterveldt et al. [24] excluded trials using injury- or joint-specific exercises and reviewed the efficacy of generic exercise interventions. Contradicting evidence of efficacy of these interventions was attributed to differences in study samples, design, and compliance. Included trials focused predominantly on adolescent female footballers. Four of the six included trials investigated only female participants, and one trial included only male participants. Five of the trials assessed footballers under the age of 19 years.

The high proportion of injury-prevention research in adolescent females is likely to be due to their increased risk of severe injury, such as ACL rupture [25-27]. Also, the positive influence of neuromuscular training has been attributed to improvements in kinematics of movement, which may be more apparent in females due to gender-related differences in limb biomechanics, neuromuscular/strength imbalances, and hormonal influences [28-31]. These gender-related differences imply that injury-prevention research in female footballers may not be extrapolated to males. Males represent the largest group of participants in football, accounting for 90% of players internationally, and it has been reported that they may have an injury incidence similar to or higher than that of females [1,32,33]. There are currently no high-quality systematic reviews evaluating the efficacy of all forms of exercise intervention in reducing the risk of injury in adult male footballers.

Objectives

The objective of this systematic review is to evaluate the efficacy of exercise in preventing injury in adult male football.

Methods

This systematic review conforms to the Preferred Reporting Items for Systematic Reviews and Meta-Analyses (PRISMA) statement [22].

Protocol

This systematic review was completed according to predefined protocols that followed the method guidelines from the *Cochrane Handbook* [20] and the Centre for Reviews and Dissemination's *Guidance for Undertaking Reviews in Healthcare* [34].

Eligibility criteria

The following criteria were used to inform study selection, with reference to participants, interventions, comparators, outcomes, and study design (PICOS) [23,34].

Studies

Studies included were randomized controlled trials (RCTs) with at least one comparison group continuing with regular training. Limiting the comparison to regular training rather than non-exercise interventions allowed a pragmatic analysis of the efficacy of exercise used as an alteration or addition to regular training. Articles not written in English were excluded, rather than not included, to ensure that the risk of language bias could be assessed [35,36]. There were no restrictions on publication date up to 1 March 2013.

Participants

Male footballers competing at any level of adult football were included [37]. The age used for inclusion was 16 years, as adult teams often include players of this age [8,38-41]. This is also in accordance with the *FIFA Laws of the Game*, which are rules for players aged 16 and over and may be adjusted for those under 16 [37]. To ensure that the efficacy of exercise in injury prevention rather than rehabilitation was evaluated, only footballers uninjured at the start of a study were included. Mixed populations were included if there was a separate analysis of footballers meeting these criteria.

Interventions

Interventions were required to be exclusively exercise based. Studies assessing multiple interventions were included if there was a separate analysis of an exclusively exercise-based intervention.

Outcome measures

Included were outcome measures determining injury incidence. This could be a measure of injury rate or risk. Three often utilized measures of injury incidence are the incidence of injury per unit of athlete time (incidence rate), the number of injured athletes divided by the number of athletes at risk (epidemiologic incidence proportion), or the number of injuries divided by the number of athletes at risk (clinical incidence) [42].

Information sources

Electronic databases including CINAHL (Cumulative Index to Nursing and Allied Health Literature), MEDLINE, Embase, AMED (The Allied and Complementary Medicine Database), the Cochrane Central Register of Controlled Trials, PEDro (The Physiotherapy Evidence Database), SPORTDiscus™, the National Research Register, Current Controlled Trials website (York), and http://www.ClinicalTrials.gov were searched for relevant studies. The National Technical Information Service, System for Information on Grey Literature, and Index to Scientific and Technical Proceedings were searched for unpublished research [34]. All searches were conducted using sensitive search strategies to 1 March 2013.

Literature search

The search strategies were created by one reviewer and modified as required for each database. Table 1 demonstrates an example of search terms used. Screening of references listed in relevant systematic reviews and hand searches of journals that were the source of at least 10% of the relevant articles were also employed. The searches were performed independently by two reviewers.

Study selection

The two reviewers independently screened the title and abstract of all identified studies, assessing the studies for inclusion using the grades 'eligible', 'may be eligible', or 'not eligible' [43] for each criterion on a standardized form. Studies that did not meet the inclusion criteria were excluded. If a study could not be unequivocally excluded, if there was disagreement between reviewers, or if there was insufficient information in the title and abstract, the full text of the study was obtained. The full texts were

Table 1 Example of a search strategy (the Medline OvidSP search)

1	(Football* OR Soccer).ti,ab
2	exp FOOTBALL/
3	exp SOCCER/
4	1 OR 2 OR 3
5	(injur* OR ruptur* OR sprain* OR strain* OR disloc* OR accident* OR trauma* OR tendin* OR tendon* OR tear* OR fractur* OR break*).ti,ab
6	exp WOUNDS AND INJURIES/
7	exp RUPTURE/
8	exp SPRAINS AND STRAINS/
9	exp ACCIDENTS/
10	exp TENDINOPATHY/OR exp TENDON INJURIES/
11	exp ATHLETIC INJURIES/
12	exp SOFT TISSUE INJURIES/
13	exp KNEE INJURIES/
14	exp FRACTURES, BONE/
15	exp ANKLE INJURIES/
16	exp HIP INJURIES/
17	exp BACK INJURIES/
18	5 OR 6 OR 7 OR 8 OR 9 OR 10 OR 11 OR 12 OR 13 OR 14 OR 15 OR 16 OR 17
19	(exercis* OR neuromuscular OR proprio* OR strength* OR stretch* OR "warm-up" OR balance OR flexibility OR training OR intervention* OR kinesiotherapy OR program*).ti,ab
20	exp EXERCISE/OR exp EXERCISE MOVEMENT TECHNIQUES/OR exp EXERCISE THERAPY/OR exp PLYOMETRIC EXERCISE/
21	exp MUSCLE STRETCHING EXERCISES/OR exp PHYSICAL EDUCATION AND TRAINING/
22	19 OR 20 OR 21
23	(prevent* OR protect* OR risk* OR reduc* OR avoid* OR prehab* OR reccuren*).ti,ab
24	exp ACCIDENT PREVENTION/
25	exp RECURRENCE/
26	23 OR 24 OR 25
27	22 OR 26
28	(trial* OR random* OR control* OR rct).ti,ab
29	(trial* OR random* OR control* OR rct).pt
30	exp RANDOMIZED CONTROLLED TRIAL/
31	28 OR 29 OR 30
32	4 AND 18 AND 27
33	31 AND 32

independently reviewed, and a study was included if both reviewers were satisfied that it met the eligibility criteria. If there was disagreement between the reviewers, agreement was sought by consensus after consulting the protocol, with a third reviewer mediating in the event of on-going disagreement. The level of agreement between reviewers was evaluated using Cohen's weighted κ [44], and using the Landis and Koch criteria for interpretation [45].

Data collection process

Data from each included trial were independently extracted by the two reviewers using a standardized form based on the guidance in the *Cochrane Handbook* [20].

Data items

The extracted data included characteristics of the study and participants, details regarding interventions, outcome measures, duration until follow-up assessments, compliance, subject numbers, withdrawals, and intention to treat (ITT) analyses. For the purpose of this review, ITT analyses were defined as a complete assessment of outcomes of all randomized trial participants, regardless of withdrawal from the trial or adherence to the treatment regime [46]. This approach was taken because, without ITT analyses, there is potential for overoptimistic results of intervention efficacy [47].

Risk of bias in individual studies

The internal validity of the included trials was independently appraised by the two reviewers using the Cochrane Collaboration's tool for assessing risk of bias [20]. This tool was used as each of its domains is supported by empirical research, as is the use of the component rather than the scale approach [20,48]. This flexible, adaptive tool also fits well where the intervention cannot be blinded, as the potential influence of findings is considered in the appraisal. The reviewers used standardized forms to document each component of the risk-of-bias appraisal, and inter-observer agreement between reviewers was evaluated using Cohen's weighted κ [44], again using the Landis and Koch criteria for interpretation [45]. If reviewers disagreed, agreement was sought by consensus after consulting the Cochrane tool guidance [20], with a third reviewer mediating in the event of on-going disagreement. Risk-of-bias scores were summarized in line with Rushton et al. [49]. The study selection and risk of bias assessment processes were initially piloted by the two reviewers.

Summary measures

If feasible, a common measure of injury risk reduction would have been used to facilitate data synthesis across trials with similar interventions.

Synthesis of results

Comparability of interventions, outcomes and timing of assessments, and risk of bias were considered to determine potential for appropriate quantitative synthesis of the trials. If the trials were sufficiently comparable and had a low risk of bias, meta-analyses would be performed and if not, a qualitative data synthesis produced.

Risk of bias across studies

A summary of risk of bias across trials was tabulated, and the overall risk of bias was agreed by consensus. Differences in trial design, intervention, and outcome, and the inclusion of fewer than ten trials rendered it not helpful to produce a funnel plot to visualize potential publication bias [20,34].

Additional analyses

If at least two trials were available with comparable study design, interventions, and outcomes, subgroup analyses would have been used to examine the implications of heterogeneity.

Results

Study selection

Eight trials from five countries were included [12,50-56]. Database and hand searches provided a total of 1,942 citations. After removal of duplicates, 763 remained. Following screening of titles and abstracts, 744 studies were excluded as they did not meet the eligibility criteria. Of the remaining 19 studies, attempts to obtain the full texts of two unpublished studies were unsuccessful. The full texts of the remaining 17 studies were reviewed. Of these, nine did not meet the inclusion criteria. The study selection flow diagram shows the number of studies at each stage of selection (Figure 1). Using weighted κ, substantial inter-reviewer agreement was achieved on trial inclusion (Cohen κ 0.638, 95% confidence interval [CI] −0.003 to 1.280) [44,45]. Less than perfect agreement arose from the evaluation of one study due to the definition of injury. The study was included after discussion [51].

Trial characteristics

Methods

Five trials investigated an exercise intervention group compared to a control group [50-54]. Two trials assessed exercise or orthotic intervention groups compared with a control group [55,56]. One trial divided participants into high- or low-risk subgroups for specific injuries and assigned the high-risk players to either an injury-specific exercise intervention group or a control group [12]. All control groups continued with their usual warm-up and training. Table 2 shows the main characteristics of the included trials.

Participants

The eight trials included a total of 3,355 participants meeting the eligibility criteria. Five trials [50-54] and 2,647 participants had no reported history of injury or increased risk of injury; 200 participants with a history of injury were recruited in two trials [55,56]. A further trial included assessment of 388 participants reported to be at high risk of injury [12].

Interventions

A range of exercise interventions were used, including specific targeted muscle strengthening and/or stretching [50-52,55], proprioceptive exercise [55,56], and multi-faceted exercise intervention regimes [12,53,54]. Most trials used supervised exercise intervention as part of or in addition to regular training [12,50,51,53,54]. One trial used four supervised and then largely independent exercise sessions [52].

Outcomes

A range of injury types were assessed. Several trials investigated the incidence of specific injuries, including hamstring [50,52], ankle [55,56], Achilles and/or patellar tendon [51] or groin injuries [53]. Engebretsen et al. [12] assessed the incidence of injuries to the ankle, knee, groin, or hamstring, and van Beijsterveldt et al. [54] investigated all injuries.

Three trials reported a primary outcome on which a power calculation was based [50,53,54]. For each of these, the primary outcome was injury, defined as a physical complaint obtained during training or match play irrespective of the need for medical attention or time loss from football activities. This was also the main outcome of a further two trials [51,55]. The three remaining trials had a main outcome of time loss injuries, defined as an injury that results in a player missing training or match play [12,52,56].

Table 2 demonstrates that measures used for reporting injury incidence varied. The use of time until first injury [53] and total number of injured players rather than number of injuries in two trials [51,53] resulted in an inability to create a common measure of risk reduction for all of the trials. Several trials used further outcomes, including changes to athletic ability [52] and ultrasound assessment of structural changes to a tendon [51]. Other injury-related outcomes, such as severity of injury, were used by a number of trials [12,50,51,54].

Risk of bias within studies

Using weighted κ, moderate inter-reviewer agreement was achieved on evaluating trial risk of bias (Cohen κ 0.602, 95% CI 0.402–0.788), with 100% agreement following discussion [44,45]. All eight trials were evaluated as high risk of bias (Table 3), which impacts on the interpretation of results [20].

Results of individual studies

Two of the four trials reporting a statistically significant reduction in injury related to hamstrings. Each showed a significantly lower incidence of hamstring strain with eccentric exercise intervention. Petersen et al. [50] reported 3.8 acute hamstring injuries per 100 player seasons in the intervention group and 13.1 in the control group (rate

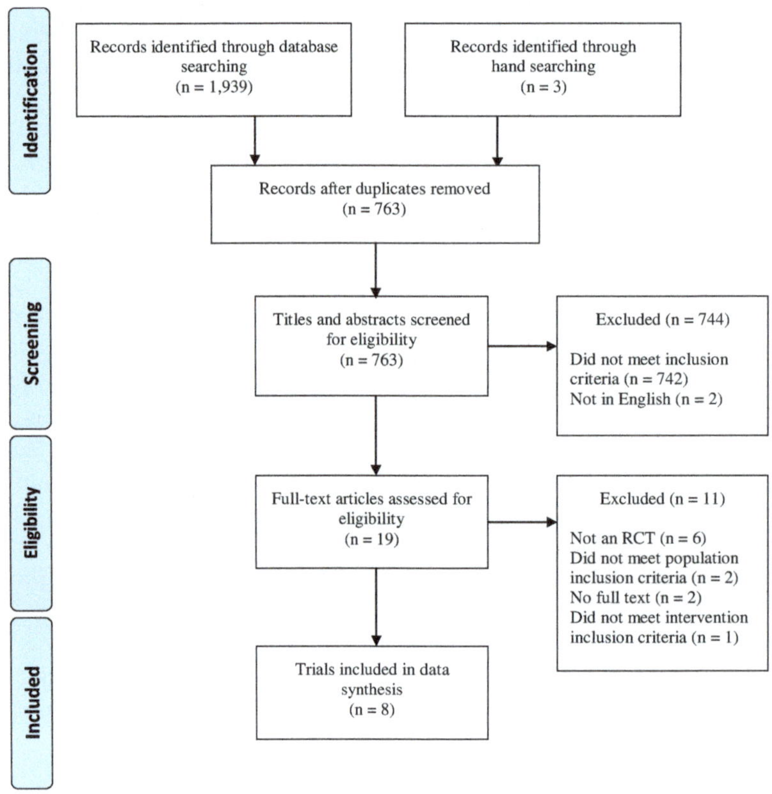

Figure 1 Study selection flow diagram [22].

ratio 0.292; 95% CI 0.136–0.631; $p < 0.001$); Askling et al. [52] reported 20% of players experienced hamstring injuries in the intervention group and 67% in the control group ($p < 0.05$).

Two of the four trials reporting a statistically significant reduction in injury related to ankle injuries in those with history of injury, with proprioception training [55,56]. Mohammadi [55] reported a reduced risk of re-injury in a proprioception training intervention group (relative risk of injury 0.13; 95% CI 0.003–0.93; $p = 0.02$) and no reduced risk in a strength training group (0.5; 95% CI 0.11–1.87; $p = 0.27$). Tropp et al. [56] showed that significantly fewer of the proprioception intervention group experienced re-injuries (5%) compared with the control group (25%) ($p < 0.01$).

Four trials showed no statistically significant difference in injury incidence between control and exercise intervention groups [12,51,53,54].

Synthesis of results

All trials were of high risk of bias and were not sufficiently homogenous for meta-analysis. When grouping trials according to injury type, two trials evaluated hamstring injuries, two trials evaluated ankle sprain re-injuries, and four trials were not comparable. No further analyses were conducted owing to differences in study design, intervention, and outcomes across the trials. The two hamstring trials used different interventions, duration of intervention period, and outcomes (injury definition), and also had differences in study design, notably with use of clustering [50,52]. The ankle trials were not comparable on intervention, outcomes (injury definition), and timing of outcomes [55,56]. A qualitative analysis was conducted.

Risk of bias across studies

Table 3 shows consistent components of risk of bias across the trials, including performance and detection bias due to inadequate blinding in all of the trials, and selection bias due to a lack of transparency regarding sequence generation in most trials [12,51,52,55,56] and of allocation concealment in all trials. There was a lack of blinding of outcome measurement, with evidence of injury registration being performed by personnel providing the intervention in all of the included trials in which the injury registration process is reported [12,50-54]. There were also issues regarding blinding of research staff, with staff visiting intervention groups during the study period in two of the trials [52,55]. Only one trial had a published protocol demonstrating pre-defined study goals [50], introducing a risk of selective reporting of outcomes in the other trials. Two trials were poorly reported, limiting accurate assessment of their internal validity [55,56]. A

Table 2 Summary of trial characteristics

References country	Primary outcome measure/means of reporting	Participants	Intervention	Follow-up period	Compliance	Effect of intervention (95% CI)	Conclusion	Comments
Askling et al. [52] Sweden	Time loss Injuries to the hamstring% Injury occurrence	IG: 15 CG: 15 Mean age IG: 24 CG: 26	10 weeks preseason intervention encompassing 16 sessions of hamstring training using concentric and eccentric actions, after a standardized warm-up	1 season of 10 months	NR	IG 20% CG 67% Significantly fewer injuries in the IG ($p < 0.05$)	Eccentric hamstring training may result in a lower occurrence of hamstring strains	High injury rate in the CG (67%) No loss to FU
Engebretsen et al. [12] Norway	Time loss Injuries to the ankle, knee, groin, or hamstring in high-risk players Mean injury Incidence per 1,000 h/RR)	High-risk players IG: 193 CG: 195 Mean age NR	Progressive exercise program for the ankle, knee, groin, and/or hamstring 3 × a week for 10 weeks then × 1 a week for the rest of the season	1 season of 7 months	19–30% during the preseason intervention	IG = 4.9 CG = 5.3 RR 0.93 (0.71–1.21) This was NS ($p = 0.50$)	The risk of injury in players deemed at higher risk was not changed with a targeted training program	19 of the 31 teams already performed preventive exercises in regular training ITT analysis conducted 3% players lost to FU
Fredberg et al. [51] Denmark	All injuries to the Achilles and/or patellar tendon% Injury risk/RD	IG: 98 CG: 146 Mean age 25	Eccentric exercise and stretching program of Achilles and patellar tendons All exercises performed for 10 min 3 times a week	12 months	2.25/week	Patella = RD 0% ($p = 1.0$) Achilles = RD 2% ($p = 0.86$) These were NS	Eccentric exercise had no positive effects on the risk of Achilles or patella tendon injury	CG 'allowed to continue with the different types of flexibility training that they all used' No ITT analysis 17% team withdrawn
Hölmich et al. [53] Denmark	All injuries to the groin Time to first groin injury/HR	IG: 524 CG: 453 Mean age IG: 24 CG: 25	6 exercises including hip adduction and abdominal strengthening, coordination and stretching, 2–4 times a week	1 season of 10 months	NR	HR 0.69 (0.40–1.19) This was NS ($p = 0.18$)	Intervention resulted in no significant reduction in groin injury risk	No ITT analysis Injured players censored 56% teams and 7% of remaining players withdrawn
Mohammadi [55] Unclear	All ankle inversion sprain re-injuries RR of injury per 1,000 h	Each IG: 20 CG: 20 Mean age 25	Progressive ankle disc training for 30 min daily (PT) Isometric and dynamic specific evertor strength training (ST).	1 season after injury	NR	PT – RR 0.13 (0.003–0.93) significantly fewer injuries in the IG ($p = 0.02$) ST – RR 0.5 (0.11–1.87) This was NS ($p = 0.27$)	Progressive ankle disc training may reduce the risk of recurrent ankle inversion injuries	Information on much of the study design is lacking No ITT analyses No loss to FU
Petersen et al. [50] Denmark	All hamstring injuries Injury rates per 100 player seasons/rate ratio	IG: 461 CG: 481 Mean age IG: 23 CG: 24	10 weeks of progressive eccentric hamstring training followed by a weekly program	1 season (2 half seasons over 12 months)	91% of the initial 27 sessions	IG 3.8 CG 13.1 Rate ratio 0.292 (0.136–0.631) Significantly fewer injuries in the IG ($p < 0.001$)	Additional eccentric hamstring training significantly reduced the risk of hamstring strain	No ITT analysis 7% teams and 8% of remaining players withdrawn
Tropp et al. [56] Sweden	Time loss ankle sprains in those with a history of sprain% Injury risk	CG: 75 IG: 65 Mean age NR	10 min of ankle disc training 5 times a week for 10 weeks. Then 5 min, 3 times a week	6 months	NR	IG 5% CG 25% Significantly fewer re-injuries in the IG ($p < 0.01$)	In players with a history of ankle sprain, ankle disc training is indicated to reduce the risk of re-injury	Information on key aspects of study design lacking No loss to FU
van Beijsterveldt et al. [54] Holland	All injury incidences Injury incidence per 1,000 sports h	IG: 223 CG: 233 Mean age IG: 24 CG: 25	10 exercises, used at each training session, 2/3 times a week. Included core stability, muscle strengthening, proprioceptive, stabilization and plyometric exercises	1 season of 9 months	71% player compliance	IG: 9.6 (8.4–11.0) CG: 9.7 (8.5–11.1) This was NS ($p > 0.05$)	No significant differences found in the overall injury incidence or injury severity between the IG and CG	No ITT analysis 6% players lost to FU

***CG* control group, *CI* confidence interval, *FU* follow-up, *HR* hazard risk, *IG* intervention group, *ITT* intention-to-treat analysis, *NR* not reported, *NS* not significant, *RD* risk difference, *RR* relative risk, *ST* strength training, *PT* proprioceptive training.**

Table 3 Summary of risk of bias scores [20], reported in line with Rushton et al. [49]

References	Components of risk of bias[a]						Overall	Comments, high-risk components
	1	2	3	4	5	6		
Askling et al. [52]	U	U	H	U	U	U	High 1 Unclear 5 Low 0	High-risk components: 1 No participant, intervention provider, or outcome assessor blinding
Engebretsen et al. [12]	U	U	H	L	U	U	High 1 Unclear 4 Low 1	High-risk components: 1 No participant, intervention provider, or outcome assessor blinding
Fredberg et al. [51]	U	U	H	U	U	U	High 1 Unclear 5 Low 0	High-risk components: 1 No participant, intervention provider, or outcome assessor blinding
Hölmich et al. [53]	L	U	H	U	U	L	High 1 Unclear 3 Low 2	High-risk components: 1 No participant, intervention provider, or outcome assessor blinding
Mohammadi [55]	U	U	U	L	U	H	High 1 Unclear 4 Low 1	High-risk components: 1 Inadequate reporting of many aspects of study design
Petersen et al. [50]	L	U	H	L	L	L	High 1 Unclear 1 Low 4	High-risk components: 1 No participant, intervention provider, or outcome assessor blinding
Tropp et al. [56]	U	U	U	L	U	H	High 1 Unclear 4 Low 1	High-risk components: 1 Inadequate reporting of many aspects of study design
van Beijsterveldt et al. [54]	L	U	H	L	U	U	High 1 Unclear 3 Low 2	High-risk components: 1 Insufficient participant, intervention provider, and outcome assessor blinding

[a]Components of risk of bias: 1, random sequence generation; 2, allocation concealment; 3, blinding of participants, personnel, and outcome assessors; 4, incomplete outcome data; 5, selective reporting; 6, other bias. Levels of risk of bias: H, high risk of bias; U, unclear risk of bias; L, low risk of bias.

number of trials did not present complete outcome data, using available case analyses rather than including all randomized participants. Three of the trials had full data on all randomized subjects [52,55,56] and one of the remaining trials conducted an ITT analysis [12]. A high rate of withdrawals introduced a risk of attrition bias to the trial by Hölmich et al. [53], and the reliability of several of the trials was impaired by low cohort sizes or evidence of insufficient power [50,52,55,56]. Compliance was poorly reported and, of the four trials in which compliance with at least part of the intervention is documented [12,50,51,54], lower compliance than pre-defined targets was reported in two [12,51].

Discussion

Summary of evidence

This systematic review evaluated the efficacy of exercise for injury prevention in adult male football. The eight included trials, with 3,355 participants, used a range of exercise interventions and outcome measures. Disappointingly, despite a number of trials being recent, all trials were assessed as having a high risk of bias. Four trials demonstrated statistically significant reductions in the incidence of injury: two relating to hamstring strains and two relating to recurrent ankle sprains. These findings are of interest, given that hamstring and ankle injury are two areas most prone to injury in footballers [5,57].

Hamstring strains are one of the most common injuries at professional football clubs, accounting for 12–16% of all injuries [5,39,58,59]. It is believed that they often occur during rapid eccentric loading when they are stretched beyond the optimal torque for generating tension, notably during sprinting [52,58,60]. It has been suggested that eccentric exercise increases this angle of optimal torque and may reduce the risk of injury [61-65]. There was some evidence demonstrating a reduction of the incidence of hamstring injury over the course of a season as an outcome of pre-season eccentric hamstring training, with two trials showing statistically significant reductions [50,52]. Although these findings are interesting, both trials were assessed as having a high risk of bias due to inadequate blinding, notably lacking blinding of staff registering injuries. The positive findings of these trials are consistent with those evaluating male athletes from different sports [66,67]; however, these trials are also of poor quality. These findings from trials with a high risk of bias demonstrate the need for an adequately powered trial with a low risk of bias to evaluate the efficacy of eccentric hamstring exercises on hamstring injury incidence. Future research should also consider whether participants have a history of injury, as both of the included trials demonstrated a reduction of hamstring injury recurrence with eccentric training [50,52]. Notably, Petersen et al. [50] demonstrated a significant reduction of approximately 85%. This is particularly relevant given that previous injury is the greatest risk factor for hamstring strain [68] and that re-injuries cause longer absences from sport [5].

History of injury is also a key risk factor for other football injuries [69,70], including ankle injuries, which account for 11% of injuries to footballers and have a high recurrence rate of up to 34% [38,71]. The high risk of recurrence has been associated with impaired sensorimotor function after injury in the form of proprioceptive deficits, such as muscle reaction timing [72]. Balancing exercises are purported to improve these deficits [73]. There was some evidence of reduced incidence of ankle sprain re-injury as an outcome of balancing exercises using an unstable surface, with two trials showing statistically significant reductions [55,56]. Although these findings are interesting, the trials were assessed as having a high risk of bias due to poor reporting. There is not sufficient evidence to reach a clear conclusion regarding the efficacy of proprioceptive training on ankle injury recurrence in adult male football. An adequately powered trial with a low risk of bias is required, particularly considering a recent meta-analysis including male and female, athletic and non-athletic populations that found no statistically significant difference in risk of ankle re-injury with proprioceptive training [74].

Four trials, each evaluating different injuries, were unable to provide evidence of efficacy of exercise intervention for injury prevention, with each reporting no statistically significant benefit. One of these trials identified footballers at increased risk of injury, but the targeted exercise intervention did not reduce the incidence of common football injuries [12]. A major limitation of this trial was low compliance with the intervention (19–30%), which increased the risk of type II error. Groin injuries are common in football and can lead to prolonged periods away from play, hence a program to reduce the risk of groin injury could be of great benefit to football clubs [40]. However, the trial by Hölmich et al. [53] that evaluated a groin injury prevention program also showed no statistically significant effect on injury incidence. One further trial did not provide support for the prophylactic use of eccentric exercise for preventing Achilles or patellar tendon injuries [51], despite some evidence supporting the use of eccentric exercise for the treatment of tendon injuries [75]. A further finding was that a general injury prevention program evaluated in the trial by van Beijsterveldt et al. [54], which included a range of exercises in the form of a warm-up, did not show statistically significant effects on injury incidence over a season. Their finding of no effect on overall injury incidence was similar to the findings of trials using the same program, 'The 11' or the modified version 'The 11+' in adolescent female football players [76,77].

The key finding of this review is that, based on the current level of evidence, it is not possible to evaluate whether exercise is efficacious in the prevention of injuries in adult male football. A lack of high-quality RCTs of injury prevention in the adult male football population is contradictory to the number of publications on injury epidemiology and risk factors in this population. The findings are similar to those of van Beijsterveldt et al. [24], who reviewed general exercise programs for injury prevention in footballers, finding conflicting and weak evidence to support their use. However, the findings are in contrast to the systematic review by Kirkendall and Dvorak [21], which uses findings, including those from studies with male participants, to support the use of a range of exercises in an injury-prevention program. The latter review demonstrates a number of methodological flaws; hence, the findings must be extrapolated with caution. Findings of this review also contrast with those in adolescent female footballers, where positive effects of neuromuscular exercise programs on injury incidence have been found [17]. This could be due to a number of reasons, including a difference in the intervention type or compliance, or a disparity in the quantity and quality of research. It could also be due to age- or sex-related differences in study participants [28,29]. It is possible that neuromuscular programs are more effective in reducing the risk of injury in female footballers because they address neuromuscular imbalances and movement patterns that have been associated with an increased risk of severe injury, such as ACL rupture, in females [28,78]. Corresponding with this, it has been suggested that programs designed to target gender-related differences in injury risk and incidence may be warranted [28].

Two definitions of injury were used by the trials, either 'any injury' or 'time loss injury', both of which correspond with those recommended by the consensus statement published in 2006 by Fuller et al. [79]. Consensus should be found regarding the use of specific outcome measures, such as injury definition, which would allow the use of data pooling in the future. Wider reporting of injury severity and duration of time loss from football would also benefit future research in this field, allowing the impact of injuries to be assessed. Also, incidence of adverse effects should be more widely reported, as demonstrated by the findings of Fredberg et al. [51] where, contrary to expectation, eccentric exercise increased patella tendon injury incidence in footballers with degenerate tendons.

Strengths and limitations

Strengths of this review are its rigorous methodology based on a pre-defined protocol. Its main limitation was the finding of poor reporting of included trials and high risk of bias components. These findings are particularly disappointing considering a number of trials were published after the Consolidated Standards of Reporting Trials (CONSORT) statement, which supports explicit reporting of trials [80,81]. High risk of bias components included randomization and concealment of allocation, processes that, if inadequately performed, may lead to an overestimation of treatment effect [82,83]. The nature of the interventions may preclude blinding of the participants; however, this also introduced a risk of bias, particularly with the use of subjective measures such as self-reporting of injury [84] as used in the trials by Askling et al. [52] and Fredberg et al. [51]. There was also little evidence of predefined outcomes, partly due to a lack of published protocols. Issues relating to compliance are also notable, as direct correlations between compliance and the efficacy of injury prevention programs have been found [85].

Using GRADE [86] (the Grading of Recommendations Assessment, Development and Evaluation system), based on the eight trials included in the qualitative synthesis, the quality of evidence evaluating the efficacy of exercise intervention on injury prevention in adult male football was 'very low'. This level of evidence is defined as "very little confidence in the effect estimate: the true effect is likely to be substantially different from the estimate of effect" [86]. The quality of evidence was downgraded due to high risk of bias, inconsistent results, indirectness of evidence, and imprecision [86].

Conclusions

This rigorous systematic review has identified very low-quality evidence on the efficacy of exercise on prevention of injuries in adult male football. There is some support for the use of eccentric hamstring exercise for hamstring injury prevention and proprioceptive training to reduce the incidence of recurrent ankle sprains; however, sufficient evidence is lacking to reach a clear conclusion regarding their efficacy. There is a need for low risk of bias, comprehensively reported and properly powered trials evaluating the efficacy of generic and specific exercise interventions for injury prevention. Notable areas of future research may relate to the prevention of ankle and hamstring injuries. Future research should also be considered regarding the efficacy of exercise in preventing groin injuries and knee sprains, for these are also major injury burdens in male adult football and lack high-quality trials evaluating efficacy of preventive interventions [4,5,12,69].

Acknowledgments

Tom Porter and Dr Alison Rushton declare that they have no conflicts of interest. The authors gratefully acknowledge the assistance of reviewer David Hunt for his contributions. No financial support was received for the conduct of this study or preparation of this manuscript.

References

1. FIFA. FIFA Big Count 2006: 270 million people active in football. FIFA, Zurich. 2008. http://www.fifa.com/mm/document/fifafacts/bcoffsurv/bigcount.statspackage_7024.pdf. Accessed 16 Feb 2013.
2. Parry L, Drust B. **Is injury the major cause of elite soccer players being unavailable to train and play during the competitive season?** *Phys Ther Sport.* 2006; **7(2)**:58–64.
3. Schmikli SL, Backx FJ, Kemler HJ, van Mechelen W. **National survey on sports injuries in the Netherlands: target populations for sports injury prevention programs.** *Clin J Sports Med.* 2009; **19(2)**:101–06.
4. Ekstrand J, Hägglund M, Kristenson K, Magnusson H, Waldén M. Fewer ligament injuries but no preventive effect on muscle injuries and severe injuries: an 11-year follow-up of the UEFA Champions League injury study. Br J Sports Med. 2013. doi:10.1136/bjsports-2013-092394.
5. Ekstrand J, Hägglund M, Waldén M. **Injury incidence and injury patterns in professional football: the UEFA injury study.** *Br J Sports Med.* 2011; **45(7)**:553–58.
6. Hägglund M, Waldén M, Magnusson H, Kristenson K, Bengtsson H, Ekstrand J. Injuries affect team performance negatively in professional football: an 11-year follow-up of the UEFA Champions League injury study. Br J Sports Med. 2013. doi:10.1136/bjsports-2013-092215.
7. van Beijsterveldt AMC, Krist MR, Schmikli SL, Stubbe JH, de Wit GA, Inklaar H, et al. Effectiveness and cost-effectiveness of an injury prevention programme for adult male amateur soccer players: design of a cluster-randomised controlled trial. Inj Prev. 2011. doi:10.1136/ip.2010.027979.
8. Woods C, Hawkins R, Hulse M, Hodson A. **The football association medical research programme: an audit of injuries in professional football—analysis of preseason injuries.** *Br J Sports Med.* 2002; **36(6)**:436–41.
9. Appaneal RN, Levine BR, Perna FM, Roh JL. **Measuring postinjury depression among male and female competitive athletes.** *J Sport Exerc Psychol.* 2009; **31(1)**:60–76.
10. Mujika I, Padilla S. **Detraining: loss of training-induced physiological and performance adaptations. Part II: long term insufficient training stimulus.** *Sports Med.* 2000; **30(3)**:145–54.
11. Myklebust G, Bahr R. **Return to play guidelines after anterior cruciate ligament surgery.** *Br J Sports Med.* 2005; **39(3)**:127–31.
12. Engebretsen AH, Myklebust G, Holme I, Engebretsen L, Bahr R. **Prevention of injuries among male soccer players: a prospective, randomized intervention study targeting players with previous injuries or reduced function.** *Am J Sports Med.* 2008; **36(6)**:1052–60.
13. Hewett TE, Lindenfeld TN, Riccobene JV, Noyes FR. **The effect of neuromuscular training on the incidence of knee injury in female athletes. A prospective study.** *Am J Sports Med.* 1999; **27(6)**:699–706.
14. Mandelbaum BR, Silvers HJ, Watanabe DS, Knarr JF, Thomas SD, Griffin LY, et al. **Effectiveness of a neuromuscular and proprioceptive training program in preventing anterior cruciate ligament Injuries in female athletes.** *Am J Sports Med.* 2005; **33(7)**:1003–10.
15. Heidt RS, Sweeterman LM, Carlonas RL, Traub JA, Tekulve FX. **Avoidance of soccer injuries with preseason conditioning.** *Am J Sports Med.* 2000; **28(5)**:659–62.
16. Gilchrist J, Mandelbaum BR, Melancon H, Ryan GW, Silvers HJ, Griffin LY, et al. **A randomized controlled trial to prevent noncontact anterior cruciate ligament injury in female collegiate soccer players.** *Am J Sports Med.* 2008; **36(8)**:1476–83.
17. Grindstaff TL, Hammill RR, Tuzson AE, Hertel J. **Neuromuscular control training programs and noncontact anterior cruciate ligament injury rates in female athletes: a numbers-needed-to-treat analysis.** *J Athl Train.* 2006; **41(4)**:450–56.
18. Sadoghi P, von Keudell A, Vavken P. **Effectiveness of anterior cruciate ligament injury prevention training programs.** *J Bone Jt Surg Am.* 2012; **94(9)**:769–76.
19. Caraffa A, Cerulli G, Projetti M, Aisa G, Rizzo A. **Prevention of anterior cruciate ligament injuries in soccer. A prospective controlled study of proprioceptive training.** *Knee Surg Sports Traumatol Arthrosc.* 1996; **4(1)**:19–21.
20. Higgins J, Green S. Cochrane handbook for systematic reviews of interventions version 5.0.2 [updated September 2009]. The Cochrane Collaboration. 2009. http://www.cochrane-handbook.org. Accessed 31 March 2013.
21. Kirkendall DT, Dvorak J. **Effective injury prevention in soccer.** *Phys Sportsmed.* 2010; **38(1)**:147–57.
22. Moher D, Liberati A, Tetzlaff J, Altman DG. Preferred reporting items for systematic reviews and meta-analyses: the PRISMA statement. BMJ. 2009. doi:10.1136/bmj.b2535.
23. Liberati A, Altman DG, Tetzlaff J, Mulrow C, Gøtzsche PC, Ioannidis JPA, et al. The PRISMA statement for reporting systematic reviews and meta-analyses of studies that evaluate healthcare interventions: explanation and elaboration. BMJ. 2009. doi:10.1136/bmj.b2700.
24. van Beijsterveldt AMC, Horst N, Port IL, Backx FJ. **How effective are exercise-based injury prevention programmes for soccer players?** *Sports Med.* 2013; **43(4)**:257–65.
25. Prodromos CC, Han Y, Rogowski J, Joyce B, Shi K. **A meta-analysis of the incidence of anterior cruciate ligament tears as a function of gender, sport, and a knee injury-reduction regimen.** *Arthroscopy.* 2007; **23(12)**:1320–25.
26. Waldén M, Hägglund M, Werner J, Ekstrand J. **The epidemiology of anterior cruciate ligament injury in football (soccer): a review of the literature from a gender-related perspective.** *Knee Surg Sports Traumatol Arthrosc.* 2011; **19(1)**:3–10.

27. Arendt EA, Agel J, Dick R. **Anterior cruciate ligament injury patterns among collegiate men and women.** *J Athl Train.* 1999; **34(2)**:86–92.
28. Hewett TE, Ford KR, Hoogenboom BJ, Myer GD. **Understanding and preventing ACL injuries: current biomechanical and epidemiologic considerations—update 2010.** *N Am J Sports Phys Ther.* 2010; **5(4)**:234–51.
29. Alentorn-Geli E, Myer GD, Silvers HJ, Samitier G, Romero D, Lazaro-Haro C, et al. **Prevention of non-contact anterior cruciate ligament injuries in soccer players. Part 1: mechanisms of injury and underlying risk factors.** *Knee Surg Sports Traumatol Arthrosc.* 2009; **17(7)**:705–29.
30. Smith HC, Vacek P, Johnson RJ, Slauterbeck JR, Hashemi J, Shultz S, et al. **Risk factors for anterior cruciate ligament injury: a review of the literature: part 2: hormonal, genetic, cognitive function, previous injury, and extrinsic risk factors.** *Sports Health.* 2012; **4(2)**:155–61.
31. Smith HC, Vacek P, Johnson RJ, Slauterbeck JR, Hashemi J, Shultz S, et al. **Risk factors for anterior cruciate ligament injury: a review of the literature: part 1: neuromuscular and anatomic risk.** *Sports Health.* 2012; **4(1)**:69–78.
32. Hagglund M, Walden M, Ekstrand J. **Injuries among male and female elite football players.** *Scand J Med Sci Sports.* 2009; **19(6)**:819–27.
33. Junge A, Dvorak J. Injury surveillance in the world football tournaments 1998–2012. Br J Sports Med. 2013. doi:10.1136/bjsports-2013-092205.
34. Tacconelli E. **Systematic reviews: CRD's guidance for undertaking reviews in health care.** *Lancet Infect Dis.* 2010; **10(4)**:226.
35. Egger M, Zellweger-Zähner T, Schneider M, Junker C, Lengeler C, Antes G. **Language bias in randomised controlled trials published in English and German.** *Lancet.* 1997; **350(9074)**:326–29.
36. Vickers A, Goyal N, Harland R, Rees R. **Do certain countries produce only positive results? A systematic review of controlled trials.** *Control Clin Trials.* 1998; **19(2)**:159–66.
37. FIFA. Laws of the Game 2013/2014. FIFA, Zurich. 2013. http://www.fifa.com/mm/document/footballdevelopment/refereeing/81/42/36/log2013en_neutral.pdf. Accessed 09 Oct 2013.
38. Woods C, Hawkins R, Hulse M, Hodson A. **The football association medical research programme: an audit of injuries in professional football: an analysis of ankle sprains.** *Br J Sports Med.* 2003; **37(3)**:233–38.
39. Hawkins RD, Hulse MA, Wilkinson C, Hodson A, Gibson M. **The association football medical research programme: an audit of injuries in professional football.** *Br J Sports Med.* 2001; **35(1)**:43–7.
40. Werner J, Hägglund M, Waldén M, Ekstrand J. **UEFA injury study: a prospective study of hip and groin injuries in professional football over seven consecutive seasons.** *Br J Sports Med.* 2009; **43(13)**:1036–40.
41. Ekstrand J, Hagglund M, Walden M. **Epidemiology of muscle injuries in professional football (soccer).** *Am J Sports Med.* 2011; **39(6)**:1226–32.
42. Knowles SB, Marshall SW, Guskiewicz KM. **Issues in estimating risks and rates in sports injury research.** *J Athl Train.* 2006; **41(2)**:207–15.
43. Furlan AD, Pennick V, Bombardier C, van Tulder M. **2009 updated method guidelines for systematic reviews in the Cochrane Back Review Group.** *Spine.* 2009; **34(18)**:1929–41.
44. Cohen J. **A coefficient of agreement for nominal scales.** *Educ Psychol Meas.* 1960; **20(1)**:37–46.
45. Landis JR, Koch GG. **The measurement of observer agreement for categorical data.** *Biometrics.* 1977; **33(1)**:159–74.
46. Fisher L, Dixon D, Herson J, Frankwski R, Hearron M, Peace K. **Intention to treat in clinical trials.** In: Peace K, editor. *Statistical issues in drug research and development.* New York: Marcel Dekker; 1990: p. 331–50.
47. Heritier SR, Gebski VJ, Keech AC. **Inclusion of patients in clinical trial analysis: the intention-to-treat principle.** *Med J Aust.* 2003; **179(8)**:438–40.
48. Jüni P, Witschi A, Bloch R, Egger M. **The hazards of scoring the quality of clinical trials for meta-analysis.** *JAMA.* 1999; **282(11)**:1054–60.
49. Rushton A, Wright C, Heneghan N, Eveleigh G, Calvert M, Freemantle N. Physiotherapy rehabilitation for whiplash associated disorder II: a systematic review and meta-analysis of randomised controlled trials. BMJ. 2011. doi:10.1136/bmjopen-2011-000265.
50. Petersen J, Thorborg K, Nielsen MB, Budtz-Jorgensen E, Holmich P. **Preventive effect of eccentric training on acute hamstring injuries in men's soccer: a cluster-randomized controlled trial.** *Am J Sports Med.* 2011; **39(11)**:2296–303.
51. Fredberg U, Bolvig L, Andersen NT. **Prophylactic training in asymptomatic soccer players with ultrasonographic abnormalities in Achilles and patellar tendons: the Danish Super League Study.** *Am J Sports Med.* 2008; **36(3)**:451–60.
52. Askling C, Karlsson J, Thorstensson A. **Hamstring injury occurrence in elite soccer players after preseason strength training with eccentric overload.** *Scand J Med Sci Sports.* 2003; **13(4)**:244–50.
53. Hölmich H, Larsen P, Krogsgaard K, Gluud C. **Exercise program for prevention of groin pain in football players: a cluster randomized trial.** *Scand J Med Sci Sports.* 2010; **20(6)**:814–21.
54. van Beijsterveldt AMC, van de Port IGL, Krist MR, Schmikli SL, Stubbe JH, Frederiks JE, et al. Effectiveness of an injury prevention programme for adult male amateur soccer players: a cluster-randomised controlled trial. Br J Sports Med. 2012. doi:10.1136/bjsports-2012-091277
55. Mohammadi F. **Comparison of 3 preventive methods to reduce the recurrence of ankle inversion sprains in male soccer players.** *Am J Sports Med.* 2007; **35(6)**:922–26.
56. Tropp H, Askling C, Gillquist J. **Prevention of ankle sprains.** *Am J Sports Med.* 1985; **13(4)**:259–62.
57. Inklaar H. **Soccer injuries. I: incidence and severity.** *Sports Med.* 1994; **18(1)**:55–73.
58. Woods C, Hawkins RD, Maltby S, Hulse M, Thomas A, Hodson A. **The football association medical research programme: an audit of injuries in professional football—analysis of hamstring injuries.** *Br J Sports Med.* 2004; **38(1)**:36–41.
59. Arnason A, Andersen TE, Holme I, Engebretsen L, Bahr R. **Prevention of hamstring strains in elite soccer: an intervention study.** *Scand J Med Sci Sports.* 2008; **18(1)**:40–8.
60. Arnason A, Gudmundsson A, Dahl HA, Johannsson E. **Soccer injuries in Iceland.** *Scand J Med Sci Sports.* 1996; **6(1)**:40–5.
61. Brughelli M, Cronin J. **Preventing hamstring injuries in sport.** *Strength Cond J.* 2008; **30(1)**:55–64.
62. Mendiguchia J, Brughelli M. **A return-to-sport algorithm for acute hamstring injuries.** *Phys Ther Sport.* 2011; **12(1)**:2–14.
63. Brockett CL, Morgan DL, Proske U. **Predicting hamstring strain injury in elite athletes.** *Med Sci Sports Exerc.* 2004; **36(3)**:379–87.
64. Proske U, Morgan DL, Brockett CL, Percival P. **Identifying athletes at risk of hamstring strains and how to protect them.** *Clin Exp Pharmacol Physiol.* 2004; **31(8)**:546–50.
65. Brughelli M, Cronin J. **Altering the length-tension relationship with eccentric exercise: implications for performance and injury.** *Sports Med.* 2007; **37(9)**:807–26.
66. Gabbe BJ, Branson R, Bennell KL. **A pilot randomised controlled trial of eccentric exercise to prevent hamstring injuries in community-level Australian Football.** *J Sci Med Sport.* 2006; **9(1–2)**:103–09.
67. Brooks JHM, Fuller CW, Kemp SPT, Reddin DB. **Incidence, risk, and prevention of hamstring muscle injuries in professional rugby union.** *Am J Sports Med.* 2006; **34(8)**:1297–306.
68. Mendiguchia J, Alentorn-Geli E, Brughelli M. Hamstring strain injuries: are we heading in the right direction? Br J Sports Med. 2011. doi:10.1136/bjsm.2010.081695.
69. Hägglund M, Waldén M, Ekstrand J. **Risk factors for lower extremity muscle injury in professional soccer: the UEFA injury study.** *Am J Sports Med.* 2013; **41(2)**:327–35.
70. Arnason A, Sigurdsson SB, Gudmundsson A, Holme I, Engebretsen L, Bahr R. **Risk factors for injuries in football.** *Am J Sports Med.* 2004; **32(1 suppl)**:5S–16S.
71. van Rijn RM, van Os AG, Bernsen RM, Luijsterburg PA, Koes BW, Bierma-Zeinstra SM. **What is the clinical course of acute ankle sprains? A systematic literature review.** *Am J Med.* 2008; **121(4)**:324–31.
72. Munn J, Sullivan SJ, Schneiders AG. **Evidence of sensorimotor deficits in functional ankle instability: a systematic review with meta-analysis.** *J Sci Med Sport.* 2010; **13(1)**:2–12.
73. Osborne MD, Chou LS, Laskowski ER, Smith J, Kaufman KR. **The effect of ankle disk training on muscle reaction time in subjects with a history of ankle sprain.** *Am J Sports Med.* 2001; **29(5)**:627–32.
74. Postle K, Pak D, Smith TO. **Effectiveness of proprioceptive exercises for ankle ligament injury in adults: a systematic literature and meta-analysis.** *Man Ther.* 2012; **17(4)**:285–91.
75. Rees JD, Wolman RL, Wilson A. **Eccentric exercises; why do they work, what are the problems and how can we improve them?** *Br J Sports Med.* 2009; **43(4)**:242–46.
76. Steffen K, Myklebust G, Olsen OE, Holme I, Bahr R. **Preventing injuries in female youth football—a cluster-randomized controlled trial.** *Scand J Med Sci Sports.* 2008; **18(5)**:605–14.

77. Soligard T, Myklebust G, Steffen K, Holme I, Silvers H, Bizzini M, et al. **Comprehensive warm-up programme to prevent injuries in young female footballers: cluster randomised controlled trial.** *BMJ.* 2008; **337:**a2469.
78. Alentorn-Geli E, Myer G, Silvers H, Samitier G, Romero D, Lázaro-Haro C, et al. **Prevention of non-contact anterior cruciate ligament injuries in soccer players. Part 2: a review of prevention programs aimed to modify risk factors and to reduce injury rates.** *Knee Surg Sports Traumatol Arthrosc.* 2009; **17(8):**859–79.
79. Fuller CW, Ekstrand J, Junge A, Andersen TE, Bahr R, Dvorak J, et al. **Consensus statement on injury definitions and data collection procedures in studies of football (soccer) injuries.** *Br J Sports Med.* 2006; **40(3):**193–201.
80. Altman DG, Schulz KF, Moher D, Egger M, Davidoff F, Elbourne D, et al. **The revised CONSORT statement for reporting randomized trials: explanation and elaboration.** *Ann Intern Med.* 2001; **134(8):**663–94.
81. Moher D, Schulz KF, Altman DG. **The CONSORT statement: revised recommendations for improving the quality of reports of parallel-group randomised trials.** *Lancet.* 2001; **357(9263):**1191–94.
82. Schulz KF, Chalmers I, Hayes RJ, Altman DG. **Empirical evidence of bias. Dimensions of methodological quality associated with estimates of treatment effects in controlled trials.** *JAMA.* 1995; **273(5):**408–12.
83. Moher D, Pham B, Jones A, Cook DJ, Jadad AR, Moher M, et al. **Does quality of reports of randomised trials affect estimates of intervention efficacy reported in meta-analyses?** *Lancet.* 1998; **352(9128):**609–13.
84. Wood L, Egger M, Gluud LL, Schulz KF, Jüni P, Altman DG, et al. **Empirical evidence of bias in treatment effect estimates in controlled trials with different interventions and outcomes: meta-epidemiological study.** *BMJ.* 2008; **336(7644):**601–05.
85. Soligard T, Nilstad A, Steffen K, Myklebust G, Holme I, Dvorak J, et al. **Compliance with a comprehensive warm-up programme to prevent injuries in youth football.** *Br J Sports Med.* 2010; **44(11):**787–93.
86. Balshem H, Helfand M, Schünemann HJ, Oxman AD, Kunz R, Brozek J, et al. **Rating the quality of evidence. J Clin Epidemiol.** *J Clin Epidemiol.* 2011; **64(4):**401–06.

3

The acute effect of exercise modality and nutrition manipulations on post-exercise resting energy expenditure and respiratory exchange ratio in women: a randomized trial

Hailee L Wingfield[1], Abbie E Smith-Ryan[1*], Malia N Melvin[1], Erica J Roelofs[1], Eric T Trexler[1], Anthony C Hackney[1,2], Mark A Weaver[3] and Eric D Ryan[1]

Abstract

Background: The purpose of this study was to examine the effect of exercise modality and pre-exercise carbohydrate (CHO) or protein (PRO) ingestion on post-exercise resting energy expenditure (REE) and respiratory exchange ratio (RER) in women.

Methods: Twenty recreationally active women (mean ± SD; age 24.6 ± 3.9 years; height 164.4 ± 6.6 cm; weight 62.7 ± 6.6 kg) participated in this randomized, crossover, double-blind study. Each participant completed six exercise sessions, consisting of three exercise modalities: aerobic endurance exercise (AEE), high-intensity interval running (HIIT), and high-intensity resistance training (HIRT); and two acute nutritional interventions: CHO and PRO. Salivary samples were collected before each exercise session to determine estradiol-β-17 and before and after to quantify cortisol. Post-exercise REE and RER were analyzed via indirect calorimetry at the following: baseline, immediately post (IP), 30 minutes (30 min) post, and 60 minutes (60 min) post exercise. A mixed effects linear regression model, controlling for estradiol, was used to compare mean longitudinal changes in REE and RER.

Results: On average, HIIT produced a greater REE than AEE and HIRT ($p < 0.001$) post exercise. Effects of AEE and HIRT were not significantly different for post-exercise REE ($p = 0.1331$). On average, HIIT produced lower RER compared to either AEE or HIRT after 30 min ($p < 0.001$ and $p = 0.0169$, respectively) and compared to AEE after 60 min ($p = 0.0020$). On average, pre-exercise PRO ingestion increased post-exercise REE ($p = 0.0076$) and decreased post-exercise RER ($p < 0.0001$) compared to pre-exercise CHO ingestion.

Conclusion: HIIT resulted in the largest increase in REE and largest reduction in RER.

Key points

- HIIT elicited the largest increase in post-exercise energy expenditure.
- HIIT resulted in the largest reduction in post-exercise RER, increasing fat oxidation, compared to AEE and HIRT.
- In combination with varying exercise modalities, PRO intake elevated post-exercise REE and fat oxidation (via RER) to a greater extent than CHO.
- Integrating HIIT and pre-exercise PRO intake into exercise routines for women, may have positive implications on weight and body composition.

* Correspondence: abbsmith@email.unc.edu
[1]Department of Exercise and Sport Science, University of North Carolina, 209 Fetzer Hall, CB #8700, Chapel Hill, NC 27599-8700, USA
Full list of author information is available at the end of the article

Background

More than 60% of women in the United States are overweight, and 1/3 of those women are obese [1]. In addition, 75% of normal weight women believe they are overweight and 90% overestimate their body size [2]. With such high obesity and body dissatisfaction rates, it is important for women to receive reliable health and weight loss recommendations. In addition, lack of time has shifted the focus on more practical time-efficient strategies for exercise.

For health and weight maintenance, aerobic endurance exercise (AEE) is usually prescribed [3]. However, more recently, higher-intensity exercise modalities have been suggested as more time-efficient strategies for improvements in health and energy expenditure [4-6]. Post-exercise resting energy expenditure (REE) has been reported to increase following a 20-min treadmill run [4], while high-intensity interval training (HIIT) has increased total caloric energy expenditure (EE) in half the time [7]. In addition, high-intensity resistance training (HIRT) with short rest intervals has been shown to enhance post-exercise REE above that seen with more commonly prescribed resistance training [8] of lesser intensity and longer rest periods. While these three common exercise modes seem to be successful at expending calories, previous research has indicated that high-intensity exercise stimulates similar increases in post-exercise REE in comparison to lower intensity exercise, in half the time [9,10]. Research is still conflicted on whether aerobic or resistance exercise is more effective for augmenting EE. Higher intensity exercise has also been linked to higher rates of fat oxidation, measured by respiratory exchange ratio (RER) [6,11,12].

The combined effect of varying exercise modalities and pre-workout nutrition on energy substrate utilization and EE in women is limited. Pre-exercise ingestion of protein (PRO) has been found to increase post-exercise REE more than that of pre-exercise ingestion of carbohydrate (CHO) [13,14]. While women rely heavily on fat as an energy substrate during exercise, previous data has demonstrated the importance of pre-exercise feedings on augmenting lipolysis [15]. In addition, a higher rate of fat oxidation in women than men in the fasted state, but not in the postprandial state, has been reported [16]. Pre-exercise nutrient timing and content may be important when evaluating exercise substrate utilization in women.

When evaluating exercise and nutritional responses in women, it is important to consider hormonal variances, such as the sex-specific hormone estradiol that varies throughout the menstrual cycle. Estradiol has been shown to have an impact on REE [17-19]. Controlling for estradiol concentrations in metabolic evaluations is crucial for determining the practical effects an intervention may have [18]. High-intensity aerobic exercise has been shown to stimulate increases in cortisol [20], a stress hormone that regulates energy substrate utilization by mobilizing amino acids from skeletal muscle and promoting gluconeogenic activity [21]. Elevated cortisol concentrations have been reported as a primary hormonal factor augmenting exercise adaptations from high-intensity exercise, as well as impacting rates of lipolysis [20].

To date, no investigations have evaluated the combined effects of varying exercise modalities and acute nutritional supplementation in women. Therefore, the purpose of the current study was to examine the effect of common exercise modalities, AEE, HIIT, and HIRT, combined with pre-exercise CHO or PRO ingestion, on post-exercise REE and RER in women.

Methods

Experimental design

To test the study hypotheses, a randomized, crossover, factorial design was used. After preliminary resting heart rate, body composition, and strength testing, each participant completed six randomly ordered exercise sessions consisting of three exercise modalities: AEE, HIIT, and HIRT; and two acute randomized nutritional interventions: CHO and PRO (Figure 1). Participants performed each exercise mode twice, with a different nutritional intervention each time. Salivary samples were collected before each exercise session to determine estradiol and cortisol concentrations and after each exercise session to determine cortisol concentrations. Exercise sessions were performed at the same time of day, within 2 h, with at least 48 h between each session, and the order was randomly assigned using random allocation software (version 1.0.0; Isfahan, Iran). Subjects were instructed to stay well hydrated, to be 3 h postprandial, to refrain from caffeine 5 h prior, and to refrain from strenuous exercise 24 h prior to all exercise sessions.

Participants

Twenty-one eumenorrheic, college-aged, recreationally active women were enrolled to participate in this study; one participant withdrew due to unrelated injury. Twenty women ($n = 20$) completed the study (Table 1) and were included in the statistical analyses. The study protocol was approved by the University's Institutional Review Board, and all procedures followed were in accordance with the Helsinki Declaration of 1975, as revised in 2008. Prior to participation, all participants provided written informed consent and completed a health history questionnaire. To be included in this study, participants had to be a woman between the ages of 18 and 35 and be recreationally active, defined as accumulating 1 to 5 h per week of aerobic and/or resistance exercise, excluding competitive athletes. Participants were excluded if they were unfit, pregnant, had any cardiovascular or neuromuscular health risks, had injuries, or had any heart, lung, kidney, or liver disease.

Heart rate reserve measurement and body composition assessment

Participants reported to the Applied Physiology Laboratory after an 8-h fast, where they rested for 15 min. Resting heart rate (RHR) was measured using a polar heart rate monitor (Polar FT1, Polar USA, Port Washington, NY, USA), while age-predicted maximal heart rate (MHR) was

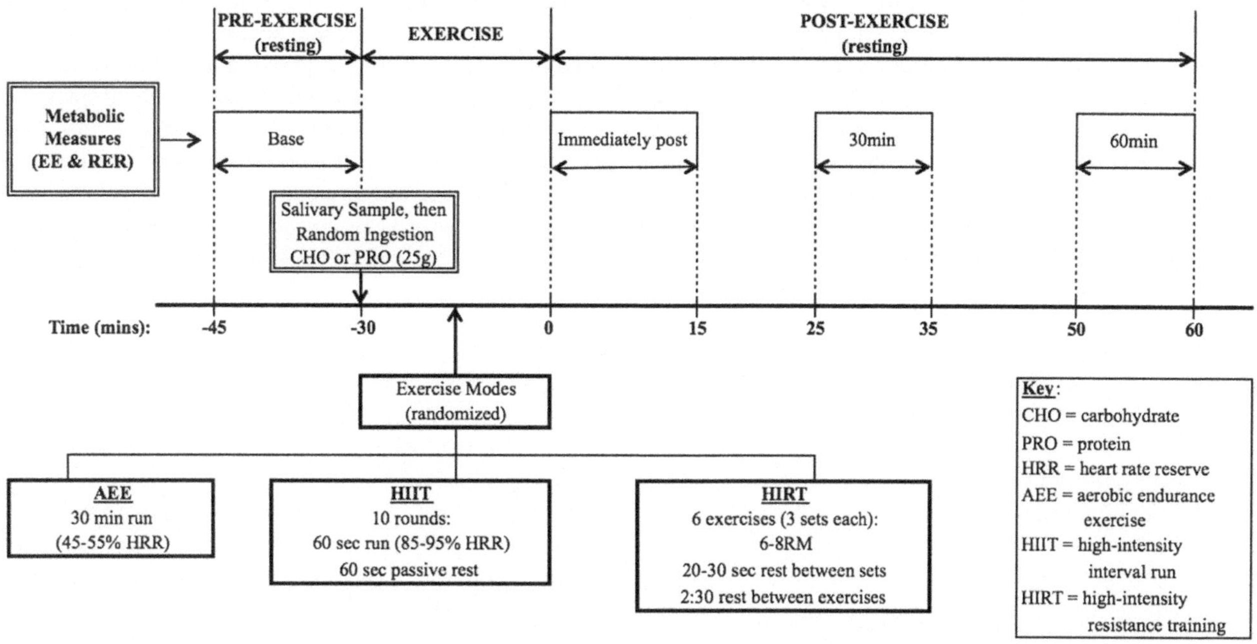

Figure 1 Experimental protocol schematic. REE, resting energy expenditure (kcal/day); RER, respiratory exchange ratio; CHO, carbohydrate; PRO, protein; HRR, heart rate reserve; AEE, aerobic endurance exercise; HIIT, high-intensity interval run; HIRT, high-intensity resistance training.

determined. Exercise target heart rate (THR) was calculated using the Karvonen equation [THR = ((MHR − RHR) % intensity) + MHR] [3]. During each exercise bout, heart rate (HR) was measured using the aforementioned HR monitor. Exercises were matched for caloric expenditure (pilot data not published), opposed to time, in order to control for exercise length.

For baseline data, whole body composition was measured using a Hologic Dual Energy X-ray Absorptiometer (DEXA, Hologic Discovery W, Bedford, MA, USA) using the device's default software (Apex software version 3.3). The device uses rectilinear fan beam acquisition to give a three-compartment assessment of body composition, including fat mass (FM), lean mass (LM), and percent body fat (% fat). After removing all metal objects, subjects laid supine in the middle of the platform with hands facedown near their sides. Subjects were instructed to remain still and breathe normally for the duration of the scan. All scans were performed by the same DEXA-certified technician. The device was calibrated according to the manufacturer recommendations before testing to ensure valid results. Previous test-retest reliability in our lab were FM: ICC = 0.98, SEM = 0.85 kg; LM: ICC = 0.99, SEM = 1.07 kg; % fat: ICC = 0.98, SEM = 1.0%.

Table 1 Descriptive statistics for all subjects ($n = 20$) at baseline

	Mean ± SD
Age (years)	24.6 ± 3.9
Height (cm)	164.4 ± 6.6
Weight (kg)	62.7 ± 6.6
Fat mass (kg)	17.6 ± 4.0
Lean mass (kg)	42.5 ± 4.4
Percent body fat (%)	28.2 ± 4.8

Maximal strength test

In a standard post-absorptive state, each participant performed a one-repetition maximum (RM) strength test for bench press and leg press, using free weights and a spotter, according to standard guidelines previously used in this laboratory. After a 5-min warm-up and light stretching, participants were familiarized with the equipment and the motion of the movements. Each participant then performed eight to ten repetitions at 50% of their predicted 1RM. After a 1-min rest period, each participant performed four to six repetitions at 80% of their predicted 1RM. Following a 1-min rest period, the weight was increased to an estimated 1RM load, which participants lifted one time. After each successful set of one repetition, the weight was increased until a failed attempt occurred, within four attempts. Two to three minutes of rest was given between 1RM attempts.

After the 1RM tests, participants performed a multiple-RM strength test for four accessory exercises: alternating stationary lunge, overhead shoulder press, biceps curls, and overhead triceps extension. With free weights and a spotter, participants performed each exercise with a weight they could lift for one set of no less than three, and no more than ten repetitions. The weight for each exercise, set by the lab assistants, was based on each participant's past strength training experience. If the participant was unable to perform the exercise for three repetitions or was able to perform more than ten repetitions, the weight was decreased or increased, respectively, and the test was redone. A 2- to 3-min rest was given between each exercise.

The multiple RM obtained from the strength tests was used to estimate 1RM for the accessory exercises using the following equation [22]:

$$1RM = \frac{RepWt}{0.522 + 0.419^{(-0.055 \times RTF)}}$$

where RepWt = amount of weight lifted (lbs) with each repetition and RTF = amount of repetitions to fatigue.

Once the participant's 1RM was determined for all exercises, 80% to 85% was calculated for the 6RM to 8RM used for the HIRT sessions.

Energy intake assessment

All participants completed a baseline 3-day food record to assess their regular nutrient intake. Participants were educated on food portions and were asked to eat similar diets the day prior to each exercise session to facilitate similar macronutrient profiles. Nutrition intake was analyzed using a nutrition software program (The Food Processor, version 10.12.0, Esha Research, Salem, OR, USA). On average, subjects ingested 2,078.7 ± 679.9 kcal, 253.7 ± 97.6 g CHO (approximately 48.8% CHO), 84.3 ± 29.9 g PRO (approximately 16.2% PRO), and 80.9 ± 36.7 g of fat (approximately 35.0% fat) per day.

Saliva collection and analysis

In order to account for possible energy substrate utilization differences between the exercise sessions, estradiol was measured. Estradiol concentrations were determined by a 2.5 to 5.0 mL saliva sample prior to each exercise bout, using an ELISA assay for salivary estradiol-β-17 (estrogen) (Salivary 17β-Estradiol Enzyme Immunoassay Kit, Salimetrics, LLC, State College, PA, USA). To ensure valid saliva collection results, participants were asked to avoid drinking alcohol for 12 h and eating a major meal for 3 h prior to giving saliva samples. Participants were asked to rinse their mouth with water 10 min prior to saliva collection, to remove food residue. To avoid blood in saliva collections, participants were asked to avoid brushing teeth for 45 min and obtaining dental work for 48 h prior to giving saliva samples. All samples were maintained at 4°C no longer than necessary before freezing them at −20°C. Intra-assay precision coefficient of variation (CV) for estrogen was 8.7% to 18.6%; inter-assay precision CV was 3.9%. Due to the physiological role of estradiol-β-17 on energy substrate utilization in women [17,19], baseline estradiol levels were used as covariates in the REE and RER analyses.

Cortisol was measured to account for the stress response from each modality of exercise. Cortisol concentrations were determined by a 2.5 to 5.0 mL saliva sample prior to and following each exercise bout, using an ELISA Assay for salivary cortisol (Salivary Cortisol Enzyme Immunoassay Kit, Salimetrics, LLC, State College, PA, USA); the aforementioned protocol for collection and storage was used. Once all samples were collected, smaller subsamples were pooled between the two supplements to produce one pre- and one post-exercise sample to determine the effect of each modality on cortisol, independent of treatment. Intra-assay precision CV for cortisol was 12.0% to 17.1%; inter-assay precision CV was 4.9%.

Nutritional intervention

After providing a saliva sample and immediately prior to beginning each exercise session, in a double-blind fashion, participants orally ingested 25 g of CHO (maltodextrin) or PRO (whey isolate; Elite Whey Protein Isolate, Dymatize Nutrition, Farmers Branch, TX, USA) mixed with 6 oz of water in an opaque bottle. Treatment order was randomly assigned using random allocation software. In accordance to the CONSORT guidelines, nutritional products were blinded by the company prior to arrival to the laboratory. All participants and research team members were blinded to the treatment, until after the statistical analyses.

Aerobic endurance exercise (AEE)

An AEE bout consisted of a self-selected 5-min warm-up, followed by a 30-min treadmill (Q65 Series 90, Quinton Instrument Co., Seattle, WA, USA) jog at 45% to 55% HRR [4]. RPE (Borg scale) was recorded, and HR was measured at the end of each minute; both were averaged over the 30-min exercise period.

High-intensity interval running (HIIT)

A HIIT bout consisted of a self-selected 5-min warm-up, followed by ten rounds of a 60-s treadmill run at 85% to 95% HRR with a 60-s passive rest period. The entire exercise bout lasted approximately 20 min. RPE was recorded, and HR was measured at the end of each interval; and an average of the ten 60-s exercise intervals was used for statistical analysis.

High-intensity resistance training (HIRT)

Data obtained from the strength assessment were used to determine an appropriate weight load for the HIRT session. Exercises were performed in the following order: leg press and bench press (York Barbell Co., York, PA, USA), lunges, shoulder press, biceps curl, and triceps extension using free weights. Subjects performed a self-selected warm-up prior to starting. A HIRT bout consisted of three sets of 6RM to 8RM followed by a 20- to 30-s rest for each exercise. There was a rest period of 2.5 min between each exercise [8]. The average length of HIRT sessions was approximately 25 min. HR was measured at the end of each set, and RPE was recorded at the end of each exercise; the average of HR and RPE of each of the six exercises was used in the statistical analyses.

Metabolic measurements

REE and RER were analyzed using a metabolic cart and internal software (TrueOne 2400, ParvoMedics, Inc., Sandy, UT, USA). Indirect assessments of oxygen uptake (VO_2) and carbon dioxide production (VCO_2) were measured and used in the following equations to calculate REE [23] and RER [24], respectively:

$$\text{REE (kcal/day)} = [(3.9 * (\text{VO}_2\ (L * \text{min}^{-1}))) + (1.1 * (\text{VCO}_2\ (L * \text{min}^{-1})))] * 1440\ \text{min}$$

$$\text{RER} = \frac{\text{VCO}_2\ (L * \text{min}^{-1})}{\text{VO}_2\ (L * \text{min}^{-1})}$$

The gas analysis was performed via a mouthpiece and hose immediately prior to each exercise session, for 15 min, to obtain resting measures (base). Immediately after the conclusion of the exercise sessions, participants were seated and reconnected to the metabolic cart for 15 min to obtain immediately post- (IP) exercise measures. The participants were then disconnected from the cart and remained quietly seated. Measurements were taken again during minutes 25 to 35 (30 min) and 50 to 60 (60 min).

Statistical analyses

A one-way repeated measures ANOVA was performed to determine baseline differences in salivary estradiol and cortisol levels. An analysis of covariance (ANCOVA) mixed effects linear model was used to compare mean longitudinal changes in REE and RER. Initial models included fixed effects for nutritional treatment (CHO vs. PRO), exercise modality (AEE vs. HIIT vs. HIRT), time (baseline vs. IP vs. 30 min vs. 60 min), two-way and three-way interactions, as well as baseline salivary estradiol level. The three-way interaction was tested first; if non-significant, a reduced model was fit without the three-way interaction. Multiple degree of freedom contrasts were then used to test for any evidence of differences between nutritional interventions or exercise modalities over time. Only if those overall contrasts were significant, pairwise comparisons were completed. An ANCOVA was performed on the change in cortisol, covaried for baseline differences. A repeated measures ANOVA was performed on HR and RPE differences in modalities. SPSS version 20 (IBM; Armonk, NY, USA) was used to perform the statistical analyses. All tests were conducted at the 5% significance level.

Results

Estradiol

There was no significant difference ($p = 0.636$; ES = 0.035) between baseline estradiol concentrations for each exercise session. While this p value was not significant, the concentrations obtained were physiologically different between and within subjects. Concentrations spanned from 0.00 to 5.04 pg/mL between subjects, with one subject ranging 0 to 4.70 pg/mL between testing days.

REE (kcal/day)

The three-way interaction for REE was non-significant ($p = 0.634$), so it was removed from the model. The modality and treatment interaction was not significant ($p = 0.060$) (Additional file 1: Appendix 1), so main effects over time are reported. Significant two-way interactions were found between modality and time ($p < 0.001$) and time and treatment ($p = 0.008$), indicating differential changes over time.

Significant modality differences were found between HIIT and AEE ($p < 0.001$), and HIIT and HIRT ($p < 0.001$) over time, but not between AEE and HIRT ($p = 0.133$). Mean REE significantly increased more with HIIT compared to AEE from baseline to IP exercise ($p < 0.001$), 30 min post ($p = 0.002$), and 60 min post ($p = 0.002$); (Additional file 1: Appendix 1 and Figure 2A). Mean REE significantly increased more with HIIT than HIRT from baseline to IP exercise ($p < 0.001$) but was not significantly different at 30 min ($p = 0.335$) or 60 min ($p = 0.143$). Mean REE significantly increased more following PRO compared to CHO IP ($p = 0.007$), 30 min ($p = 0.010$), and 60 min ($p = 0.002$) (Figure 2B).

RER

The three-way interaction for RER was non-significant ($p = 0.161$), so it was removed from the model. The interaction between modality and treatment was not significant ($p = 0.650$), so main effects were over time. Significant two-way interactions were found between modality

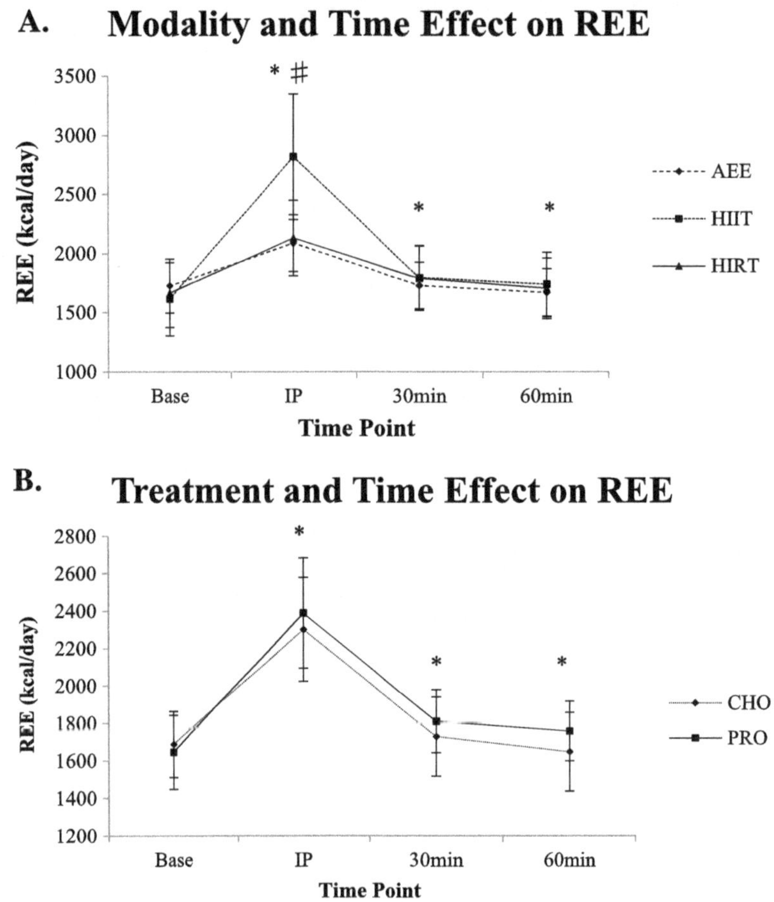

Figure 2 Energy expenditure (REE; kcal/day) as a result of A) modality and time and B) treatment and time. Values expressed as mean ± SD. **A)** Asterisk indicates significant difference between AEE and HIIT ($p < 0.001$ to $p = 0.002$); Number sign indicates significant difference between HIIT and HIRT ($p < 0.001$). **B)** Asterisk indicates significant difference between CHO and PRO ($p = 0.002$ to $p = 0.010$). REE, resting energy expenditure (kcal/day); CHO, carbohydrate; PRO, protein; AEE, aerobic endurance exercise; HIIT, high-intensity interval run; HIRT, high-intensity resistance training; Base, baseline measurement; IP, immediately post-exercise measurement; 30 min, 30 minutes post-exercise measurement; 60 min, 60 minutes post-exercise measurement.

and time ($p < 0.001$) and time and treatment ($p < 0.001$), indicating differential changes over time.

Significant over-time differences were found between HIIT and AEE ($p < 0.001$), HIIT and HIRT ($p < 0.001$), and AEE and HIRT ($p = 0.002$). As a result of HIIT, mean RER increased significantly more than AEE and HIRT from baseline to IP exercise ($p < 0.001$) (Additional file 1: Appendix 2 and Figure 3A). However, mean RER significantly decreased more at 30 ($p < 0.001$) and 60 min post exercise ($p = 0.002$) for HIIT than AEE. Mean RER significantly reduced more from baseline to 30 min ($p = 0.017$) but was not significantly different at 60 min post ($p = 0.360$) for HIIT when compared to HIRT. When comparing HIRT and AEE, there was no significant difference from baseline to IP exercise ($p = 0.337$), but mean RER was significantly lower for HIRT to 30 ($p < 0.001$) and 60 min ($p = 0.027$). Mean RER was significantly different over time between CHO and PRO IP exercise ($p < 0.001$) and was significantly lower for PRO compared to CHO from baseline to 30 ($p = 0.001$) and 60 min post ($p < 0.001$) (Figure 3B).

Cortisol

ANCOVA change scores demonstrated no significant effect of exercise modality on cortisol values ($p = 0.168$; ES = 0.015) (Table 2).

HR and RPE

There was a modality effect on average HR ($p < 0.001$) and RPE ($p < 0.001$). Compared to HIIT, AEE produced a significantly lower mean HR ($\Delta = -58$ bpm; $p < 0.001$) and RPE ($\Delta = -6$; $p < 0.001$) (Table 3). There was no difference in HR ($\Delta = -3$ bpm; $p = 0.834$) between AEE and HIRT. Mean RPE was significantly lower for AEE

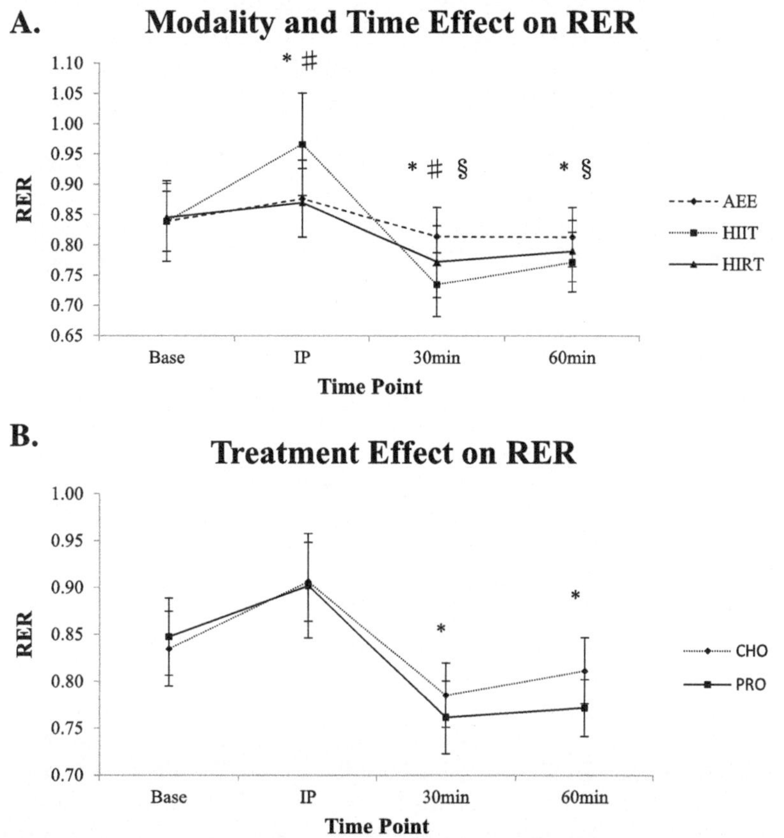

Figure 3 Respiratory exchange ratio as a result of A) modality and time and B) treatment and time. Values expressed as mean ± SD. **A)** Asterisk indicates significant difference between AEE and HIIT ($p < 0.001$ to $p = 0.002$); Number sign indicates significant difference between HIIT and HIRT ($p < 0.001$ to $p = 0.017$); Section sign indicates significant difference between AEE and HIRT ($p = 0.001$ to 0.027). **B)** Asterisk indicates significant difference between CHO and PRO ($p < 0.001$ to $p = 0.001$). RER, respiratory exchange ratio; CHO, carbohydrate; PRO, protein; AEE, aerobic endurance exercise; HIIT, high-intensity interval run; HIRT, high-intensity resistance training; Base, baseline measurement; IP, immediately post-exercise measurement; 30 min, 30 minutes post-exercise measurement; 60 min, 60 minutes post-exercise measurement.

compared to HIRT ($\Delta = -5$; $p < 0.001$). HIIT resulted in significantly higher mean HR ($\Delta = 54$ bpm; $p < 0.001$) and RPE ($\Delta = 1$; $p = 0.001$) compared to HIRT.

Discussion

Previous research evaluating the effect of AEE, HIIT, and HIRT individually on energy expenditure and energy substrate utilization have failed to provide direct comparisons between exercise modes; as well as failing to evaluate these effects in women. The current study is the first to compare common exercise modalities, with acute nutritional intake, on post-exercise REE and RER in women. Results of the current study indicate that HIIT produces a significantly higher REE than AEE up

Table 2 Change in cortisol (μg/dL) as a result of modality (mean ± SD)

Modality	Base	Post	Δ
AEE	0.39 ± 0.31	0.39 ± 0.33	0.00 ± 0.22
HIIT	0.44 ± 0.40	0.59 ± 0.50	0.15 ± 0.23
HIRT	0.35 ± 0.18	0.40 ± 0.20	0.05 ± 0.14

AEE, aerobic endurance exercise; HIIT, high-intensity interval run; HIRT, high-intensity resistance training; Base, baseline measurement; Post, post-exercise measurement; Δ, change in cortisol (μg/dL).

Table 3 Average HR and RPE during the duration of each modality (Mean ± SD)

	HR (bpm)	RPE
AEE	$126 \pm 7^{*}$	$10 \pm 1^{*\S}$
HIIT	$184 \pm 29^{\#}$	$16 \pm 1^{\#}$
HIRT	129 ± 17	15 ± 1

AEE, aerobic endurance exercise; HIIT, high-intensity interval run; HIRT, high-intensity resistance training; HR, heart rate (bpm); RPE, rating of perceived exertion (Borg scale).
*Indicates significant difference between AEE and HIIT ($p < 0.0001$).
#Indicates significant difference between HIIT and HIRT ($p < 0.0001$ to $p = 0.001$).
§Indicates significant difference between AEE and HIRT ($p < 0.0001$).

to 60 min post exercise and a significantly higher post-exercise REE than HIRT IP exercise; while AEE and HIRT produced similar post-exercise REE responses. HIIT and HIRT both also stimulated greater fat utilization (via a lower RER) when compared to AEE. In the current study, ingesting PRO prior to exercise produced an increased post-exercise resting energy expenditure, compared to CHO consumption. PRO ingestion also resulted in significantly augmented fat utilization 30 and 60 min post exercise.

REE

As hypothesized, a single bout of HIIT produced a significantly higher post-exercise REE than AEE through 60 min post exercise ($\Delta = 189.2$ kcal/day). Similar to the current study, higher post-exercise net EE with high-intensity short-duration cycling (75% VO_{2max}) compared to shorter and longer durations at a low intensity (50% VO_{2max}) has been found in men [9], indicating that exercise intensity affects the magnitude and duration of excess post-exercise oxygen consumption (EPOC). HIIT's metabolic inefficiency has been contributed to rapid changes in skeletal muscle oxidative capacity due to the high level of muscle fiber recruitment, particularly in type II fibers [25]. In contrast to the current study, bouts of 60 s of work with 60 s rest, at 90% VO_{2max}, have been found to have the same total net EE as 20-min bouts at 70% VO_{2max} [7]. Perhaps the difference in exercise intensities for the two sessions was not substantial enough to elicit significant differences, such as those found in the current study. Additionally, it is unclear if differences between exercise intensities were controlled for [7]. Subjects in the present study completed 30 min, instead of 20 min, of AEE in order to closely match EE during HIIT (determined during pilot testing; unpublished data).

In contrast to our hypothesis, when compared to HIIT, REE from HIRT was significantly lower from baseline to IP exercise ($\Delta = -169.3$ kcal/day), with no differences at 30 and 60 min post exercise. Additionally, there was no difference between AEE and HIRT ($\Delta = 19.8$ kcal/day). Research that has examined REE differences between AEE or HIIT and HIRT is limited. However, single bouts of resistance training and running performed at the same intensity have both resulted in elevated REE up to 10 h post exercise [26]. Contrary to the current study, total body circuit weight training (three sets of 15 repetitions at 65% 1RM) has been shown to elicit a higher post-exercise REE in women than a treadmill run matched for aerobic energy cost [27]. The current study also matched EE demands of AEE and HIRT during pilot testing, with HIRT being slightly lower, yet at a higher intensity than that of Braun et al. [27]. Post-exercise REE data from the current study eludes to exercise intensity, instead of duration, as the primary determinant of EPOC variance, similar to several studies [4-6]. Collectively, it seems as if HIIT is the most time-effective exercise modality for increasing EE in women.

Combined acute PRO feedings with exercise resulted in a significantly higher REE for PRO than for CHO up to 60 min post exercise ($\Delta = 59.3$ kcal/day). This is similar to previous findings [13,14] that demonstrate greater post-exercise REE and fat oxidation following a pre-exercise meal or snack with higher PRO content. The increase in post-exercise REE with PRO ingestion can be contributed to PRO's thermic effect of food, which is higher and more prolonged than that of CHO and fat [28]. In women, higher PRO diets have elicited an increased effect on diet-induced EE, in comparison to a lower PRO diet [28,29], which may be explained by amino acid absorption and disposal costs [29]. Consuming an additional 100 kcal of PRO prior to exercise, as done in the current study, may increase EE up to an hour after exercise.

RER

Exercise intensity has previously been shown to be a driving factor for energy substrate utilization during and after exercise. Immediately after HIIT, RER was significantly increased compared to AEE, indicating a higher utilization of CHO during and immediately after exercise. Within 25 min afterward, RER was significantly lower than AEE ($p < 0.001$), demonstrating higher fat utilization, which was maintained up to 60 min post. Similar to the current study, previous studies have reported a significantly lower RER post exercise with repeated bouts of moderate intensity cycling, compared to a single bout [12] and a lower RER with a lower vs. higher intensity cycle bout (50% and 70% VO_{2max}) through 3 h post exercise, indicating increased fat utilization [11]. Previous data demonstrates differing exercise intensity can augment post-exercise REE and fat oxidation, but intervals do not produce differences compared to continuous exercise if total EE, duration, and intensity between the two remain the same throughout the exercise bout. In contrast to the current study, exercise bouts at 45% and 65% VO_{2max} resulted in similar RER values when EE of exercise was matched [30]. Although diets were kept constant, residual effects of pre-exercise meals could cause similar RER values, since a fasting period of only 2 h was implemented prior to exercise.

During the post-exercise period, oxygen consumption is elevated for a period of time as a result of homeostasis disruption caused by exercise. Physiological changes, such as those in cellular ion concentrations, tissue temperatures, and metabolite and hormone levels, take place into recovery, disabling oxygen consumption to lower back to resting levels [24]. This process of EPOC is related to exercise duration and intensity and can be influenced by sex-based hormones (estrogen) and macronutrient availability, among other things [24]. CHO is the primary fuel used during moderate- to high-intensity exercise; but post exercise, the body shifts from CHO to lipid energy sources, which lowers RER [30]. The current study demonstrates the fuel shift within 25 min post exercise, indicating greater post-exercise fat utilization with HIIT. When comparing HIIT and HIRT, RER was significantly higher IP, significantly lower at 30 min, but similar 60 min after exercise. RER was lower for HIRT than AEE at 30 ($p < 0.001$) and 60 min post exercise ($p = 0.027$). Little research has compared RER between aerobic and resistance training, but investigations that have been done present conflicting results. In contrast to this study, no post-exercise differences in RER were found between a 60-min circuit weight training bout (four sets of ten repetitions, 70% 1RM) and a cycling bout (70% VO_{2max}) in men [31]. Similar to the current study, a lower RER was demonstrated 22 h after HIRT compared to more traditional resistance training (four sets of 8 to 12 repetitions, 1- to 2-min rest) [8]. In relation to sex, no differences were reported in post-circuit weight training RER between men and women [32]. It is important to examine the menstrual cycle due to the effects estrogen may have on energy substrate utilization, as the mid-luteal phase is characterized by high estrogen levels, which can enhance lipid utilization with exercise in women [19,33].

In the present study, no differences were found in RER between CHO and PRO IP exercise; but supporting our hypothesis, RER was significantly decreased for PRO compared to CHO at 30 min ($\Delta = 0.036$; $p = 0.001$) and 60 min post exercise ($\Delta = 0.052$; $p < 0.001$). Similarly, higher fat oxidation has been reported with a low CHO diet compared to a moderate CHO diet at 1 h post exercise [14]. Substrate oxidation can be influenced by substrate availability from dietary intake and physical activity. While this study only evaluated acute feedings, low CHO diets have been shown to decrease circulating insulin levels, which promotes fatty acid utilization in skeletal muscle [14], perhaps supporting the lower RER for PRO ingestion in the current study.

Dietary intake

Chronic dietary manipulations have an impact on substrate utilization. Based on 3-day diet logs, participants consumed on average 48.8% CHO, 16.8% PRO, and 34.2% fat daily. Although intakes were within the Acceptable Macronutrient Distribution Ranges for Americans, average baseline PRO intake was 1.3 $g{\cdot}kg^{-1}$ day^{-1} (0.5 $g{\cdot}kg^{-1}$ day^{-1} higher than the Recommended Dietary Allowance) [34]. Interestingly, while average PRO intake was relatively high, an additional acute feeding of 25 g of PRO significantly augmented REE in the current study, perhaps supporting the suggestion that higher protein needs (1.63 $g{\cdot}kg^{-1}$ day^{-1}) may be necessary for women to maintain nitrogen balance [35]. While the importance of chronic dietary manipulations is apparent, the current study supports the benefit of acute PRO feedings on EE, in healthy women eating within dietary guidelines. Acute pre-exercise feedings have positively influenced fat oxidation, in comparison to a fasted state that blunted fat oxidation [16]. Future long-term studies identifying the acute effects on weight loss and body composition improvements in women would be valuable.

Limitations

A limitation in the current study was the use of indirect calorimetry to measure REE and RER, rather than whole body direct calorimetry, which is considered the gold standard. Also, excluding the acute PRO and CHO supplementation, no dietary modifications were made, which could have a potential effect on the acute RER measurement. However, because no modifications were made, the study results may be more practical for a woman who only wants to change her pre-workout nutrition rather than her whole diet. In addition, since this was an acute intervention, and post-exercise measurements were only conducted for 60 min, it is difficult to predict longer term EE and energy substrate utilization. Specifically, EE calculations extrapolate our 60-min findings to a 24-h period (using Weir et al. [23] equation), potentially elevating the actual caloric differences (i.e. approximately 800 kcal). Future research should focus on determining the effects of chronic exercise and nutrition modifications in women using whole body calorimetry.

Conclusion

This study indicates that HIIT elicited the largest increase in post-exercise REE, as well as augmented RER, compared to AEE and HIRT. Immediately post exercise, there was a heightened caloric effect from the HIIT bout stimulating approximately 800 kcal/day more than HIRT and AEE. Beginning around 30 min post exercise, HIIT and HIRT both had a higher fat utilization than AEE; at 60 min post, HIIT and HIRT resulted in similar energy substrate utilization in comparison to each other. In combination with varying exercise modalities, PRO intake elevated post-exercise REE and fat oxidation to a greater extent than CHO. PRO ingestion prior to exercise may help further maximize the caloric effect, with an additional approximately 90 kcal/day expended compared to CHO. Around 30 min post exercise, PRO increased fat utilization compared to CHO. Collectively, these findings suggest a potential benefit of integrating HIIT and pre-exercise PRO intake into exercise routines. Specifically in women, this strategy may have positive implications on their health, weight, and body composition.

Competing interests
The authors declare that they have no competing interests.

Authors' contributions
HWL assisted with study design, carried out data collection, and drafted manuscript; ASR conceived study design, carried out statistical analysis, and drafted manuscript; EJR and ETT carried out data collection, reviewed results, and manuscript draft; MAW assisted with study design and statistical analysis; ACH assisted with biochemical analyses; EDR contributed to study design and reviewed results and manuscript draft. All authors read and approved the final manuscript.

Acknowledgements
This study was supported by the National Strength and Conditioning Association Foundation. CHO and PRO were blinded and donated by Dymatize Nutrition (Farmers Branch, TX, USA). ASR and MW declare that they were supported by the National Center for Advancing Translational Sciences, National Institutes of Health, through Grants *1KL2TR001109* and *1UL1TR001111*. The content is solely the responsibility of the authors and does not necessarily represent the official views of the NIH.

Author details
[1]Department of Exercise and Sport Science, University of North Carolina, 209 Fetzer Hall, CB #8700, Chapel Hill, NC 27599-8700, USA. [2]Department of Nutrition - Gillings School of Global Public Health, University of North Carolina, Chapel Hill, NC, USA. [3]Departments of Medicine and Biostatistics, University of North Carolina, Chapel Hill, NC, USA.

References
1. Overweight, obesity, and weight loss [Internet]. U.S. Department of Health and Human Services, Office on Women's Health. 2009 [cited 2014 Mar 7]. Available from: http://www.womenshealth.gov/publications/our-publications/fact-sheet/overweight-weight-loss.pdf
2. Eating disorders: body image and advertising [Internet]. Healthy Place. 2013 [cited 2014 Mar 7]. Available from: http://www.healthyplace.com/eating-disorders/main/eating-disorders-body-image-and-advertising/menu-id-58/
3. Pescatello LS, Arena R, Riebe D, Thompson PD, editors. ACSM's guidelines for exercise testing and prescription. 9th ed. Philadelphia, PA: Wolters Kluwer Health; 2013.
4. Gore CJ, Withers RT. The effect of exercise intensity and duration on the oxygen deficit and excess post-exercise oxygen consumption. Eur J Appl Physiol Occup Physiol. 1990;60(3):169–74.
5. Smith J, Naughton LM. The effects of intensity of exercise on excess postexercise oxygen consumption and energy expenditure in moderately trained men and women. Eur J Appl Physiol Occup Physiol. 1993;67(5):420–5.
6. Warren A, Howden EJ, Williams AD, Fell JW, Johnson N a. Postexercise fat oxidation: effect of exercise duration, intensity, and modality. Int J Sport Nutr Exerc Metab [Internet]. 2009;19(6):607–23.
7. Gosselin LE, Kozlowski KF, DeVinney-Boymel L, Hambridge C. Metabolic response of different high-intensity aerobic interval exercise protocols. J Strength Cond Res. 2012;26(10):1866–2871.
8. Paoli A, Moro T, Marcolin G, Neri M, Bianco A, Palma A, et al. High-intensity interval resistance training (HIRT) influences resting energy expenditure and respiratory ratio in non-dieting individuals. J Transl Med [Internet]. Journal of Translational Medicine; 2012 Jan [cited 2014 Jan 22];10(1):237. Available from: http://www.ncbi.nlm.nih.gov/pubmed/23176325
9. Sedlock DA, Fissinger JA, Melby CL. Effect of exercise intensity and duration on postexercise energy expenditure. Med Sci Sports Exerc. 1989;21(6):662–6.
10. Elliot DL, Goldberg L, Kuehl KS. Effect of resistance training on excess post-exercise oxygen consumption. J Appl Sport Sci Res. 1992;6(2):77–81.
11. Chad KE, Quigley BM. Exercise intensity: effect on postexercise O_2 uptake in trained and untrained women. J Appl Physiol. 1991;70:1713–9.
12. Goto K, Tanaka K, Ishii N, Uchida S, Takamatsu K. A single versus multiple bouts of moderate-intensity exercise for fat metabolism. Clin Physiol Funct Imaging [Internet]. 2011;31(3):215–20. Available from: http://www.ncbi.nlm.nih.gov/pubmed/21470361.
13. Hackney KJ, Bruenger AJ, Lemmer JT. Timing protein intake increases energy expenditure 24 h after resistance training. Med Sci Sports Exerc [Internet]. 2010;42(5):998–1003. Available from: http://www.ncbi.nlm.nih.gov/pubmed/19997003.
14. Patterson R, Potteiger J a. A comparison of normal versus low dietary carbohydrate intake on substrate oxidation during and after moderate intensity exercise in women. Eur J Appl Physiol [Internet]. 2011;111(12):3143–50. Available from: http://www.ncbi.nlm.nih.gov/pubmed/21479654.
15. Wenz M, Berend J, Lynch N, Chappell S, Hackney A. Substrate oxidation at rest and during exercise: effects of menstrual cycle phase and diet composition. J Physiol Pharmacol. 1997;48:851–60.
16. Henderson GC, Alderman BL. Determinants of resting lipid oxidation in response to a prior bout of endurance exercise. J Appl Physiol [Internet]. 2014;116(1):95–103. Available from: http://www.ncbi.nlm.nih.gov/pubmed/24235102.
17. Campbell SE, Febbraio MA. Effects of ovarian hormones on exercise metabolism. Curr Opin Clin Nutr Metab Care. 2001;4(6):515–20.
18. Isacco L, Duché P, Boisseau N. Influence of hormonal status on substrate utilization at rest and during exercise in the female population. Sport Med [Internet]. 2012;42(4):327–42. Available from: http://www.ncbi.nlm.nih.gov/pubmed/22380007.
19. Nicklas BJ, Hackney AC, Sharp RL. The menstrual cycle and exercise: performance, muscle glycogen, and substrate responses. Int J Sports Med. 1989;10(4):264–9.
20. Wahl P, Zinner C, Achtzehn S, Bloch W, Mester J. Effect of high- and low-intensity exercise and metabolic acidosis on levels of GH, IGF-I, IGFBP-3 and cortisol. Growth Hormone Research Society [Internet]. 2010;20(5):380–5. Available from: http://www.ncbi.nlm.nih.gov/pubmed/20801067.
21. Fry AC, Kraemer WJ. Resistance exercise overtraining and overreaching: neuroendocrine responses. Sport Med. 1997;23(2):106–29.
22. Mayhew JL, Ball TE, Arnold MD, Bowen JC. Relative muscular endurance performance as a predictor of bench press strength in college men and women. J Appl Sport Sci Res. 1992;4(6):200–6.
23. Weir JB. New methods for calculating metabolic rate with special reference to protein metabolism. J Physiol. 1949;109(1–2):1–9.
24. Brooks G, Fahey T, Baldwin K. Exercise physiology: human bioenergetics and its applications. 4th ed. New York, NY: McGraw-Hill; 2005.
25. Gibala MJ, McGee SL. Metabolic adaptations to short-term high-intensity interval training: a little pain for a lot of gain? Exerc Sport Sci Rev [Internet]. 2008;36(2):58–63. Available from: http://www.ncbi.nlm.nih.gov/pubmed/18362686.
26. Jamurtas AZ, Koutedakis Y, Paschalis V, Tofas T, Yfanti C, Tsiokanos A, et al. The effects of a single bout of exercise on resting energy expenditure and respiratory exchange ratio. Eur J Appl Physiol [Internet]. 2004;92(4–5):393–8. Available from: http://www.ncbi.nlm.nih.gov/pubmed/15205961.
27. Braun WA, Hawthorne WE, Markofski MM. Acute EPOC response in women to circuit training and treadmill exercise of matched oxygen consumption. Eur J Appl Physiol [Internet]. 2005;94(5–6):500–4. Available from: http://www.ncbi.nlm.nih.gov/pubmed/15942765.
28. Westerterp KR, Wilson SA, Rolland V. Diet induced thermogenesis measured over 24 h in a respiration chamber: effect of diet composition. Int J Obes [Internet]. 1999;23(3):287–92. Available from: http://www.ncbi.nlm.nih.gov/pubmed/10193874.
29. Luscombe ND, Clifton PM, Noakes M, Farnsworth E, Wittert G. Effect of a high-protein, energy-restricted diet on weight loss and energy expenditure after weight stabilization in hyperinsulinemic subjects. Int J Obes [Internet]. 2003;27(5):582–90. Available from: http://www.ncbi.nlm.nih.gov/pubmed/12704402.
30. Kuo CC, Fattor J a, Henderson GC, Brooks G a. Lipid oxidation in fit young adults during postexercise recovery. J Appl Physiol [Internet]. 2005;99(1):349–56. Available from: http://www.ncbi.nlm.nih.gov/pubmed/15591292.
31. Melanson EL, Sharp T a, Seagle HM, Donahoo WT, Grunwald GK, Peters JC, et al. Resistance and aerobic exercise have similar effects on 24-h nutrient oxidation. Med Sci Sports Exerc [Internet]. 2002;34(11):1793–800. Available from: http://www.ncbi.nlm.nih.gov/pubmed/12439085.

32. Ortego AR, Dantzler DK, Zaloudek A, Tanner J, Khan T, Panwar R, et al. Effects of gender on physiological responses to strenuous circuit resistance exercise and recovery. J Strength Cond Res. 2009;23(3):932–8.
33. Hackney AC. Influence of oestrogen on muscle glycogen utilization during exercise. Acta Physiol Scand. 1999;167(3):273–4.
34. Service AR. Report of the dietary guidelines advisory committee on the dietary guidelines for Americans. 2010.
35. Houltham SD, Rowlands DS. A snapshot of nitrogen balance in endurance-trained women. Appl Physiol Nutr Metab. 2014;39(2):219–25.

4

A tutorial on oxidative stress and redox signaling with application to exercise and sedentariness

Robert Buresh[1*] and Kris Berg[2]

Abstract

Oxidative stress has been shown to play a role in the etiology of several chronic diseases, including cardiovascular disease, diabetes mellitus, and cancer. Free radicals and, most prominently, the superoxide radical, result from oxidative metabolism and several enzyme-catalyzed reactions, and endogenous cellular antioxidants dismutate many reactive oxygen species (ROS). Under certain conditions, ROS production can outpace dismutation (e.g., long-term sedentariness and positive energy balance) and the result is oxidative stress, with proteins, lipids, and DNA the most common targets of radicals. However, the molecules that contribute to oxidative stress also appear to participate in vital cell signaling activity that supports health and stimulates favorable adaptations to exercise training, such that inhibiting ROS formation prevents common adaptations to training. Furthermore, researchers have recently suggested that some proteins are not as readily formed when the redox state of the cell is insufficiently oxidative. Exercise training appears to optimize the redox environment by dramatically enhancing the capacity of the cell to neutralize ROS while regularly creating oxidative environments in which membrane and secretory proteins can be synthesized. The role that exercise plays in enhancing management of ROS likely explains many of the associated health benefits.

Key points

- Reactive oxygen species (ROS) in excess are toxic and have been implicated in the development of aging and chronic disease.
- ROS have also been shown to enhance acute muscular activity, and to be required signaling molecules for favorable adaptations to exercise training.
- Long-term sedentariness is characterized by chronically elevated basal ROS production and reduced antioxidant capacity.
- The oxidative environment induced by exercise stimulates antioxidant capacity and may enhance synthesis of specific proteins.

Introduction

Oxidative stress has been implicated in the etiology of a number of chronic diseases including cardiovascular disease, diabetes mellitus, and cancer. It has been defined as an imbalance between oxidants and antioxidants in favor of oxidants, leading to the disruption of redox signaling and control and/or molecular damage [1]. Recent studies have shed a great deal of light on factors that influence oxidative stress. Exercise training is among the factors known to provide protection against oxidative stress, and understanding how exercise training improves oxidative status may be helpful to exercise professionals. The purposes of this review are to (1) explain what oxidative stress is, and how and where it occurs; (2) summarize recent studies that suggest that some minimal level of oxidative molecules are essential for cell signaling and stimulating beneficial adaptations to training; (3) explain how oxidative agents, in excess, are damaging; and (4) explain the effects of acute exercise and chronic exercise training on oxidative stress. As the major focus of this paper is exercise, we primarily consider these concepts within muscle fibers. However, exercise appears to stimulate reductions in signs of oxidative stress systemically (e.g., in brain and liver tissue), and those influences are also addressed briefly.

Oxidation, reduction, and radicals

Oxidation occurs when a molecule loses an electron. When one molecule loses an electron, another will acquire it, and the molecule that gains an electron is said to be reduced. Oxidation and reduction, then, occur

* Correspondence: rburesh@kennesaw.edu
[1]Department of Exercise Science and Sport Management, Kennesaw State University, 520 Parliament Garden Way NW, Kennesaw, GA 30144, USA
Full list of author information is available at the end of the article

together, in that whenever a molecule is oxidized, another is reduced. The fact that they occur together has led to the development of the term 'redox' being used in the context of this class of chemical reactions.

While there are countless examples of redox reactions in biochemistry, the reactions that are most closely related to oxidative stress involve molecules that are especially strong oxidizing agents, known collectively as free radicals, and include reactive oxygen species (ROS) and reactive nitrogen species (RNS) (the predominance of RNS is often referred to as nitrosative stress). These molecules are especially strong oxidizing entities because they have an unpaired electron in their outer shells. Oxygen and nitrogen are atoms that display a high level of electronegativity, owing to the size of the atoms and the number of protons in their nuclei. The result is that these atoms have a strong attraction for electrons when there are no unpaired electrons in their outer shells, and that attraction is much stronger when there is an unpaired electron.

One commonly produced radical, and one that is the basis of other oxidative agents, is the superoxide radical—molecular dioxide (O_2)—that has undergone a one-electron reduction. Superoxide reacting with other molecules can result in other radicals or oxidizing agents being produced. For example, much of the superoxide that is produced in mitochondria is dismutated or partially neutralized by an enzyme known as manganese superoxide dismutase (MnSOD), a protein that converts superoxide to hydrogen peroxide (H_2O_2). H_2O_2 is an oxidizing agent, but it does not have an unpaired electron, so it is less reactive and much more stable than superoxide. The relative stability of H_2O_2 lends to its ability to serve as a cellular signal of oxidative, or redox, state, a role that is discussed later.

The hydroxyl radical is another ROS, the neutral form of the hydroxide (OH) ion. It can result from H_2O_2 reacting with iron, or from superoxide reacting with H_2O_2 [2]. Like the superoxide radical, this molecule is extremely reactive and unstable. In fact, it is more reactive than any other known radical, reacting with nearly any molecular entity typically within two molecular diameters [3].

Biological Sources of Reactive Oxygen Species (ROS) and endogenous antioxidants

Some production of ROS appears to be an inescapable byproduct of cellular oxygen consumption, and radicals are produced in several commonly occurring biological reactions with many being quickly neutralized by various forms of antioxidants inside the cell. For example, superoxide radicals are produced in reactions of the electron transport chain (ETC.) within the mitochondria. The reduced forms of nicotinamide adenine dinucleotide (NADH) and flavin adenine dinucleotide ($FADH_2$) deliver electrons to the ETC. at specifice sites, and the electrons move down the chain from carrier to carrier, releasing energy that is used to pump protons from the mitochondrial matrix to the inter-membrane space and thereby developing an electrochemical gradient that drives adenosine triphosphate (ATP) synthesis by ATP synthase. In the process of electrons being passed down the ETC., some escape, or leak, and are delivered to molecular oxygen forming superoxide. This has been shown to happen most commonly at ETC. complex I (ROS is formed within the mitochondrial matrix) and ETC. complex III (ROS formed within the mitochondrial matrix and in the inter-membrane space) [4,5]. Basal ROS production had previously been estimated to account for between 2 and 5% of oxygen consumed, but more recent evidence suggests that it is substantially less—perhaps approximately 0.15% of consumed oxygen [6,7]—and ROS production at ETC. complex I increases by approximately 187%, and at ETC. complex III by 138% during exhaustive muscular activity [7]. Note that while this is a sizeable increase in the rate of ROS production, it may be less than one might expect given that the metabolic rate of contracting muscle fibers increases approximately 100-fold or more from resting levels [8]. This suggests that mitochondria in skeletal muscle produce ROS at a much lower rate per unit of oxygen consumption during contractile activity, and one possible explanation for that is considered later.

The increase in ROS production in the mitochondria appears to be a result of increased electron flux during muscular activity, and, as noted above, much of it is reduced by superoxide dismutase (SOD) (MnSOD is found within the mitochondrial matrix, while copper- and zinc-containing SOD [Cu/ZnSOD] is primarily in the cytosol [9]) and converted to H_2O_2. Some of the H_2O_2 is further neutralized by the activity of catalase, which converts it to water and molecular oxygen. H_2O_2 can also be reduced to water and oxygen by other enzyme-catalyzed reactions including glutathione peroxidase and the thioredoxin systems [10-12]. However, as is discussed later, H_2O_2 also serves as a signaling molecule and its oxidative nature is used to trigger events in the cell.

Another muscular source of superoxide is an enzyme called nicotinamide adenine dinucleotide phosphate (NADPH) oxidase (NOX). In the context of this discussion, one important role of NADPH involves an antioxidant. Glutathione (GSH) is a molecule that is capable of dismutating ROS, itself becoming oxidized in the process. When oxidized, it will bind with another oxidized GSH molecule, resulting in its oxidized form, GSSG. In this form, it can no longer function as an antioxidant until it is reduced, and an enzyme called GSSG reductase performs that reaction using NADPH as a cofactor and producing two reduced GSH molecules that can again quench ROS

[13]. As such, NADPH enhances the capacity of the cell to neutralize ROS through its involvement in reducing oxidized GSH.

The enzyme NOX is unique in that it is the only mammalian enzyme for which the sole purpose is ROS synthesis [14]. It functions by transferring an electron from NADPH to molecular oxygen, thereby forming superoxide [15]. NOX can be found in a number of locations, one of which is near sarcoplasmic reticulum (SR). NOX-produced ROS at the SR have been shown to enhance calcium release from the SR by oxidizing calcium release channels [16,17]. This NOX is stimulated by calcium release [18], and as such its activity is elevated during muscle contraction. Another site of NOX localization is at transverse tubules of skeletal muscle, where it is stimulated by action potentials [19,20], and it may be that the ROS synthesized in this area serve as a redox signal, either intra- or extracellularly. In any case, NOX enzymes produce ROS and do so at an increased rate during muscular contraction.

Phospholipase A2 (PLA2) is another enzyme that participates in ROS production, largely by activating NOX [21]. Some PLA2 isoforms are dependent on calcium and most are found within mitochondria, while other isoforms are calcium-independent and found mostly in the cell cytoplasm. It has been suggested that the calcium-dependent PLA2 is responsible for ROS formation during exercise, while the calcium-independent PLA2 is responsible for basal ROS production [22].

Xanthine oxidase (XO) also generates superoxide radicals while oxidizing hypoxanthine and forming xanthine [23]. Hypoxanthine is produced as a result of adenosine monophosphate (AMP) degradation, wherein AMP is first converted to inosine and then to hypoxanthine [24]. An increase in the availability of the substrate hypoxanthine may increase the rate of XO activity and, therefore, ROS production, and hypoxanthine levels increase with exercise, and especially with intense or anaerobic exercise. This possibility is supported by Radak et al. [25] who reported a linear relationship between intramuscular lactic acid concentration and XO activity during exhaustive treadmill exercise in rats.

Nitric oxide (NO) is a molecule that serves a number of functional and signaling roles. It is produced by one of three isoforms of NO synthase (NOS): endothelial NOS (eNOS), inducible NOS (iNOS), and neuronal NOS (nNOS). eNOS plays an important role in blood flow distribution to support muscular activity. Under optimal conditions (i.e., when all necessary substrates are available), eNOS produces NO, which then induces vasodilation via relaxation of vascular smooth muscle cells resulting in hyperemia to active muscle fibers. However, the lack of any requisite substrate for eNOS results in an 'uncoupled' enzyme, and in this state eNOS production of superoxide is increased [26-28]. The increase in ROS has the capacity to reduce functional NO via two related mechanisms: (1) NO can react with superoxide, which results in the formation of peroxynitrite radicals; and (2) ROS, and especially peroxynitrite, can reduce the availability of one necessary substrate of NOS, thereby further uncoupling NOS and further increasing superoxide production [26,29]. These outcomes impair the capacity for hyperemia to active skeletal muscle to support contractile activity. In addition, peroxynitrite is a particularly reactive molecule, and has been shown capable of causing oxidative injury and of triggering necrosis and apoptosis [30].

A number of additional mechanisms of ROS production are known to exist, but it appears that those described here are the most productive [31], so we confine our further discussions to these pathways. Importantly, all ROS species produced in skeletal muscle are derived from either superoxide or NO [32], and the production of, and neutralizing of, these two molecules explains most of cellular redox state at any given time.

ROS as critical signaling molecules

As discussed above, there are a number of enzyme-catalyzed pathways through which ROS are produced. While there is considerable interest in the role that oxidative stress plays in the etiology of chronic diseases, consideration of these reaction pathways is also suggestive that a threshold level of ROS must be needed for optimal cellular function. That is especially apparent when considering NOX, as the sole known purpose for this enzyme is the production of ROS, as opposed to the other reaction pathways that have been identified wherein ROS production is a by-product.

For a molecule to function effectively in a signaling role, its levels must be able to be regulated (i.e., adjusting rates of synthesis and degradation), it must have specific targets or receptors, and its signaling effect must be reversible [33]. Superoxide and hydroxyl radicals and peroxynitrite are highly reactive and unstable, and, as such, are unsuitable in a signaling role. That is, they simply cannot travel far without oxidizing some nearby molecule. However, H_2O_2 is considered to be the primary intracellular redox signaling molecule [34-36]. H_2O_2 is small and can diffuse easily, and it is stable enough to travel and oxidize specific sites on target molecules [37]. As discussed previously, superoxide and other more reactive radicals are partially neutralized by being converted to H_2O_2, allowing this molecule to be reflective of the overall oxidative state in the cell.

Several studies have produced results in support of ROS having a signaling role, both with short-term exercise and as a result of exercise training. As noted above, NOX-induced ROS contribute to increasing calcium release from SR. Reid [38,39] showed that reduction of

ROS below basal levels reduced the force production of skeletal muscle, while increasing ROS to a certain point increased force production, and ROS exposure above that point resulted in a reduction in force production [40]. Other studies have demonstrated that beneficial training adaptations are eliminated when trainees are treated with antioxidants. Gomez-Cabrera et al. [41] found that 1,000 mg per day of vitamin C supplementation attenuated increased PGC-1a (peroxisome proliferator-activated receptor-gamma coactivator-1 alpha; a transcriptional cofactor that is involved in initiating mitochondrial biogenesis) expression and, consequently, attenuated the increase in mitochondrial density that commonly occurs with aerobic exercise training. In addition, the training-induced increase in several antioxidant enzymes was inhibited with vitamin C supplementation [41]. Similarly, Ristow et al. [42] found that daily supplementation with a combination of 1,000 mg of vitamin C and 400 IU of vitamin E eliminated the training-induced increases in insulin sensitivity and PGC-1a expression, as well as levels of endogenous antioxidants SOD and glutathione peroxidase. It is noteworthy that another recent study of the effects of antioxidant supplementation on training adaptations in humans found that daily supplementation with 500 mg of vitamin C and 400 IU of vitamin E had no effect on physiological responses to 12 weeks of aerobic exercise training [43]. These contradictory findings may be attributable to the dosage of antioxidant supplement utilized, but further research in this area is merited [43].

Although how ROS signaling induces adaptations to training is not fully understood, a number of possible mechanisms have been identified. For example, certain proteins, especially those composed of sulfur-containing amino acids such as cysteine, are readily and reversibly oxidized by ROS [44,45]. In addition, the oxidation of amino acid residues containing aromatic structures (e.g., histidine, tyrosine, tryptophan, and phenylalanine) can result in protein conformational changes that alter affinity to target molecules and potentially increase or decrease binding to inhibitors or stimulators [46]. ROS have also been shown to affect the catalytic rate of kinases and phosphatases, a finding suggesting that ROS have the capacity to 'fine-tune' the magnitude and duration of inhibitory and stimulatory signals [46]. Together, these findings suggest a critical role for ROS in improving muscle function acutely, and in stimulating adaptations to exercise training, and that some critical level of ROS production may be needed to limit oxidative damage.

ROS and oxidative stress

Under conditions of chronic abundance of oxidants relative to antioxidants, oxidative damage can occur. Primary targets of excessive ROS are proteins, lipids, and DNA. As mentioned earlier in this review, oxidizing agents acquire electrons from target molecules. In proteins, this can result in conformational changes, some of which are irreversible. For example, the formation of carbonyl groups on several amino acid residues is an irreversible modification, and affected proteins are targeted for degradation [47,48]. Oxidative stress, then, is a stimulus for protein catabolism.

Lipid molecules can also be targeted by ROS, resulting in them being oxidized, a process called peroxidation. The interaction of a lipid molecule with a radical sets off a self-propagating chain reaction [49], as one radicalized lipid molecule interacts with others, a process that continues until two radicals interact with each other. This process is damaging to cells and tissue, and has been implicated in the development of atherosclerosis, asthma, Parkinson's disease, and other conditions [49].

Oxidative damage to DNA can take many forms, dependent on the portion of the DNA structure affected, and the specific ROS involved [50-52]. The details of how oxidation affects DNA is beyond the scope of this review, but, briefly, oxidative damage to DNA has been linked to cancer, with its primary role likely being the initiation of carcinogenesis rather than cancer promotion/progression [52].

Sedentariness, exercise, and oxidative stress

The association between sedentary behavior and chronic disease is well-established, and it may be that oxidative stress is a key process whereby inactivity leads to a number of chronic diseases. Specifically, oxidative stress is known to be associated with aging, cardiovascular disease, and sarcopenia, and it may be that exercise exerts its beneficial effects on each of these disease processes through its effects on redox status.

As discussed previously, the mitochondria are one source of ROS, as superoxide is produced when electrons leak from the ETC. and bind with molecular oxygen. Mitochondrial superoxide production does seem to be increased during exercise relative to a basal state [7], and while factors such as temperature [53] may also influence mitochondrial function and ROS production, it has been suggested that long-term sedentariness produces an environment conducive to high basal levels of superoxide formation. It was noted earlier that mitochondrial ROS production increases less than threefold between rest and exhaustive exercise, while metabolic rate increases approximately 100-fold. Several studies have reported that state IV mitochondrial respiration (resting) is more productive of ROS than state III mitochondrial respiration (exercise) [53-57]. Fisher-Wellman and Neufer [58] explain that the rate at which electrons flow down the ETC. is influenced by energy demand, and not energy availability. As such, sedentariness and the relative lack of adenosine diphosphate (ADP) availability results in a slower transmission of electrons through the ETC., thereby allowing for increased electron leakage. In addition, the concentration of reducing equivalents (e.g., NADH and $FADH_2$) influences the cumulative redox state, and an increase in the concentration of reducing equivalents as may be caused by over-nutrition induces a more reduced environment, which subsequently increases the driving force for electron entry into the ETC. at complex I (NADH/NAD+) and complex II ($FADH_2$/FAD+) [58]. As a result, though oxygen flux through skeletal muscle is many times higher during exercise, the rate of electron flow through the ETC. is faster due to the increased energy demand (state III respiration). This condition 'de-stresses' the mitochondria and permits less time for electron leakage, and as a result mitochondrial ROS production increases relatively little.

People who are chronically inactive also exhibit lower levels of endogenous antioxidants [59-61]. In fact, it appears that the regular inducement of exercise-mediated ROS formation stimulates an adaptation in skeletal muscle that enhances its capacity to manage oxidative stress, a finding consistent with hormesis, the concept that many biological systems respond in a bell-shaped or inverted U-shaped pattern to potential stressors [59]. For example, moderate exercise training alters oxidative homeostasis by reducing basal levels of oxidative damage [60], and by increasing resistance to oxidative stress, mediated largely through increased endogenous antioxidant defenses [60,62]. Jackson et al. [63] found that skeletal muscle contraction-induced ROS activates several identified redox-sensitive transcription factors, including nuclear factor-κB (NF-κB). This transcription factor regulates expression of cell-protective genes during adaptation to exercise [64].

Aerobic exercise training sufficient to improve cardiorespiratory fitness might also be expected to improve oxidative balance via its effects on purine metabolism. As noted previously, hypoxanthine is the substrate for XO, an enzyme that produces xanthine and superoxide. Intensive, and especially anaerobic, exercise has been shown to lead to increased XO activity [25]. Because aerobic exercise training typically increases aerobic capacity and work rate at lactate threshold, it is capable of reducing hypoxanthine levels in the plasma [65], thereby providing less substrate for XO and resulting in less ROS production at any submaximal absolute work rate.

Sirtuin 1 (SIRT1) is an enzyme that functions to remove acetyl groups from proteins involved in cellular regulation and can therefore influence expression of specific genes. Two known targets of SIRT1 are PGC-1a and FOXOs, which are Forkhead box transcription factors, some of which affect antioxidant enzyme expression (e.g., catalase and MnSOD) [66-68]. Exercise training has been shown to increase SIRT1 activity [69], and this may mediate much of the exercise-related improvement in oxidative state. Increased mitochondrial biogenesis and increased mitochondrial density alone may reduce ROS production while at rest by providing new mitochondria to supplement those that are aged or dysfunctional due to oxidative stress, as well as increasing mitochondrial membrane surface area to facilitate diffusion and dissipation of proton gradients, thereby reducing the slowing of electron flow in the ETC. during rest [68]. Additionally, long-term exercise training appears to increase the level of endogenous antioxidants in proportion to the level of ROS production, resulting in a supercompensation that affords protection from their potentially damaging effects [60,62,63].

Good evidence exists showing an inverse relationship between measures of aerobic fitness and oxidative stress [70-72], and, as has been noted, it is likely that much of the protection against oxidative stress afforded by exercise is mediated through improvements in antioxidant capacity. Mitochondrial ROS production is proportional to oxygen flux [6,7], and exercise increases ROS formation in the ETC. Likewise, ROS formation by NOX is also elevated during exercise [18], and it may be that an increase in aerobic capacity may also increase the capacity for ROS formation via these pathways. Conversely, given that improved aerobic fitness would be expected to reduce AMP levels at any given absolute exercise intensity, it may be expected that ROS synthesis by XO would be reduced with an increase in aerobic fitness. It appears that ROS production is increased during exercise, and, as such, it may be that an increase in aerobic capacity is accompanied by an increased capacity for ROS production. However, it also appears that regularly inducing an oxidative environment with exercise results in significant improvements in antioxidant levels and activity. Falone et al. [73] found that recreational runners exhibited greater serum antioxidant capacity and reduced protein carbonyl content before and after exhaustive exercise than untrained subjects. Interestingly, they also reported that, compared to pre-exercise baseline levels, exhaustive exercise resulted in reduced levels of thiobarbituric acid-reactive substances (TBARS) in trained subjects, while resulting in increased levels of TBARS in untrained subjects. (TBARS are formed as a byproduct of lipid peroxidation.) These findings support the conclusion that greater levels of aerobic fitness are accompanied by improved antioxidant capacity such that, though ROS formation is elevated with exercise, indicators of oxidative stress are reduced.

Although it appears that skeletal muscle exhibits the largest exercise-induced enhancement in controlling oxidative stress, other tissues also significantly enhance antioxidant defense mechanisms. For example, Azizbeigi et al. [74] reported that 8 weeks of progressive resistance training improved the antioxidant capacity of erythrocytes mainly through increases in SOD activity. Similarly, Metin et al. [75] reported that erythrocytes in young male soccer players exhibited greater SOD activity than controls. While there may be numerous consequences of these adaptations in the blood (e.g., less lipid oxidation in plasma), one effect that has been identified is that erythrocytes demonstrate better resistance to ROS-induced hemolysis after exercise training [76].

Another example is the liver. This organ has a high metabolic rate at rest, but it is markedly reduced during exercise as blood flow is redirected to the working muscles [77]. As such, a relative ischemia is induced in the liver during exercise. This stimulus results in xanthine dehydrogenase being converted to XO and increased ROS production via the enzyme-catalyzed mechanism described earlier. It is noteworthy that the liver contains much higher levels of XO than does skeletal muscle [58], and this pathway therefore provides a significant proportion of hepatic ROS. Radak et al. [78] showed that in rats, exercise training at 75% of maximum oxygen uptake (VO_{2max}) for 8 weeks resulted in a significant reduction in ROS production in the liver compared with non-exercised animals. They also reported that reduced GSH levels were higher, and oxidized GSH (GSSG) levels were lower in the trained group than in the sedentary group, reflecting a more favorable redox state.

Redox balance in the brain also appears to respond favorably to exercise training. Regular physical exercise results in an increase in the content of several antioxidants in the brain, including Cu/ZnSOD and glutathione peroxidase, as well as increases in PGC-1a [79]. In addition, exercise appears to stimulate an increase in the production of brain-derived neurotrophic factor (BDNF) [80], though the mechanisms are not fully understood. BDNF is a uniquely versatile substance, and has been shown to influence brain development, neuroplasticity, neurogenesis, and neuron cell survival [81], and BDNF content in the brain has been shown to increase in response to exercise and oxidative stress [82]. It appears that oxidative stress stimulates an increase in BDNF content, which subsequently stimulates increased antioxidant enzyme expression, at least in part via increased NF-κB activation [83,84]. Oxidative stress has been implicated in several disorders of the brain, including Alzheimer's disease and Parkinson's disease [85]. A number of studies have found that regular activity provides protection against acquiring these conditions, and the anti-oxidative influence of physical exercise on the brain may provide one important explanation for those findings [85,86]. Importantly, increases in BDNF production appear to depend largely on increased neural activity, which can be induced with exercise, intellectual activity, or reduced caloric intake [87].

Exercise-induced oxidative environment, ROS signaling, and protein synthesis

It was noted earlier that exercise acutely increases ROS production via increased activity of several enzyme-

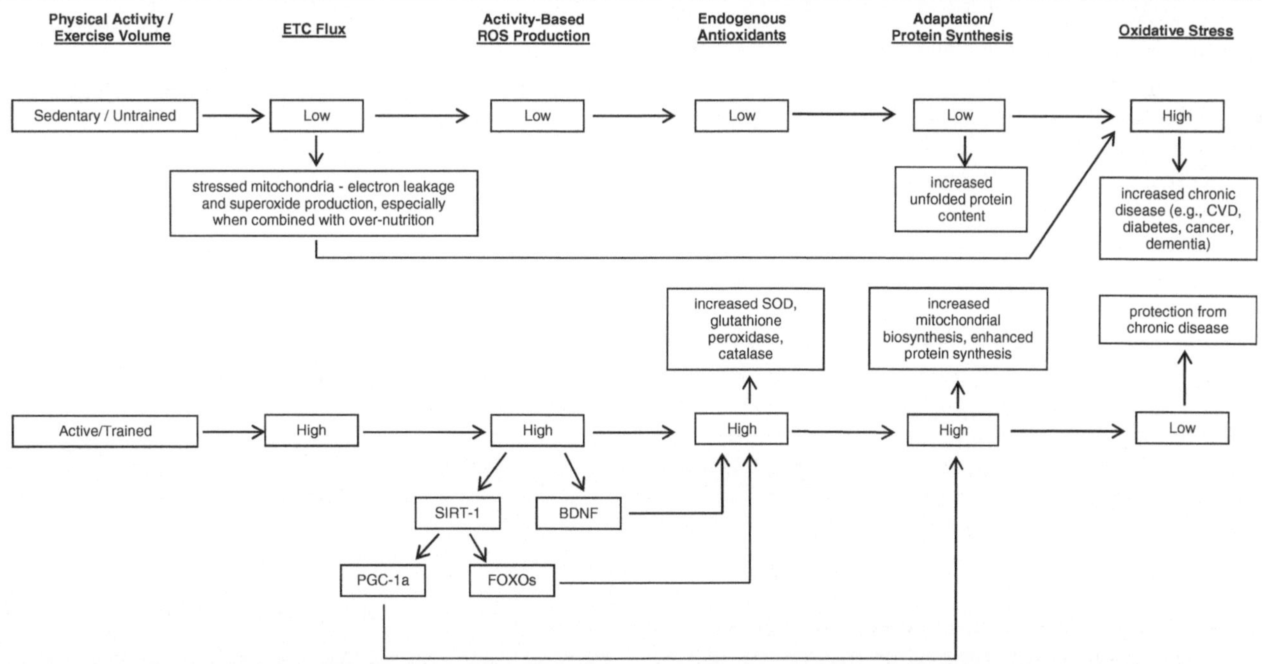

Figure 1 *BDNF* **brain-derived neurotrophic factor, ETC. electron transport chain,** *CVD* **cardiovascular disease,** *FOXOs* **forkhead box transcription factors,** *PGC-1a* **peroxisome proliferator-activated receptor-gamma coactivator-1 alpha,** *ROS* **reactive oxygen species,** *SIRT-1* **sirtuin-1,** *SOD* **superoxide dismutase.**

catalyzed processes. It was also previously noted that several studies have shown that blocking ROS formation associated with exercise also attenuates many of the key adaptations to exercise training. Taken together, these findings suggest that ROS formation is not simply a toxic byproduct of muscle contraction or oxygen metabolism, but is a key participant in stimulating beneficial adaptations to training, and, as such, regularly inducing an oxidative redox state may be important in promoting health. Several recent studies have yielded results that seem to support this position. Nyberg et al. [61] measured arteriovenous GSH and GSSG differences in the legs of young (23 ± 1 years) sedentary, old (66 ± 2 years) sedentary, and old (62 ± 2 years) active men during knee extension exercise. As noted previously, GSH is an antioxidant, and is converted to GSSG in its reduced form, so an increase in GSSG and/or an increase in the GSSG:GSH ratio would indicate a more oxidative redox state. Young sedentary men demonstrated an exercise-associated increase in GSSG and the GSSG:GSH ratio in venous blood that was correlated with intensity. Interestingly, the exercise-related increases did not occur in older sedentary or older active men, though the older active men did display higher levels of GSH and antioxidant enzymes. It appears that the oxidative stress associated with aging chronically activates NF-κB and results in increased antioxidant enzyme activity, but the capacity of aged muscle to stimulate a further increase of ROS during contraction sufficient to measurably alter the GSSG:GSH ratio is significantly reduced compared with young muscle [88-90]. Given the important signaling roles played by ROS (e.g., stimulation of mitochondrial biosynthesis, described previously), it is possible that a reduced capacity to stimulate an oxidative redox state via muscle contraction may contribute to aging and the development of chronic disease.

Recently, it has also been speculated that the oxidative environment that is associated with exercise may be critical for the synthesis of certain proteins, specifically those that exhibit disulphide bonds, many of which are membrane or secretory proteins [91]. Oxidation of cysteine residues leads to the formation of sulfenic acid intermediates, and in close proximity to other oxidized cysteine residues can result in disulphide bonds [92,93]. Said another way, these bonds cannot be formed in a reduced redox state. In fact, Ron and Harding [94] found that the endoplasmic reticulum of sedentary, insulin-resistant rats had significantly fewer disulphide bonds and, therefore, more unfolded proteins than their active, insulin-sensitive counterparts. Therefore, it may be that the transient and significant increase in ROS production and the consequent oxidative shift that results during exercise is necessary to optimize the production of these proteins, and people who are chronically inactive may not provide that environment frequently enough for optimal protein synthesis. If this is true, it provides yet one more additional mechanism whereby regular physical exercise sufficient to produce an oxidative redox state optimizes health.

Summary

Oxidative stress is a consequence of the presence of too many oxidants relative to antioxidants, and can result in cellular or tissue damage, illness, and disease. However, ROS are not entirely toxic, and research evidence indicates important healthy roles for oxidants, including cell signaling, adaptation, and inducing an environment conducive to synthesis of proteins containing disulphide bonds. Several studies report that many of the beneficial adaptations to exercise training are reduced or eliminated when ROS levels are artificially reduced, further supporting the conclusions that regularly inducing an oxidative redox state through exercise is healthful. Habitual sedentariness, especially in combination with overnutrition, may lead to chronically stressed mitochondria and increased mitochondria-sourced superoxide production, and to reduced levels of endogenous antioxidant enzymes, as well as reduced mitochondrial biosynthesis, all of which foster a vicious cycle that results in an environment that is increasingly oxidative. Conversely, regular exercise appears to produce a hormesis response, whereby the stressor (exercise) induces a transient, systemically oxidative environment that stimulates adaptations enhancing the capacity of tissues throughout the body to neutralize ROS and to more effectively regulate redox balance (see Figure 1). These adaptations provide resistance to development of a number of chronic diseases, and may explain much of the exercise-related improvement in health and longevity cited in many epidemiological studies.

Competing interests
The authors declare that they have no competing of interests.

Acknowledgments
No financial support was received for the preparation of this manuscript.

Author details
[1]Department of Exercise Science and Sport Management, Kennesaw State University, 520 Parliament Garden Way NW, Kennesaw, GA 30144, USA. [2]School of Health, Physical Education, and Recreation, University of Nebraska at Omaha, Omaha, NE, USA.

References
1. Sies H, Jones DP. *Oxidative stress.* Amsterdam: Elsevier; 2007.
2. Gutowski M, Kowalczyk S. **A study of free radical chemistry: their role and pathophysiological significance.** *Acta Biochim Pol.* 2013; **60(1)**:1–16.
3. Pryor WA. *Free radicals.* New York: McGraw-Hill; 1966.
4. Xu X, Arriaga EA. **Qualitative determination of superoxide release at both sides of the mitochondrial inner membrane by capillary electrophoretic analysis of the oxidation products of triphenylphosphonium hydroethidine.** *Free Radic Biol Med.* 2009; **46(7)**:905–13.

5. Muller FL, Liu Y, Van Remmen H. **Complex III releases superoxide to both sides of the inner mitochondrial membrane.** *J Biol Chem.* 2004; **279(47)**:49064–73.
6. St-Pierre J, Buckingham JA, Roebuck SJ, Brand MD. **Topology of superoxide production from different sites in the mitochondrial electron transport chain.** *J Biol Chem.* 2002; **277**:44784–90.
7. Saborido A, Naudi A, Portero-Otin M, Pamplona R, Megias A. **Stanozolol treatment decreases the mitochondrial ROS generation and oxidative stress induced by acute exercise in rat skeletal muscle.** *J Appl Physiol.* 2011; **110**:661–9.
8. Gaitanos GC, Williams C, Boobis LH, Brooks S. **Human muscle metabolism during intermittent maximal exercise.** *J Appl Physiol.* 1993; **75**:712–19.
9. Corbi G, Conti V, Russomanno G, Longobardi G, Furgi G, Filippelli A, Ferrara N. **Adrenergic signaling and oxidative stress—a role for sirtuins?** *Front Physiol.* 2013; **4**:324–324. doi:10.3389/fphys.2013.00324.
10. Kang SW, Chae HZ, Seo MS, Kim K, Baines IC, Rhee SG. **Mammalian peroxiredoxin isoforms can reduce hydrogen peroxide generated in response to growth factors and tumor necrosis factor-a.** *J Biol Chem.* 1998; **273**:6297–302.
11. Tao L, Gao E, Bryan NS, Qu Y, Liu HR, Hu A, et al. **Cardioprotective effects of thioredoxin in myocardial ischemia and reperfusion: role of S-nitrosation.** *Proc Natl Acad Sci U S A.* 2004; **101**:11471–6.
12. Yamawaki H, Haendeler J, Berk BC. **Thioredoxin: a key regulator of cardiovascular homeostasis.** *Circ Res.* 2003; **93**:1029–33.
13. Lu SC. **Regulation of hepatic glutathione synthesis: current concepts and controversies.** *FASEB J.* 1999; **13(10)**:1169–83.
14. Fu XJ, Peng YB, Hu YP, Shi YZ, Yao M, Zhang X. **NADPH oxidase 1 and its derived reactive oxygen species mediated tissue injury and repair.** *Oxidative Med Cell Longev.* 2014; **2014**:282854. doi:10.1155/2014/282854.
15. Halliwell B, Gutteridge J. *Free radicals in biology and medicine.* Oxford: Oxford University Press; 2007.
16. Cherednichenko G, Zima AV, Feng W, Schaefer S, Blatter LA, Pessah IN. **NADH oxidase activity of rat cardiac sarcoplasmic reticulum regulates calcium induced calcium release.** *Circ Res.* 2004; **94**:478–86.
17. Xia R, Webb JA, Gnall LL, Cutler K, Abramson JJ. **Skeletal muscle sarcoplasmic reticulum contains a NADH-dependent oxidase that generates superoxide.** *Am J Physiol Cell Physiol.* 2003; **285**:C215–21.
18. Nathan C, Cunningham-Bussel A. **Beyond oxidative stress—an immunologist's guide to reactive oxygen species.** *Nat Rev Immunol.* 2013; **13(5)**:349–61.
19. Espinosa A, Leiva A, Pena M, Muller M, Debandi A, Hidalgo C, et al. **Myotube depolarization generates reactive oxygen species through NAD (P)H oxidase: ROS-elicited Ca^{2+} stimulates ERK, CREB, early genes.** *J Cell Physiol.* 2006; **209**:379–88.
20. Hidalgo C, Sanchez G, Barrientos G, Aracena-Parks P. **A transverse tubule NADPH oxidase activity stimulates calcium release from isolated triads via ryanodine receptor type 1 S-glutathionylation.** *J Biol Chem.* 2006; **281**:26473–82.
21. Zhao X, Bey EA, Wientjes FB, Cathcart MK. **Cytosolic phospholipase A2 (cPLA2) regulation of human monocyte NADPH oxidase activity: cPLA2 affects translocation but not phosphorylation of p67(phox) and p47 (phox).** *J Biol Chem.* 2002; **277**:25385–92.
22. Gong MC, Arbogast S, Guo Z, Mathenia J, Su W, Reid MB. **Calcium independent phospholipase A2 modulates cytosolic oxidant activity and contractile function in murine skeletal muscle cells.** *J Appl Physiol.* 2006; **100**:399–405.
23. McCord JM. **Oxygen-derived free radicals in postischemic tissue injury.** *N Engl J Med.* 1985; **312**:159–63.
24. Kalyanaraman B. **Teaching the basics of redox biology to medical and graduate students: oxidants, antioxidants and disease mechanisms.** *Redox Biol.* 2013; **1**:244–57.
25. Radak Z, Asano K, Inoue M, Kizaki T, Oh-Ishi S, Suzuki K, et al. **Superoxide dismutase derivative reduces oxidative damage in skeletal muscle of rats during exhaustive exercise.** *J Appl Physiol.* 1995; **79**:129–35.
26. Sindler AL, Delp MD, Reyes R, Wu G, Muller-Delp JM. **Effects of ageing and exercise training on eNOS uncoupling in skeletal muscle resistance arterioles.** *J Physiol.* 2009; **587**:3885–97.
27. Vasquez-Vivar J, Kalyanaraman B, Martasek P, Hogg N, Masters BS, Karoui H, et al. **Superoxide generation by endothelial nitric oxide synthase: the influence of cofactors.** *Proc Natl Acad Sci U S A.* 1998; **95**:9220–5.
28. Cosentino F, Luscher TF. **Tetrahydrobiopterin and endothelial nitric oxide synthase activity.** *Cardiovasc Res.* 1999; **43**:274–8.
29. Bevers LM, Braam B, Post JA, van Zonneveld AJ, Rabelink TJ, Koomans HA, et al. **Tetrahydrobiopterin, but not L-arginine, decreases NO synthase uncoupling in cells expressing high levels of endothelial NO synthase.** *Hypertension.* 2006; **47(1)**:87–94.
30. Pacher P, Beckman JS, Liaudet L. **Nitric oxide and peroxynitrite in health and disease.** *Physiol Rev.* 2007; **87**:315–424.
31. Dikalov S. **Cross talk between mitochondria and NADPH oxidases.** *Free Radic Biol Med.* 2011; **51**:1289–301.
32. Powers SK, Jackson MJ. **Exercise-induced oxidative stress: cellular mechanisms and impact on muscle force production.** *Physiol Rev.* 2008; **88**:1243–76.
33. Bartosz G. **Reactive oxygen species: destroyers or messengers?** *Biochem Pharmacol.* 2009; **77**:1303–15.
34. Toledano MB, Planson A-G, Delaunay-Moisan A. **Reining in H(2)O(2) for safe signaling.** *Cell.* 2010; **140**:454–6.
35. Rhee SG, Kang SW, Jeong W, Chang TS, Yang KS, Woo HA. **Intracellular messenger function of hydrogen peroxide and its regulation by peroxiredoxins.** *Curr Opin Cell Biol.* 2005; **17**:183–9.
36. Bae YS, Oh H, Rhee SG, Yoo YD. **Regulation of reactive oxygen species generation in cell signaling.** *Mol Cells.* 2011; **32**:491–509.
37. Davies MJ. **The oxidative environment and protein damage.** *Biochim Biophys Acta.* 2005; **1703**:93–109.
38. Reid MB. **Nitric oxide, reactive oxygen species, and skeletal muscle contraction.** *Med Sci Sports Exerc.* 2001; **33**:371–6.
39. Reid MB. **Redox modulation of skeletal muscle contraction: what we know and what we don't.** *J Appl Physiol.* 2001; **90**:724–31.
40. Reid MB, Khawli FA, Moody MR. **Reactive oxygen in skeletal muscle. III. Contractility of unfatigued muscle.** *J Appl Physiol.* 1993; **75**:1081–7.
41. Gomez-Cabrera MC, Domenech E, Romagnoli M, Arduini A, Borras C, Pallardo FV, et al. **Oral administration of vitamin C decreases muscle mitochondrial biogenesis and hampers training-induced adaptations in endurance performance.** *Am J Clin Nutr.* 2008; **87**:142–9.
42. Ristow M, Zarse K, Oberbach A, Kloting N, Birringer M, Kiehntopf M, et al. **Antioxidants prevent health-promoting effects of physical exercise in humans.** *Proc Natl Acad Sci U S A.* 2009; **106**:8665–70.
43. Yfanti C, Akerstrom T, Nielsen S, Nielsen A, Mounier R, Mortensen OH, et al. **Antioxidant supplementation does not alter endurance training adaptation.** *Med Sci Sports Exerc.* 2010; **42**:1388–95.
44. Janssen-Heininger YM, Mossman BT, Heintz NH, Forman HJ, Kalyanaraman B, Finkel T, et al. **Redox-based regulation of signal transduction: principles, pitfalls, and promises.** *Free Radic Biol Med.* 2008; **45**:1–17.
45. Hoshi T, Heinemann S. **Regulation of cell function by methionine oxidation and reduction.** *J Physiol.* 2001; **531**:1–11.
46. Corcoran A, Cotter TG. **Redox regulation of protein kinases.** *FEBS J.* 2013; **280**:1944–65.
47. Grune T, Reinheckel T, Davies KJ. **Degradation of oxidized proteins in mammalian cells.** *FASEB J.* 1997; **11**:526–34.
48. Levine RL. **Carbonyl modified proteins in cellular regulation, aging, and disease.** *Free Radic Biol Med.* 2002; **32**:790–6.
49. Mylonas C, Kouretas D. **Lipid peroxidation and tissue damage.** *In Vivo.* 1999; **1999(13)**:295–310.
50. Szabo C, Ohshima H. **DNA damage induced by peroxynitrite: subsequent biological effects.** *Nitric Oxide.* 1997; **1(5)**:373–85.
51. Burney S, Caulfield JL, Niles JC, Wishnok JS, Tannenbaum SR. **The chemistry of DNA damage from nitric oxide and peroxynitrite.** *Mutat Res.* 1998; **424**:37–49.
52. Cooke MS, Evans MD, Dizdaroglu M, Lunec J. **Oxidative DNA damage: mechanisms, mutation, and disease.** *FASEB J.* 2003; **17**:1195–214.
53. Di Meo S, Venditti P. **Mitochondria in exercise-induced oxidative stress.** *Biol Signals Recept.* 2001; **10**:125–40.
54. Kavazis AN, Talbert EE, Smuder AJ, Hudson MB, Nelson WB, Powers SK. **Mechanical ventilation induces diaphragmatic mitochondrial dysfunction and increased oxidant production.** *Free Radic Biol Med.* 2009; **46**:842–50.
55. Herrero A, Barja G. **ADP-regulation of mitochondrial free radical production is different with complex I- or complex II-linked substrates: implications for the exercise paradox and brain hypermetabolism.** *J Bioenerg Biomembr.* 1997; **29**:241–9.
56. Adhihetty PJ, Ljubicic V, Menzies KJ, Hood DA. **Differential susceptibility of subsarcolemmal and intermyofibrillar mitochondria to apoptotic stimuli.** *Am J Physiol Cell Physiol.* 2005; **289**:C994–1001.
57. Kozlov AV, Szalay L, Umar F, Kropik K, Staniek K, Niedermuller H, et al. **Skeletal muscles, heart, and lung are the main sources of oxygen radicals in old rats.** *Biochem Biophys Acta.* 2005; **1740**:382–9.

58. Fisher-Wellman KH, Neufer PD. **Linking mitochondrial bioenergetics to insulin resistance via redox biology.** *Trends Endocrinol Metab.* 2012; **23(3):**142–53.
59. Radak Z, Chung HY, Goto S. **Systemic adaptation to oxidative challenge induced by regular exercise.** *Free Radic Biol Med.* 2008; **2008(44):**153–9.
60. Urso ML, Clarkson PM. **Oxidative stress, exercise, and antioxidant supplementation.** *Toxicology.* 2003; **2003(189):**41–54.
61. Nyberg M, Mortensen SP, Cabo H, Gomez-Cabrera MC, Vina J, Hellsten Y. **Roles of sedentary aging and lifelong physical activity in exchange of glutathione across exercising human skeletal muscle.** *Free Radic Biol Med.* 2014; **73:**166–73.
62. Sen CK. **Oxidants and antioxidants in exercise.** *J Appl Physiol.* 1995; **79(3):**675–86.
63. Jackson MJ, Papa S, Bolanos J, Bruckdorfer R, Carlsen H, Elliott RM, et al. **Antioxidants, reactive oxygen and nitrogen species, gene induction and mitochondrial function.** *Mol Aspects Med.* 2002; **23:**209–85.
64. Vasilaki A, Mansouri A, Remmen H, van der Meulen JH, Larkin L, Richardson AG, et al. **Free radical generation by skeletal muscle of adult and old mice: effect of contractile activity.** *Aging Cell.* 2006; **5:**109–17.
65. Teixeira-Lemos E, Nunes S, Teixeira F, Reis F. Regular physical exercise training assists in preventing type 2 diabetes development: focus on its antioxidant and anti-inflammatory properties. Cardiovasc Diabetol. 2011;10:12. doi:10.1186/1475-2840-10-12. http://www.cardiab.com/content/10/1/12.
66. Finkel T, Deng CX, Mostoslavsky R. **Recent progress in the biology and physiology of sirtuins.** *Nature.* 2009; **460:**587–91.
67. Haigis MC, Sinclair DA. **Mammalian sirtuins: biological insights and disease relevance.** *Annu Rev Pathol.* 2010; **5:**253–95.
68. Guarente L, Franklin H. **Epstein lecture: sirtuins, aging, and medicine.** *N Engl J Med.* 2011; **364:**2235–44.
69. Navarro-Arevalo A, Canavate C, Sanchez-del-Pino MJ. **Myocardial and skeletal muscle aging and changes in oxidative stress in relationship to rigorous exercise training.** *Mech Ageing Dev.* 1999; **108:**207–17.
70. Campbell PT, Gross MD, Potter JD, Schmitz KH, Duggan C, McTiernan A, et al. **Effect of exercise on oxidative stress: a 12-month randomized, controlled trial.** *Med Sci Sports Exerc.* 2010; **42:**1448–53.
71. Nojima H, Watanabe H, Yamane K, Kitahara Y, Sekikawa K, Yamamoto H, et al. **Effect of aerobic exercise training on oxidative stress in patients with type 2 diabetes mellitus.** *Metabolism.* 2008; **57:**170–6.
72. Elosua R, Molina L, Fito M, Arquer A, Sanchez-Quesada JL, Covas MI, et al. **Response of oxidative stress biomarkers to a 16-week aerobic physical activity program, and to acute physical activity, in healthy young men and women.** *Atherosclerosis.* 2003; **167:**327–34.
73. Falone S, Mirabilio A, Pennelli A, Cacchio M, Di Baldassarre A, Gallina S, et al. **Differential impact of acute bout of exercise on redox- and oxidative damage-related profiles between untrained subjects and amateur runners.** *Physiol Res.* 2010; **59:**953–61.
74. Azizbeigi K, Azarbayiani MA, Peeri M, Agha-alinejad H, Stannard S. **The effect of progressive resistance training on oxidative stress and antioxidant enzyme activity in erythrocytes in untrained men.** *Int J Sport Nutr Exerc Metab.* 2013; **23:**230–8.
75. Metin G, Atukeren P, Alturfan AA, Gulyasar T, Kaya M, Gumustas MK. **Lipid peroxidation, erythrocyte superoxide-dismutase activity and trace metals in young male footballers.** *Yonsei Med J.* 2003; **44:**979–86.
76. Blache D, Lussier-Cacan S, Gagnon J, Leon AS, Rao DC, Skinner JS, et al. **Effect of exercise training on in vitro LDL oxidation and free radical-induced hemolysis: the HERITAGE Family Study.** *Antioxid Redox Signal.* 2007; **9:**122–30.
77. Masud MM, Fujimoto T, Miyake M, Watanuki S, Itoh M, Tashiro M. **Redistribution of whole-body energy metabolism by exercise: a positron emission tomography study.** *Ann Nucl Med.* 2009; **23:**81–8.
78. Radak Z, Chung HY, Naito H, Takahashi R, Jung KJ, Kim HJ, et al. **Age-associated increase in oxidative stress and nuclear factor kappaB activation are attenuated in rat liver by regular exercise.** *FASEB J.* 2004; **18:**749–50.
79. Barde YA. **Trophic factors and neuronal survival.** *Neruon.* 1989; **2:**1525–34.
80. Stranahan AM, Lee K, Martin B, Maudsley S, Golden E, Cutler RG, et al. **Voluntary exercise and caloric restriction enhance hippocampal dendritic spine density and BDNF levels in diabetic mice.** *Hippocampus.* 2009; **19:**951–61.
81. van Praag H, Kempermann G, Gage FH. **Running increases cell proliferation and neurogenesis in the adult mouse dentate gyrus.** *Nat Neurosci.* 1999; **2:**266–70.
82. Mattson MP, Maudsley S, Martin B. **A neural signaling triumvirate that influences ageing and age-related disease: insulin/IGF-1.** *BDNF and Serotonin Ageing Res Rev.* 2004; **3:**445–64.
83. Mattson MP, Lovell MA, Furukawa K, Markesbery WR. **Neurotrophic factors attenuate glutamate-induced accumulation of peroxides, elevation of intracellular Ca^{2+} concentration, and neurotoxicity and increase antioxidant enzyme activities in hippocampal neurons.** *J Neurochem.* 1995; **65:**1740–51.
84. Radak Z, Marton O, Nagy E, Koltai E, Goto S. **The complex role of physical exercise and reactive oxygen species on the brain.** *J Sport Health Sci.* 2013; **2:**87–93.
85. Marques-Aleixo I, Oliveira PJ, Moreira PI, Magalhaes J, Ascensao A. **Physical exercise as a possible strategy for brain protection: evidence from mitochondrial-mediated mechanisms.** *Prog Neurobiol.* 2012; **2012:**149–62.
86. Texel SJ, Mattson MP. **Impaired adaptive cellular responses to oxidative stress and the pathogenesis of Alzheimer's disease.** *Antioxid Redox Signal.* 2011; **14(8):**1519–34.
87. Rothman SM, Mattson MP. **Activity-dependent, stress-responsive BDNF signaling and the quest for optimal brain health and resilience throughout the lifespan.** *Neuroscience.* 2013; **239:**228–40.
88. Vasilaki A, McArdle F, Iwanejko LM, McArdle A. **Adaptive responses of mouse skeletal muscle to contractile activity: the effect of age.** *Mech Ageing Dev.* 2006; **127:**830–9.
89. Cai D, Frantz JD, Tawa NE Jr, Melendez PA, Oh BC, Lidov HG, et al. **IKKbeta/NF-kappaB activation causes severe muscle wasting in mice.** *Cell.* 2004; **119:**285–98.
90. Ji LL. **Exercise-induced modulation of antioxidant defense.** *Ann N Y Acad Sci.* 2002; **959:**82–92.
91. Watson JD. **Type 2 diabetes as a redox disease.** *Lancet.* 2014; **383:**841–3.
92. Drose S, Brandt U. **Molecular mechanisms of superoxide production by the mitochondrial respiratory chain.** *Adv Exp Med Biol.* 2012; **748:**145–69.
93. Brown DI, Griendling KK. **Nox proteins in signal transduction.** *Free Radic Biol Med.* 2009; **47:**1239–53.
94. Ron D, Harding HP. **Protein-folding homeostasis in the endoplasmic reticulum and nutritional regulation.** *Cold Spring Harb Perspect Biol.* 2012; **4:**a013177. doi:10.1101/cshperspect.a013177.

Evaluation of Global Health in Master Swimmers Involved in French National Championships

François Potdevin[1*], Gilles Vanlerberghe[2], Gautier Zunquin[3], Thierry Pezé[3] and Denis Theunynck[3]

Abstract

Background: Swimming is often recommended as a means of increasing physical activity and gaining health benefits. The present study examined the psychological, social, and physical health states in competitive swimmers engaged in long-term training.

Methods: The study took place during the 4 days of the French master championships in France in 2011 (from 10 to 13 March). Global health parameters were evaluated and compared with general values reported in studies aiming to describe health standard values in France or Europe. All swimmers selected for the event were invited to participate in the study. Setting questionnaires concerning mental and social health (short form 36), physical activity (International Physical Activity Questionnaire), and medication were administered. Peak expiratory flow ($l.min^{-1}$) was measured, and body mass index ($kg.m^{-2}$) was calculated from height (m) and body mass (kg). Prevalence of overweight and obesity was calculated by age and gender. Chi-squared tests were used to compare prevalence of overweight and obesity between participants and reference values. Short form 36 scores and physical activity ($met.h.week^{-1}$) were compared with reference values by single *t*-tests. Two-way ANOVA was used to compare peak flow results with standard values. The level of significance was set at $p < 0.05$.

Results: Out of 1554 master swimmers, 490 participated in this study (rates of participation = 44.8 and 23.5 % for females and males, respectively). Data showed inequality of health indexes as compared with reference values, despite a significantly higher level of physical activity including swimming activity. The prevalence of obesity was significantly lower ($p < 0.05$), and peak expiratory flow values were higher among female swimmers (from 7.6 to 17 % higher according to the age, $p < 0.05$). Perception of vitality was significantly higher for all female swimmers and the older age groups of male swimmers ($p < 0.05$). Perception of bodily pain indicated significantly lower scores for swimmers than the reference values ($p < 0.05$). Significantly lower prevalence of swimmers taking medication was noted in comparison with the French national values ($p = 0.012$).

Conclusions: Compared with reference data from various sources, master competitive swimmers used less medication, had lower rates of obesity in most age groups, had greater peak expiratory flow values suggesting improved lung function, had higher levels of total physical activity, and had more favorable scores for various subscales of the SF-36. The results argue in favor of competitive swimming for its positive effects on health outcomes.
(Continued on next page)

* Correspondence: francois.potdevin@univ-lille2.fr
[1]Univ. Lille, EA 7369 - URePSSS - Unité de Recherche Pluridisciplinaire Sport Santé Société, F-59000 Lille, France
Full list of author information is available at the end of the article

(Continued from previous page)

Key Points:

- French master swimmers involved in national championships have many positive health outcomes in terms of weight management, respiratory function, and vitality. However, the very high physical activity level in this competitive context did not result in significantly better levels on all parameters in comparison with their national counterparts (pain perception, social, emotional, and mental health).
- Positive health outcomes were higher for female master swimmers in terms of weight management, respiratory function, and vitality.
- The fact that these benefits were not linked with medication consumption could be interesting in an economic context aimed at controlling expenditures on health. Based on these data, we can argue for promoting this form of physical activity across the lifespan.

Background

Regular physical activity throughout the lifespan improves health and decreases the prevalence of various chronic diseases and disorders [1, 2]. Accordingly, many programs to promote physical activity are being conducted around the world. The consensual recommendations state that all adults should carry out some degree of moderate or intense physical activity, preferably on a daily basis [3–5].

Among the possible kinds of physical activities, various authoritative groups and researchers often recommend swimming as a means of increasing physical activity and gaining health benefits. Swimming has proven to have multiple positive effects in the areas of the prevention and treatment of cardiovascular disease [6, 7], on cardiorespiratory fitness [8, 9], and on anthropometric measures such as body weight, fat distribution, waist circumference, body mass index [10, 11], and blood pressure [12]. Considered as an aerobic activity, swimming has been reported to have emotional state benefits among healthy people and clinical populations on anxiety depression, moods, or self-esteem [13, 14]. Despite studies showing that extensive training in swimming sometimes has detrimental effects on the respiratory system due to the chloramine context [15], and injuries involving the shoulders, spine, or blood pressure [16, 17], swimming is recognized over the world as an effective way to promote health.

Most studies aiming to assess the health benefits of swimming have focused on either physiological or psychological parameters. Experiments are often carried out in the short term (from 6 weeks to 1 year), which prevent them from measuring the long-term impact on overall health. According to the World Health Organization (WHO), the concept of health has to be defined as "a complete state of mental, physical, and social well-being" [18], suggesting that a multi-level analysis is needed to study the health benefits of swimming. Studies of overall health in a specific sample must therefore use several health indexes measuring different domains of health. In the case of a large sample, the health indexes used have to be relevant and easy to administer or measure at a given time. The body mass index (BMI; $kg.m^{-2}$) is a physical health parameter for assessing excess adipose tissue, which is associated with increased risks such as type 2 diabetes, cardiovascular disease, high blood pressure, and dyslipidemia, as well as certain types of cancer [19]. Spirometric lung function measurement is commonly used for the diagnosis, assessment, and management of lung diseases [20]. This measure could be especially relevant for swimmers who practice in a chloramine environment. The short form 36 health survey questionnaire (SF 36) is widely used to evaluate several aspects of health related to physical mobility, emotional well-being, social life, and overall well-being [21].

Competitive master swimmers appeared to be interesting subjects for studying the health benefits of swimming because they spend more time training than the average sedentary aging person and allow one to test for the long-term effects of swimming. This population can be defined as adult swimmers, older than 25 years old, engaged in a regular training, and participating in several competitions per year. Dionigi [22] suggested that older people who compete in sports resist the dominant negative stereotypes associated with aging and feel empowered to live a fulfilling and healthy life. Few studies have aimed to assess the health impact of competitive training among master swimmers. Vaccaro et al. [23] showed a significantly lower percentage of fat in female master swimmers ages 20 to 70 as compared with untrained women. Walsh et al. [24] found a lower prevalence of obesity in master swimmers involved in world swimming championships. Guthrie et al. [25] noted that master swimmers had a lower prevalence of high blood pressure and took less medication to manage it than their national counterparts. Additionally, the results showed that master swimmers suffering from high blood pressure considered themselves healthier. Using the same methodology, Erickson and Guthrie [26] found fewer physically and mentally unhealthy days and fewer inactive days due to health problems among master swimmers.

The hypothesis of this study was that with regular and serious engagement in swimming training over a long period of time at older ages, French competitive master swimmers (FCMS) will have better health indexes than reported in studies aiming to describe standard population in France or Europe. The aim of this study was to analyze the physiological and psychological health indexes of FCMS in conjunction with those of comparative general populations to gain a better understanding of the links between swimming, participation in competitive events, and health benefits.

Methods

Study Design

The research hypotheses were examined by comparing health parameters of FCMS corresponding to the physical, physiological, and psychological domains to values reported in studies aiming to define standard ones in the French or European population. Physical activity was quantified by differentiating swimming and other activities to avoid effects of any physical activity other than swimming. In order to avoid effects of medication on health parameters, prevalence of swimmers taking medication was measured and compared with national French values.

Setting

The study took place during the 4 days of the French master championships in France in 2011 (from 10 to 13 March). During the event, a team of five researchers and ten students had two rooms available in the aquatic center to administer questionnaires. Firstly, swimmers were invited to room 1 where questionnaires pertaining to mental health, physical activity, and medication consumption were administered. Then, they were asked to come to room 2 where height (m), body mass (kg), and peak expiratory flow (PEF; $l.min^{-1}$) were measured. These rooms were attached to the warm-up and recovery pool.

Participants

All of the 1554 swimmers selected for the event were eligible for the study. They were invited via posters, press conferences, website of the event, and speakers to participate in the study. Because of the research team's location near the warm-up and recovery pool, it was easy to communicate about the main objective and the design of the study with the swimmers.

At their convenience during the event, swimmers were encouraged to meet the research team. They were asked to participate in the protocol when they had at least a break of 4 h between two races in order to limit stress effects due to the races.

All procedures followed were in accordance with the ethical standards of the responsible committee on human experimentation (institutional and national) and with the Helsinki Declaration of 1975, as revised in 2008. Informed consent was obtained from all patients for being included in the study. Ethics consent was granted through the French National Committee on data processing and freedoms (number 1487869v0).

Data Collection and Variables

In the first room, one experimenter for four swimmers was present to supervise the written responses to questionnaires. The experimenter invited participants to ask questions in the case of lack of clarity and verify that all items were fully answered. Mental health and social health were evaluated via the SF 36 survey [21]. Seven of the current eight multi-item variables were measured: social functioning, role limitations due to physical problems, role limitations due to emotional problems, mental health, energy and vitality, pain, and general perception of health. Each item was scored out of a total of 100. The higher the score, the better the health parameter.

Physical activity was measured by using the long last 7 days self-administered version of the International Physical Activity Questionnaire (IPAQ) [27]. Each activity related to the workplace, transportation, housework, leisure time physical activity (LTPA), and time spent sitting were measured in duration and frequency to calculate metabolic equivalent tasks per week ($MET\text{-}h.week^{-1}$) based on Ainsworth et al.'s proposal [28]. Concerning LTPA, recreation and sports, subjects were asked to not include swimming in this category. Swimming activity was measured in terms of the kind of weekly training and intensity level. Distance was calculated in $MET\text{-}h.week^{-1}$, using the same scale. This differentiation between LTPA with and without swimming activity allowed evaluation of the ratio of swimming training on overall physical activity.

Medication consumption was taken into account by asking whether medical treatment in relation with categories found in French national reports was undergone: disease of bones and joints, cardiovascular disease, respiratory and ear noise and throat disease, digestive disease, and mental illness [29–35]. Ophthalmological problems and other reasons for taking medication were not measured in this study. Percentages of master swimmers taking the different types of medication were quantified.

In room 2, body mass (kg) and height (m) were directly measured by an experimenter because self-reported data gave underestimated values [36]. Body mass index ($kg.m^{-2}$) was used to measure overweight and obesity. Prevalence of overweight and obesity in FCMS was calculated according to the WHO cutoff, that is, 25 ≤ BMI < 30 kg.m^{-2} and BMI ≥30 kg.m^{-2}, respectively [37].

Lung function was assessed in PEF (l.min^{-1}) for all subjects who had not smoked or used inhalers 1 h prior to the test. One of the experimenters demonstrated the correct manner for performing the test in a standing position. Subjects were observed while they made three trial attempts in order to detect faulty technique. Recovery of 30 s between trials was respected to avoid respiratory fatigue. Once they were able to perform the test correctly, they were asked to exert as much effort as possible. The highest value reached on three correct and reproducible tests (difference lower than 40 l.min^{-1}) was recorded.

Limiting Bias and Missing Data

In order to check the representativeness of the convenient sample, proportions by gender and age were compared with the rates of all swimmers selected for the event at the end of the third day of the competition. During the last day of the event, speakers encouraged specific age and gender low-participation classes to participate in the study. They were encouraged to participate in the study only when there was a break of 4 h between two races to limit stress or fatigue due to the events. Finally, the presence of a supervisor during the data collection by questionnaires allowed avoidance of missing data and lack of clarity of the questions.

Statistical Methods

Standard statistical methods were used to calculate the means and standard deviations of the data. Normal Gaussian distribution and homoscedasticity were verified using Shapiro-Wilk's and Levene's tests. Age and gender classifications of FCMS were adjusted according to age classifications used in reference studies. For BMI and PEF results, ages were classified according to 25–29, 30–39, 40–49, 50–59, 60–69, and superior than 70 classes. For physical and SF 36 results, ages were classified according to 25–34, 35–44, 45–54, 55–64, and superior than 65 classes.

Representativeness of the sample was checked by two chi-squared tests in order compare the sample's rates by age of each gender with rates in the whole population selected for the event. Prevalence of overweight and obesity in FCMS was compared with results obtained by Charles et al. [38] in the year 2006 in a French sample of 22,374 people using the chi-squared test. The authors kindly sent us the proportion by age and gender in order to compare with our data. Short form 36 scores were compared with values from Jenkinson et al. [39] using a single-sample *t*-test. Cronbach alpha coefficients were calculated for each section (social functioning, role limitations due to physical problems, role limitations due to emotional problems, mental health, energy and vitality, pain, and general perception of health). Peak expiratory flow (l.min^{-1}) scores were compared with predicted values resulting from Nunn and Greg's equations [40] using a two-way ANOVA (age-gender). International Physical Activity Questionnaire scores were compared with results from Rütten and Abu-Omar's study [41] using a single-sample *t*-test. The prevalence of FCMS taking medications for each kind of disease was compared with French national references (bone and joint [30], cardiovascular [31], respiratory, ear noise and throat [34], digestive [35], mental illness [29]) using Wilcoxon's test. For all tests used, the significance level was set at 0.05. Statistica software was used to perform statistical procedures.

Results

Four hundred and ninety master swimmers (227 females and 263 males) participated in the study. The rates of participation for female and male and swimmers were 44.8 and 23.5 %, respectively. Chi-squared tests by age classes between samples of participants and all swimmers selected for the event showed no significant difference ($\chi^2 = 5.26$, $p = 0.38$; $\chi^2 = 5.02$, $p = 0.41$; for female and male swimmers, respectively). The age range was 25 to 95 years (45.9 ± 13.2 for women and 45.6 ± 12.9 for men), and the mean number of years of swimming training was 21 ± 13.5. Demographic description of the participants is presented in Table 1.

The physical activity levels of master swimmers are presented in Table 2. When swimming activity was included in the quantification, the physical activity of master swimmers was significantly higher than the reference values, whatever the age group (from 94 to 205 % according to the age group, $p < 0.05$). When swimming activity was excluded from the quantification, master swimmers had a significantly higher physical activity level in age groups 25–34 ($p = 0.\ 002$) and 45–54 ($p = 0.002$).

Results for the prevalence of participants categorized as overweight (25–29.99 kg.m^{-2}) indicated no significant difference between FCMS and the French population (Table 3). Results for the prevalence of participants categorized as obese (≥30 kg.m^{-2}) was significantly different for female swimmers in age groups 50–59 (1.8 % vs 16.6 %, $p = 0.02$) and 60–69 (3.8 % vs 17.7 %, $p = 0.04$) and for male swimmers in age groups 30–39 (1.6 % vs 9.3 %, $p = 0.02$) and 60–69 (4.2 % vs 20.9 %, $p = 0.03$).

The results for PEF are presented in Table 4 and showed significantly higher PEF values for female FCMS from 25 to 60 years of age in comparison with the reference values (from 7.6 to 17 % higher according to the age classes, $p < 0.05$). Men between 40 and 50 years old only had significantly higher PEF scores than the reference values (5.6 %, $p = 0.012$).

Perceptions of overall health in the physical, social, and psychological areas and Cronbach alpha coefficients

Table 1 Demographics of the participants (height (cm), body mass (kg), distance training a week (km), years of training in swimming, and years competing in master championships) by age group and gender

Age (years)		Height (cm)	Weight (kg)	Distance training per week in 2010	Years of training in swimming	Years competing in master championships
25–29	Females ($n = 24$, $N = 71$)	165 ± 0.1	63 ± 9.0	9.04 ± 4.9	15.15 ± 4.77	2.29 ± 1.1
	Males ($n = 22$, $N = 99$)	181 ± 0.1	77.3 ± 9.5	9.4 ± 4.9	15.7 ± 5.1	2.5 ± 1.3
30–39	Females ($n = 64$, $N = 167$)	167 ± 0.1	65.8 ± 13.0	8.0 ± 6.4	18.3 ± 7.5	5.6 ± 3.7
	Males ($n = 59$, $N = 292$)	180 ± 0.1	79.3 ± 9.1	9.9 ± 6.6	18 ± 7.7	6.8 ± 6.6
40–49	Females ($n = 83$, $N = 176$)	164 ± 0.1	63.3 ± 10.5	8.6 ± 4.5	18.6 ± 10.4	8.4 ± 6.0
	Males ($n = 64$, $N = 286$)	178 ± 0.1	79.6 ± 9.6	9.8 ± 5.2	20.3 ± 10.4	8.6 ± 7.7
50–59	Females ($n = 57$, $N = 112$)	164 ± 0.1	62.9 ± 7.8	9.1 ± 5.6	21.8 ± 14.6	12.8 ± 9.4
	Males ($n = 45$, $N = 147$)	177 ± 0.1	81.8 ± 10.6	10.4 ± 6.4	21.2 ± 14.2	12.0 ± 10.4
60–69	Females ($n = 23$, $N = 48$)	161 ± 0.1	62.6 ± 9.6	7.8 ± 4.63	27.2 ± 14.0	16.3 ± 11.8
	Males ($n = 27$, $N = 91$)	173 ± 0.0	75.6 ± 6.5	9.8 ± 5.01	33.2 ± 17.8	16.5 ± 16.6
>70	Females ($n = 12$, $N = 16$)	160 ± 0.0	68.6 ± 11.1	7.1 ± 5.03	46.3 ± 24.5	26.1 ± 12.4
	Males ($n = 10$, $N = 49$)	171 ± 0.1	73.4 ± 9.1	9.3 ± 5.52	41.7 ± 21.5	30.9 ± 25.0

n represents sample size and *N* represents total swimmers selected in French master championships by age and gender. Means and standard deviations were calculated for the sample size (*n*)

are presented in Fig. 1. The results indicated significantly higher perceived health scores for female FCMS in terms of physical limitations (age groups 45–54 and 55–64, $p = 0.002$ and $p = 0.003$, respectively), vitality (all age groups, $p < 0.05$), and lower scores for pain perception (age group 35–45, $p = 0.008$). For male FCMS, the results indicated higher health scores for general health perception (age group 55–64, $p = 0.03$), for vitality (age groups 45–54 and 55–64, $p = 0.001$ and $p = 0.001$, respectively), and lower scores for pain perception (age 35 to 55, $p < 0.05$).

Prevalence of FCMS medication consumption is presented in Table 5. A significantly lower score was for medication consumption by swimmers in comparison with the national values for France ($p = 0.012$).

Discussion

The aim of the present study was to determine whether master swimmers involved in French national championships exhibit better overall health when compared with the general population. The study assesses various health indexes to compare them with studies aiming to describe standard health values in French or European populations. The hypothesis was that competitive swimming increases all health indexes. Due to the large sample of participants ($n = 490$) with no significant difference in proportion with all swimmers selected for the event, this subsample can be considered as a representative of swimmers in French championships.

Interpretation of the Main Results

As expected, overall physical activity was much greater in all age groups of master swimmers in comparison with the reference values in Europe [41]. Competitive swimming was associated with a large benefit in physical activity for older age groups (55–65 and over 65 years old) and for the 35–44 age group. For the older age groups, competitive swimming helped prevent the decline in physical activity with age [42]. It is worth noting that for two of our age groups (25–34 and 45–54), the physical activity of these master swimmers was higher than the reference values even when swimming was not taken into account.

Table 2 Comparison of mean (±SD) MET-hours per week reported by individuals age 25 or older between master swimmers (with and without swimming) and European reference values [41]

Age (years)	Physical activity excluding swimming activity (MET-h.week^{-1})	Physical activity including swimming activity (MET-h.week^{-1})	European reference values (MET-h.week^{-1})
25–34	83 ± 154.4* (127.1 %)	111.5 ± 159.2* (205.1 %)	36.5
35–44	48.5 ± 93.7 (32.3 %)	79.7 ± 96.5* (117.4 %)	36.6
45–54	64.5 ± 110.7* (87.2 %)	96.5 ± 113.4* (180.1 %)	34.5
55–64	41.1 ± 62.8 (28.1 %)	75.1 ± 67.3* (134.3 %)	32.1
>65	24 ± 33.7 (−4 %)	48.8 ± 42.2* (94.9 %)	25.1

% represents the ratio between master values and the European reference values. MET corresponds to Metabolic Equivalent Tasks (MET-h.week^{-1})
*Significant differences with European normative data at $p < 0.05$

Table 3 Prevalence of overweight and obesity by age group and gender for FCMS and French reference values [38]

	Females		Males	
Age	FCMS (%)	RF (%)	FCMS (%)	RF (%)
25–29 years				
Overweight (%)	11.5	13.6	20.0	19.7
Obesity (%)	3.8	7.2	4.0	5.2
30–39 years				
Overweight (%)	22.4	20.2	31.3	33.9
Obesity (%)	6.1	13.7	1.6*	9.3
40–49 years				
Overweight (%)	16.4	22.1	41.2	40.6
Obesity (%)	6.6	13.7	7.1	13.4
50–59 years				
Overweight (%)	28.1	29.2	45.6	45.1
Obesity (%)	1.8*	16.6	10.5	15.6
60–69 years				
Overweight (%)	34.6	33.6	54.2	47.5
Obesity (%)	3.8*	17.7	4.2*	20.9
70–79 years or older				
Overweight (%)	16.7	35.2	37.5	50.0
Obesity (%)	33.3	16.8	12.5	17.1

*Significant difference between French master swimmers (FCMS) and reference values (RF) at $p < 0.05$, according to overweight and obesity ($25 \leq$ body mass index < 30 kg.m^{-2} and body mass index ≥ 30 kg.m^{-2})

The results for BMI (kg.m^{-2}) indicated significantly lower prevalence of obese people among male and female swimmers in certain age groups. These results corroborate those obtained by Walsh et al. [24] showing a lower prevalence of obesity in master world game swimmers than in the national population of Australia. In our study, no significant difference in the prevalence of overweight people was noted between master swimmers and the French population, suggesting that swimming training is not linked to high weight loss. According to Gwinup [43], swimming is not the most effective form of physical activity for losing weight, which could explain the lower prevalence of obese people because of their high physical activity level, but not high enough to decrease weight to the point defined by the WHO (BMI <25 kg.m^2). It is possible that, due to athletic activity, the French national master swimmers had a lower fat-to-lean body mass ratio than that of their national counterparts. Moreover, swimmers could benefit from a buoyancy advantage with fat deposits in certain regions of the body, and it is possible that swimmers may have tapered their diet and/or training to attain optimal body composition and physical performance for the competitive swimming event. The issue of causation must also be considered, that is, the question of whether participating in national French master swimming competitions promotes reduced obesity and lowers associated health risks or whether individuals with a lower BMI participate in master swimming championships by preference.

The PEF (l.min^{-1}) results yielded significantly higher values for female master swimmers than for the theoretical values. For male master swimmers, no significant difference was noted, although all mean values were higher than the reference values. It is worth noting that the predictive values corresponded to a healthy level of lung function. Despite the chloramine environment, competitive swimming appeared to be effective at developing respiratory functions. These results corroborate the conclusions of several studies [44–46] showing the effect of swimming training on respiratory muscles. Swimming exercise affects lung volume measurements because the respiratory muscles of swimmers are used to develop greater pressure as a consequence of immersion in water during the respiratory cycle. This may lead to functional improvement in these muscles and a subsequent improvement in lung function. The fact that only female swimmers exhibited breathing performance above the predictive values could be due to the addition of this kind of exercise and a higher physical activity level than their European counterparts. However, more investigations are needed to explore respiratory functions because PEF (l.min^{-1}) is only one parameter among the many indexes of respiratory health. In that way, the use of force expiratory volume in 1 s (FEV 1) and its ratio with force vital capacity (FVC) would be relevant in

Table 4 Peak expiratory flow (PEF; l.min^{-1}): comparison between master swimmers and theoretical values by age group and gender [40]

	Females		Males	
Age (years)	Measured PEF (l.min^{-1})	Reference values (l.min^{-1})	Measured PEF (l.min^{-1})	Reference values (l.min^{-1})
25–29	493 ± 70*	441 ± 8	641 ± 81	627 ± 11
30–39	479 ± 66*	445 ± 8	643 ± 74	643 ± 13
40–49	482 ± 77*	429 ± 10	658 ± 74*	623 ± 32
50–59	476 ± 71*	407 ± 11	622 ± 99	598 ± 17
60–69	434 ± 89	377 ± 9	599 ± 107	540 ± 20
>70	305 ± 107	334 ± 17	529 ± 104	468 ± 42

*Significant difference between measured peak expiratory flow (PEF) and estimated PEF at $p < 0.05$

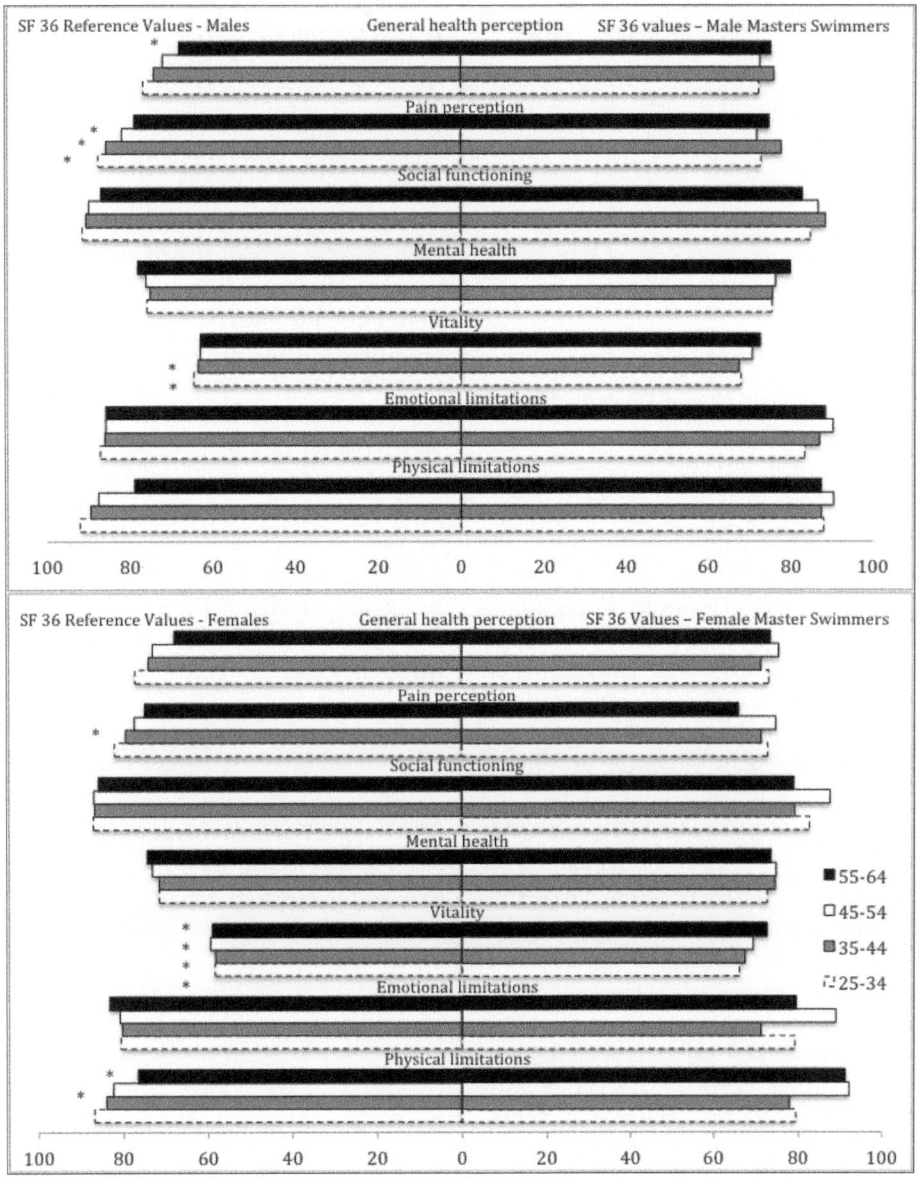

Fig. 1 Short form 36 (SF 36) score comparison between French competitive master swimmers (FCMS) and reference values taken from Jenkinson et al. (1993). Alpha Cronbach coefficient values were 0.70 for physical limitations, 0.77 for emotional limitations, 0.72 for vitality, 0.78 for mental health, 0.75 for social functioning, 0.71 for pain perception, and 0.70 for general health perception. *Significant difference between FCMS and the reference values at $p < 0.05$

future research to assess both restrictive and obstructive lung disorders [47].

Short form 36 tests were conducted in order to evaluate psychological and social health. The results showed no significant difference between master swimmers and reference values for social functioning, emotional problems, mental health, and perception of overall health. Self-perception of vitality was significantly higher for all female swimmers and for the older age groups of male swimmers (from 45 to 65 years old). These results partially corroborate Acree et al.'s [48] study showing better scores on bodily pain, vitality, and social functioning for active as opposed to sedentary old people. Competitive swimming seems to impact vitality in the same way, but gave rise to the opposite effect on perception of bodily pain, with significantly lower scores for both female and male swimmers. Further investigation is needed to determine whether the higher self-perception of pain was due to a high physical activity level in an anti-gravity context or whether a sport involving a substantial proprioception of the body would increase the perception of pain.

Table 5 Prevalence of medication consumption by disease category between participants and values reported in French national reports [29–31, 34, 35]

Drug consumption	Prevalence of master swimmers (%)	French national values (%)
Bones and joints	3.5	23
Cardiovascular	3.5	29
Respiratory, ear noise, and throat	4	10.2
Digestive	1.4	20
Mental	2	13
Probability	*	

*Significant difference ($p < 0.05$) in comparison across all disease categories between prevalence of master swimmers and French values

Master swimmers took significantly less medication than their national counterparts (Table 5). In a study at population level, drug consumption had a positive and statistically significant effect on health status among middle-age individuals (ages 40 and 60 years) [49]. However, studies aimed at measuring the effects of drug consumption on population health have used macroscopic health indexes such as morbidity, life expectancy at different ages, or infant mortality [50, 51]. The results of the present study showed good health for master swimmers involved in French championships, with significantly lower intake of medication than their national counterparts (Table 5). From this point of view, competitive swimming at the national level appears to be a good way to improve health by increasing physical activity without managing health by means of medication.

Limitations of the Study

As several cross-sectional studies have compliant samples, some results have to be taken into account with caution. The low rate of male master swimmer participation (24 %) could affect specific results concerning this gender. The free participation has limited master swimmers involved in a lot of races or selected only for 1 day of the event. It is difficult to consider that the male sample was representative of all male swimmers, even if the chi-squared test showed that the sample was not significantly different from the male master population. The second limit of this study was the old reference studies used to define standard values of health parameters. Unfortunately, our research in the standard baselines did not find more recent studies with standard values in France or Europe by age and gender. In this way, we had to adjust the age classes in our statistical methodology, which could affect statistical significance. Finally, the competitive context could affect some behavior such as anxiety, pain perception, or physical activity 7 days before the event, which could affect some health parameter values.

Conclusions

It is a commonly held conception that adherence to an exercise regime improves all indexes of general health. The results of French master swimmers involved in national championships indicated unequal indexes to the reference values, despite their greater physical activity. Based on this data from French master swimmers, we can argue for promoting this form of physical activity across the lifespan, insofar as our participants had many positive health outcomes in terms of weight management, respiratory function, and vitality. The fact that these benefits were not linked with medication consumption could be interesting in an economic context aimed at controlling expenditures on health. However, the very high physical activity level in this competitive context did not result in better levels on all parameters. Indexes of the subjective perception of body pain were lower, and the impacts on social, emotional, and mental health were not statistically different. Further investigations are needed to explore in depth the outcomes of participating in a competitive sport that requires a high physical activity throughout life.

Competing Interests

The authors declare that they have no competing interests.

Authors' contributions

FP supervised the study and the drafting of the manuscript. GV and GZ carried out data collection. TP carried out statitical analysis. DT supervised data collection. All authors read and approved the final manuscript.

Acknowledgements

The authors thank the French Swimming Federation and the master swimmers for their kind participation. No financial support was received for the conduct of this study or preparation of this manuscript.

Author details

[1]Univ. Lille, EA 7369 - URePSSS - Unité de Recherche Pluridisciplinaire Sport Santé Société, F-59000 Lille, France. [2]Univ. Littoral Côte d'Opale, Département STAPS, F- 62100 Calais, France. [3]Univ. Littoral Côte d'Opale, EA 7369 - URePSSS - Unité de Recherche Pluridisciplinaire Sport Santé Société, F-59144 Dunkerque, France.

References

1. Williamson J, Pahor M. Evidence regarding the benefits of physical exercise. Arch Intern Med. 2010;170(2):124–5. doi:10.1001/archinternmed.2009.491.
2. Ryan A. Exercise in aging: it's important role in mortality, obesity and insulin resistance. Aging health. 2010;6(5):551–63. doi:10.2217/ahe.10.46.
3. Haskell WL, Lee IM, Pate RR, Powell KE, Blair SN, Franklin BA, et al. Physical activity and public health: updated recommendation for adults from the American College of Sports Medicine and the American Heart Association. Med Sci Sports Exerc. 2007;39(8):1423–34.
4. Cabezas PC, Robledo de Dios T, Marqués F, Sanchez PR, Nemot AR, Megido BM, et al. Recomendaciones sobre el estilo de vida. Aten Primaria. 2007;39(3):27–46.
5. Tabata I. Exercise and physical activity reference for health promotion 2006: exercise guide 2006. National Institute of Health and Nutrition. 2008. http://www0.nih.go.jp/eiken/programs/pdf/exercise_guide.pdf. Accessed June 2015.

6. European Society of Cardiology guidelines for the management of arterial hypertension. Guidelines Committee. J Hypertens. 2003;21:1011–53. doi:10.1097/01.hjh.0000059051.65882.32.
7. Joint National Committee on Prevention, Detection, Evaluation, and Treatment of High Blood Pressure and the National High Blood Pressure Education Program Coordinating Committee. The sixth report of the joint national committee on prevention, detection, evaluation and treatment of high blood pressure. Arch Int Med. 1997;157:2413-2446.
8. Rezaimanesh D, Amiri-Farsani P. The effect of a six weeks aerobic and anaerobic intermittent swimming on VO2 max and some lung volumes and capacities in student athletes. Procedia Soc Behav Sci. 2011;15:2054–7.
9. Sieverdes JC, Sui X, Blair SN. Associations between physical activity and submaximal cardiorespiratory and pulmonary responses in men. J Sports Med Doping Stud. 2011;1(1):102.
10. Cox KL, Burke V, Beilin LJ, Puddey IB. A comparison of the effects of swimming and walking on body weight, fat distribution, lipids, glucose, and insulin in older women: the Sedentary Women Exercise Adherence Trial 2. Metabolism. 2010;59:1562–73.
11. Sacher PM, Kolotourou M, Chadwick PM, Cole PM, Lawson TJ, Lucas A, et al. Randomized controlled trial of the MEND program: a family-based community intervention for childhood obesity. Obesity. 2010;18(1):62–8.
12. Tanaka H, Bassett DR, Howley ET, Thompson DL, Ashraf M, Rawson FL. Swimming training lowers the resting blood pressure in individuals with hypertension. J Hypertens. 1995;15(6):651–7.
13. Guszkowska M. Effects of exercise on anxiety, depression and mood. Psychiatr Pol. 2004;38(4):611–20.
14. Saiiaria A, Moslehi M, Sajadiyan M. Effects of crawl swimming on depression in type 2 diabetic patients. Procedia Soc Behav Sci. 2011;30:2156–60.
15. Bougault V, Turmel J, Levesque B, Boulet LP. The respiratory health of swimmers. Sports Med. 2009;39(4):295–312. doi:10.2165/00007256-200939040-00003.
16. Gaunt T, Mafulli N. Soothing suffering swimmers: a systematic review of the epidemiology, diagnosis, treatment and rehabilitation of musculoskeletal injuries in competitive swimmers. Br Med Bull. 2011;4:1–44.
17. Cox KL, Burke V, Beilin LJ, Grove JR, Blanksby BA, Puddey IB. Blood pressure rise with swimming versus walking in older women: the sedentary women exercise adherence trial 2 (SWEAT 2). J Hypertens. 2006;24(2):307–14.
18. World Health Organization. Preamble to the Constitution of the World Health Organization as adopted by the International Health Conference, New York, 19–22 June 1946, and entered into force on 7 April 1948. http://www.who.int/about/definition/en/print.html. Accessed March 2014.
19. World Health Organization. The world health report: reducing risks, promoting healthy life. 2003. http://www.who.int/whr/2002/en/summary_riskfactors_chp4.pdf. Accessed April 2014.
20. Schunemann HJ, Dorn J, Grant BJ, Winkelstein W, Trevisan M. Pulmonary function is a long-term predictor of mortality in the general population: 29-year follow-up of the Buffalo Health Study. Chest. 2000;118(3):656–64.
21. Ware JE, Sherboume CD. The MOS 36-item short-form health survey (SF-36): conceptual framework and item selection. Med Care. 1992;30:473–83.
22. Dionigi R. Competitive sport as leisure in later life: negotiations, discourse, and aging. Leis Sci. 2006;28:181–96.
23. Vaccaro P, Ostrove SM, Vandervelden L, Goldfarb AH, Clarke DH. Body composition and physiological responses of masters female swimmers 20 to 70 years of age. Res Q Exercise Sport. 1984;55(3):278–84.
24. Walsh J, Climstein M, Heazlewood IT, Kettunen J, Burke S, Debeliso M, et al. Body mass index for athletes participating in swimming at the world master games. J Sports Med Phys Fitness. 2012;53:162–8.
25. Guthrie SK, Erickson SK, Lau MS. Comparison of the prevalence and treatment of hypertension in two populations in the United States: masters swimmers versus the NHANES population. J Sport Sci. 2013;31(9):930–5.
26. Erickson SR, Guthrie SK. Health status of USMS swimmers compared with a representative sample of the general population. IJARE. 2012;6(3):226–34.
27. Craig CL, Marshall AL, Sjöström M, Bauman AE, Booth ML, Ainsworth BE, et al. International physical activity questionnaire: 12-country reliability and validity. Med Sci Sports Exerc. 2003;35(8):1381–95.
28. Ainsworth BE, Haskell WL, Whitt MC, Irwin ML, Swartz AM, Strath SJ, et al. Compendium of physical activities: an update of activity codes and MET intensities. Med Sci Sports Exerc. 2000;32(9):498–504.
29. French Health Gouvernement. French population health status 2009–2010 report. 2011. http://www.sante.gouv.fr/IMG/pdf/Etat_sante-population_2011.pdf. Accessed 5 June 2014.
30. Allonier C, Boisguérin B, Le Fur P. The beneficiaries of the CMU report are more illnesses than the rest of the population. Questions d'économie et de la santé. 2012. http://www.irdes.fr/Publications/2012/Qes173.pdf. Accessed June 2014.
31. Godet-Thobie H, Vernay M, Noukpoape A, Salanave B, Malon A, Castetbon K, et al. Mean blood pressure level and prevalence of hypertension in 18 to 74 year-old adults. In: Weekly epidemiological bulletin. 2008. http://www.invs.sante.fr/beh/2008/49_50/beh_49_50_2008.pdf. Accessed June 2014.
32. Lang T, de Gaudemaris R, Chatellier G, Hamici L, Diène E. Prevalence and therapeutic control of hypertension in 30,000 subjects in the workplace. Hypertension. 2001;38(3):449–54.
33. Afrite A, Allonier C, Com-Ruelle L, Le Guen N. Asthma in France in 2006: prevalence, control and determinants. In: Institute of research and documentation in French health economy report. 2011. http://www.irdes.fr/Publications/Rapports2011/rap1820.pdf. Accessed June 2014.
34. Delmas MC, Fujrman C. Asthma in France: a review of descriptive epidemiological data. Rev Mal Respir. 2010. doi:10.1016/j.rmr.2009.09.001
35. French national society of gastroenterology disease website. 2001. http://www.snfge.org/sites/default/files/SNFGE/Rubrique_Professionnels/livre_blanc_HGE/chapitre2.pdf. Accessed June 2014.
36. Gorber S, Tremblay M, Moher D, Gorber B. A comparison of direct vs self-report measures for assessing height, weight and body mass index: a systematic review. Obes review. 2007;8:307–26.
37. Chalmers J, MacMahon S, Mancia G, Whitworth J. World Health Organization - International Society of Hypertension Guidelines for the Management of Hypertension. J Hypertens. 1999;17:151–85.
38. Charles MA, Eschwège E, Basdevant A. Monitoring the obesity epidemic in France: the Obepi surveys 1997–2006. Obesity. 2008;16(9):2182–6. doi:10.1038/oby.2008.285.
39. Jenkinson C, Coulter A, Wright L. Short form 36 (SF 36) health survey questionnaire: normative data for adults of working age. Brit Med J. 1993;306:1437–40.
40. Nunn AJ, Gregg I. New regression equations for predicting peak expiratory flow in adults. Br Med. 1989;298:1068–70.
41. Rütten A, Abu-Omar K. Prevalence of physical activity in the European Union. Soz Praventivmed. 2004;49:281–9.
42. Caspersen CJ, Pereira MA, Curran KM. Changes in physical activity patterns in the United States, by sex and cross-sectional age. Med Sci Sports Exerc. 2000;32:1601–9.
43. Gwinup G. Weight loss without dietary restriction: efficacy of different forms of aerobic exercise. American J Sports Med. 1987;15(3):275–9.
44. Courteix D, Obert P, Lecoq AM, Guenon P, Koch G. Effect of intensive swimming training on lung volumes, airway resistances and on the maximal expiratory flow-volume relationship in prepubertal girls. Eur J Applied Physiol. 1997;76(3):264–9.
45. Mehrotra PK, Verma N, Yadav R, Tewari S, Shukla N. Study of pulmonary functions in swimmers of Lucknow city. Indian J Physiol Pharmacol. 1997;41(1):83–6.
46. Doherty M, Dimitriou L. Comparison of lung volume in Greek swimmers, land based athletes, and sedentary controls using allometric scaling. Br J Sports Med. 1997;31(4):337–41.
47. Swanney MP, Ruppel G, Enright PL, Pedersen OF, Crapo RO, Miller MR, et al. Using the lower limit of normal for the FEV1/FVC ratio reduces the misclassification of airway obstruction. Thorax. 2008. doi:10.1136/thx.2008.098483.
48. Acree LS, Longfors J, Fjeldstad AS, Fjeldstad C, Shank B, Nickel KJ, et al. Physical activity is related to quality of life in older adults. Health Qual Life Outcomes. 2006. doi:10.1186/1477-7525-4-37.
49. Miller RD, Frech HE. Is there a link between pharmaceutical consumption and improved health in OECD countries? Pharmaco Economics. 2000;18(1):33–45.
50. Miller RD, Frech HE. The productivity of health care and pharmaceuticals: quality of life, cause of death and the role of obesity. In: Departmental working paper, University of California. 2002. http://escholarship.org/uc/item/4b55f1xp. Accessed March 2014.
51. Frech HE, Miller RD. The effects of pharmaceutical consumption and obesity on the quality of life in the OECD countries. Pharmacoeconomics. 2004;22:25–36.

6

Muscle Cramping During a 161-km Ultramarathon: Comparison of Characteristics of Those With and Without Cramping

Martin D Hoffman[1*] and Kristin J Stuempfle[2]

Abstract

Background: This work sought to identify characteristics differing between those with and without muscle cramping during a 161-km ultramarathon.

Methods: In this observational study, race participants underwent body weight measurements before, during, and after the race; completed a post-race questionnaire about muscle cramping and "near" cramping (controllable, not reaching full-blown cramping), drinking strategies, and use of sodium supplementation during four race segments; and underwent a post-race blood draw for determination of serum sodium and blood creatine kinase (CK) concentrations.

Results: The post-race questionnaire was completed by 280 (74.5 %) of the 376 starters. A post-race blood sample was provided by 181 (61.1 %) of the 296 finishers, and 157 (53.0 %) of finishers completed the post-race survey and also provided a post-race blood sample. Among those who completed the survey, the prevalence of cramping and near cramping was 14.3 and 26.8 %, respectively, with greatest involvement being in the calf (54 %), quadriceps (44 %), and hamstring (33 %) muscles. Those with cramping or near cramping were more likely to have a prior history of muscle cramping during an ultramarathon ($p < 0.0001$) and had higher blood CK concentrations ($p = 0.001$) than those without cramping. Weight change during the race, use of sodium supplements, intake rate of sodium in supplements, and post-race serum sodium concentration did not differ between those with and without cramping.

Conclusions: Muscle cramping is most common in those with a prior history of cramping and greater muscle damage during an ultramarathon, suggesting an association with relative muscular demand. Impaired fluid and sodium balance did not appear to be an etiology of muscle cramping during an ultramarathon.

Keywords: Creatine kinase; Endurance exercise; Exercise; Muscle cramp; Muscle fatigue; Running; Sodium; Water-electrolyte imbalance

Key points

- Muscle cramping and near cramping is common in a 161-km ultramarathon and largely involves the most active muscles (calves, quadriceps and hamstrings).
- Those with cramping or near cramping are more likely to have a prior history of muscle cramping during an ultramarathon and greater muscle damage during the event than those without cramping. Hydration status, intake rate of sodium in supplements and serum sodium concentration do not differ between those with and without cramping.
- The findings do not support an electrolyte depletion and/or dehydration basis for muscle cramping in ultramarathon running.

Background

Exercise-associated cramping of skeletal muscles is common among participants in numerous sports and other physical activities [1–4]. For instance, one study showed that the prevalence of muscle cramping during or within 6 h after an Ironman triathlon was 23 % among study participants [5], and the prevalence was 41 % at a 56-km ultramarathon [6]. In another study, muscle cramping during or immediately after a 100-km ultramarathon was

* Correspondence: mdhoffman@ucdavis.edu
[1]Department of Physical Medicine & Rehabilitation, Department of Veterans Affairs, Northern California Health Care System, and University of California Davis Medical Center, 10535 Hospital Way, Sacramento, CA, USA
Full list of author information is available at the end of the article

present in 23 % of study participants [7]. We have previously reported that muscle cramping was the main reason for dropping out of a 161-km ultramarathon by 5 % of those failing to finish, and muscle cramps were indicated to have adversely affected performance in 11 and 16 % of finishers and non-finishers, respectively [8]. Muscle cramping has also been shown to be a cause for 1–3 % of athletes to seek medical attention during ultra-endurance footraces [9, 10].

Despite the high prevalence and negative impact on performance from muscle cramping during endurance activities, controversy continues about the underlying pathophysiology [1–4, 11–13]. Two distinct theories have emerged for the cause of exercise-associated muscle cramps: (1) altered neuromuscular control from muscular fatigue resulting in increased excitatory and decreased inhibitory afferent inputs to motor neurons, and (2) hyperexcitability of motor neuron axon terminals induced by mechanical deformation and exposure to increased levels of excitatory extracellular constituents in the surrounding extracellular space [2, 12, 13]. The latter theory depends on a presumption that there is electrolyte depletion and/or dehydration. Since the prevention and treatment strategies are quite dissimilar between these potential underlying causes, further exploration into the pathophysiology of exercise-associated muscle cramping is important and carries practical implications.

Prior studies of muscle cramping associated with endurance activities up to ~18 h have shown a higher likelihood of cramping among those with a prior history of cramping [5, 6] and those racing at a relatively higher intensity [5, 6, 14]. Muscle cramping has not been related to serum sodium concentration [5, 15–17]. The purpose of this study was to learn about muscle cramping during an ultramarathon lasting up to 30 h, including the prevalence, muscle groups involved, distance at which cramping tends to occur, characteristics of those who have muscle cramping, and whether muscle cramping is related to weight change, sodium supplementation, post-race serum sodium, or extent of muscle injury as defined by serum creatine kinase (CK) concentration. It was anticipated that this new information would offer additional insight into the underlying pathophysiology of exercise-associated muscle cramping in this environment. Based on prior findings from endurance events [2–6, 8, 15–18], we hypothesized that muscle cramping would be common and more likely among those with a prior history of muscle cramping and is unrelated to hydration status, intake rate of sodium in supplements, or post-race serum sodium concentration.

Methods

The study was performed at the 2014 Western States Endurance Run, a 161.3-km ultramarathon through the Sierra Nevada Mountains of Northern California with 5500 m of cumulative climb and 7000 m of cumulative descent. Additional race details have been provided elsewhere [8, 19–23]. Nearby ambient temperatures during the competition ranged from a low of 0 °C just after the start to a high of 31.7 °C in the afternoon, which was close to the historical median high temperature for this event, but our on-course measurements (Vantage Vue Wireless Weather Station, Davis Instruments, Vernon Hills, IL) recorded a maximum air temperature of 39 °C at which time the relative humidity was 13 %. The research was approved by the institutional review boards of the Veterans Affairs Northern California Health Care System and Gettysburg College with electronic consent obtained from those participating in the questionnaire.

Body weight measurements were performed on all race participants within 1.5 h before the start of the race; when reaching the 47.8, 89.6, and 125.5 km aid stations during the race; and again immediately after finishing the race. All weight measurements were made with calibrated scales (Health O Meter, model 349KLX, Boca Raton, FL) that were on firm, level surfaces. The runners were clothed in running wear and shoes, but jackets and other items such as waist packs and hydration vests were removed, and nothing was permitted in the runner's hands. Prior to the event, the scales were examined for consistency, and though the maximum variation between scales was less than 0.5 % across the weight range of our subjects, correction equations were developed to standardize all weight measurements to a single scale.

Blood samples were drawn from willing runners within a few minutes after finishing the race. Runners were seated while blood was drawn into heparinized tubes via an antecubital vein. Samples were stored in a cooler until analyzed by a clinical laboratory for serum sodium, blood urea nitrogen (BUN), creatinine, and CK concentrations (Seimens Aktiengesellschaft, Dimension EXL, Munich, Germany).

Race participants were alerted before the race that they would be asked to complete a post-race web-based questionnaire. The invitation to the questionnaire was sent electronically to all race starters during the event. Those who had not completed the survey were sent reminder emails 7 and 12 days later, and the survey was closed 15 days after the race. The questionnaire requested information on running background and training during the 3 months prior to the race. It requested the number and brand of sodium supplements used (if any) during each of four segments of the race defined by the sites where body weights were measured. A list of the most commonly used commercially available products was provided, and the runner also had the opportunity to specify other forms of sodium supplementation. From the known sodium content of each brand of sodium supplement and official split times, the rate of sodium intake in supplements was calculated.

The questionnaire also asked whether or not the runner had experienced muscle cramping during prior ultramarathons and if they had had muscle cramping during this event, with answer options of yes, no, and "almost, but was able to control any full-blown cramping" (subsequently referred to as "near cramping"). The answer option of near cramping was included because we are aware that runners sometimes sense impending muscle cramping that can be aborted with various interventions, such as altering gait pattern. Those with cramping or near cramping were asked which muscle groups were involved and in which of the four course segments they experienced the cramping.

Between-group comparisons of categorical data were made with Fisher's exact test or chi-square test. Continuous data underwent normality testing with the D'Agostino-Pearson test. Group comparisons of continuous data were made with one-way analysis of variance and Tukey post-test, or the Kruskal-Wallis test and Dunn's multiple comparison test depending on whether or not the data passed normality testing. When two groups were compared, the unpaired *t* test or Mann Whitney test was used depending on findings from normality testing. Spearman correlation analysis was used for the single correlation performed since the data were not normally distributed. Statistical significance was set at $p < 0.05$.

Results

The race had 376 starters and 296 (78.7 %) finishers. The post-race survey was completed by 280 (74.5 %) of the starters. Survey completion rate was similar ($p = 0.46$) between men and women, but was greater ($p = 0.0005$) among finishers (78.7 %) than non-finishers (58.8 %). Of those completing the survey, 55.7 % did so within 7 days of the end of the race and 88.9 % did so within 10 days. A post-race blood sample was provided by 181 (61.1 %) finishers. There were 157 (53.0 %) finishers who completed the post-race survey and also provided a post-race blood sample.

Muscle cramping at some time during the race was reported by 40 (14.3 %) runners completing the survey. An additional 75 (26.8 %) indicated they had experienced near cramping. The frequencies of muscle cramping, near cramping, and either cramping or near cramping during the four course segments are shown in Fig. 1. The frequency of cramping (5.0–8.9 %) and near cramping (5.4–14.4 %) did not vary across segments ($p = 0.99$ and $p = 0.64$, respectively). The frequency of combined cramping or near cramping (10.4–23.2 %) was also not different across segments ($p = 0.35$).

The frequency distribution of muscle cramping in different body locations or muscle groups is shown in Table 1. The calf, quadriceps, and hamstrings were the most common muscle groups involved. Involvement of the quadriceps and forearm was less common ($p < 0.05$) for those with near cramping than for those with cramping.

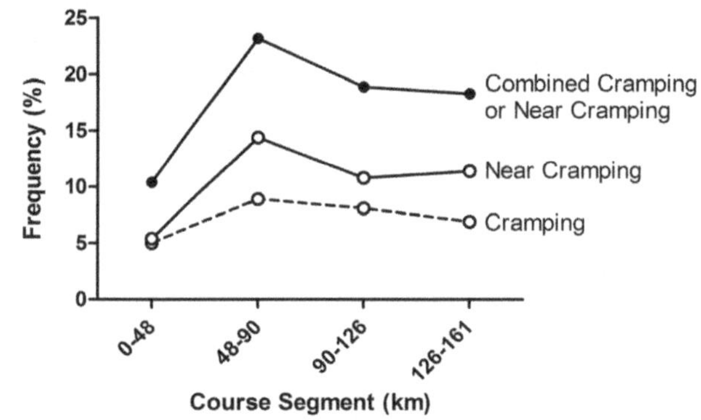

Fig 1 Frequencies of muscle cramping, near cramping, and either cramping or near cramping (combined cramping or near cramping) during the four course segments. Frequencies are shown relative to the number of race participants who ran the specified course segment. Within groups, there were no differences in frequencies across course segments

Characteristics of runners with cramping, near cramping, and no cramping are compared in Table 2. These three groups did not differ by age, sex, ultramarathon running experience, number of prior 161-km ultramarathon running finishes or drops, running training distance, finish status or time, use of sodium supplementation, rate of sodium intake in supplements, minimum weight during the

Table 1 Frequency of muscle cramping in different body locations or muscle groups among those with cramping ($n = 40$), those with near cramping ($n = 75$), and those with either cramping or near cramping ($n = 115$)

Body location or muscle group	Combined cramping or near cramping (%)	Cramping (%)	Near cramping (%)	*p* value
Calf	53.9	57.5	52.0	0.69
Quadriceps	43.5	57.5	36.0	0.031
Hamstrings	33.0	45.0	26.7	0.061
Hip flexors	15.7	17.5	14.7	0.79
Trunk	6.1	10.0	4.0	0.23
Hip adductors	4.3	2.5	5.3	0.66
Ankle dorsiflexors	3.5	7.5	1.3	0.12
Forearm	2.6	7.5	0.0	0.040
Feet	2.6	5.0	1.3	0.28
Upper arm	1.7	2.5	1.3	1.00
Hands	0.9	2.5	0.0	0.35

Values are expressed as percentages of those reporting they had experienced muscle cramping or near cramping. Since some runners had multiple areas with muscle cramping, the summation of percentages is greater than 100 %. The statistical comparison is between the cramping and near cramping groups for each body location or muscle group

Table 2 Comparison of characteristics among runners with cramping, near cramping, and no cramping, as well either cramping or near cramping

Variable	Combined cramping or near cramping	Cramping	Near cramping	No cramping	*p* value[a]
Age (years)	42 ± 9	43 ± 10	42 ± 9	42 ± 9	0.84
Sex (*n*, % men)	97, 84.3	32, 80.0	65, 86.7	126, 76.4	0.18
Ultramarathon running experience (years)	5 (3–8)	4 (3–8)	5 (3–8)	5 (3–9)	0.45
Prior 161-km ultramarathon finishes (*n*)	2 (1–4)	1 (1–3)	2 (1–4)	2 (0–5)	0.46
Prior 161-km ultramarathon drops (*n*)	0 (0–1)	0 (0–1)	0 (0–1)	0 (0–2)	0.94
Average running distance (km/week)[b]	97 (80–113)	89 (80–120)	97 (75–113)	97 (80–121)	0.70
Highest running distance in 1 week (km)[b]	145 (125–169)	142 (124–167)	145 (126–169)	140 (118–166)	0.61
Longest single run (km)[b]	80 (68–100)	80 (56–100)	80 (72–100)	80 (65–100)	0.46
Prior history of cramping (*n*, %)	94, 81.7[†]	32, 80.0*	62, 82.7*	86, 52.1	<0.0001
Finish status (*n*, % finished)	97, 84.3	31, 77.5	66, 88.0	136, 82.4	0.33
Finish time (h)	26.52 (23.37–28.61)[†]	26.60 (22.02–28.83)	26.41 (23.56–28.48)	25.06 (22.16–27.98)	0.14
Sodium supplementation (*n*, % using)	109, 94.8	38, 95.0	71, 94.7	154, 93.3	0.88
Sodium supplement intake (mg/h)	145 (59–295)	128 (35–261)	147 (66–328)	132 (62–235)	0.46
Minimum weight (% of start weight)	−3.0 (−4.3 to −2.0)	−3.3 (−4.4 to −2.5)	−2.9 (−4.0 to −1.9)	−3.1 (−4.1 to −2.1)	0.23
Post-race serum sodium (mmol/L)	139 ± 4	138 ± 5	140 ± 4	140 ± 3	0.055
Post-race blood CK (IU/L)	19,458 (10,098–46,887)[†]	35,265 (14,755–53,567)*	15,149 (9120–38,920)	11,862 (5951–24,615)	0.0010
Post-race BUN (mg/dL)	29 (22–36)[†]	35 (26–39)*	29 (20–34)	25 (20–33)	0.023
Post-race blood creatinine (mg/dL)	1.30 (1.12–1.53)	1.32 (1.15–1.60)	1.26 (1.04–1.48)	1.18 (1.03–1.41)	0.19

Values are reported as mean ± SD when data were normally distributed for the cramping, near cramping, and no cramping groups; median and interquartile range if not normally distributed for these groups; or group count (*n*) and percentage within the study group providing data for the variable
*Indicates statistical difference on post-test compared with the no cramping group
[†]Indicates statistical difference in the two-group comparison with the no cramping group
[a]*p* value for the comparison of cramping, near cramping, and no cramping groups
[b]During the 3 months prior to the event

race, and post-race serum sodium and blood creatinine. A prior history of muscle cramping during an ultramarathon was more common among those with cramping ($p = 0.0013$) and near cramping ($p < 0.0001$) than those with no cramping. In fact, those with a prior history of muscle cramping during an ultramarathon were 2.5 times more likely to have had cramping or near cramping during the present event than those without a prior history of muscle cramping (94 of 180 or 52.2 % compared with 21 of 100 or 21.0 %). Post-race BUN and blood CK concentrations were higher for the cramping group than the group without cramping ($p < 0.05$ and $p < 0.001$, respectively), as well as for the combined cramping or near cramping group compared with the group without cramping ($p = 0.030$ and 0.0013, respectively). Finish time was also slower ($p = 0.048$) for the combined cramping or near cramping group compared with the no cramping group.

Post-race serum sodium was further compared among those with cramping (mean ± SD value 138 ± 5 mmol/L), near cramping (140 ± 4 mmol/L), and no cramping (140 ± 3 mmol/L) during the last segment of the race and was found to not be different among groups ($p = 0.51$). Additionally, the proportion of runners with a serum sodium concentration at the finish below 135 mmol/L (reference range for normal is 135–145 mmol/L) was similar ($p = 0.43$) for those with cramping or near cramping (11.5 %) and those without cramping (7.0 %) during the final segment of the race, and the serum sodium concentrations for these two groups (range 125–133 and 131–134 mmol/L, respectively) were also similar ($p = 0.16$).

The relationship of post-race BUN with change in body weight is shown in Fig. 2. A significant inverse relationship ($r = -0.33$, $p < 0.0001$) was identified.

Comparison of weight change across the course between those with cramping or near cramping and those without cramping is shown in Fig. 3. Weight change did not differ between groups whether comparing the weight change at the end of the course segment in which the symptoms were considered or the weight change at the end of the segment prior to that for which the symptoms were considered.

Comparison of rate of sodium intake in supplements during each course segment between those with cramping or near cramping and those without cramping is shown in Fig. 4. The rate of sodium intake in supplements did not differ between groups whether comparing intake during the course segment where cramping or

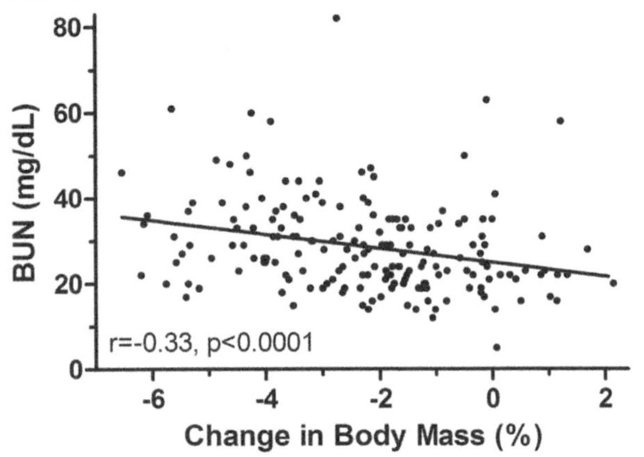

Fig 2 Relationship of post-race BUN concentration with percent change in body weight from the start to finish

near cramping occurred or the intake during the prior segment. Two runners with cramping and two with near cramping reported taking sodium in supplements at an average rate of 772–872 mg/h. Both runners also reported they were consuming electrolyte-containing energy drinks. Also, 12 runners (11 finishers) without cramping were taking no sodium in supplements throughout the race, and 1 (a finisher) indicated he also used no electrolyte-containing energy drinks for hydration purposes.

Discussion

The key findings of this study are that (1) cramping and near cramping were common in this 161-km ultramarathon; (2) the most commonly involved muscles were the calf, quadriceps, and hamstrings; (3) those with cramping or near cramping were more likely to have a prior history of muscle cramping during an ultramarathon and greater muscle damage during the race than those without cramping; and (4) hydration status, intake rate of sodium in supplements, and

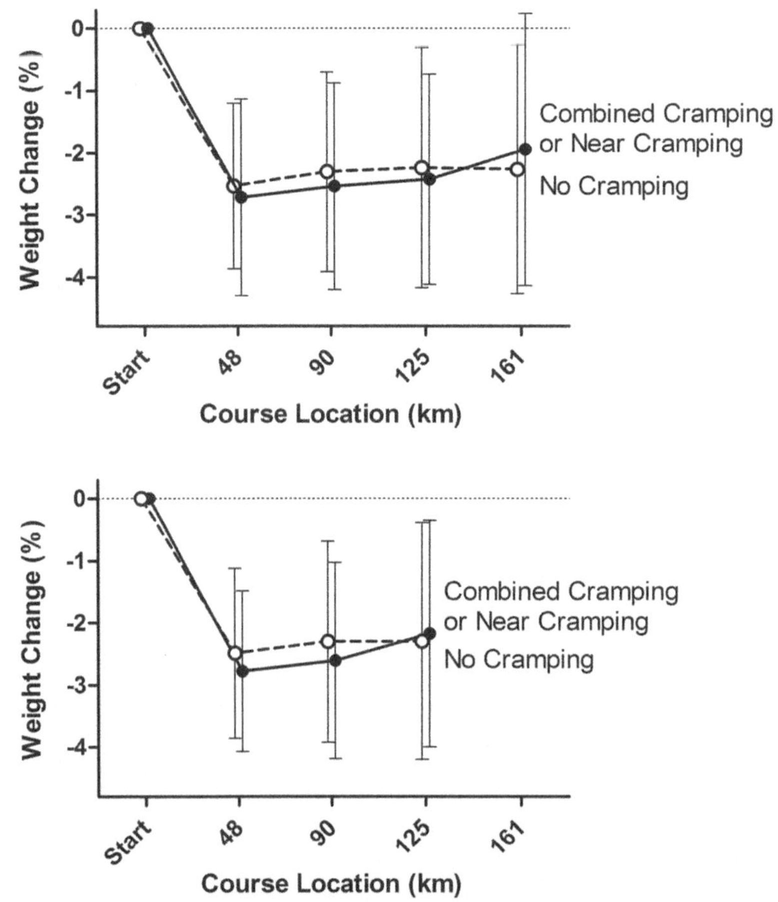

Fig 3 Mean weight change at course locations where weights were obtained for those with either cramping or near cramping (*closed circles* and *solid lines*) and those without cramping (*open circles* and *dashed lines*) during the race segment ending where weight was measured (*upper graph*) and during the subsequent course segment (*lower graph*). Data include finishers and non-finishers. *Error brackets* represent 1 SD. Data points are offset slightly along the horizontal axis for clarity of the error brackets

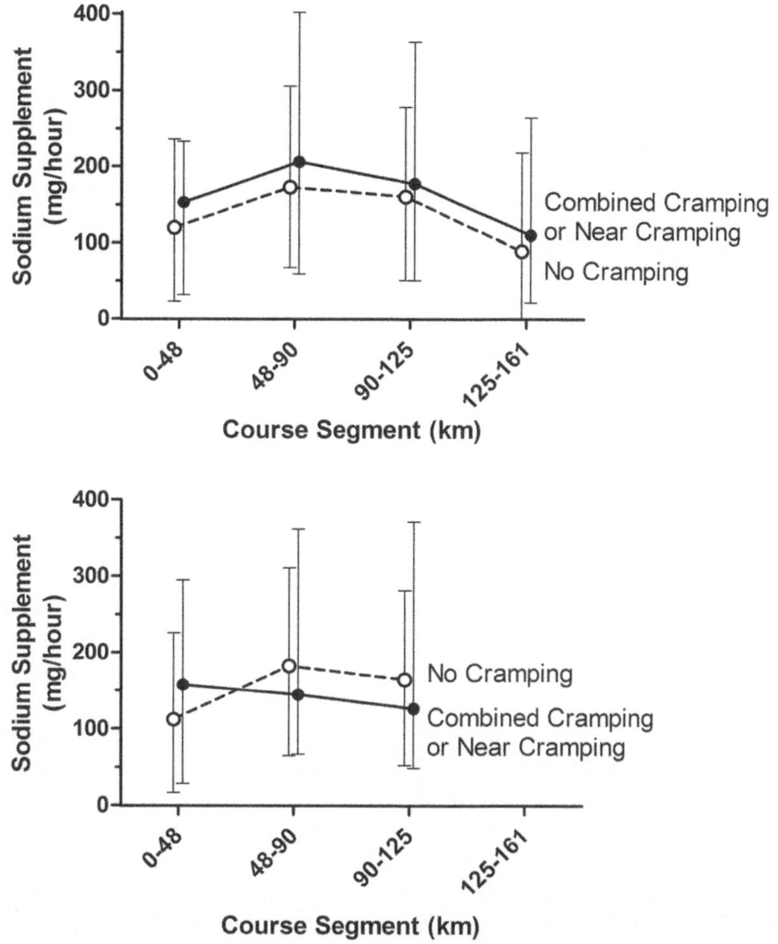

Fig 4 Median rate of intake of sodium in supplements during each course segment for those with either cramping or near cramping (*closed circles* and *solid lines*) and those without cramping (*open circles* and *dashed lines*) during the same segment (*upper graph*) and during the subsequent segment (*lower graph*). Data include finishers and non-finishers. *Error brackets* represent interquartile range. Data points are offset slightly along the horizontal axis for clarity of the error brackets

serum sodium concentration did not differ between those with cramping and those without cramping.

Prior work has demonstrated that muscle cramping is common in 161-km ultramarathons [8]. Prevalence rates of muscle cramping during or within 6 h after an Ironman triathlon were reported at 23 % [5], and the prevalence rate was 41 % at a 56-km ultramarathon [6]. While the present study did not include a post-race assessment for muscle cramping prevalence, and considered both cramping and near cramping, the 14 % prevalence of cramping and 41.1 % prevalence with inclusion of those with near cramping offer further support for this being a common phenomenon in ultramarathon running.

Muscle cramping was most commonly experienced in the large muscle groups primarily involved in running (i.e., calf, quadriceps, hamstrings) and subject to overload and fatigue during an ultramarathon. The lesser involved muscle groups and body locations could have also been subject to fatigue. This would even be true for muscles in the upper extremity, especially considering that many of the runners in these events carry fluid bottles in their hands while running. Nevertheless, since most of the cramping involved those muscle groups primarily subject to fatigue, a mechanism for cramping that involves muscle overload and fatigue seems to be supported.

Unfortunately, a formal assessment of muscular fatigue was not made in this study, so the extent of muscular fatigue across the course is not known. Although progressive muscular fatigue might be expected during a continuous event, that does not appear to be the case as muscular fatigue has been found to stabilize by around 12 h during a 24-h treadmill run [24]. Indeed, runners may accommodate by slowing as has been previously demonstrated to begin around 70 km in the present event [22, 25] and after approximately 6 h during a 24-h treadmill run [24, 26]. Variation in course profile, ambient temperature conditions, visibility impairment from darkness, and available energy sources contribute to these changes in speed during the Western States Endurance Run, making it difficult to know the extent of muscular fatigue throughout the event. Such factors may contribute to our finding that muscle cramping did not vary statistically across the course segments, although inspection of the data suggests that cramping and near cramping tended to be most common after the first course segment.

Runners developing muscle cramping during the ultramarathon were distinguished from those without cramping by more commonly having a prior history of muscle cramping during an ultramarathon and having higher post-race blood CK and BUN concentrations. A prior history of muscle cramping has previously been found to be a characteristic of those developing cramping during endurance events [5, 6], so this finding is not surprising. However, as far as we are aware, higher blood CK and BUN concentrations among those with cramping are new findings. While numerous factors account for variability in post-race blood CK concentrations, our interpretation of the finding that those with cramping had a higher blood CK relates to an association of muscle injury with relative exercise demand. In other words, we presume that the higher CK concentrations indicate that the group with cramping was placing greater demands on their muscles during the race relative to their current state of training than those without cramping. This provides additional support to the prior observation that those developing muscle cramping are racing at a relatively higher intensity than those without cramping [5, 6, 14] and that cramping in this environment may be due to muscle overload and fatigue rather than a fluid and/or electrolyte imbalance.

Interpretation of the present finding of a higher BUN concentration among those with cramping compared with those without cramping requires some exploration. In general, BUN concentration is related to hydration status. Similar to the present work, we have previously demonstrated a relationship between BUN and change in body weight such that BUN is higher among those with greater body weight loss during the event [27]. Yet for that study and the present study, weight change only explained 11–13 % of the variability of BUN concentration. It is likely because of this relatively weak relationship that the present work showed no evidence that cramping was related to percent weight change. In other words, while the post-race BUN concentrations were statistically higher among those with cramping than those without cramping, closer inspection of hydration status by weight change showed no evidence that those with cramping were more likely to have an issue with fluid balance. This finding that muscle cramping is not related to hydration level supports prior findings from observational studies of runners and triathletes [5, 15–17] as well as controlled laboratory studies [28, 29].

Runners developing muscle cramping during the ultramarathon did not have a statistically different post-race serum sodium compared with those without cramping, but the statistical effect was close to significant ($p = 0.055$). To further investigate whether a low serum sodium (below the reference range for normal of 135–145 mmol/L) might be linked to a higher incidence of cramping, we performed additional analyses. The serum sodium concentration among those with cramping, near cramping, and no cramping during the final segment of the race was compared and found to not be different. We also compared the proportion of runners with serum sodium concentrations below normal among those with cramping or near cramping and those without cramping during the final segment of the race and found no difference between groups. These analyses were performed under the presumption that the serum sodium concentration at the finish would relate best to any symptoms during the final segment of the race. Given the findings from these analyses, we conclude that cramping is not related to serum sodium concentration in this environment, a conclusion that supports prior studies of runners and triathletes [5, 15–17].

The use of sodium supplementation is common during 161-km ultramarathons. In fact, our prior work at this same event has demonstrated that 90–96 % of runners use sodium supplements [30, 31], which is comparable to the overall use by 94 % in the present work. Despite such high use of sodium supplements, we have found that they have little or no effect on hydration status [30] or the prevention of hyponatremia [31, 32]. Furthermore, total sodium intake has no relationship with the common symptoms of nausea and vomiting [33]. The present work further demonstrates that the use of sodium supplements and the rate of intake of sodium in supplements are not related to muscle cramping. Interestingly, it has been shown that pickle juice can inhibit electrically induced muscle cramps in mildly dehydrated humans; however, the effect was evident before absorption could have occurred [34]. It was speculated that some component (not necessarily the electrolyte content) of the pickle juice might trigger a reflex from the oropharyngeal region that inhibits alpha motor neurons [34].

The present findings offer some insight into the underlying pathophysiology of exercise-associated muscle cramping. Key findings in this regard were that (1) the cramping involved muscle groups under high demand during the activity; (2) cramping appeared most prevalent, though not statistically different, after the early portion of the race; (3) those with cramping had higher blood CK concentrations than those without cramping; and (4) cramping was not related to serum sodium concentration or hydration status. Considering the two main theories for the pathophysiology of exercise-associated muscle cramping, these findings seem most consistent with muscle fatigue as an underlying mechanism for muscle cramping in this environment rather than an electrolyte or fluid balance issue.

The theory of exercise-associated cramping being due to hyperexcitability of motor neuron axon terminals relies on the premise that there is a loss in plasma volume during exercise from sweating that causes a shift of water from the interstitial compartment to the intravascular space [12]. Increased local concentrations of excitatory extracellular constituents such as acetylcholine, electrolytes, and exercise-related metabolites are thought to then provide an environment for hyperexcitability of neuromuscular junctions. While plasma volume was not measured in the present study, the findings of similar serum sodium concentrations and weight changes between those with and without cramping suggest that there was no difference in the level of plasma volume contraction or fluid shift from the interstitial compartment between groups.

The study is limited in some regards, largely due to the restraints of performing research at a competitive event. Such work generally requires an observational design, which makes it challenging to specifically examine underlying pathophysiology. Furthermore, since the current beliefs among most participants in the present event is that sodium supplementation is important, we had to accept that most subjects would be using sodium supplements. This means that the number of subjects with muscle cramping who did not use sodium supplements was small. We were also limited by an inability to quantify total sodium intake which requires a full dietary analysis and is not feasible with a large sample size. Another limitation is that the study depended on subject willingness to provide a post-race blood sample and to complete the post-race questionnaire. The latter depended on subject recall, although runners were alerted in advance that they would be asked to provide information about hydration strategies. Furthermore, significant memory distortion was likely limited since most study participants completed the survey within a few days of the race and since most runners avoid adopting new hydration approaches for an event of this nature. Because the study was performed at a competitive event, the blood work was only performed at the finish, although it would have been optimal to know the intermediate values in order to more closely examine relationships with cramping during each race segment. Finally, a formal measurement of muscular fatigue during each race segment would have been valuable, but was not feasible on a large scale in a competitive event.

Conclusions

From this work, we conclude that muscle cramping and near cramping are common in a 161-km ultramarathon, largely involve the most active muscles, and tend to occur after the early segment of the race. Compared with those not having cramping, those with cramping or near cramping are more likely to have a prior history of muscle cramping during an ultramarathon, and evidence suggests that they are placing greater demands on their muscles during the race relative to their current state of training. Hydration status, intake rate of sodium in supplements, and serum sodium concentration do not differ between those with and without cramping. Of the two main theories for the pathophysiology of exercise-associated muscle cramping, the present findings support a muscle fatigue basis for muscle cramping during ultra-endurance exercise over the theory based on hyperexcitability of motor neuron axon terminals due to an electrolyte or fluid imbalance.

Abbreviations

BUN: Blood urea nitrogen; CK: Creatine kinase.

Competing interests

The authors declare that they have no competing interests.

Authors' contributions

MDH and KJS participated in the design of the study and carried out the data collection. MDH performed the statistical analysis and drafted the manuscript. Both authors read and approved the final manuscript.

Authors' information

MDH is Director of Research and KJS is a member of the Research Committee of the Western States Endurance Run.

Acknowledgements

This material is the result of work supported with resources and the use of facilities at the VA Northern California Health Care System. The work was also supported by the Western States Endurance Run Foundation. We thank Sutter Auburn Faith Hospital for laboratory services, Lodi Health and James Milner for phlebotomy services, and the following individuals for assistance with data collection: Dr. Jim Agnew, Maddison Bowles, Dr. Jeffrey A. Chan, Colleen Conners-Pace, Ali Etemady-Deylamy, Dr. Keith George, Dr. Steve Hammer, Dr. Tracy Beth Høeg, Samuel Jurek, Rachel Lord, Dr. Christine Mathiesen, Dr. David Oxborough, Dr. David Paris, Emily Pearce, Peter K. Raisanen, Professor John Somauroo, Taylor Valentino, Lisa Weiss, and Casey Westbrooke. The contents reported here do not represent the views of the Department of Veterans Affairs or the United States Government.

Author details

[1]Department of Physical Medicine & Rehabilitation, Department of Veterans Affairs, Northern California Health Care System, and University of California Davis Medical Center, 10535 Hospital Way, Sacramento, CA, USA. [2]Health Sciences Department, Gettysburg College, Gettysburg, PA, USA.

References

1. Eichner ER. The role of sodium in 'heat cramping'. Sports Med. 2007;37:368–70.
2. Schwellnus MP. Cause of exercise associated muscle cramps (EAMC)—altered neuromuscular control, dehydration or electrolyte depletion? Br J Sports Med. 2009;43:401–8.
3. Schwellnus MP. Muscle cramping in the marathon: aetiology and risk factors. Sports Med. 2007;37:364–7.
4. Schwellnus MP, Drew N, Collins M. Muscle cramping in athletes—risk factors, clinical assessment, and management. Clin Sports Med. 2008;27:183–94.

5. Schwellnus MP, Drew N, Collins M. Increased running speed and previous cramps rather than dehydration or serum sodium changes predict exercise-associated muscle cramping: a prospective cohort study in 210 Ironman triathletes. Br J Sports Med. 2011;45:650–6.
6. Schwellnus MP, Allie S, Derman W, Collins M. Increased running speed and pre-race muscle damage as risk factors for exercise-associated muscle cramps in a 56 km ultra-marathon: a prospective cohort study. Br J Sports Med. 2011;45:1132–6.
7. Kao WF, Hou SK, Chiu YH, Chou SL, Kuo FC, Wang SH, et al. Effects of 100-km ultramarathon on acute kidney injury. Clin J Sport Med. 2015;25:49–54.
8. Hoffman MD, Fogard K. Factors related to successful completion of a 161-km ultramarathon. Int J Sports Physiol Perform. 2011;6:25–37.
9. McGowan V, Hoffman MD. Characterization of medical care at the 161-km Western States Endurance Run. Wilderness Environ Med 2015;26:29–35
10. Scheer BV, Murray A. Al Andalus Ultra Trail: an observation of medical interventions during a 219-km, 5-day ultramarathon stage race. Clin J Sport Med. 2011;21:444–6.
11. Eichner ER. The salt paradox for athletes. Curr Sports Med Rep. 2014;13:197–8.
12. Bergeron MF. Muscle cramps during exercise—is it fatigue or electrolyte deficit? Curr Sports Med Rep. 2008;7:S50–5.
13. Minetto MA, Holobar A, Botter A, Farina D. Origin and development of muscle cramps. Exerc Sport Sci Rev. 2013;41:3–10.
14. Shang G, Collins M, Schwellnus MP. Factors associated with a self-reported history of exercise-associated muscle cramps in Ironman triathletes: a case-control study. Clin J Sport Med. 2011;21:204–10.
15. Maughan RJ. Exercise-induced muscle cramp: a prospective biochemical study in marathon runners. J Sports Sci. 1986;4:31–4.
16. Schwellnus MP, Nicol J, Laubscher R, Noakes TD. Serum electrolyte concentrations and hydration status are not associated with exercise associated muscle cramping (EAMC) in distance runners. Br J Sports Med. 2004;38:488–92.
17. Sulzer NU, Schwellnus MP, Noakes TD. Serum electrolytes in Ironman triathletes with exercise-associated muscle cramping. Med Sci Sports Exerc. 2005;37:1081–5.
18. Schwellnus MP, Derman EW, Noakes TD. Aetiology of skeletal muscle 'cramps' during exercise: a novel hypothesis. J Sports Sci. 1997;15:277–85.
19. Hoffman MD, Ingwerson JL, Rogers IR, Stuempfle KJ, Hew-Butler T. Increasing creatine phosphokinase concentration at the 161-km Western States Endurance Run. Wilderness Environ Med. 2012;23:56–60.
20. Hoffman MD, Stuempfle KJ, Rogers IR, Weschler LB, Hew-Butler T. Hyponatremia in the 2009 161-km Western States Endurance Run. Int J Sports Physiol Perform. 2011;7:6–10.
21. Hoffman MD, Wegelin JA. The Western States 100-Mile Endurance Run: participation and performance trends. Med Sci Sports Exerc. 2009;41:2191–8.
22. Parise C, Hoffman MD. Influence of temperature and performance level on pacing a 161-km trail ultramarathon. Int J Sports Physiol Perform. 2011;6:243–51.
23. Rogers IR, Hook G, Stuempfle KJ, Hoffman MD, Hew-Butler T. An intervention study of oral versus intravenous hypertonic saline administration in ultramarathon runners with exercise-associated hyponatremia: a preliminary randomized trial. Clin J Sports Med. 2011;21:200–3.
24. Martin V, Kerhervé H, Messonnier LA, Banfi JC, Geyssant A, Bonnefoy R, et al. Central and peripheral contributions to neuromuscular fatigue induced by a 24-h treadmill run. J Appl Physiol (1985). 2010;108(5):1224–33.
25. Hoffman MD. Pacing by winners of a 161-km mountain ultramarathon. Int J Sports Physiol Perform. 2014;9(6):1054–6.
26. Gimenez P, Kerhervé H, Messonnier LA, Féasson L, Millet GY. Changes in the energy cost of running during a 24-h treadmill exercise. Med Sci Sports Exerc. 2013;45(9):1807–13.
27. Hoffman MD, Stuempfle KJ, Fogard K, Hew-Butler T, Winger J, Weiss RH. Urine dipstick analysis for identification of runners susceptible to acute kidney injury following an ultramarathon. J Sports Sci. 2013;31:20–31.
28. Braulick KW, Miller KC, Albrecht JM, Tucker JM, Deal JE. Significant and serious dehydration does not affect skeletal muscle cramp threshold frequency. Br J Sports Med. 2013;47:710–4.
29. Miller KC, Mack GW, Knight KL, Hopkins JT, Draper DO, Fields PJ, et al. Three percent hypohydration does not affect threshold frequency of electrically induced cramps. Med Sci Sports Exerc. 2010;42:2056–63.
30. Hoffman MD, Stuempfle KJ. Hydration strategies, weight change and performance in a 161 km ultramarathon. Res Sports Med. 2014;22:213–25.
31. Winger JM, Hoffman MD, Hew-Butler TD, Stuempfle KJ, Dugas JP, Fogard K, et al. Physiology and hydration beliefs affect race behavior but not post-race sodium in 161-km ultramarathon finishers. Int J Sports Physiol Perform. 2013;8:536–41.
32. Hoffman MD, Stuempfle KJ. Sodium supplementation and exercise-associated hyponatremia during prolonged exercise. Med Sci Sports Exerc 2014. [Epub ahead of print]
33. Stuempfle KJ, Hoffman MD, Weschler LB, Rogers IR, Hew-Butler T. Race diet of finishers and non-finishers in a 100 mile (161 km) mountain footrace. J Am Coll Nutr. 2011;30:529–35.
34. Miller KC, Mack GW, Knight KL, Hopkins JT, Draper DO, Fields PJ, et al. Reflex inhibition of electrically induced muscle cramps in hypohydrated humans. Med Sci Sports Exerc. 2010;42:953–61.

7

The impact of trunk impairment on performance of wheelchair activities with a focus on wheelchair court sports: a systematic review

Viola C Altmann[1*], Anne L Hart[2], Yves C Vanlandewijck[3], Jacques van Limbeek[4] and Miranda L van Hooff[5]

Abstract

Background: Trunk impairment seems to impact significantly on performance in wheelchair court sports, but evidence to support this impression has never been systematically assessed. The objective of this study is to systematically review, describe and synthesise the literature investigating the impact of trunk impairment on wheelchair activities in court sports.

Methods: This systematic review was performed according to the consensus statement for the meta-analysis of observational studies in epidemiology (MOOSE). The search strategy for original articles comprised Medline (1950- November 2014), Cinahl (1981-November 2014), and Embase (1980- November 2014), using the search terms: trunk, trunk muscles, postural balance, posture and wheelchair.
Eligibility criteria for further review were 1) participants included experienced wheelchair users, 2) comparisons were made between a) participants with different levels of trunk impairment or b) between able bodied participants and participants with trunk impairment, or c) between participants with trunk impairment with and without compensatory equipment, and 3) outcome measures were quantitative data on wheelchair activities. For methodological quality assessment, the STROBE (Strengthening the reporting of observational studies in epidemiology) checklist was used.

Results: After assessment of 358 potentially relevant studies for the eligibility criteria, 25 studies were appropriate for methodological assessment. Twelve articles fulfilled the predetermined minimum of 15 reported items on the 22-item STROBE checklist. These studies were limited to observational studies with small populations. All but one study were restricted to patients with spinal cord injury (SCI).

Conclusions: Limited evidence was found about the impact of trunk impairment on wheelchair activities. Reach to the front and multidirectional reach was further in able bodied persons than in persons with SCI. In a perturbation that equals deceleration in wheelchair court sports, able bodied persons maintain balance, whereas persons with SCI lose balance. No evidence was found to support a difference in acceleration between persons with partial trunk muscle strength and persons with full trunk muscle strength. For future research, there is a need for a test that includes all types of trunk impairment and identification of activities that determine performance in wheelchair court sports. Furthermore, populations of athletes with all trunk impairment types should be included.

* Correspondence: v.altmann@maartenskliniek.nl
[1]Rehabilitation Centre, Sint Maartenskliniek, P.O. Box 90116500 GM Nijmegen, The Netherlands
Full list of author information is available at the end of the article

Background

Classification is a process in which a single group of entities are ordered into a number of smaller groups on the basis of observable properties. In health and health-related domains, this basis for classification is impairment in body structure and function [1,2]. In paralympic sports, classification of impairment in athletes is vital to minimise the impact of impairment on the outcome of competition. Without classification, paralympic sport competition could potentially have a one-sided and predictable outcome, in which athletes with the least impairment would have the best chance to win. Classification systems have been developed and applied since the founding of the paralympic movement [3]. All paralympic classification systems evolved from a medical assessment model, developed based on expert opinion by classifiers. Typically, these individuals are volunteers with medical or health-related professional training and/or sport-specific expertise. In 2007, the International Paralympic Committee (IPC) published the *IPC Classification Code and International Standards* to provide a structure for classification principles for all paralympic sports [4]. The IPC Classification Code states that classification in the paralympic movement should be based on eligible impairment types per sport and the effect of these impairments on sport-specific activity, irrespective of the health condition causing the impairment. An important purpose of the *Classification Code* is to charge international sports federations with the development of evidence-based classification systems through research. An evidence-based classification system is a requirement for each sport federation to maintain compliance with the code and, consequently, preserve membership in the paralympic movement. The IPC position stand, published in 2009, defined evidence-based classification and provided guidelines on how an evidence-based classification system may be achieved [2].

Similar to other paralympic sports, the classification system in wheelchair rugby is based on expert opinion. Wheelchair rugby is a sport originally developed for athletes with tetraplegia due to complete spinal cord injury (SCI). The fast-paced sport has grown to include athletes with all biomechanical impairment types as defined by IPC: impaired muscle strength, impaired passive range of motion, limb deficiency, leg length difference, short stature, hypertonia, ataxia and athetosis [2,5]. An increasing number of athletes with eligible impairment types resulting from health conditions such as incomplete SCI, congenital or acquired limb deficiencies and cerebral palsy entered the sport. These athletes differ in the type and degree of impairment from those of the pioneers in the sport. These athletes have partial to no impairment in muscle strength, coordination and range of motion of the trunk. By observing athletes with and without trunk impairment, classifiers, athletes and stakeholders in wheelchair rugby perceived a significant impact of trunk impairment on performance in wheelchair activities. Trunk impairment did not seem adequately considered in the classification system [6].

To incorporate the principles of evidence-based practice to improve classification of trunk impairment, an exploration of the available literature was deemed necessary. Although classification systems for other paralympic sports, including wheelchair basketball, Nordic skiing and athletics, examine trunk impairment, these systems are largely based on expert opinion, similar to the classification system for wheelchair rugby [7-9]. Previous research indicates trunk muscle strength, trunk coordination and trunk range of movement determine: a) trunk position which impacts on force application on the hand rims, b) trunk stability which decreases paradoxical movements, making arm movements and force application more effective and c) trunk movement which determines the range of the push rim that can be used in each push stroke. Therefore, trunk impairment may impact significantly on wheelchair propulsion, especially in high resistance wheeling such as accelerating from standstill [10,11]. However, some significant activities determining wheelchair sport performance were not assessed (e.g. reach, turning and maintaining balance after perturbation). Furthermore, the impact of impairment on performance in wheelchair sports can be modified by equipment [12]. Athletes in wheelchair court sports always perform using equipment. The minimum equipment is a sports wheelchair that is usually custom made. In addition, many athletes use belts and straps to improve force generation. Athletes who have trunk impairment also use straps to increase stability. The use of equipment is not considered in determining the sports class according to the IPC classification code [4]. Therefore, to support evidence-based classification, the impact of equipment should be treated as a covariate.

The goal of the present study is to systematically review, describe and synthesise literature investigating the impact of impairment in muscle strength, coordination and range of movement of the trunk on performance in wheelchair activities, with a focus on wheelchair court sports. The primary question was proposed in wheelchair rugby; however, because wheelchair rugby has many commonalities with other court sports [12-14], the scope of this study includes all wheelchair court sports (including wheelchair rugby, basketball and tennis). There is no evidence-based set of tests that determines the performance in wheelchair activities in general or in any wheelchair sport [15]. Therefore, the existing literature about wheelchair activities that determine performance in wheelchair court sports was analysed [12-14,16-18]. This review resulted in the following activities: maintaining balance after perturbation, reach, propulsion, acceleration, change of direction and specific for wheelchair basketball and wheelchair rugby, tilting the chair. These activities matched those previously used in earlier research to assess the performance in wheelchair rugby [19-21]. The impact of equipment on performance in the presence of trunk impairment was dealt with as a covariate.

Methods

This systematic review was conducted and reported according to the specifications referred to in the consensus statement for the meta-analysis of observational studies in epidemiology (MOOSE) [22]. Two independent researchers, VA and AH, performed the search for articles. Both are experienced wheelchair rugby classifiers; VA is a medical doctor and AH is a physiotherapist, PhD.

Data sources

The search strategy for original articles was comprised of Medline (1950 to November 2014), Cinahl (1981 to November 2014) and Embase (1980 to November 2014). The following three groups of search terms were used: trunk/trunk muscles (replaced by torso and abdominal muscles as the closest matching MeSh terms in Medline), postural balance/posture and wheelchair. The terms within each group were concatenated by the Boolean OR and were performed independently of one another before each group was concatenated by the Boolean AND with the relevant health conditions of athletes playing wheelchair rugby: spinal cord injury, poliomyelitis, neuromuscular disease, cerebral palsy and amputation.

The search was extended using the option "related articles" in Medline and a manual search of all references of the included articles. First, the titles of the "related articles" and the references were screened. Only if the title indicated potential relevance, the abstract was further assessed and added to the numbers of identified records. To assess if any relevant unpublished research was available, one of the authors (VA) screened all abstracts over the past 8 years of several conferences, which were relevant in relation to the objectives of the review: the IPC Vista conferences in 2006, 2011 and 2013, the fourth and the fifth international state-of-the-art congress Rehabilitation: Mobility, Exercise and Sports 2009 and 2014 and the 2012 International Convention on Science, Education & Medicine in Sport. For any abstracts that matched the inclusion criteria, author VA contacted the authors to obtain unpublished manuscripts.

Study selection

Studies were selected for further review if the following criteria met clinical relevance: 1) participants included experienced wheelchair users; 2) comparisons were made a) between participants with different levels of trunk impairment or b) between able bodied persons and persons with trunk impairment or c) between persons with trunk impairment with and without compensation by equipment and 3) if the outcome measures were wheelchair activities, presented in quantitative data. Furthermore, articles written in English were selected as well as German, French or Dutch, if the abstract was in English.

Studies were excluded: 1) if only able-bodied persons participated, 2) if no comparison of trunk impairment or compensation for trunk impairment was made, 3) if no definition of trunk impairment was reported or 4) also excluded were articles containing only qualitative data, expert opinions or case reports.

To identify potentially relevant articles, two reviewers (VA and AH) independently screened titles and abstracts. If one reviewer found an article, both reviewers screened for the inclusion criteria. If the inclusion criteria were met, the full text of the potential article was assessed. In case of disagreement between the reviewers about the inclusion criteria, a consensus procedure was used with four authors of the review (VA, AH, JvL and MvH). This consensus procedure consisted of an open discussion and a vote, if no consensus was reached after discussion. In case of a tie vote, the study would be included. Articles found more than once using the search strategies (doubles) were only included once.

Quality assessment

Two reviewers (VA and AH) independently assessed the methodological quality of each study using the Strengthening The Reporting of Observational Studies in Epidemiology (STROBE) checklist for reports of observational studies [23]. The STROBE checklist consists of 22 items. Each item was scored as present ('1') or absent ('0'). If an item contained sub items, the concerning item was scored present if at least 50% of the sub items were scored present. The STROBE recommendations do not provide a guideline or threshold for including meaningful studies in a systematic review. However, in a study performed on the methodological quality of observational studies published in high-quality journals, these authors found on average 69% of the STROBE items were reported [24]. Consistent with this study and with others using quantitative cut-off scores for observational studies, we decided that a minimum of 15 reported items (69%) indicated "good quality", whereas 14 reported items or less indicated "moderate to low quality" [25].

When disagreement existed on any item of the STROBE checklist, the same consensus procedure applied for inclusion criteria was used with four authors of the review (VA, AH, JvL and MvH).

Results

Search results

Figure 1 shows the number of articles found following each step of the search strategy.

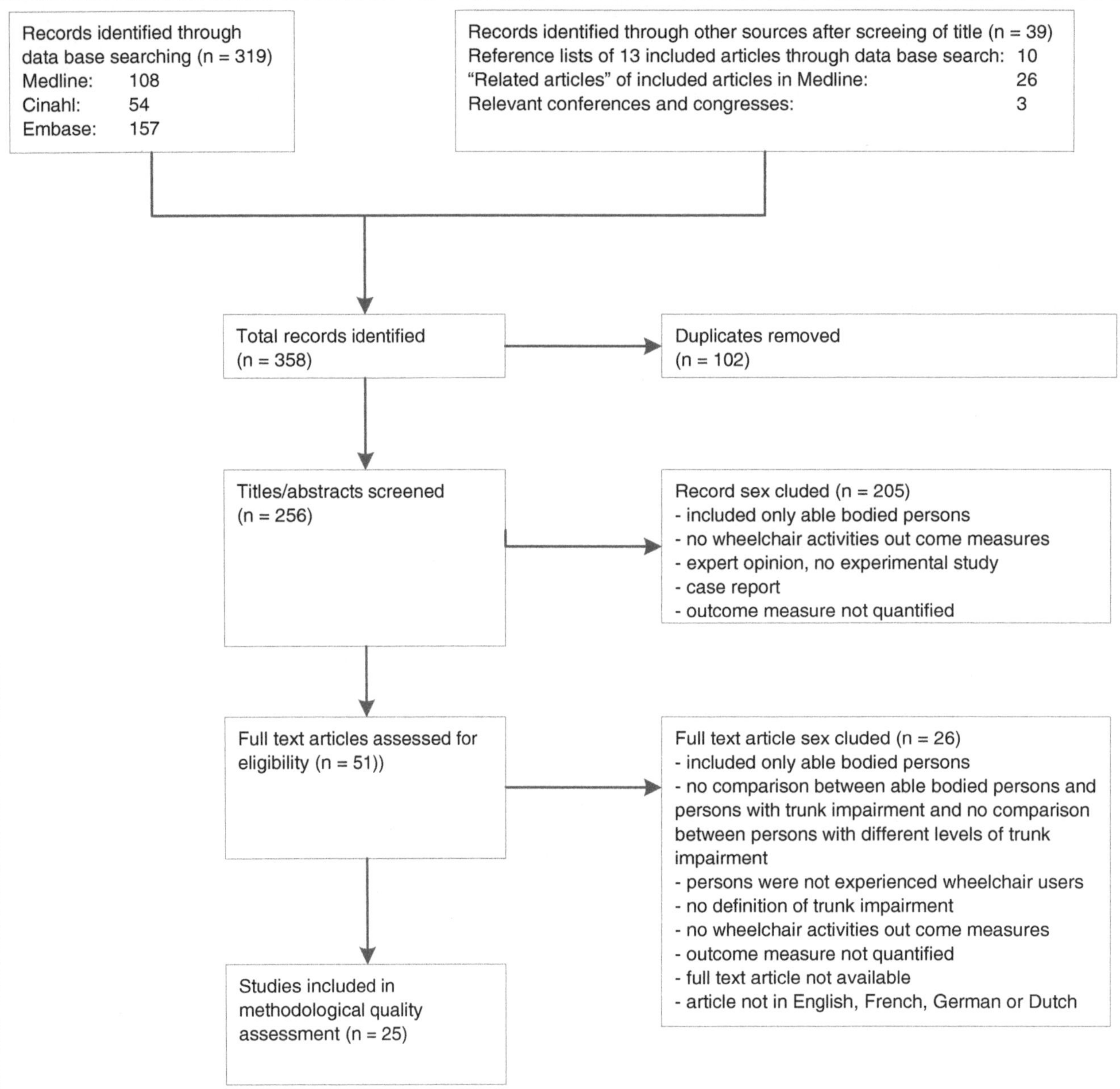

Figure 1 Flow diagram of the literature search.

After database searching, the researchers found 319 studies, which were potentially relevant. After assessment for the eligibility criteria based on screening of titles and the abstracts and if indicated, assessment of the full article, the researchers reached consensus that 13 articles were eligible for methodological quality assessment. Most articles were excluded because the population did not consist of experienced wheelchair users, there was no definition of trunk impairment or the outcome measures did not include wheelchair activities. One article was excluded based on language. All references of the 13 articles that were eligible after the database searching were searched manually. Furthermore, those articles in Medline with the option "related articles" were screened. The 36 potentially relevant studies found by this manual search were also assessed for eligibility. After cross checking for duplicates with the 13 articles that were already eligible, 12 studies were added, so a total of 25 studies were eligible for methodological assessment.

The search for unpublished manuscripts resulted in three relevant abstracts: one abstract in which the reach in a seated position of wheelchair slalom athletes with cerebral palsy was compared to the reach of persons without any health condition [26], one abstract about static and dynamic sitting balance in wheelchair rugby and wheelchair basketball athletes [27] and one abstract about the relation to trunk muscle strength and sprinting performance [28]. Full text manuscripts were not available; therefore, these studies were excluded.

Methodological quality

The results of the quality assessment of the 25 articles, eligible based on the inclusion criteria, are shown in Table 1.

Findings of the review

Twelve articles fulfilled the predetermined minimum of 15 reported items on the STROBE checklist (see Table 1) [29-40]. All 12 used a cross-sectional design. All but one study [40] was restricted to patients with SCI. And trunk impairment was defined by the America Spinal Injury Association (ASIA) score [41] in nine of the 12 studies [31,32,40].

In relation to activities determining proficiency in wheelchair court sports, the following three activities were described in the included articles: reach, maintaining balance after external perturbation and acceleration. No studies were found that assessed steady state propulsion, change of direction or tilting the chair.

Reach was assessed in a total of nine studies [29-34,37-39]: forward reach in five studies [33,34,37-39] and multidirectional reach in four studies [29-32]. Persons who were able bodied could reach further than those with SCI [33,34,37,38]. No distinction was found in forward reaching distance between persons with different levels of SCI as determined by the ASIA score (high thoracic T2-T8, low thoracic T9-T12 and lumbar L1-L5) [33,34,37]. Only one study reported further displacement of the centre of pressure (CoP) in persons with low thoracic SCI (T9-12) compared to persons with high thoracic SCI (T2-8) [38]. In multidirectional reach, differences in reaching in all directions summed in a single measure were found, with better reach in able bodied persons than in persons with SCI [32]. If a single measure for each direction was given, there was better reaching in almost all single directions in able-bodied persons compared to persons with SCI [31,32]. Also, there was better reach in persons low thoracic SCI than in persons with high SCI [30]. Similarly, persons with SCI with voluntary trunk muscle contractions could reach further than persons with SCI without trunk muscle contractions [32]. No difference was found in single direction measures between subgroups of persons with SCI for reaching in the lateral directions to both sides [29,31], to the left side [32] and for oblique directions to the left side [29,32].

Maintaining balance after external perturbation by tilting a platform on which the person was seated in a wheelchair, was described in two studies [35,36]. In tilting the platform in the sagittal or the frontal directions, those who were able bodied did not lose balance in any of the tilting accelerations (2 and 4 m/s^2) or at any of the tilting angles. Persons with SCI all lost balance; the tilting angle in which balance loss occurred was higher in the low accelerations than in the high accelerations for all persons with SCI. Persons with paraplegia (T2-9) lost balance at a larger tilting angle in both directions than persons with tetraplegia (C5-7).

Only one included study explored acceleration in wheelchair racing [40]. This was the only study that included persons with other health conditions than SCI. More important, this was the only study that assessed the relation between impairment, irrespective of the health condition causing the impairment and activities. Trunk impairment was defined by a clinical test for trunk muscle strength. No difference in acceleration was found between athletes with full trunk muscle strength and those without full trunk muscle strength.

Four studies assessed the impact of equipment on performance in individuals with trunk impairment. Two studies assessed wheelchair set up, chair inclination [33] and the use of a rigid versus an elastic footrest [42] in relation to forward reach. No difference in reach was found for any of these adaptations to chair set up for either persons who were able bodied or those with SCI. One study examined the effect of thigh and chest belts on multidirectional reach [31]. In persons with SCI, reach increased in all directions by using a chest belt and to a lesser extent by using a thigh belt. Reach decreased by using a belt in persons who were able bodied. One study examined the use of functional electro stimulation (FES) and reported an increase in reach with FES application with both lifting a light and lifting a heavier object [40].

Discussion

Summary of evidence

In this systematic review, the authors synthesised the evidence available in the literature on the impact of trunk impairment on the execution of wheelchair activities that determine the performance in court sports. As expected, all identified studies were observational studies. All but three studies defined trunk impairment based on SCI lesion level and not on the biomechanical impairment types consisting of trunk muscle strength, coordination of the trunk and range of movement of the trunk. The evidence reported in the included studies indicates that persons who are able bodied can reach further forward than persons with SCI [33,34,37,38]. The difference in forward reaching distance between persons with different levels of SCI was conflicting, with no difference found in three studies [33,34,37] and larger reach found in one study in persons with low thoracic SCI compared to those with high thoracic SCI [38].

Table 1 Participants, interventions, comparison and outcome measures of all studies and quality score STROBE checklist

Reference no.	Study	Participants	Intervention	Comparison	Outcome measure	Total score STROBE	Methodological quality
[49]	Bernard et al.	Six SCI T4-8 (high), six SCI T11-L5 (low) and six AB	Perturbation on moving platform for wheelchair	High SCI, low SCI, AB 4 oscillation levels	Damping factor of head	4	Moderate-poor
[29]	Boswell Ruys et al.	30 SCI C5-L2 AIS-D, 14 high level and 16 low level	Upper body sway = sit still unsupported for 30 sMaximal balance range forwards and backwardsCoordinated stability = follow track with pencil by adjusting trunk position in bending and rotating. Alternating reach test = tapping table eight times fast with and without arm supportSeated reach distance lateral left and rightUpper body dressing	New (<1 year post injury) vs. old (>1 year post injuryHigh level = C6-T7 AIS A vs. low level = T8-L2 AIS A or incomplete AIS B-D with abdominal innervation	Reliability and validity of the tests	15	High
[30]	Chen et al.	Eight SCI T1-6 (high thoracic)22 SCI T7-12 (low thoracic)	Sitting stability static (unsupported 30 s) and dynamic (30 s maximum leaning to four sides)Time needed for functional activities: upper body dressing, lower body dressing and transfer.	Low versus high thoracic SCITrunk strength (hand held dynamometry), lesion level and trunk length in relation to sitting balance. Sitting balance in relation to functional tasks.	CoP displacement static and dynamic (sum score for all directions)Time to complete functional tasks	16	High
[31]	Curtis et al.	Seven athletes with spinal cord injury; four in IWBF class 1 and three in IWBF class 2, nine AB	Reaching in sagittal and transverse plane	IWBF class 1 and 2, ABBelt at thigh and trunk versus no belt	Reaching distance in sagittal and transverse plane	16	High
[50]	De Abreu et al.	11 SCI T2-L2, AIS A-C, six AB	Reaching in anterior-posterior direction seated on different cushion types	AB versus SCIDifferent cushion types	Maximum reachAnterior displacement of the trunkReaching time for 50%, 75% and 90% and maximum reach	13	Moderate-poor
[32]	Gauthier et al.	15 SCI: 9 "Abdo" (levelT7 or lower or active contraction abdominals to generate trunk flexion) 6 "No Abdo" (level higher than T7, no active contraction abdominals to generate trunk flexion)15 AB	Move CoP to eight directions with 45° interval	AB vs SCI "Abdo" versus SCI "No Abdo"	OSI (Overall Stability Index)DSI (Direction Specific Index of Stability)	17	High
[51]	Harel et al.	Seven SCI T1-T11 AIS A-BSeven AB	Static balance with eyes open (EO) and eyes closed (EC) Dynamic balance: leaning in multiple directions	AB versus SCI	Sitting items Berg Balance ScaleModified functional reach test Seated posturography: postural sway EO and ECMaximum	14	Moderate-poor

Table 1 Participants, interventions, comparison and outcome measures of all studies and quality score STROBE checklist *(Continued)*

					excursion centre of gravity (CoG) and directional control		
[33]	Janssen-Potten et al.	Ten SCI T2-8 (high)Ten SCI T9-12 (low)Ten AB	Bimanual forward reaching task 15%, 30%, 75% and 90% of maximum	Standard chair (S)7° tilt (7 T)12° tilt (12 T)22° recline (22R)	Maximum reaching distanceCoP displacement EMG erector spinae T3, erector spinae T9, erector spinae L3, latissimus dorsi, trapezius pars ascendens, pectoralis major, serratus anterior, oblique abdominal musclesReaction time and movement time	14	Moderate-poor
[33]	Janssen-Potten et al.	Ten SCI T2-8 (high) Ten SCI T9-12 (low) Ten AB	Bimanual forward reaching task 90% of maximum	High and low SCI Standard chair and 10° forward inclination	CoP displacement EMG erector spinae T3, erector spinae T9, erector spinae L3, latissimus dorsi, trapezius pars ascendens, pectoralis major, serratus anterior, oblique abdominal musclesKinematics pelvis (tilt)	15	High
[34]	Janssen-Potten et al.	Ten SCI T9-12 (low T)Ten SCI L1-5 (L)Ten AB	Bimanual forward reaching task 90% of maximum	Low T, L and ABWith and without rigid footrest	Maximum displacement CoP (CoP max)Movement time EMG erector spinae T9, erector spinae L3, rectus abdominis, oblique abdominals, gluteus max, tensor fascia lata, rectus femoris, vastus lateralis, biceps femoris, semitendinosus, tibialis anterior, gastrocnemius medialis	15	High
[35]	Kamper et al.	Four SCI C5-7 (tetraplegia) Four SCI T2-9 (paraplegia) Five AB	Tilting movement in frontal plane on servo controlled platform in standard WC	Tetraplegia-paraplegia-ABAnd tilting movements with high and low amplitude and acceleration	Balance lossFLCP = fraction of limit of CoP movementVelocity of CoP displacementKinematic dataKinetic data (torque of pelvis, lower trunk and upper trunk)	17	High
[36]	Kamper et al.	Four SCI C5-7 (tetraplegia) Four SCI T2-9 (paraplegia) Five AB	Tilting movement in sagittal plane on servo controlled platform in standard WC	Tetraplegia-paraplegia-ABAnd tilting movements with high and low amplitude and acceleration	Balance lossFLCP = fraction of limit of CoP movementKinematic data	17	High
[52]	Kerk et al.	Six SCI T3-6, absent abdominal muscles	Sub maximal and maximal exercise test on wheelchair roller in own WC	With and without elastic abdominal binder	Pushing stroke parameters, physiologic parameters, trunk movement	12	Moderate-poor
[37]	Potten et al.	Ten SCI T2-8 (high)Ten SCI T9-12 (low)Ten AB	Bimanual forward reaching task 15%, 30%, 75% and 90% maximum	High SCI, low SCI and AB	CoP displacementEMG serratus anterior, m. pectoralis major, latissimus dorsi, erector spinae T3, trapezius pars ascendens	16	High
[53]	Requejo et al.		Three pushing speeds (0.85, 1.03 and 1.21 m/s) and one	Low and high SCI, wheelchair with rear suspension (three	Self-selected speedVertical seat reaction forceHead acceleration	10	Moderate-poor

Table 1 Participants, interventions, comparison and outcome measures of all studies and quality score STROBE checklist *(Continued)*

		Five SCI T4 and higher (high), five SCI T12 and lower (low)	self-selected speed, administering frequent small bumps	types), and without rear suspension			
[46]	Schantz et al.	Four SCI low thoracic, three SCI cervical	Comfortable and maximum pushing speed, maximum acceleration on gymnasium wooden floor	SCI low thoracic and SCI cervical	Maximum velocity and acceleration, EMG activity of arm muscles, trunk position and movement	8	Moderate-poor
[54]	Seelen et al.	15 SCI T4-T1215 AB	Reaching forward 30%, 60% and 90% of maximum after warning signal with and without cue	SCI and AB	Reaction timeMovement timeEMG activity latissimus dorsi and trapezius pars ascendens	11	Moderate-poor
[55]	Seelen et al.	15 SCI T2-8 (high)15 SCI T9-12 (low) 15 AB	Bimanual forward reaching task 15%, 30%, 75% and 90% of maximum	High and low SCI in experiment 1; none (only AB) in 2	CoP displacementEMG erector spinae T3, erector spinae T9, erector spinae L3, latissimus dorsi, trapezius pars ascendens, pectoralis major, serratus anterior, oblique abdominal muscles Antero-posterior force component	14	Moderate-poor
[56]	Seelen et al.	Five SCI T4-T8 (high), seven SCI T9-T12 (low)	Releasing push button on lapReaching forward bilaterally	15%, 30%, 75% and 90% of maximum reachhigh and low SCIduration since SCI	Reaction timeMovement time	13	Moderate-poor
[47]	Seelen et al.	Five SCI T4-8 (high)Seven SCI T9-12 (low)	Bimanual forward reaching task 15%, 30%, 75% and 90% of maximum	High and low SCI, different points in timeBraced vs. non braced (post hoc)	CoP displacementEMG erector spinae T3, erector spinae T9, erector spinae L3, latissimus dorsi, trapezius pars ascendens, pectoralis major, serratus anterior, oblique abdominal muscles	13	moderate-poor
[38]	Seelen et al.	15 SCI T2-8 (high)15 SCI T9-12 (low)15 AB	Bimanual forward reaching task 15%, 30%, 75% and 90% of maximum	High and low SCI	Reaction time, movement timeCoP displacement	15	High
[44]	Serra-Anno et al.	24 SCI higher than T9 (high); T9 and lower (low) 24 AB	Static sitting balance (ST) with eyes open (EO) and eyes closed (EC)Dynamic sitting balance (SLT)	High SCI, low SCI, AB	ST: signal amplitude, range, frequency spectrum in anterior-posterior and medial-lateral directions.SLT: maximum CoP displacement, efficient CoP displacement and normalised total excursion of CoP	13	Moderate-poor
[57]	Shin et al.	Seven SCI T10 and higher (high)11 SCI T10-L1 (low) 18 AB	Functional reach test: reaching as far as possible with dominant hand	High SCI, low SCI, AB	Functional reach, velocity and CoP trajectory, functional boundary	13	Moderate-poor
[39]	Triolo et al.	Eight SCI low (T5-10) and high (C6-7) with implanted neuroprosthesis.	Seated bimanual reach: 30 in. = desktop and 48 in. = high shelf, loaded (20% of unilateral shoulder flexion strength) lifting a light or an heavier object	High and low SCI Stimulation on and off, Strong and weak based on volitional trunk extension strength with stimulation	Unsupported bimanual reaching distance with and without stimulation.	17	High

Table 1 Participants, interventions, comparison and outcome measures of all studies and quality score STROBE checklist *(Continued)*

[40]	Vanlandewijck et al.	13 track athletes, three female no full trunk function, four male no full trunk function, six male full trunk function. Diagnosis: SCI, spina bifida, arthrogryposis, amputation	Maximum acceleration track and treadmill with 4× resistance	Male athletes full trunk function versus male athletes no full trunk function	Distance on track after 1, 2 and 3 s (m) and distance on ergometer after 1, 2 and 3 s (m)	19	High

STROBE, strengthening the reporting of observational studies in epidemiology; SCI, patients with spinal cord injury; WC, wheelchair; AB, able bodied persons; C, cervical level; T, thoracic level; L, lumbar level; IWBF class, International Wheelchair Basketball Federation class; CoP, centre of pressure; AIS, American Spinal Injury Association (ASIA) Impairment Scale [54].
Articles with a total STROBE score ≥15 were included in the analysis.

For multidirectional reach, if a sum measure for all directions was used, the following differences were found: (1) those who were able bodied showed better reach than persons with SCI. (2) Persons with SCI who could partially use their trunk muscles had better reach than those who had paralysed trunk muscles [31,32]. If separate directions were analysed, persons who were able bodied showed a larger reach than persons with SCI in almost all directions. For subgroups of persons with SCI, two studies found no differences in the left-right direction [29,31] and one did not find a difference in the left direction [32]. Two studies reported no differences in left oblique directions, but did find differences in the right oblique directions [29,32]. Consequently, oblique directions seem to be the most sensitive directions to discriminate in dynamic balance between persons with different levels of SCI. The difference between left and right oblique directions may be explained because reaching to the dominant right side is a more practised movement. Because of the limited number of participants per study, the power may have been too low to detect smaller differences to the non-dominant side. As a result, the authors suggest all reaching directions could possibly be affected by lesion level of SCI in optimally trained athletes.

There was also evidence to support that persons who are able bodied do not lose balance in perturbation with any force impact through acceleration in the lateral and forward direction in a seated position. The force impact that was applied (maximum acceleration of 4 m/s^2) seems to match the impact of deceleration from maximum speed to stop in wheelchair court sports [12-14]. Persons with thoracic SCI do lose balance in perturbations in both the frontal and the lateral directions with this impact. Moreover, persons with cervical SCI lose balance with a lower impact than persons with thoracic SCI [35,36].

The only study exploring the relationship between trunk muscle strength and acceleration in wheelchair racing found no difference between athletes with full trunk muscle strength and athletes without full trunk muscle strength [40]. No literature was found for all other wheelchair activities of interest for this review, steady state propulsion, change of direction or tilting the chair.

The limited findings of this systematic review are difficult to generalise to athletes who compete in wheelchair court sport, because almost all study participants had complete SCI with trunk impairment defined according to the ASIA score [41]. The ASIA score is based on medical examination of strength and sensation. However, the trunk level (thoracic) is defined according to impairment in sensation only. The ASIA score only reflects impairment in trunk muscle strength in athletes with complete SCI in whom the level of impaired sensation equals the level of motor impairment. For impairment types other than trunk muscle strength (range and coordination), no information was found. The distribution of impairment in trunk muscle strength is typical for those with SCI, depending on lesion level [41]. However, impairment in trunk muscle strength can have a different distribution in individuals with other medical conditions, which may result in a different impact on activities. The authors of this systematic review could only report on evidence of effect of lesion level in SCI on reach and balance after external perturbation and not for any other activities that determine performance in wheelchair court sports.

A growing issue in the paralympic movement is the impact of equipment on performance. In this systematic review, equipment was defined as a covariate in relation to the study goal. Athletes are competitive by nature and will try to enhance their performance as well as limit the impact of impairment on performance by using optimised equipment. This use of equipment is sport specific and often based on experience. However, the equipment permitted in wheelchair court sports shows similarities across sports [12-14]. Studies in this review explored the use of belts and straps, wheelchair set up, seating configuration and functional electrical stimulation (FES). Two studies assessed the possible influence of equipment in relation to trunk impairment [36,38] though equipment that is not used for wheelchair court sports was tested [13,16]. The only study that assessed equipment used in court sports found that multidirectional reach improves in athletes with SCI by the use of a thigh or trunk belt [31]. Reach is only one of the many relevant activities for wheelchair court sport, and in addition to belting, the chair set up (position of the seat and the backrest and height of the backrest) is also believed to impact on reach [16]. In one study, FES of the trunk extensor muscles was used to improve unsupported seating and to lift objects with different weights [39]. Functional electrical stimulation primarily impacts on impairment in muscle strength. The use of implanted electrodes as a piece of equipment is new to moment in the paralympic movement. So far, there is no consensus if this equipment should be allowed during sport performance and whether or not this equipment should be part of athlete evaluation in classification [43]. On the other hand, in the study exploring the effect of trunk impairment on acceleration in wheelchair racing, athletes used their own custom designed wheelchair. It must be noted that a racing wheelchair seating configuration is quite different from the configuration of a wheelchair for court sports. Opposite to wheelchairs used for court sports, the racing wheelchair does not have rear castor wheels to prevent tipping when maximum force is applied on the wheel [44]. As a consequence of the absence of the castor wheel, the racing athletes in this study may not have been able to use maximum force in accelerating, because of the risk of tipping backward. This limits the generalisation of the results of this study regarding the impact of trunk impairment on acceleration to wheelchair court sports. Additional research is necessary to examine the acceleration in a court sports wheelchair with the typical rear castor wheels to determine if trunk muscle strength does impact on acceleration when tipping of the chair is prevented.

So far, the findings of this review provide limited support to the experience of wheelchair athletes and empirical information, supporting there is a significant impact of equipment on performance in wheelchair sport [18,45].

Strengths and limitations

This systematic review has number of strengths. First, this study synthesised existing literature about the impact of trunk impairment on performance in wheelchair court sports using a strict set of inclusion and exclusion criteria. The methodological quality of all relevant studies was assessed using the STROBE checklist which is accepted as international standard for reporting of observational research [22]. The study was reported according to the MOOSE [21], which is accepted as a standard for meta-analysis. This strict approach enables replicating the study and extending it in the future if new evidence becomes available. Second, several types of potential bias were acknowledged and addressed in selecting studies for this review prior to the quality assessment, including publication bias, selection bias and quality assessment bias. The authors tried to minimise publication bias by manually searching abstracts of all conferences over the past 8 years that were relevant in relation to the objectives of this review. Only three potentially relevant abstracts were identified. Based on the lack of relevant unpublished information, it is unlikely that publication bias played a major role in this review. Furthermore, selection bias for study inclusion was addressed by independent literature searches in multiple databases completed individually by the two researchers using the same search terms. Bias in methodological quality assessment was minimized by the independent assessment of study quality by the two researchers (VA and AH). If there was no consensus between the two researchers, a consensus procedure with all authors was used for the final decision. Finally, bias in results and conclusions could have been introduced by the choice of method for quality assessment. By the authors' knowledge, the STROBE guideline provides the only checklist available for methodological assessment of observational studies. The authors of the STROBE checklist state that "good reporting reveals the strengths and weaknesses of a study and facilitates sound interpretation and application of study results". "The aim of the STROBE guideline is to ensure clear presentation of what was planned, done and found in observational studies" [23]. However, the STROBE recommendations do not provide a guideline or threshold for making decisions on inclusion of studies in a systematic review. In this systematic review, the authors chose a cut-off score for sufficient methodological quality for inclusion based on a study that determined the average score of present items in observational studies in high-quality medical journals, i.e., 69% [24].

There are several limitations to be considered when interpreting the results. All studies included small populations, which limited the study power. Possible effects of trunk impairment on the execution of wheelchair activities are not likely detected based on this limited power per study. Because the definition of trunk impairment and the outcome measures were different for each study, pooling of data to increase the power was not possible.

There are several aspects in the way tests were executed in the selected studies that may have caused bias in the results, including differences in measuring sitting balance, seating positions, use of belts and the experience level of the study participants. There were differences in the position of the arms during the measurement of sitting balance. One study allowed arm movements to compensate during trunk movements [29]. Most studies had a prescribed position of the arms, but they differed from a hand on the thighs position, which can support to some extent in forward movements [32], actively reaching with one [29] or both arms to a target [33,34,38,42], lifting a ball [31], or lifting objects with low and higher weight [39], to crossing the arms in front of the chest [35,36]. It is known that persons with a lack of trunk muscle strength can compensate with the recruitment of shoulder and arm muscles [37,46,47]; therefore, the difference in arm position can have caused bias in these results. Also, there were differences in seating position from the use of a flat surface with the knees and the hips in 90° flexion with feet supported [29,30] to sitting in a standardised wheelchair [35,36]. Although no evidence for the impact of seating position was found in the present review, there is anecdotal evidence suggesting that seating position does impact on the execution of wheelchair activities [18]. Last but not least, contrary to most studies where persons perform without a belt, in two studies, persons were provided with a lap belt [35,36]. Because of the possible impact of different arm and seating positions and the use of a lap belt on reach and perturbation, the results should be interpreted with caution. For future research on trunk impairment in wheelchair activities, the positioning of the athlete, the positioning of the arms and the use of equipment should be standardised. Preferably for application to classification in sport, these positions and equipment should be relevant to the sport of which the activities are assessed.

Finally, the majority of studies included patients while only one study included trained athletes [40]. Experience in using a wheelchair is known to have a significant impact on the execution of wheelchair activities; consequently, studies including participants with very limited experience in manual wheelchair use were excluded [48]. Nevertheless, a significant difference in skills between patients from a hospital or rehabilitation centre and optimally trained athletes is well established [15]. Consequently, there are limitations in deducting the impact of trunk impairment on performance in athletes from the included studies, using patients or persons who had limited experience in wheelchair mobility. Additional research using athletes is required to generalise the results to wheelchair court sports. There are important obstacles being able to obtain appropriate samples in classification research in wheelchair court sports. These obstacles include the limited number of athletes, spread over large areas and limited financial resources for athlete training and research. Consequently, adequate populations of athletes cannot likely be tested or studied outside of major competitions. To overcome these obstacles, effort should be given to promote future testing around these competitions and to enable athlete participation in research.

Conclusions

The literature provided limited information to aid in the development of evidence-based classification of trunk impairment in wheelchair court sports. As expected, additional research is needed, particularly for athletes with other health conditions than SCI resulting in impairment types other than trunk muscle strength. However, deficits in the current evidence were defined and can be used to guide future research in this field. The authors recommend the following for further research in wheelchair court sports: 1) Development of a test or scale for trunk impairment, comprising all biomechanical impairments of the trunk (trunk muscle strength, trunk coordination and trunk range of motion) [2]. This test needs to provide clear data for trunk impairment independent of the health condition causing the impairment. 2) Development of standardised tests for wheelchair activities that impact on wheelchair court sports performance. 3) Controlling for other factors that can impact on performance in wheelchair activities in sport, such as wheelchair configuration, positioning and strapping. 4) Facilitation of networking between researchers in several wheelchair sports needs to be facilitated to overcome limitations in resources and numbers of participants.

Statement of ethics

The manuscript does not contain clinical studies or patient data.

Competing interests

The authors declare that they have no competing interests.

Authors' contributions

VA initiated the study, designed the study, conducted the databases search, scored methodological quality and wrote the paper. AH conducted the databases search, scored methodological quality and contributed to the writing of the paper. YV initiated and designed the study, monitored the progress and contributed to the discussion of the results. JvL designed the study, participated in the consensus procedure for the inclusion criteria and the STROBE checklist and contributed to the discussion of the results. MvH designed the study, participated in the consensus procedure for the inclusion criteria and the STROBE checklist, contributed to the discussion of the results and contributed to the writing of the paper. All authors read and approved the final manuscript.

Acknowledgements

No funding was awarded for the completion of this review.

Author details

[1]Rehabilitation Centre, Sint Maartenskliniek, P.O. Box 90116500 GM Nijmegen, The Netherlands. [2]Department of Physical Therapy and Athlete Training, Northern Arizona University, Flagstaff, Arizona, USA. [3]Department of Rehabilitation sciences, Katholieke Universiteit Leuven, Leuven, Belgium. [4]Achmea Health Insurance Company, Amersfoort, The Netherlands. [5]Sint Maartenskliniek, Research, Nijmegen, The Netherlands.

References

1. International Classification of Functioning, Disability and Health 2001. In: http://apps.who.int/classifications/icfbrowser/. Accessed November 2014.
2. Tweedy SM, Vanlandewijck YC. International Paralympic Committee position stand- Background and scientific rationale for classification in Paralympic sport. Br J Sports Med. published online 22 Oct 2009;doi:10.1136/bjsm.2009.065060.
3. Tweedy S, Howe PD. Introduction to the Paralympic Movement. In: Vanlandewijck YC, Thompson W, editors. The Paralympic Athlete. UK: Wiley-Blackwell; 2011. p. 3–30.
4. IPC Classification Code and International Standards. 2007 [internet]. Available from: http://www.paralympic.org/Classification/Code.
5. Malone LA, Morgulec-Adamowics N, Orr K. Contribution of sport science to performance- wheelchair rugby. In: Vanlandewijck YC, Thompson W, editors. The Paralympic Athlete. UK: Wiley-Blackwell; 2011. p. 249–63.
6. Altmann VC, Hart AL, van Limbeek J, Vanlandewijck YC. Improvement of the classification system for wheelchair rugby: athlete priorities. Adapt Phys Activ Q. 2014;31(4):377–89. Doi: 10.1123/apaq. 2013-0064.
7. Pernot HFM, Lannem AM, Geers RPJ, Ruijters EFG, Bloemendal M, Seelen HAM. Validity of the test-table-test for Nordic skiing for classification of paralympic sit ski sports participants. Spinal Cord. 2011;49(8):935–41. doi: 10.1038/sc.2011.30. Epub 2011 May.
8. Strohkendl H. Funktionelle Klassifizierung für den Rollstuhlsport. Berlin, Heidelberg, New York: Springer; 1978.
9. Beckman EM, Tweedy SM. Towards evidence based classification in Paralympic athletics: evaluating the validity of activity limitation tests for use in classification of Paralympic running events. Br J Sports Med. 2009;43(13):1067–72. Doi: 10.1136/bjsm.2009.061804. Epub 2009 Oct 12.
10. Vanlandewijck Y, Theisen D, Daly D. Wheelchair propulsion biomechanics. Implications for wheelchair sports. Sports Med. 2001;31(5):339–67.
11. Chow JW, Millikan TA, Carlton LG, Chae WS, Lim YT, Morse MI. Kinematic and electromyographic analysis of wheelchair propulsion on ramps and slopes for young men with paraplegia. Arch Phys Med Rehabil. 2008;90(2):271–8. doi: 10.1016/j.apmr.2008.07.019.
12. Orr K, Malone LA. Wheelchair Rugby. In: Vicky G-T, editor. Wheelchair Sport. A complete guide for athletes, coaches and teachers. USA: Human Kinetics; 2010. p. 155.
13. Frogley M. Wheelchair Basketball. In: Vicky G-T, editor. Wheelchair Sport. A complete guide for athletes, coaches and teachers. USA: Human Kinetics; 2010. p. 120–2.
14. Newbery D, Richards G, Trill S, Whait M. Wheelchair Tennis. In: Vicky G-T, editor. Wheelchair Sport. A complete guide for athletes, coaches and teachers. USA: Human Kinetics; 2010. p. 176–83.

15. Fliess-Douer O, Vanlandewijck YC, Lubel Manor G, Van Der Woude LHV. A systematic review of wheelchair skills for manual wheelchair users with spinal cord injury: towards a standardised outcome measure. Clin Rehabil. 2010;24(10):867–86. doi: 10.1177/0269215510367981.
16. Rice I, Hettinga FJ, Laferrier J, Sporner ML, Heiner CM, Burkett B, et al. Biomechanics. In: Vanlandewijck YC, Thompson W, editors. The Paralympic Athlete. UK: Wiley-Blackwell; 2011. p. 41–2.
17. Mason BS, van der Woude LHV, Goosey-Tolfrey VL. The ergonomics of wheelchair configuration for optimal performance in the wheelchair court sports. Sports Med. 2013;43(1):23–38. doi: 10.1007/s40279-012-0005-x.
18. Mason BS, Porcellato L, van der Woude LHV, Goosey-Tolfrey V. A qualitative examination for optimal mobility performance in wheelchair sports: a pilot study. J Rehabil Med. 2010;42(2):141–9. doi: 10.2340/16501977-0490.
19. Morgulec-Adamowicz N, Kosmol A, Molik B, Yilla AB, Laskin JJ. Aerobic, anaerobic, and skill performance with regard to classification in wheelchair rugby athletes. Res Q Exerc Sport. 2011;82(1):61–9.
20. Mason B, van der Woude L, Tolfrey K, Goosey-Tolfrey V. The effects of rear-wheel camber on maximal effort mobility performance in wheelchair athletes. Int J Sports Med. 2012;33(3):199–204. doi: 10.1055/s-0031-1295443. Epub 2011 Dec 20.
21. Mason BS, van der Woude LH, Goosey-Tolfrey VL. Influence of glove type on mobility performance for wheelchair rugby players. Am J Phys Med Rehabil. 2009;88(7):559–70. doi: 10.1097/PHM.0b013e3181aa41c5.
22. Stroup DF, Berlin JA, Morton SC, Olkin I, Williamson GD, Rennie D, et al. Meta-analysis of Observational Studies in Epidemiology: A proposal for reporting. Meta-analysis of Observational Studies in Epidemiology (MOOSE) group. JAMA. 2000;283(15):2008–12. Review.
23. Vandenbroucke JP, von Elm E, Altman DG, Gotzsche PC, Mulrow CD, Pocock SJ, et al. Strengthening the reporting of observational studies in epidemiology (STROBE): Explanation and elaboration. PLoS Med. 2007;4(10):e297. Review. doi:10.1371/journal.pmed.0040297.
24. Poorolajal J, Cheraghi Z, Doosti Irani A, Rezaeian S. Quality of Cohort Studies Reporting Post the Strengthening the Reporting of Observational Studies in Epidemiology (STROBE) Statement. Epidemiol Health. 2011;33:e2011005. Published online Jun 7, 2011. doi: 10.4178/epih/e2011005.
25. Wong W, Cheung WC, Hart CSK, Graham J. Development of a quality assessment tool for systematic reviews of observational studies (QATSO) of HIV prevalence in men having sex with men and associated risk behaviours. Emerg Themes Epidemiol. 2008;5:23. Published online Nov 17, 2008. doi.
26. Guzmán-Morales S, Reina R, Elvira JLL, López-Valenciano A, Vera-Garciá FJ. Comparison of trunk sagittal displacement control in sitting position between slalom athletes with cerebral palsy and controls. IPC Vista conference 2011 August 31- September 3. "A multidisciplinary approach to Paralympic Succes." Bonn, Germany. Retrieved from: http://www.paralympic.org/pidas/vista/2011_08_VISTA2011_Booklet.pdf
27. Altmann VC, Groen BE, Keijsers NLW, Hart AL, Vanlandewijck YC. Moving towards evidence based classification in wheelchair rugby: classification of trunk impairment in relation to static sitting balance measures. Retrieved from: http://www.paralympic.org/sites/default/files/document/130424165020623_vista+booklet.pdf
28. Keijsers NLW, Altmann VC, Limbeek J, Groen BE, Vanlandewijck YC. Sprint performance, trunk muscle strength and trunk classification in wheelchair rugby and basketball athletes. Retrieved from: http://www.paralympic.org/sites/default/files/document/130424165020623_vista+booklet.pdf
29. Boswell-Ruys CL, Sturnieks DL, Harvey LA, Sherrington C, Middleton JW, Lord SR. Validity and reliability of assessment tools for measuring unsupported sitting in people with spinal cord injury. Arch Phys Med Rehabil. 2009;90(9):1571–7. doi:10.1016/j.apmr.2009.02.016.
30. Chen CL, Yeung KT, Bih LI, Bih LI, Wang CH, Chen MI, et al. The relationship between sitting stability and functional performance in patients with paraplegia. Arch Phys Med Rehab. 2003;84:1276–81. doi:10.1016/S0003-9993(03)00200-4.
31. Curtis KA, Kindlin CM, Reich KM, White DE. Functional reach in wheelchair users: the effects of trunk and lower extremity stabilization. Arch Phys Med Rehabil. 1995;76(4):360–7.
32. Gauthier C, Gagnon D, Grangeon M, Jacquemin G, Nadeau S, Masani K, et al. Comparison of multidirectional seated postural stability between individuals with spinal cord injury and able-bodied individuals. J Rehabil Med. 2013;45(1):47–54. doi: 10.2340/16501977-1066.
33. Janssen-Potten YJ, Seelen HA, Drukker J, Huson T, Drost MR. The effect of seat tilting on pelvic position, balance control and compensatory postural muscle use in paraplegic subjects. Arch Phys Med Rehabil. 2001;82:1393–1402. doi:10.1053/apmr.2001.25989.
34. Janssen-Potten YJ, Seelen HA, Drukker J, Spaans F, Drost MR. The effect of footrest on sitting balance in paraplegic subjects. Arch Phys Med Rehabil. 2002;83:642–8. doi:10.1053/apmr.2002.32437.
35. Kamper D, Barin K, Parnianpour M, Reger S, Weed H. Preliminary investigation of the lateral postural stability of spinal cord injured individuals subjected to dynamic perturbations. Spinal Cord. 1999;37:40–46.
36. Kamper D, Parnianpour M, Barin K, Adams T, Linden M, Hemami H. Postural stability of wheelchair users exposed to sustained external perturbations. J Rehabil Res Dev. 1999;36:121–32.
37. Potten YJM, Seelen HAM, Drukker J, Reulen JPH, Drost MR. Postural muscle responses in the spinal cord injured persons during forward reaching. Ergonomics. 1999;42(9):1200–15.
38. Seelen HAM, Janssen-Potten YJM, Adam JJ. Motor preparation in postural control in seated spinal cord injured people. Ergonomics. 2001;44(4):457–72.
39. Triolo RJ, Nogan Bailey S, Miller ME, Lombardo LM, Audu ML. Effects of Stimulating Hip and Trunk Muscles on Seated Stability, Posture and Reach after Spinal Cord Injury. Arch Phys Med Rehabil. 2013;94(9):1766–75. Published online Mar 13, 2013. doi:10.1016/j.apmr.2013.02.023.
40. Vanlandewijck YC, Verellen J, Beckman E, Connick M, Tweedy SM. Trunk strength effect on track wheelchair start: implications for classification. Med Sci Sports Exerc. 2011;43(12):2344–51. doi:10.1249/MSS.0b013e318223af14.
41. American Spinal cord Injury Association Impairment Scale. Available from http://www.asia-spinalinjury.org/elearning/ISNCSCI_Exam_Sheet_r4.pdf
42. Janssen-Potten YJ, Seelen HA, Drukker J, Reulen JPH. Chair configuration and balance control in persons with spinal cord injury. Arch Phys Med Rehabil. 2000;81:401–8. doi:10.1053/mr.2000.3859.
43. Vanlandewijck YC, Verellen J, Tweedy S. Towards evidence-based classification in wheelchair sports: impact of seating position on wheelchair acceleration. J Sports Sci. 2011;29(10):1089–96. doi: 10.1080/02640414.2011.576694.
44. Serra-Ano P, Pellicer-Chenoll M, Garcia-Massó X, Brizuela G, Garcia-Lucerga C, González L-M. Sitting balance and limits of stability in persons with paraplegia. Spinal Cord. 2013;51:267–72.
45. French J. On my feet again: My journey out of the wheelchair using neurotechnology. San Francisco USA: Neurotech Press; 2012.
46. Schantz P, Björkman P, Sandberg M. Movement and muscle activity pattern in wheelchair ambulation by persons with para- and tetraplegia. Scand J Rehabil Med. 1999;31(2):67–76.
47. Seelen HAM, Potten YJM, Drukker J, Reulen JPH, Pons C. Development of new muscle synergies in postural control in spinal cord injured subjects. J electromyogr kinesiol. 1998;8:23–34.
48. Liu HY, Rice IM, Laferrier JZ, Cooper R, Boninger M, Cooper R. Sport Wheelchair set up and selection. In: Vicky G-T, editor. Wheelchair Sport. A complete guide for athletes, coaches and teachers. USA: Human Kinetics; 2010. p. 30–45.
49. Bernard PL, Peruchon E, Micallef JP, Hertog C, Rabischong PR. Balance and stabilization capability of paraplegic wheelchair athletes. J Rehabil Res Dev. 1994;31(4):287–96.
50. De Abreu DCC, Takara K, Metring NL, Reis JG, Cliquet A. Interference of different types of seats on postural control system during a forward-reaching task in individuals with paraplegia. Int J Rehabil Res. 2012;35(3):208–13. Doi: 10.1097/MRR.0b013e328353353c.
51. Harel NY, Asselin PK, Fineberg DB Pisano TJ, Bauman WA, Spungen AM. Adaptation of computerized posturography to assess seated balance in persons with spinal cord injury. J Spinal Cord Med. 2013;36(2):127–33. Doi 10.1179/2045772312Y.0000000053.
52. Kerk JK, Clifford PS, Snyder AC, Prieto TE, O'Haggan KP, Schot PK, et al. Effect of an abdominal binder during wheelchair exercise. Med Sci Sports Exerc. 1995;27(6):913–9.
53. Requejo PS, Kerdanyan G, Minkel J, Adkins R, Waters R. Effect of rear suspension and speed on seat forces and head accelerations experienced by manual wheelchair riders with spinal cord injury. J Rehabil Res Dev. 2008;45(7):985–996. doi:10.1682/JRRD.2008.01.0006.
54. Seelen HAM, Vuurman EFPM. Compensatory muscle activity for sitting posture during upper extremity task performance in paraplegic persons. Scand J Rehab Med. 1991;23:89–96.
55. Seelen HAM, Potten YJM, Huson A, Spaans F, Reulen JPH. Impaired balance control in paraplegic subjects. J electromyogr kinesiol. 1997;7(2):149–60.
56. Seelen HAM, Potten YJM, Adam JJ, Drukker J, Spaans F, Huson A. Postural motor programming in paraplegic patients during rehabilitation. Ergonomics. 1998;41(3):302–16.

57. Shin S, Sosnoff JJ. Spinal Cord Injury and time to instability in seated posture. Arch Phys Med Rehab. 2013;94:1615–20. doi:10.1016/j.apmr.2013.02.008.
58. Kilkens OJ, Dallmeier AJ, Nene AV, Post MW, van der Woude LH. The longitudinal relation between physical capacity and wheelchair skill performance during inpatient rehabilitation of people with spinal cord injury. Arch Phys Med Rehabil. 2005;86(8):1575–81. doi: 10.1016/j.apmr.2005.03.020.

8

'Aerobic' and 'Anaerobic' terms used in exercise physiology: a critical terminology reflection

Karim Chamari[1] and Johnny Padulo[2,3*]

Abstract

The purpose of this Current Opinion article is to focus on the appropriate use of the terms 'aerobic'- and 'anaerobic'-exercise in sports medicine, in order to try to unify their use across coaches/athletes and sport scientists. Despite the high quality of most of the investigations, the terms aerobic/anaerobic continue to be used inappropriately by some researchers in exercise science. Until late 2014, for instance, 14,883 and 6,136 articles were cited in PubMed, in the field of 'exercise science', using the words 'aerobic' or 'anaerobic', respectively. In this regard, some authors still misuse these terms. For example, we believe it is wrong to classify an effort as 'anaerobic lactic exercise' when other metabolic pathways are also simultaneously involved. It has extensively been shown that the contribution of the metabolic pathways mainly depends on both exercise intensity and duration. Therefore, it is our intent to further clarify this crucial point and to simplify this terminology for coaches and sports scientists. In this regard, several research articles are discussed in relation to the terminology used to describe the predominant metabolic pathways active at different exercise durations and the oversimplification this introduces. In conclusion, we suggest that sports scientists and field practitioners should use the following terms for *all-out ('maximal')* efforts based on *exercise duration*: (a) 'Explosive Efforts' (duration up to 6 s, with preponderance of the 'phosphagens' metabolic pathway'); (b) 'High Intensity Efforts' (efforts comprised between >6 s and 1 min, with preponderance of the 'glycolytic pathway'), and (c) 'Endurance Intensive Efforts' (for exercise bouts longer than 1 min, with preponderance of the 'oxidative phosphorylation pathway').

Key Points

- Appropriate use of terms 'aerobic' and 'anaerobic' in Exercise Science is discussed.
- Metabolic contributions to exercise cannot be so easily separated or categorized; therefore, it is advisable to remove them when naming physical efforts.
- The *All-out* ('maximal') efforts could be categorized in 'Explosive', 'High-Intensity', or 'Endurance-Intensive' - Efforts based on exercise duration.

Background

Sport science and sport practice on the field are tightly linked. Indeed, researchers are often inspired by sport performance and training facts, while sport practitioners (athletes, coaches, physicians, physiotherapists...) extensively use sport science in their daily practice. Ideally, both sides should use common terms to avoid any misunderstanding that could be translated to, among other things, inappropriate training. In that regard, in 1978, Knuttgen [1] published a pioneering study which proposed the term 'intensity' to describe the hardness with which the exercise is performed or perceived as percentage of the external load. Some 30 years later, a book by Winter and MacLaren [2] highlighted this paradigm using '*maximal-intensity exercise*' to describe the exercise physiology related to aerobic/anaerobic metabolism's contribution to energy supply. In this context, we believe that describing efforts/exercise based on their 'physiological pathway' could lead to mistakes. Indeed, many authors describe short-duration exercise as '*anaerobic*' [3-6] and longer efforts as '*aerobic*' [3-7]. Nevertheless, exercise physiology has evolved during the last decade, and technology has contributed to evolve from Douglas bags in the laboratory to portable gas analyzers in the field to assess cardiorespiratory responses to exercise [8]. Moreover, invasive methods such as muscle biopsies allow for researchers to clarify the kinetics of the aerobic/anaerobic metabolism during exercise [9,10].

* Correspondence: sportcinetic@gmail.com
[2]University e-Campus, Via Isimbardi, 10-22060 Novedrate, CO, Italy
[3]Tunisian Research Laboratory "Sports Performance Optimization", National Center of Medicine and Science in Sports, Tunis, Tunisia
Full list of author information is available at the end of the article

Henceforth, portable and affordable blood lactate analyzers [11] allow the researchers to easily measure lactate (a metabolite of glycolysis) and to assess the extent of 'anaerobic' contribution to exercise, in the field within seconds [12]. Despite that, some recent publications still report nomenclatures that are not up to date [13].

The purpose of the present 'Current Opinion article' is therefore to highlight the errors underlying particular nomenclature. This should help to standardize the terminologies published by scientists across the world. In that regard, the aerobic/anaerobic terminology in sport science (Figure 1) raises some issues for the following reasons:

(a) The term 'anaerobic' is misunderstood - some think it refers to the absence of O_2. The term 'aerobic' also seems implying an absence of any 'anaerobic' contribution.
(b) Metabolic contributions to exercise cannot be so easily separated or categorized.
(c) The intensity of the exercise highly impacts upon the metabolic contribution of the energy pathways; therefore, a clarification should be done in that regard.
(d) Some sport practitioners could have a limited 'physiology background' and, therefore, increases the likelihood of misusing terms and concepts in their field practice.

In recent times, a number of key publications have challenged former concepts resulting in a change in opinions and understandings. For example, Racz et al. (2002) [14] investigated muscle contraction and brought new data to the view-point of muscle contraction as represented by Hill in 1938 [15]. In the same context, a number of recent articles highlighted in this 'Current Opinion Article' have allowed us to 'consider' efforts in a different way than the way they were first described some decades ago.

It is important to note that the 'anaerobic' metabolism is not a pathway that functions in the absence of oxygen but rather it 'does not use oxygen'. The 'anaerobic' metabolism that transforms adenosine triphosphate (ATP) and phosphocreatine (CrP) should therefore not be termed 'anaerobic' but rather 'independent of oxygen' or 'non-mitochondrial' [16]. Thus, instead of calling it the 'anaerobic a-lactic pathway', it should be termed the 'phospagens' pathway'. Likewise, 'glycolysis' should simply replace the 'anaerobic lactic pathway', as again although not directly involved in this pathway, oxygen is still present. For the third metabolic energy pathway, 'oxidative phosphorylation' should replace the term 'aerobic pathway'. Furthermore, at the laboratory, attempts to quantify contributions from anaerobic/aerobic metabolisms are bedevilled by technical and theoretical challenges that have been addressed quite successively by several research groups [7,10,17]. For instance, Medbo et al. (1988) have presented a method to assess anaerobic metabolism capacity [17]. This method, even though being based on sound theory, has been further criticized for the fact that over VO_{2max}, the power/VO_2 relationship is no longer linear [17,18].

Discussion

Very short all-out efforts (lasting less than 1 s to around 6 s) are not only dependent on the phosphagen pathway, but also partially on glycolysis [19,20]. For example, one single 'maximal' 6-s sprint is in fact performed with approximately half the energy originating from 'phosphagens' while the other half is originating from 'glycolytic' pathways [20]. This finding of Gaitanos et al. [20] was published more than 20 years ago, and we believe it is time to take it into account when understanding short 'all-out' efforts. The latter efforts are exercise bouts during which the athlete tries to reach the highest performance possible for the pre-determined effort duration [21]. Therefore, instead of calling these efforts as 'anaerobic a-lactic exercises', they should be called, for example, 'short-term high intensity efforts' or, in a shorter way, 'explosive efforts'. These explosive efforts are performed at power outputs approximately sixfold higher than that of 'maximal aerobic power (MAP; which is discussed in further detail below)' [2]. Moreover, years ago, longer all-out efforts of less than 1-min duration were described as 'anaerobic'; a claim based on (a) a theoretical equation [22] and (b) on the oxygen uptake measured during the first minute of exercise [23]. However, Spencer et al. [21], amongst others, demonstrated mixed anaerobic/aerobic contributions in different exercise durations (from 20 to 234 s) corresponding to racing distances ranging from 200 to 1,500 m. Several authors [6,7] showed that even in very short all-out field and laboratory efforts a significant contribution from 'oxidative phosphorylation' (which is also called 'aerobic metabolism') was also present [16]. In particular, this relative contribution increases further when sprints are repeated [24].

On the field, endurance efforts are often described as 'aerobic'. However, purely aerobic exercise does not exist as long as a minimum of intensity is put into the efforts. In this context, it is incorrect to call the considered 'gold-standard' test used for assessing aerobic capability/ fitness, i.e., 'the maximal oxygen uptake (VO_{2max}) test', an 'aerobic test'. In this regard, recent studies challenge the concept of VO_{2max} after modifications to the test protocol allowed attainment of different VO_{2max} values [25]. Indeed, one of the criteria for the attainment of the VO_{2max} plateau is to reach a minimum value for Lactate of 6 to 9 mmol L^{-1} (depending on the authors and the age of the subjects). This clearly shows a significant participation of 'Glycolysis' prior to the cessation of exercise. This is not surprising, as a maximal effort at the end of a 'VO_{2max} test' occurs at intensities well beyond the second ventilatory threshold (which is also described as respiratory compensation threshold [26]). Therefore, we believe that every exercise should be described for what it is specifically assessing thereby avoiding erroneously describing particular metabolic pathway(s) involved. For instance, to describe an incremental test (VO_{2max}) outcome, one cannot speak of the 'maximal aerobic speed' reached, but of the 'peak speed reached at VO_{2max}' or '*vpeak*VO_{2max}' as justly used by Billat et al. [27].

Moreover, there have been lacks of quantification of the contribution of the anaerobic energy [2] to discriminate percentage of anaerobic versus aerobic metabolism during an effort. To clarify this gap, 40 years ago, Hermansen proposed for the first time an indirect estimation of anaerobic capacity by the '*maximal accumulated oxygen deficit* (MAOD) assessment' based on maximal intensity exercise and gas exchange measures [28]. Several years later, the MAOD method was further experimented by Mebdo et al. [17], even though this method also raises some small methodological issues (mentioned above), it is now possible to estimate anaerobic and aerobic contributions to exercise. In that regard, it has been too often suggested that 'aerobic' metabolism contributes to the provision of exercise energy several seconds/minutes after the start of exercise. However, Granier et al. (1995) showed that for a 30-s *all-out* exercise (Wingate-test, firstly presented as a way of assessing anaerobic capacity [29]), the contribution of this pathway varies from 28% to 45% of total energy production (depending on the profile of the athletes [7]), showing again a misnomer in exercise physiology/testing [2]. Furthermore, during a 400-m *all-out* run of about 52-s, the last 20-s of effort is performed at VO_{2max}, showing that the activation of 'oxidative phosphorylation' is much faster than previously thought [21]. Today, it is accepted that the energy provision for every effort relies on the simultaneous participation of all three energy pathways with a predominant pathway working above the others [21]. Therefore, describing the efforts should not be based on their 'physiological processes', but rather they should be called in accordance to their duration/intensity. More specifically, for 'all-out efforts' (maximal effort for the pre-determined duration), we propose to call

1. 'Explosive Efforts': all-out exercises with a duration of up to 6 s (predominance of 'phosphagens' pathway').
2. 'High Intensity Efforts': all-out efforts lasting from 6 s to 1 min [21] (predominance of the 'glycolytic pathway' in addition to the 'phosphagen's pathway' and 'oxidative phosphorylation'); and finally,
3. 'Endurance Intensive Efforts': exercise with a duration exceeding 1 min (predominance of 'oxidative phosphorylation').

For sub-maximal intensity exercise, other definitions also need to be proposed. In that regard, the paradigm of aerobic and anaerobic metabolism is in need of further research, with both systems complementing each other. In fact, 'aerobic' is often intended as 'uses oxygen', whereas 'anaerobic' as 'does not use oxygen'. That's why any misuse of the terms may lead to misleading concepts and misunderstanding for the readers, and potential mistakes on the field for training prescription. We believe that some other concepts of exercise physiology in *sport science* still need similar clarification, and we encourage expert colleagues to clarify these points in relevant consensus statements. This would help sport and exercise science evolve in the right direction, using

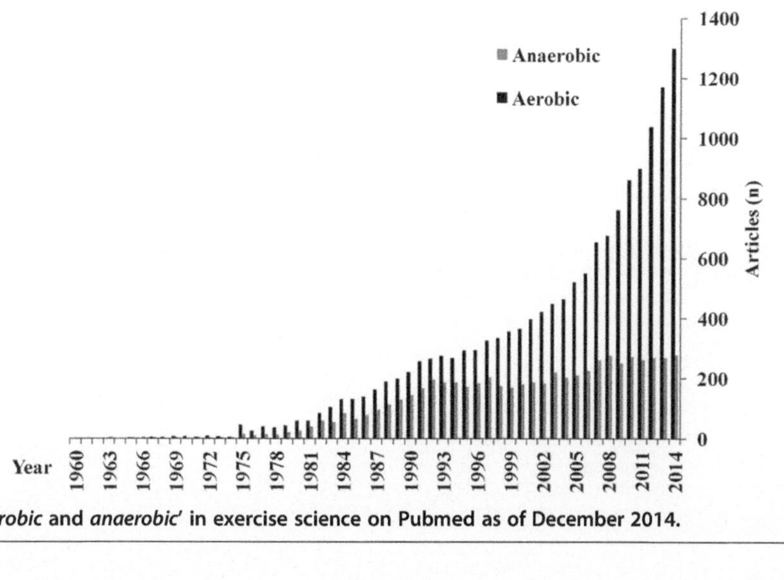

Figure 1 Use of terms *'aerobic* and *anaerobic*' in exercise science on Pubmed as of December 2014.

appropriate terminology that helps scientists, coaches, teachers, and students to speak the same language [30].

Conclusions

In summary, instead of calling an exercise effort anything related to 'aerobic' and/or 'anaerobic' physiological pathways, even if a further research studies might be needed to improve our proposal, we suggest that sports scientists should use the following terms for *all-out* (maximal) efforts based on *exercise duration*:

1. 'Explosive Efforts' (duration up to 6 s)
2. 'High Intensity Efforts' (efforts comprised between >6 s to 1 min)
3. 'Endurance Intensive Efforts' (for exercise bouts longer than 1 min)

Competing interests

The authors declare that they have no competing interests.

Authors' contributions

KC and JP have contributed equally to this manuscript. All authors read and approved the final manuscript.

Acknowledgements

The authors would like to thank Ms *Sabra Hammoudi* and *Gavin Travers* for the language editing of the manuscript.

Author details

[1]Athlete Health and Performance Research Centre, ASPETAR, Qatar Orthopaedic and Sports Medicine Hospital, Doha, Qatar. [2]University e-Campus, Via Isimbardi, 10-22060 Novedrate, CO, Italy. [3]Tunisian Research Laboratory "Sports Performance Optimization", National Center of Medicine and Science in Sports, Tunis, Tunisia.

References

1. Knuttgen HG. Force, work, power, and exercise. Med Sci Sports. 1978;10(3):227–8.
2. Winter EM, MacLaren DP. Assessment of maximal-intensity exercise. In: Eston R, Reilly T, editors. Kinanthropometry and Exercise Physiology Laboratory Manual Volume 2: Physiology (third edition). Routledge: Abingdon; 2009. p. 307–33.
3. Chaouachi A, Coutts AJ, Chamari K, Wong DP, Chaouachi M, Chtara M, et al. Effect of Ramadan intermittent fasting on aerobic and anaerobic performance and perception of fatigue in male elite judo athletes. J Strength Cond Res. 2009;23(9):2702–9.
4. Chtourou H, Hammouda O, Chaouachi A, Chamari K, Souissi N. The effect of time-of-day and Ramadan fasting on anaerobic performances. Int J Sports Med. 2012;33(2):142–7.
5. Rodriguez-Marroyo JA, Garcia-Lopez J, Chamari K, Cordova A, Hue O, Villa JG. The rotor pedaling system improves anaerobic but not aerobic cycling performance in professional cyclists. Eur J Appl Physiol. 2009;106(1):87–94.
6. Billat V, Renoux JC, Pinoteau J, Petit B, Koralsztein JP. Times to exhaustion at 90, 100 and 105% of velocity at VO2 max (maximal aerobic speed) and critical speed in elite long-distance runners. Arch Physiol Biochem. 1995;103(2):129–35.
7. Granier P, Mercier B, Mercier J, Anselme F, Prefaut C. Aerobic and anaerobic contribution to Wingate test performance in sprint and middle-distance runners. Eur J Appl Physiol Occup Physiol. 1995;70(1):58–65.
8. McLaughlin JE, King GA, Howley ET, Bassett Jr DR, Ainsworth BE. Validation of the COSMED K4 b2 portable metabolic system. Int J Sports Med. 2001;22(4):280–4.
9. Bangsbo J, Gollnick PD, Graham TE, Juel C, Kiens B, Mizuno M, et al. Anaerobic energy production and O2 deficit-debt relationship during exhaustive exercise in humans. J Physiol. 1990;422:539–59.
10. Bangsbo J. Oxygen deficit: a measure of the anaerobic energy production during intense exercise? Can J Appl Physiol. 1996;21(5):350–63.
11. Baldari C, Bonavolonta V, Emerenziani GP, Gallotta MC, Silva AJ, Guidetti L. Accuracy, reliability, linearity of Accutrend and Lactate Pro versus EBIO plus analyzer. Eur J Appl Physiol. 2009;107(1):105–11.
12. Hertogh C, Chamari K, Damiani M, Martin R, Hachana Y, Blonc S, et al. Effects of adding a preceding run-up on performance, blood lactate concentration and heart rate during maximal intermittent vertical jumping. J Sports Sci. 2005;23(9):937–42.
13. Wells GD, Selvadurai H, Tein I. Bioenergetic provision of energy for muscular activity. Paediatr Respir Rev. 2009;10(3):83–90.
14. Racz L, Beres S, Hortobagyi T, Tihanyi J. Contraction history affects the in vivo quadriceps torque-velocity relationship in humans. Eur J Appl Physiol. 2002;87(4–5):393–402.
15. Hill AV. The heat of shortening and the dynamic constants of muscle. Proceedings of the Royal Society of London Series B, Biological Sciences. 1938;126:136–95.
16. Baker JS, McCormick MC, Robergs RA. Interaction among skeletal muscle metabolic energy systems during intense exercise. J Nutr Metab. 2010;2010:905612.
17. Medbo JI, Mohn AC, Tabata I, Bahr R, Vaage O, Sejersted OM. Anaerobic capacity determined by maximal accumulated O2 deficit. J Appl Physiol (1985). 1988;64(1):50–60.
18. Chamari K, Chaouachi A, Racinais S. Anaerobic power and capacity. In: P Connes OHaSP, editor. Exercise Physiology: from a Cellular to an Integrative Approach. 2010.
19. Chamari K, Ahmaidi S, Blum JY, Hue O, Temfemo A, Hertogh C, et al. Venous blood lactate increase after vertical jumping in volleyball athletes. Eur J Appl Physiol. 2001;85(1–2):191–4.
20. Gaitanos GC, Williams C, Boobis LH, Brooks S. Human muscle metabolism during intermittent maximal exercise. J Appl Physiol (1985). 1993;75(2):712–9.
21. Spencer MR, Gastin PB. Energy system contribution during 200- to 1500-m running in highly trained athletes. Med Sci Sports Exerc. 2001;33(1):157–62.
22. Hartree W, Hill AV. The anaerobic processes involved in muscular activity. J Physiol. 1923;58(2–3):127–37.
23. Astrand PO, Saltin B. Oxygen uptake during the first minutes of heavy muscular exercise. J Appl Physiol. 1961;16:971–6.
24. Glaister M. Multiple sprint work: physiological responses, mechanisms of fatigue and the influence of aerobic fitness. Sports Med. 2005;35(9):757–77.
25. Beltrami FG, Froyd C, Mauger AR, Metcalfe AJ, Marino F, Noakes TD. Conventional testing methods produce submaximal values of maximum oxygen consumption. Br J Sports Med. 2012;46(1):23–9.
26. Beaver WL, Wasserman K, Whipp BJ. A new method for detecting anaerobic threshold by gas exchange. J Appl Physiol (1985). 1986;60(6):2020–7.
27. Billat VL, Blondel N, Berthoin S. Determination of the velocity associated with the longest time to exhaustion at maximal oxygen uptake. Eur J Appl Physiol Occup Physiol. 1999;80(2):159–61.
28. Hermansen L. Anaerobic energy release. Med Sci Sports Exerc. 1969;1:32–8.
29. Bar-Or O. The Wingate anaerobic test. An update on methodology, reliability and validity. Sports Med. 1987;4(6):381–94.
30. Winter EM, Fowler N. Exercise defined and quantified according to the Systeme International d'Unites. J Sports Sci. 2009;27(5):447–60.

9

Effect of Segment-Body Vibration on Strength Parameters

Ruben Tobias Goebel[1*], Heinz Kleinöder[2], Zengyuan Yue[3], Ranajay Gosh[4] and Joachim Mester[2]

Abstract

Background: In this study, we examine the biomechanical advantage of combining localized vibrations to hamstring muscles involved in a traditional resistance training routine.

Methods: Thirty-six male and female participants with at least 2 years of experience in resistance training were recruited from the German Sport University Cologne. The participants were randomized into two training groups: vibration training group (VG) and traditional training group (TTG). Both groups underwent a 4-week training phase, where each participant worked out at 70 % of the individual 1 repeat maximum (RM—maximum load capacity of a muscle for one lift to fatigue) (4 sets with 12 repetitions each). For participants in the VG group, local vibration was additionally applied directly to hamstring muscles during exercise. A 2-week examination phase preceded the pretests. After the pretests, the subjects underwent a prescribed training for 4 weeks. At the conclusion of the training, a 2-week detraining was imposed and then the study concluded with posttests and retest.

Results: The measured parameters were maximum isometric force of the hamstrings and maximum range of motion and muscle tension at maximum knee angle. The study revealed a significant increase in maximum isometric force in both training groups (VG = 21 %, TTG = 14 %). However, VG groups showed an increase in their range of motion by approximately 2 %. Moreover, the muscle tension at maximum knee angle increased less in VG (approximately 35 %) compared to TG (approximately 46 %).

Conclusions: We conclude that segment-body vibrations applied in resistance training can offer an effective tool to increase maximum isometric force, compared to traditional training. The cause for these findings can be attributed to the additional local vibration stimulus.

Keywords: Segment-body vibration; Strength training; Maximum isometric force; Maximum range of motion; Maximum muscle tension

Key Points

- Maximum isometric force, range of motion, and muscle tension of hamstring muscle were compared between training regimes incorporating localized vibrations and traditional leg curl.
- The vibrational training group showed statistically significant improvements in maximum isometric force after the first week of training compared to 3 weeks for the traditional training regimen.
- The vibrational training group retained gain in performance for a longer time after the testing regimen than traditional training.
- The range of motion was improved, and muscle tension increase was less for the vibrational training group compared to the traditional training group.

Background

Resistance training is considered as the bedrock for improving neuromuscular performance for both athletic and preventive health [1–7]. Over the recent past, establishing additional training protocols over a traditional resistance training routine has been a key focus of sports and conditioning experts [8–11]. In this paper, we specifically focus on enhancement through vibration

* Correspondence: ruben.goebel@qu.edu.qa
[1]Sport Science Program, Qatar University, P.O. Box 2713, Doha, Qatar
Full list of author information is available at the end of the article

training method which has recently emerged as an effective and convenient technique in improving neuromuscular performance especially when combined with a strength training program. Underscoring this trend, whole-body vibration, which is easy to administer through a vibrating platform, has gained tremendous popularity over the last decade for neuromuscular improvements [12–14]. For instance, it was found that when whole-body vibrations were induced through the feet using a vibrating platform into resistance training individuals, maximum isometric force of the corresponding muscle group improved between 6.5 % and approximately 40 % (for example, see [15, 16]). Two effects are believed to be the primary reasons for the increase of maximum force of vibration training compared to traditional training. First, Martin and Park [17] and Mester et al. [18] found that reflectory muscle contractions take place during the vibration stimulus. The sensitivity of muscle spindles increases during vibration training, and their effects on the stretch-shortening cycle are acute responses of the skeleton muscles to vibration training. It is assumed that consequently the reaction time and the threshold to create an action potential are decreased [19 21]. Park and Martin [22] identified an increase of muscle strength in hand flexor muscles while introducing segment-body vibrations to the tendons of the same muscles. Second, Eklund and Hagbarth [23] showed the antagonistic muscle relaxation during vibration, which improves motor coordination between agonist and antagonist [17]. As a consequence, the synchronization of neuronal activity between the muscles was improved, which resulted in increased maximum force [24, 25]. Rehn et al. [20] showed in their rating of 19 studies " [...] that there is strong to moderate evidence that long-term whole body vibrations can have positive effects regarding leg muscular performance" ([20], p. 4–5). It is furthermore reported that muscle tension (MT) increases after a traditional resistance training program [26]. No publication in English language could be identified to correlate muscle tension and vibration training.

In contrast to whole-body vibration, which only indirectly influences the training muscle groups, direct stimulation of a specific muscle group can be a good alternative candidate due to specificity and greater control. Only few studies examined the effect of vibration training called segment-body vibration on muscle strength and athletic performance [27]. These studies have reported an increase of the maximum force between 5 and 50 % (e.g., [24, 28, 29]). Therefore, the present study examined the effects of a special local vibration training, in which local segment-body vibrations were directly induced into the belly of the hamstring muscles in comparison to an identical training regime without vibrations. Both maximum isometric force and maximum flexibility as well as MT of the trained muscles were measured following a predefined period and regimen of training. Approved by the Ethics-Committee of the German Sport Univeristy Cologne.

Methods

In the present intervention study, the leg flexor muscles were strengthened unilaterally. A total of 36 healthy subjects with at least 2 years' experience in resistance training were selected for the study and randomized into a vibration training group (VG) and traditional training group (TTG). Note that no special prescriptions on diet and other behavioral activities were imposed for this study on any of the subjects. Additional informed consent was obtained from all patients for whom identifying information is included in this article. All procedures followed were in accordance with the ethical standards of the responsible committee on human experimentation (institutional and national) and with the Helsinki Declaration of 1975, as revised in 2008 [5].

The matched-pair technique [30] has been applied after the sixth pretest measurement to establish the two training groups. This technique assigned eight female subjects (44 %) to the VG and six female subjects (33 %) to the TTG. Both study groups performed the same exercise (leg curl) for the hamstrings on the right leg only. The setup of the leg curl machine in combination with the vibration generator physically only allowed superimposed vibrations during exercise of the right leg. The leg curl was performed on a lying leg curl machine (Gym 80, Signum Standart line, International Products, Gelsenkirchen, Germany [31]) with a standardized deadweight of 320 kg and a serially standardized weight stack of 85 kg. The weight stack did not limit the training load of any of the subjects. In addition to the regular resistance training machine, vibration was administered using a Medic Swing vibration generator (Mechatronic, Hamm, Germany). The device was convex and could be adjusted in height and angle, which allows its usage for local vibrations of lower body segments. Before participation, all subjects were fully informed of the purpose, experimental procedures, possible risks, and their rights and gave their written consent to participate.

Variables and Statistics

The comparative performance metric for the current experiment was set to the following variables: isometric force, maximum range of motion (ROM), and maximum MT. The reliability of the measurements was measured beforehand in a test-retest design with 12 test persons during the pretests. The results of the test-retest scenario are as follows: isometric force $r = 0.75$, ROM $r = 0.79$, and MT $r = 0.69$ where r describes the correlation coefficient. Means and standard deviations were calculated by ANOVA with repeated measurements. Differences were tested with the Tukey post hoc test. Moreover, the different values between pre- and posttests were examined by dependent *t* test as well. The progression from pretest to retest (six measurements) within the two study groups was also recorded. Finally, the 1-Pearson correlation as a measure of similarity between the time course of the individual changes has been calculated at VG and TTG to present the means of maximum isometric force development from pretest to retest. Ward's cluster algorithm has been applied at VG and TTG to present individual cases [32]. Sociometrical and anthropometrical data for this experiment are displayed in Table 1.

Testing

During the 2 weeks of pretesting phase, each subject additionally performed six measurements of all variables in order to exclude adaptations due to the familiarization of the testing protocol by the subjects. These test results are not part of the pretest. The actual pretest was performed prior to the first training with a rest interval of 72 h before the first session of training commenced. First, second, and third measurements and posttest have been performed after each training week with at least 24 h rest after the last training session. After 2 weeks of detraining, the same tests were repeated during the retest to measure changes in performance. Note that during this phase of testing, no vibrations were provided to the VG.

The maximum isometric force of the leg flexors was measured using a leg curl machine (Gym 80 International, Gelsenkirchen, Germany), which was equipped with a force sensor (Mechatronic) (see Fig. 1, right part). The sample rate of the force sensor was 100 Hz, and the accuracy of measurement was 0.01 N. The time frame, during which the force was recorded, covered 5 s. Subjects took a facedown position during the measurement. The inner knee angle during measurements was 160° (see Fig. 1, left part).

In order to determine the range of motion of the knee joint, the following novel setup has been applied considering the anatomical structures of the knee joint. To the best of our knowledge, no references record this setup. Subjects lay on their backs with the counter-lateral knee

Table 1 Sociometrical and anthropometrical data of the subjects in study 1 ($\bar{x}$ = mean, s_x = standard deviation)

	Females (n = 14)		Males (n = 22)	
	$\bar{x}$	s_x	$\bar{x}$	s_x
Age (years)	23.9	3.2	23.3	2.6
Height (cm)	165.6	8.9	188.7	8.2
Mass (kg)	63.0	3.7	83.5	6.9

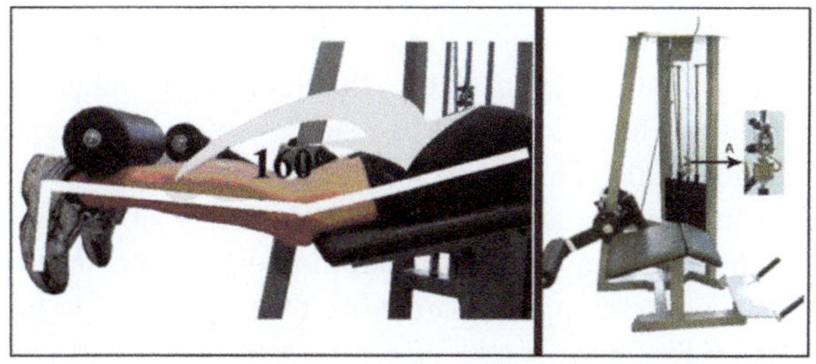

Fig. 1 Measurement of maximum isometric force. *Left*: measurement position; *right*: leg curl machine with force sensor

protruding over the edge of the bench. This leg was fixed with a belt (see Fig. 2b) to avoid evasive movement of the hip joint. The leg to be studied was brought to maximum flexion in the hip joint (hip angle β; see Fig. 2). The two-joint hamstring muscles (m. semitendinosus, m. semimembranosus, m. biceps femoris (caput longum)) were fixed in their final position at the hip joint (see Fig. 2a). The hip angle β was measured taking the horizontal plane and the distal end of the condylus lateralis as reference points and trochanter major as pivot point. The maximum hip angle β of the pretest is re-established during all following measurements and therefore standardized the measurement. While the hip joint angle is fixed, subjects used a cable winch to bring the leg to be studied into a stretching position. Consequently, the hamstring muscles experience an extension. The distal end of the condylus lateralis, the trochanter major of the hip joint, and the malleolus lateralis of the ankle form the reference points for the knee angle α (see Fig. 2). The measurement accuracy of the goniometer was 1°. Angles were recorded after 3 s in the maximum joint angle. The maximum knee angle was self-determined by the subjects and defined as a position which the volunteer felt discomfort, but no pain. The

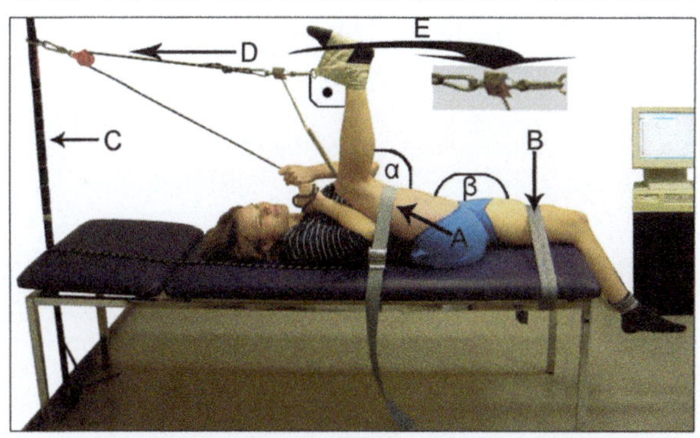

Fig. 2 Measurement station and measurement procedure of muscle tension. *A*: fixation of the leg to be tested, *B*: fixation of the counter-lateral leg, *C*: adjustment pole, *D*: direction of traction, *E*: force sensor, target angle *α*, hip angle *β*, 90° between lower leg and cable winch

knee angle α of the pretest served as reference value for the muscle tension and therefore was established in all following measurements. After this standard value was achieved, subjects are asked to reach their maximum possible knee angle. This novel setup to measure the ROM of the knee joint to determine the extensibility of the hamstring muscles was applied to eliminate the pain that occurs while stretching the hamstring muscles with full knee extension [33–36].

While stretching the hamstrings, the muscle tension was measured using a force sensor (Mechatronic), which was located between the cable winch and foot loop. The force sensor and the lower leg of the subject were in a rectangular position. The force was recorded over a period of 5 s. The effect of gravity and the weight of the leg were eliminated from the maximum value measured in Newton. The following formula was used to calculate the actual muscle tension (the symbols explained in Table 2):

$$\text{Muscle Tension} = \frac{F1 * L + f * L * \cos(\alpha + \beta)}{\delta}.$$

Training

Both study groups performed the same exercise (leg curl) for the hamstrings on the right leg only. The subjects executed 4 training sets of 12 repetitions with 90 s pause between sets for all individuals of both groups. A total of three training sessions per week was carried out for a total of 4 weeks. The resistance progression was tracked using repeated measurements of the maximum isometric force as the test progressed. The VG group, in addition to the abovementioned protocol, also underwent vibrational loading on their hamstring. For the test persons in VG, the vibration area was placed directly on the center of the hamstrings (Fig. 3, right part). This device worked with a constant amplitude of 4 mm and allows a variable frequency between 18 and 38 Hz. Only the VG group trained with additional segment-body vibrations. Table 3 describes and summarizes in greater detail the training parameters for hamstring strengthening in both groups.

The initial training load was determined at the end of the pretest phase, applying a test procedure previously described in detail [37]. The relative resistance was kept at 70 % of 1 RM for the whole training period in order to maintain a training load recommended for hypertrophy in resistance training [37, 38]. Consequently, the effective training load was adjusted according to the weekly measured maximum isometric force of the subject.

The resistance training followed a 5-min general warm-up procedure for both groups which included 3 min of treadmill running at 8 km/h, stretching of quadriceps and hamstring muscles (twice holding each stretch for 15 s alternating between each leg), and jumping exercises, which included skipping (6 m), two foot ankle hops (6 reps), and split squat jump (5 reps) [39].

Results and Discussion

Maximum Isometric Force

The progression of the mean maximum isometric force (in percent) over the duration of the study is plotted in Fig. 4. The mean of the pretest values for both groups was normalized to 100 %. The force (*F*) values of 10.22 in the VG and 8.19 in the TTG became significant in the one-way ANOVA with repeated measurements. Thus, both interventions, i.e., strengthening with and without vibration, produced a significant increase on maximum force. However, more useful information could be gleaned using the post hoc test (Tukey) which provides information about the effects of the training time on maximum force.

Next, we studied at the *t* test for dependent samples for the changes in the groups from pretest to posttest (see Table 4). Both training groups showed significant changes between pretest and posttest. The mean maximum isometric force in the VG was 523 N in the pretest and 636 N in the posttest. For the TTG, the values were 567 N (pretest) and 648 N (posttest), respectively.

Table 2 Explanation of the parts of the formula used to convert the measured muscle tension into the actual muscle tension and their units

F1	Measured muscle tension in Newton (N)
L	Length of lower leg in centimeters (cm)
f	Weight of lower leg in Newton[a] (N)
α	Knee angle in degrees (°)
β	Hip angle in degrees (°)
δ	Lever arm of force (60) = 0.035 m

[a]According to Leva (1996), with reference to studies by Zatsiorsky V and Seluyanov V [62], the percentage of the lower leg relative to the total body mass is 4.33 % in females and 4.81 % in males. The appraisal of the weight of the lower leg was based on these data

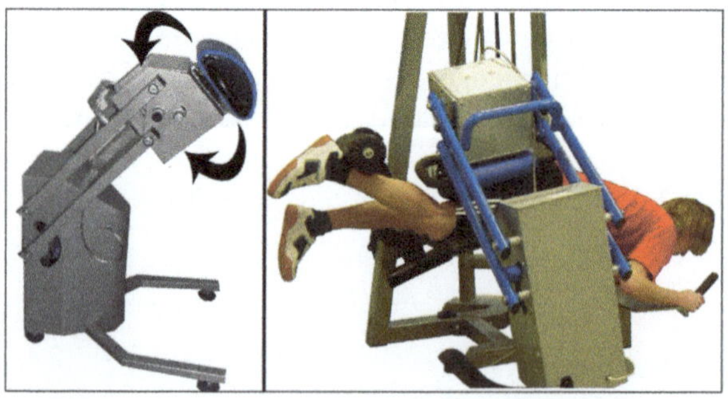

Fig. 3 *Left*: vibration trainer Medic Swing (Mechatronic). *Right*: vibration training of the hamstrings

Table 3 Training parameters

Hamstring training	
Training load	4 series, 12 repetitions; with 70 % 1 RM for each arm
Pause	90 s between series
Training sessions per week	3
Training period	4 weeks
Hamstring training with additional vibration	
Frequency	18, 24, 30, and 36 Hz (1st, 2nd, 3rd, and 4th training week)
Amplitude	4 mm

Results for Maximum Knee Angle

The variance analyses only revealed one significant F value (2.69) for the VG. The value calculated for the TTG (1.53) was not significant. Based on this result, we can assume that vibration-supported maximal strength training has an impact on the maximum knee angle. For the TTG, neither time of measurement nor training stimuli influenced the development of the maximum knee angle significantly.

The Tukey post hoc test for the VG showed that the development of maximum ROM shows only one significant difference. Thus, we can conclude that a vibration training of the hamstrings only has a limited impact on the maximum flexibility of the same musculature. The following t test for dependent samples provides more information about the development of the maximum knee angle over the duration of the training period (see Table 5).

Maximum Muscle Tension

Figure 5 illustrates the course of the mean muscle tension (MT) at maximum knee angle over the duration of the study. The conclusion we can draw from the significant F values for both groups ($F = 8.1$ for the VG; $F = 6.91$ for the TTG) is that maximal strength training with

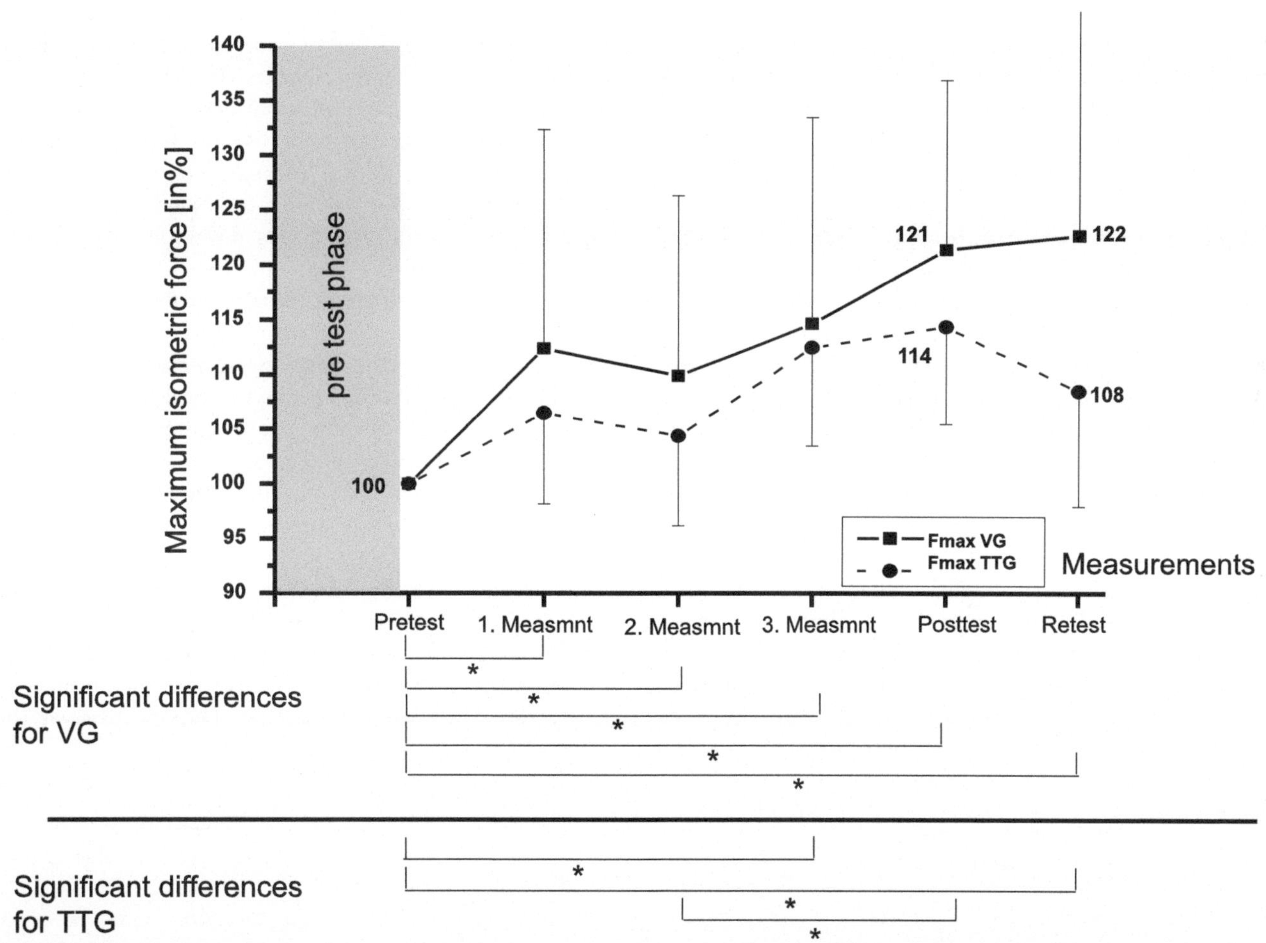

Fig. 4 Development of maximum isometric force (Fmax) in VG and TTG (Tukey post hoc test). Significant differences ($\alpha = 5$ %) between mean values of measurements were marked with an *asterisk*

Table 4 Result of the *t* test for dependent samples for VG and TTG with increases of isometric maximum force

	MV	SD	Number	Diff	SoD	*t*	*df*	*p*	Fmax increase in %
VG pretest	523	193							21.4
VG posttest	635	196	18	−112	69	6.84	17	<0.05	
TTG pretest	567	194							14.2
TTG posttest	648	218	17	−81	57	4.89	16	<0.05	

MV mean value, *SD* standard deviation, *Diff* difference, *SoD* standard deviation of differences, *t* t value, *df* degrees of freedom, *p* probability, two-sided

and without vibration influences the maximum ROM and maximum MT of the trained musculature. The Tukey post hoc test showed that the increase of MT in the posttest differed significantly from all previous measurements of VG. This is also true for the retest values of VG when compared to all other measurements except for the pretest. Similarly, we cannot assess any changes in MT for the TTG's first 3 weeks of training (i.e., the pretest period). Statistically significant differences were measured between the pretest, first and third measurements, and posttest. These changes indicate an increase in MT at maximum knee angle. Finally, a significant decrease in MT can be ascertained between posttest and retest. The significant changes from the post hoc analysis were illustrated in Fig. 5. The subsequent *t* test for dependent samples showed the changes in both groups from pretest to posttest (see Table 6).

Conclusions

These results, on maximum isometric force illustrated in Fig. 4, indicated significant variations over the whole training period. The results indicate that the maximum isometric force of the VG increased significantly from the pretest value even after the first training week. Thereafter, compared to the pretest, all the following measurements became significant. This can be contrasted with the TTG which achieved statistically relevant maximal force improvements only between the last three measurements and the pretest. Furthermore, the first significant difference in TTG is between the second measurement and posttest. This indicates that—in comparison to the VG—the improvement of maximum force occurred at a later time in the TTG. A possible reason for the faster response can be explained by an acute increase of training intensity through superimposed segment-body vibrations in VG [22]. The resulting higher load on the neuromuscular system in VG explained by the reflectory response forced by the vibration stimulus [18] may have caused a faster neuromuscular adaptation in VG compared to TTG.

The *t* test (Table 4) shows that the mean increases in maximum force of 21.4 % (VG) and 14.2 % (TTG) were significant. A possible cause for this higher improvement rate of the VG likely stems from the additional vibration stimulus. In order to work out the practical relevance of this study, a cluster analysis was performed, and the results are summarized in Figs. 6 and 7. As a result, three groups (see Fig. 6, right) with distinct development levels became visible. The different courses of the mean values of all groups [1–3] are presented in Fig. 6 (right). For group A (four subjects), an initial decrease in maximum isometric force after the first week of training was observed. From the second measurement onwards, the maximum force value steadily increased compared to the posttest. In contrast to this development, group B (five subjects) showed a steady increase of the maximum force from pretest to retest. Finally, group C (nine subjects) experienced an initial steep increase in maximum force compared to the first measurement, which was subsequently followed by stagnation until the posttest.

The results for TTG subjects are plotted in Fig. 7 (left) with the dividing line at 0.9. Similar to VG subjects, TTG subjects were split up into three observational groups. The mean values for group A (two subjects) revealed an initial increase in maximum isometric force until the values dropped below the initial level in the post- and the retest. The slope of group B (four subjects) first showed a decrease in maximum isometric force to the second measurement. Afterwards, the maximum isometric force increased until it reached the peak at the

Table 5 Result of the *t* test for dependent samples for the VG and TTG with increases in maximum knee angle (ROM)

	MV	SD	Number	Diff	SoD	*t*	*df*	*p*	Increase in max. ROM %
VG pretest	114	11							
VG posttest	116	11	18	−2	4	2.38	17	<0.05	2
TTG pretest	116	19							
TTG posttest	119	17	17	−3	6	2.01	16	n.s.	

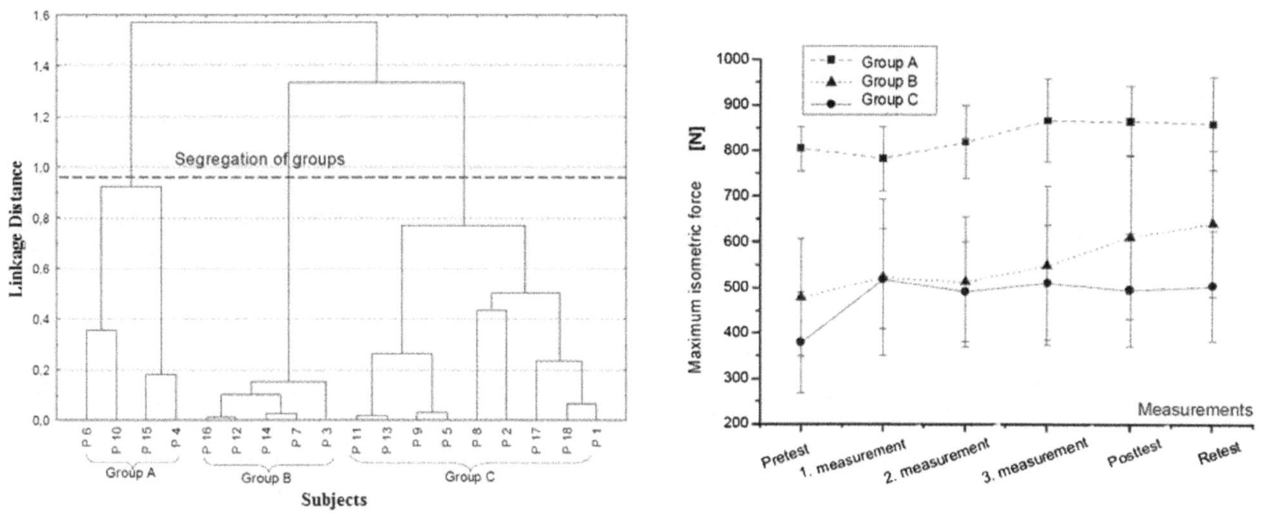

Fig. 5 Development of maximum MT (muscle tension) of VG and TTG and results of the Tukey post hoc test. Significant differences ($\alpha = 5$ %) between mean values of measurement are marked with an *asterisk*

posttest. Similar to group B of the VG, group C of the TTG (12 subjects) showed a continuously increasing maximum isometric force until the posttest. In summary, superimposed vibration during a submaximal resistance training on individuals with a comparably high strength level in hamstring muscles can initially decrease isometric force. A possible reason for this development is to be found in the higher absolute load of this training group, which might have caused an initial musculoskeletal overtraining to muscles, bones, and joints of the subjects [40]. In contrast, the same training method applied to individuals with a comparably average or lower strength level leads to an increase of isometric force after three training units. The effect of vibration training lasts also after 2 weeks of detraining for individuals of all entry levels. In comparison, a traditional submaximal strength training improves isometric force initially but reveals a potential loss of isometric force for comparably well-trained individuals after the third training week. Those results have to be treated with care, because the subjects have not been distributed equally in numbers to the groups A–C. The cluster analysis gives an overview about possible inter-individual different adaptations to a submaximal resistance training with and without superimposed segment-body vibrations. Further studies have to reveal the physiological reasons behind those differences.

Finally, the increase of maximum isometric force after 2 weeks of detraining at the retest remains significant at 22 % for the VG. Those results are in accordance with other findings [41–43], although little is known about the effects of segment vibration training on the magnitude and rate of strength loss during detraining. In contrast, the TTG significantly decreases the maximum isometric force during the same time period by 6 %. It is possible that the cause of the sustainability of the isometric maximum force level in VG can be found in the higher training intensity through the superimposed vibrations, and therefore a different regeneration time compared to the TTG of this population. It can be assumed that a change in isometric force manifested either earlier or later to the retest. Future studies should provide evidence for the effects of different detraining phases of vibration training. With regard to the maximum knee angle, from Table 5, a significant change from pretest to posttest can be noticed in the VG. Maximal strength training with induced vibration causes a higher increase in maximum ROM than traditional

Table 6 Results of the *t* test for dependent samples for VG and TTG with increases in MT

	MV	SD	Number	Diff	SoD	*t*	*df*	*p*	Increase in MT in %
VG pretest	1205	606							34.3
VG posttest	1618	603	18	−413	394	4.45	17	<0.05	
TTG pretest	1156	681							46.0
TTG posttest	1688	864	17	−532	442	4.96	16	<0.05	

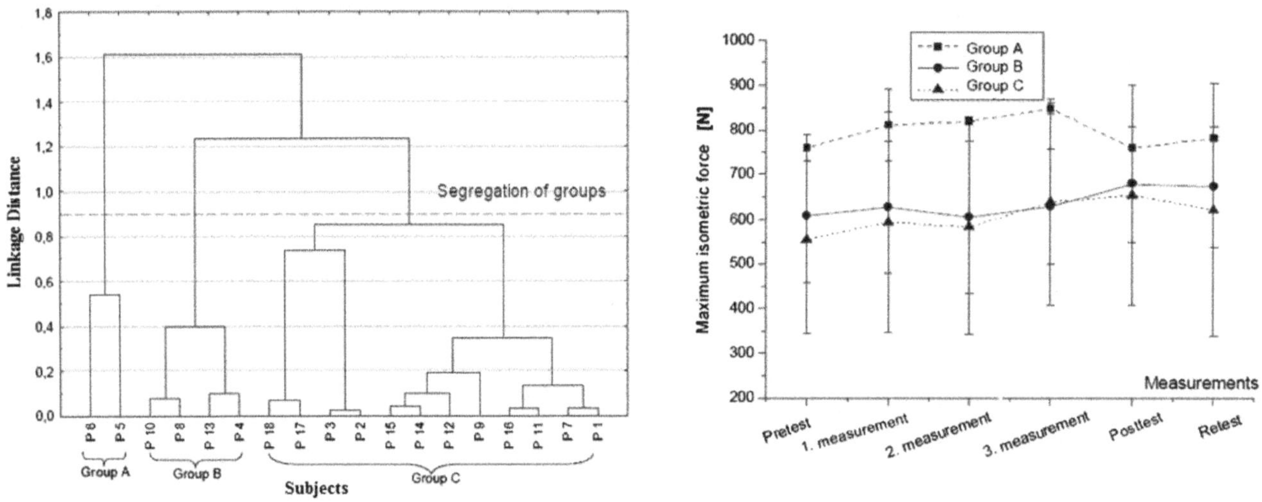

Fig. 6 *Left*: tree diagram of Ward's cluster analysis. Representation of groups of subjects (groups A, B, C) with similar maximum isometric force development from pre-retest of VG—group segregation after cluster analysis. *Abscissa* lists the subjects; *ordinate* shows the 1-Pearson correlation coefficient value (*r*) [31]. *Segregation line* was set at linkage distance 0.95. *Right*: presentation of mean maximum isometric force development of the three groups

resistance training. However, the statistically relevant increase in the range of motion of 2 % plays a minor role in sports practice. Finally, for the maximum muscle tension, the data from Table 6 shows that the significant difference between pretest and posttest values becomes obvious in both groups. The mean increases in MT at maximum knee angle in VG (34.3 %) and TTG (46.0 %) were significant. This study reveals that a maximal strength training of the hamstrings brings about a significant increase of MT of this musculature.

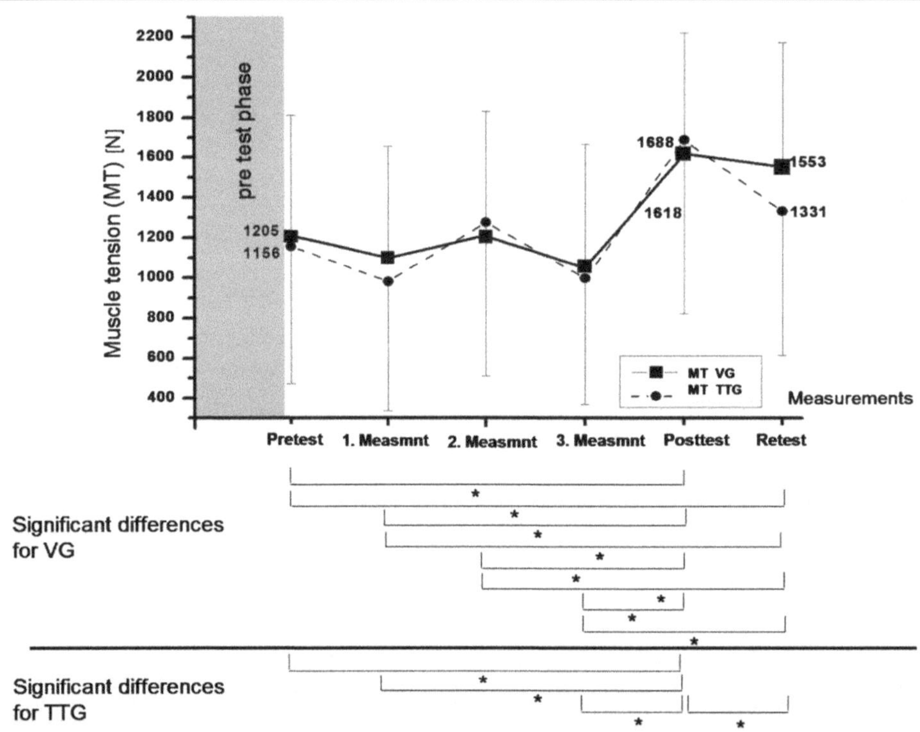

Fig. 7 *Left*: tree diagram of Ward's cluster analysis. Representation of groups of subjects (groups A, B, C) with similar maximum isometric force development from pre-retest of TTG—group segregation after cluster analysis. *Abscissa* lists the subjects; *ordinate* shows the 1-Pearson correlation coefficient value (*r*) [31]. *Segregation line* was set at linkage distance 0.9. *Right*: presentation of mean maximum isometric force development of the three groups

These results thus indicate that dynamic strength training with additional local vibration stimulation represents an effective means to an increase of maximum isometric force of the hamstrings. In the VG, 21.4 % (112 N) of maximum isometric force was gained from pretest to posttest in contrast to 14.2 % (81 N) in the TTG. This vast increase of the VG is consistent with results reported in different sources (e.g., [44]; Knauf 1999, unpublished). Single cases with additional vibration stimulation show even higher increases between 13 % and 60 % of this parameter (e.g., [45, 16]). Clearly, the additional local vibration stimulus can be considered to be the reason for the much higher increase of maximum isometric force compared to the TTG. The fact that the vibrations are induced directly into the target muscle ensures that the generated amplitude and frequency reached the trained muscle without major transmission loss [46]. Moreover, since the frequency in the present study ranged between 18 and 36 Hz, a harmonic reflectory response of the involved muscles seems plausible [17] as well as a substantial relaxation of the antagonist [23]. Another explanation for the higher force development can be attributed to the reflectory contractions which lead to higher muscular activity [18]. In combination with submaximal loads (e.g., 70 % of the 1 RM), this causes an increase in force in the stimulated muscles [17] and a synchronization of muscular activity [24, 25].

Another important finding of this study was the long-term effects due to vibration training. In the retest, the maximum isometric force of the VG was still 22.7 % higher than at the time of the pretest (Römpke 2004 unpublished, [41]). In contrast to this, maximum isometric force of the TTG was 4 % lower in the retest than in the pretest. Since the training load was comparable in both groups, the increased intensity, which results from the additionally induced segment-body vibrations, obviously triggers a memory effect in the nerve-muscle system. The cluster analysis illustrated differences in the development of maximum isometric force between vibration training and traditional strengthening. Subjects of VG with high maximum force values in the pretest experience an initial decrease before they reach their late maximum in the retest. In contrast to this, the maximum force of the hamstrings of the subjects with high force values within TTG increased remarkably already after the first week of training. Another difference within TTG was the considerable decrease in the last week of training below the pretest value. Subjects with a low maximum isometric force showed an increase of this parameter within the first week of training (VG) and subsequently stagnated until the posttest, whereas the TTG revealed a continuous increase until the posttest. Obviously, the weaker athletes have difficulties coping with the vibration training stimulus. In the VG, the maximum knee angle increased significantly 2 % (2°) from pretest to posttest. The results of the TTG are almost identical (2.5 %, 3°). As a consequence, there were no better results produced using the additional vibration input. Among other factors, submaximal strength training generally improves recruitment, frequency (e.g., [47–49]), and synchronization of muscles and muscle groups. If the relaxation potential of the hamstrings can be thus enhanced, we can assume that the maximum range of motion increases. For the purpose of this study, the development of flexibility was of great importance. By means of repeated measurement, Mall et al. [50] were able to prove an increase in range of motion of 3.4°. Likewise, a study by Wydra et al. [51] showed an increase in passive range of motion of 8° within 2 weeks time. In this study, the tested leg performed a total number of 12 muscle stretches with a small improvement of 2°–2.5°. So the main reason for changes in maximum knee angle in this study can be found in the total number of 6 measurements during the whole study. MT at maximum knee angle also developed similarly in both training groups. MT remained almost unaltered from pretest until the third measurement, but increased afterwards. The increase increment of 34.3 % in the VG and 46.0 % in the TTG between pretest and posttest became significant in the *t* test. Since the maximum range of motion does not increase considerably between the third measurement and posttest, the development of MT must have a different cause. Submaximal strength training leads to both neuronal and structural adaptation processes in the musculature [52]. One of the results of muscle hypertrophy is an increase in parallel or serial sarcomere number, and thus an increase in the number of titin-myosin-complex filaments in the musculature which are part of every sarcomere [53]. The effects are supposedly related to an activation of more titin-myosin-complex filaments within one muscle (-group) which themselves increase the maximum MT [53]. As the maximum isometric force increases from the pretest to every measurement that follows and the MT increases after the third measurement, it is safe to assume that the process of muscle hypertrophy (consequently the changes in muscle structure) occurs following after the second training week. Since the time of the increase in MT is the same in both groups, it is also safe to assume that muscle hypertrophy occurs independently of the different training stimuli.

To the best of our knowledge, this is the first study to explore the effects of segment muscle vibrations superimposed to the muscle belly of the agonist muscle. The findings demonstrated that segment-body vibrations may improve muscle coordination, increasing the activation of the agonist muscle, resulting in an increase of maximum force. Therefore, we conclude that initially, the neuronal adaptations to submaximal strength training lead to an increase in maximum isometric force, but not to a significant increase in MT before the third measurement. This method thus offers to athletes a short-term increment of maximum force, which has the potential to improve overall performance in force-dependent sports. Resistance training in sports already covers a significant part of the training schedule. The application of segment muscle vibration in the present study increases the quality of the resistance training by achieving the same effects with segment muscle vibrations in shorter training time or achieving a higher isometric muscle force in the same training time. Moreover, evidence of positive effects of the application of whole-body vibrations in rehabilitations has been reported. Vibration training has been successfully applied in the rehabilitation process of anterior cross-ligament injuries [54–56], in treatment of knee ostearthritis [57], in rehabilitation of spina bifida [58], etc. In contrast, no evidence can be found that supports the use of vibration training in the rehabilitation process of stroke patients [59]. Those above rehabilitation applications are based on whole-body vibration. To the best of our knowledge, no studies about segment-body vibrations and rehabilitation exist. It is to be assumed that similar and more specific effects in rehabilitation can be achieved with segment-body vibrations. The role of muscle tension in static and dynamic force development is still under investigation. Force measurement under isometric conditions is influenced by muscle properties and neural factors [60]. The key limitation brought about due to lack of a control group can be alleviated if more studies are conducted, which include a control group and EMG. This can further reveal the role of muscle tension and would be the subject of future research. We will also like to point out another limitation of the study which stems from the fact that the bilateral effects of two different training methods of the two arms have not been controlled. It is known that unilateral resistance training of the elbow flexor muscles of the non-dominant arm of a test person can have a significant increase of isometric maximum force of 5.3 % at the contralateral elbow flexor muscles [61]. Thus, in summary, we conclude that segment-body vibrations applied in resistance training can offer an effective tool to increase maximum isometric force, compared to traditional training. Thus, as the training quality improves, higher benchmarks can be realized in the same period of training time compared to regular strength straining. The results of this study show the practical application of training method which is superior to traditional training by 7 % compared to traditional training.

Competing interests

The authors declare that they have no competing interests.

Authors' Contributions

RG is the main and corresponding author of this publication. He carried out the studies on the effects of segment-body vibrations on resistance training parameters of the hamstring muscles. He made substantial contribution in all areas of the published study, such as conception, design, data acquisition, analysis, and interpretation. Furthermore, he drafted and finalized the manuscript. HK contributed substantially to the concept of the study and the study design. He conceptualized the training intervention protocol and the measurement protocol. He furthermore has been involved in revising the manuscript critically for important intellectual content. ZY contributed specifically in data acquisition, statistical analysis, and result presentation. In particular, he developed the mathematical formula to calculate the muscle tension. RG has been involved in drafting and critically revising the manuscript's content and participated in the sequence alignment. JM conceived the study, supervised and coordinated the study, and helped to draft the manuscript. All authors read and approved the final manuscript.

Authors' Information

Dr. RG is the Acting Director of the Sport Science Program, College of Arts and Sciences, Qatar University, Doha, Qatar. Dr. HK is the Head of Strength Diagnostics and Motion Analysis in the Institute of Training Sciences and Sport Informatics, German Sport University Cologne, Cologne, Germany. Dr. ZY is from The German Research Center, Center of Elite Sport, Cologne, Germany. Dr. RG is an associate research scientist in Mechanical and Industrial Engineering, Northeastern University, Boston, MA, USA. Univ.-Prof. JM is the Director of the Institute of Training Sciences and Sport Informatics, German Sport University Cologne, Cologne, Germany, and the Chairman of The German Research Center, Center of Elite Sport, Cologne, Germany.

Acknowledgements

This report was made possible by a NPRP award NPRP 05-086-2-031 from the Qatar National Research Fund (a member of The Qatar Foundation). The statements made herein are solely the responsibility of the authors.

Author details

[1]Sport Science Program, Qatar University, P.O. Box 2713, Doha, Qatar. [2]Institute of Training Science and Sport Informatics, German Sport University Cologne, Cologne, Germany. [3]The German Research Center, Center of Elite Sport, German Sport University Cologne, Cologne, Germany. [4]Department of Mechanical and Industrial Engineering, Northeastern University, Boston, MA, USA.

References

1. Veliz RR, Requena B, Suarez-Arrones L, Newton RU, de Villarreal ES. Effects of 18-week in-season heavy-resistance and power training on throwing velocity, strength, jumping, and maximal sprint swim performance of elite male water polo players. J Strength Cond Res. 2014;28(4):1007–14.
2. Fleck SJ, Kraemer W. Designing resistance training programs, 4th ed. Human Kinetics. 2014.
3. Deschenes MR, Judelson DA, Kraemer WJ, Meskaitis VJ, Volek JS, Nindl BC, et al. Effects of resistance training on neuromuscular junction morphology. Muscle Nerve. 2000;23(10):1576–81.
4. Behm DG. Neuromuscular implications and applications of resistance training. J Strength Cond Res. 1995;9(4):264–74.
5. Winett RA, Carpinelli RN. Potential health-related benefits of resistance training. Prev Med. 2001;33(5):503–13.
6. Braith RW, Kerry JS. Resistance exercise training its role in the prevention of cardiovascular disease. Circulation. 2006;113(22):2642–50.
7. Harries SK, Lubans DR, Callister R. Resistance training to improve power and sports performance in adolescent athletes: a systematic review and meta-analysis. J Sci Med Sport. 2012;15(6):532–40.
8. Anagnostakou V, Chatzimichail K, Dimopoulos S, Karatzanos E, Papazachou O, Tasoulis A, et al. Effects of interval cycle training with or without strength training on vascular reactivity in heart failure patients. J Card Fail. 2011;17(7):585–91.
9. Sharp CPM, Pearson DR. Amino acid supplements and recovery from high-intensity resistance training. J Strength Cond Res. 2010;24(4):1125–30.

10. Katsura Y, Takahiro Y, Shin-Ya U, Tatsuya U, Daisuke S, Hayato N, et al. Effects of aquatic exercise training using water-resistance equipment in elderly. Eur J Appl Physiol. 2010;108(5):957–64.
11. Artero EG, Espada-Fuentes JC, Argüelles-Cienfuegos J, Román A, Gómez-López PJ, Gutiérrez A. Effects of whole-body vibration and resistance training on knee extensors muscular performance. Eur J Appl Physiol. 2012;112(4):1371–8.
12. Jones MT. Progressive-overload whole-body vibration training as part of periodized, off-season strength training in trained women athletes. J Strength Cond Res. 2014;28(9):2461–9.
13. Preatoni E, Colombo A, Verga M, Galvani C, Faina M, Rodano R, et al. The effects of whole-body vibration in isolation or combined with strength training in female athletes. J Strength Cond Res. 2012;26(9):2495–506.
14. Roelants M, Verschueren SM, Delecluse C, Levin O, Stijnen V. Whole body-vibration-induced increase in leg muscle activity during different squat exercises. J Strength Cond Res. 2006;20(1):124–9.
15. Berschin G, Schmiedeberg I, Sommer HM. Zum Einsatz von Vibrationskrafttraining als spezifisches Schnellkrafttrainingsmittel in Sportspielen. Leistungssport. 2003;4:11–22.
16. Spitzenpfeil P. Vibrationsbelastungen im alpinen Skilauf. Diss: Deutsche Sporthochschule Köln; 2000.
17. Martin BJ, Park HS. Analysis of the tonic vibration reflex: influence of vibration variables on motor unit synchronisation and fatigue. Eur J Appl Physiol. 1997;75:504–11.
18. Mester J, Spitzenpfeil P, Yue Z. Vibration loads: potential for strength and power development. In: Komi PV, editor. Strength and power in sport. Oxford: Blackwell Scientific; 2003. p. 488–501.
19. Cardinale M, Bosco C. The use of vibration as an exercise intervention. Exerc Sport Sci Rev. 2003;31:3–7.
20. Rehn BB, Lidström JJ, Skoglund JJ, Lindström BB. Effects on leg muscular performance from whole-body vibration exercise: a systematic review. Scandinavian J Med & Sci In Sports. 2007;17(1):2–11.
21. Martínez Sánchez F, Rubio J, Ramos D, Esteban P, Mendizábal S, Jiménez F. Effects of 6 week whole body vibration training on the reflex response of the ankle muscles: a randomized controlled trial. Intern J Sports Physical Therapy [serial online]. 2013;8(1):15–24.
22. Park HS, Martin BJ. Contribution of the tonic vibration reflex to muscle stress and muscle fatigue. Scan J Work Environment and Health. 1993;19:35–42.
23. Eklund G, Hagbarth KE. Normal variability of tonic vibration reflexes in man. Exp Neurol. 1966;16:80–92.
24. Bosco C, Colli R, Introni E, Cardinale M, Tsarpela O, Madella A, et al. Adaptive responses of human skeletal muscle to vibration exposure. J Clin Physiol. 1999;19:183–7.
25. Lippold OCJ, Redfearn JWT, Vuco J. The rhythmical activity of groups of motor units in the voluntary contraction of muscles. Physiol Rev. 1957;137:473–87.
26. Erskine RM, Jones DA, Williams AG, Stewart CE, Degens H. Resistance training increases in vivo quadriceps femoris muscle specific tension in young men. Acta Physiol. 2010;199(1):83–9.
27. Scheibe W, Schwarzlose H. Mechanische Schwingungen. In: Rohmert W, Rutenfranz J, editors. Praktische Arbeitsphysiologie. Stuttgart, New York: Thieme; 1983. p. 258–97.
28. Becerra-Motta, Becker R. Die Wirksamkeit der biomechanischen Stimulation (BMS) in Verbindung mit traditionellen Methoden der Kraftausdauerentwicklung im Schwimmsport. Leistungssport. 2001;2:29–35.
29. Issurin VB, Liebermann DG, Tenenbaum G. Effect of vibratory stimulation training on maximal force and flexibility. J Sport Sci. 1994;12:561–6.
30. Thomas JR, Nelson JK, Silverman SJ. Research methods in physical activity. 6th ed. Champaign, IL: Human Kinetics; 2011.
31. GYM 80. GYM 80 International - products. 2015. http://www.gym80.de/pages/de/sygnum_standards_detail.php?line=2&pid=7. Accessed January 2nd 2015.
32. Tabachnik BG, Fidell LS. Using multivariate statistics. 6th ed. Boston: Pearson Education; 2013.
33. Law RYW, Harvey LA, Nicholas MK, Tonkin L, De Sousa M, Finniss DG. Stretch exercises increase tolerance to stretch in patients with chronic musculoskeletal pain: a randomized controlled trial. Phys Ther. 2009;89(10):1016–26.
34. Magnusson SP, Aagaard P, Simonsen EB, Bojsen-Moller F. Biomechanical evaluation of cyclic and static stretch in human skeletal muscle. Int J Sports Med. 1998;19:310–6.
35. Marshall PWM, Cashman A, Cheema BS. A randomized controlled trial for the effect of passive stretching on measures of hamstring extensibility, passive stiffness, strength, and stretch tolerance. J Sci Med Sport. 2011;14(6):535–40.
36. Ylinen J, Kankainen T, Kautiainen H, Rezasoltani A, Kuukkanen T, Häkkinen A. Effects of stretching on hamstring muscle compliance. J Rehabil Med. 2009;41(1):1937–44.
37. Baechle T, Earle R. Essentials of strength training and conditioning. 3rd ed. Champaign, IL: Human Kinetics; 2008.
38. Kenney W, Wilmore J. Physiology of sport and exercise. 5th ed. Champaign, IL: Human Kinetics; 2012.
39. Sotiropoulos K, Smilios I, Christou M, Barzouka K, Spaias A, Douda H, et al. Effects of warm-up on vertical jump performance and muscle electrical activity using half-squats at low and moderate intensity. J Sports Sci & Med. 2010;9(2):326–31.
40. Figoni SF, Morse M, Hedrick B. Sports overtraining. Sports 'N Spokes Magazine. 2005;31(2):41–2.
41. Goebel RT, Kleinöder H, Mester J. Effects of local body vibrations on the triceps brachii on maximal force of the biceps brachii. J Sport Sci Health. 2012;13 Supplement 1:86.
42. Hakkinen K, Alen M, Kallinen M, Newton RU, Kraemer WJ. Neuromuscular adaptation during prolonged strength training, detraining and re-strength-training in middle-aged and elderly people. Eur J Appl Physiol. 2000;83:51–62.
43. Ivey FM, Tracy BL, Lemmer JT, Nessaiver M, Metter EJ, Fozard JL, et al. Effects of strength training and detraining on muscle quality: age and gender comparisons. J Gerontol A Biol Sci Med Sci. 2000;55:B152–7. discussion B158-159.
44. Becerra L, Becerra M, Becker R. Die biomechanische Stimulation beim Muskeltraining. Leistungsport. 2002;5:38–43.
45. Weber R. Muskelstimulation durch vibration. Leistungssport. 1997;1:53–6.
46. Yue Z, Kleinöder H, Mester J. A model analysis of the effects of wobbling mass on whole-body vibration. Europ J of Sport Sci. 2001;1(1):1–19.
47. Rabita G, Perot C, Lensel-Corbeil G. Differential effect of knee extension isometric training on the different muscles of the quadriceps femoris in humans. Europ J Applied Physiol. 2000;83:531–8.
48. Häkkinen A, Häkkinen K, Hannonen P, Alen M. Strength training induced adaptations in neuromuscular function of premenopausal women with fibromyalgia: comparison with healthy women. Ann Rheum Dis. 2001;60:21–6.
49. Rutherford OM, Purcell C, Newham DJ. The human force: velocity relationship; activity in the knee flexor and extensor muscles before and after eccentric practise. Eur J of Appl Physiol. 2001;84:133–40.
50. Mall NN, Mall T, Sharma SN. Comparative effectiveness of static stretching and PNF stretching for improving hip joint flexibility. Snipes J. 1984;7:14–20.
51. Wydra G, Bös K, Karisch G. Zur Effektivität verschiedener Dehntechniken. Dtsch Zs Sportmed. 1991;42(9):386–400.
52. MacDougal JD. Hypertrophy and hyperplasia. In: Komi PV, editor. Strength and Power in Sport. Oxford: Blackwell Scientific; 2003. p. 252–64.
53. Wiemann K, Klee A, Startmann M. Filamentäre Quellen der Muskel-Ruhespannung und die Behandlung muskulärer Dysbalancen. Dtsch Zs Sportmed. 1998;4:111–8.
54. Fu CLA, Yung SHP, Law KYB, Leung KHH, Lui PYP, Siu HK, et al. The effect of early whole-body vibration therapy on neuromuscular control after anterior cruciate ligament reconstruction a randomized controlled trial. Am J Sports Med. 2013;41(4):804–14.
55. Moezy A, Olyaei G, Hadian M, Razi M, Faghihzadeh S. A comparative study of whole body vibration training and conventional training on knee proprioception and postural stability after anterior cruciate ligament reconstruction. Br J Sports Med. 2008;42(5):373–85.
56. Berschin G, Sommer B, Behrens A, Sommer H. Whole body vibration exercise protocol versus a standard exercise protocol after ACL reconstruction: a clinical randomized controlled trial with short term follow-up. J Sports Sci Med. 2014;13(3):580–9.
57. Wang P, Yang X, Yang Y, Yang L, Zhou Y, Liu C, Reinhardt JD, He C. Effects of whole body vibration on pain, stiffness and physical functions in patients with knee osteoarthritis: A systematic review and meta-analysis Clin Rehabil 0269215514564895, first published on December 18, 2014 doi:10.1177/026921551456489.
58. Stark C, Hoyer-Kuhn HK, Semler O, Hoebing L, Duran I, Cremer R, Schoenau E. Neuromuscular training based on whole body vibration in children with spina bifida: a retrospective analysis of a new physiotherapy treatment program. Childs Nerv Syst. 2015;31:301–9.

59. Ling-Rong L, Meizhen H, Lam FH, Pang MC. Effects of whole-body vibration therapy on body functions and structures, activity, and participation post-stroke: a systematic review. Phys Ther. 2014;94(9):1232–51.
60. Đorđević S, Tomažič S, Narici M, Pišot R, Meglič A. *In-vivo* measurement of muscle tension: dynamic properties of the MC sensor during isometric muscle contraction. Sensors. 2014;14(9):17848–63. doi:10.3390/s140917848.
61. Hubal MJ, Gordish-Dressman HEATHER, Thompson PD, Price TB, Hoffman EP, Angelopoulos TJ, et al. Variability in muscle size and strength gain after unilateral resistance training. Med Sci Sports Exerc. 2005;37(6):964–72.
62. Zatsiorsky V, Seluyanov V, The mass Inertia Characteristics of the Main Segment of the Human Body. Matsui, H. & Kobayashi, K. (Ed.): Biomechanics (1983). VIII-B, 1152-1159.

10

Single parent status and children's objectively measured level of physical activity

John Singhammer[1*], Mathias Ried-Larsen[2], Niels Christian Møller[2], Peter Lund-Kristensen[2], Karsten Froberg[2] and Lars Bo Andersen[2]

Abstract

Background: Single-parent family status has been investigated as a possible psychosocial determinant of children's level of physical activity (PA)—although with mixed and inconclusive results. Prevailing evidence of the importance of two-parent family status as a resource for children's PA is based on a mix of subjective and objective measurements of PA.

Objectives: To investigate if the level of PA among children living with a single parent was lower compared to children living with two parents by means of a meta-analysis of published and unpublished studies. We restricted our analysis to studies with objective measurements of PA.

Methods: Data sources: The databases, Social Science Citation Index, PsycINFO, PubMed, and EBSCO were searched (1987–2013).

Study eligibility criteria: Observational studies comparing objectively measured PA between single-parent children and children from two-parent families.

Study appraisal and synthesis methods: We used guidelines from the *Cochrane Handbook of Systematic Reviews of Interventions* and a modified version of the Newcastle–Ottawa Scale overall to assess the quality of the included studies. We refrained from calculation of summary scores.

Results: Twelve studies met the following inclusion criteria of which six were unpublished: (a) child age (6–18 years) and (b) objectively measured level of PA. Meta-analysis revealed pooled estimates of −0.01 for boys (95 % CI −0.04–0.03, $p = 0.77$, $I^2 = 6.5$ %, $p = 0.38$) and 0.01 for girls (95 % CI −0.03–0.04, $p = 0.62$, $I^2 = 21.0$ %, $p = 0.24$), respectively. Estimates show no differences in objectively measured physical activity between children living in single-parent families compared to children living with two parents. Analyses investigating seven potential moderators did not yield any statistical significant effect size estimates. No evidence of heterogeneity between studies was observed.

Limitations: Retrieved articles were assessed by several of the authors. Blinding of the authors was not feasible, as most of the authors have been involved in the studies.

Conclusions: No evidence was found suggesting that children of single-parent families are in special need of extraordinary measures to facilitate their level of PA.

Keywords: Physical activity; Children; Adolescents; Family status; Meta-analysis

* Correspondence: josi@via.dk
[1]Department of Physiotherapy, VIA University College, Hedeager 2, DK8200 Aarhus, Denmark
Full list of author information is available at the end of the article

Key points

- Single-parent family status has been investigated as a possible determinant of children's physical activity. The available studies that have used accelerometer-based measurements of physical activity are diverse and generally of poor quality.
- Pooled estimates show no differences in objectively measured physical activity between children living in single-parent families compared to children living with two parents.
- There is no evidence to conclude that children of single-parent families are in special need of extraordinary measures to facilitate their level of physical activity.

Background

Children's level of physical activity (PA) declines from adolescence [1] and remains low throughout adulthood for many individuals [2], thereby increasing the risk for later cardio-metabolic diseases (CMD) [3]. It has been suggested that children with single-parent family status (SPFS) are less physically active compared to children from dual-parent households [4, 5]. Studies investigating the association between family status and children's PA are based on the hypothesis that children living with a single parent have less access to the beneficial entities of parental influence (e.g., role modeling and support) compared to children living in a two-parent home [4, 6–8]. However, past reviews have reported mixed findings, with some scholars reporting no evidence of an association between SPFS and children's PA [9] and others reporting inconclusive findings [6]. With one out of every fourth child living with one parent in Europe and USA (24 and 25 %, respectively) [10, 11], SPFS may be an important factor that contributes to increased CMD risks through a low level of PA. An understanding of the social and contextual factors that influence PA is an important prerequisite for the design and implementation of PA-promoting interventions, and the association between SPFS and children's PA has been of interest to scholars for decades [9, 6, 12, 13].

However, the methods used to evaluate the evidence of an association between SPFS and children's level of PA may be flawed. For example, the vote-counting method used by Van der Horst et al. [13] and Sallis et al. [9] is based on the evaluation of (1) the number of studies included in their reviews, (2) the presence of a statistically significant association, and (3) consistency of the direction of the association in some, but not all of the included studies. One caveat of this approach is the lack of a quantification of the magnitude of evidence in terms of an overall effect size, which also takes the sample size of the included studies into account. As information of an overall effect size and the relative weight of each study included in the review (e.g., in terms of sample size) is not included in the study by Van der Horst et al. [13], the premise behind the reported conclusion is not transparent. More seriously, conclusions are based on a mixture of studies that measure children's PA either objectively (e.g., by accelerometers) or subjectively by self-report. It has been argued that self-reported PA is vulnerable to culturally different interpretations, and hence, that the validity and reliability of objective measures of PA is superior to subjective measures [14]. Thus, comparison across studies that measures PA differently increases the possibility for misclassification of the outcome, which in turn may bias any estimate of an overall association between SPFS and children's PA. Furthermore, conclusions on the SPFS-PA association do not include unpublished studies, which may otherwise change the bulk of available knowledge that is used to reach conclusions. The present study addresses these caveats by restricting the assessment of the SPFS-PA to studies that measure children's PA objectively. Our overall objective was to investigate if the level of PA among children living with a single parent was lower compared to children living with two parents by means of a meta-analysis of results from published studies and from six studies that have not been published before. In line with the overall majority of studies investigating the association between SPFS and children's PA, we report gender-separated results.

Methods

We included cross-sectional studies and prospective observational studies with information on the level of PA for children, separately, by single- versus two-parent families. Inclusion criteria were studies comparing objectively measured PA between single-parent children and children from two-parent families. We explicitly choose studies that measured PA with accelerometers. Exclusion criteria were as follows: lacking information on parental status, insufficient information to calculate an effect size, self-reported PA estimates or cardio-respiratory fitness as the outcome measure (e.g., VO_{2max}), and sedentary behavior or inactivity as the outcome measure. A protocol of this review was not registered prior to commencement.

The literature search was performed from March to November 2013. The literature search was limited to 1987 as studies using accelerometers for obtaining measures of PA conducted before 1987 are rare [15]. Participants were restricted to children aged 6 to 18 years, stratified by family status (single- versus two-parent families). In studies with estimates separated by age groups within family status, estimates were calculated separately for each group and combined to a single estimate as the number of studies available permitting calculation of age-separate effect size estimates were too low.

Outcome

Objectively measured levels of PA were compared between children of single- and those of two-parent families and were either reported in tabular form or in the text.

Search Strategy

The following electronic databases were searched: Social Sciences Citation Index [16], PsycINFO, PsycArticles, Journals OVID Full Text [17], Medline [18], and EBSCO [19], including the databases SportDiscus, CINAHL, Academic Search Premier, and ERIC. The following search terms were used: Physical activity, Accelerometry, Parents OR Family, Relations, Marital OR Status, Children OR Adolescents. The search term "psychosocial" was used with Journals OVID Full Text. Search terms including Boolean phrases were entered both separately and in combination. All terms were treated as separate blocks and were finally entered simultaneously using the separator AND. Duplicates across databases were identified with the EndNote software (version X4.0.2). The reference lists of primary studies and reviews identified from the literature search were scanned for other relevant studies. Searches were limited to studies published in English, Danish, Swedish, or Norwegian. This process revealed 16 studies suitable for investigating the association between SPFS and PA. Fourteen authors of these studies were contacted by email for information on unpublished studies, details of sampling methodology, sample size and attrition, and for further information necessary to compute effect sizes.

Unpublished Studies

Raw data from the European Youth Heart Study (EYHS) from Denmark (1997 and 2003), Estonia (EYHS 1997), Portugal (EYHS 1997), and Norway (EYHS 1997) were available to the authors of the present study and were included for calculation of an overall effect size. Methods for the EYHS studies are reported elsewhere [20, 21].

Unpublished data from the Copenhagen School Child Intervention Study (CoSCIS) [22,23] were also available and included in the present analysis. A description of the methods, including sample size and measures of PA, are reported elsewhere [23].

Information on children's PA, parental status, and mothers' educational level was used for children aged from 9 to 15 years between 1997 and 1999 from the EYHS (1997, Denmark, Estonia, Portugal, and Norway $n = 4515$) and for 9-year-old children included in the Danish arm of the EYHS study in 2003 ($n = 419$) (Table 1). From CoSCIS, an analysis was conducted on 419 children with information on their level of PA and SPFS. Study protocols for the EYHS and CoSCIS studies conformed to international guidelines on biomedical research and were approved by the ethical board of University of Southern Denmark. The Danish Data Inspectorate approved the studies. The studies are conducted in accordance with the World Medical Association Declaration of Helsinki. Written informed consent was obtained from the children's parent or legal guardian.

Data Extraction

Forty-eight retrieved articles were independently assessed by two authors (JS and MRL). Of these, 12 studies (of which six were unpublished) were selected for further assessment. Blinding of the authors was not feasible, as most of the authors have been involved in the unpublished studies. We extracted the following characteristics: methods (study design, sampling strategy, sample size, location, publication status), participants (recruitment, gender, age, proportion of SPFS), and outcome (accelerometer model used, number of days measured, cut-point used to define level of measurement, percentage respondents with valid measurements). Any discrepancies were resolved with mutual agreement among reviewers.

Assessing Risk of Bias

Prior to assessment, consensus was reached among all authors about the criteria for assessing risk of bias. We used the guidelines from the *Cochrane Handbook of Systematic Reviews of Interventions* [24] and the Newcastle–Ottawa Scale [25], although some criteria had to be modified for the specific topic. We assessed risk of bias by the following criteria: Selection (potential selection bias due to non-response, ascertainment of exposure), Comparability (adjustment for potential confounding factors (e.g., parental age and parental socioeconomic status)), and Outcome (incomplete outcome data with less than 75 % of the study sample, information on number of days assessing participant's PA with accelerometers, length of epoch specified by the authors, and the cut-points used to define moderate to vigorous physical activity (MVPA)). The first author (JS) assessed the full text of the included studies and discussed the assessment with the other authors. Disagreement was resolved by consensus. Quality assessment was completed before data extraction was started. Currently, no evidence-based algorithm exists to quantify and evaluate the quality of the studies, and we refrained from calculation of summary scores that are often used to weight the studies in a later meta-analysis [24]. Hence, the quality of the included studies rest on our subjective assessment, and this may introduce selection bias to the meta-analysis. Therefore, all studies were used for analysis, irrespective of the quality assessment.

Analyses

We used meta-analysis to calculate pooled gender-separated random effect size from all 12 studies. Effect size estimates were calculated for studies with detailed information on measurement of SPFS [5, 8, 20, 26] and

Table 1 Characteristic of studies included in the meta-analysis

Studies	*n*	Response rate (%)	Sampling strategy	Age	Percentage of single-parent families (%)	Publication status
Bagley et al. [27]	1215	35	STRS	7 and 11	13	Published
Bradley et al. [28]	1364	28	I/N	9	I/N	Published
Hesketh et al. [5]	2458	40	SRS	6 and 11	16	Published
Sallis et al. [30]	200	66	STRS	6 to 18	I/N	Published
Sallis et al. [29]	732	53	RA	10	22	Published
Sallis et al. [9]	297	40	I/N	9	13	Published
CoSCIS, Eiberg Hansen et al. [22]	411	52	CS	9	18	Unpublished
Riddoch et al. [20], EYHS Denmark, first cohort	1019	75	CRS	12	20	Unpublished
McMinn et al. [26], EYHS Denmark, second cohort	419	65	CRS	9	22	Unpublished
EYHS Estonia	1122	76	CRS	13	24	Unpublished
Riddoch et al. [20], EYHS Norway	754	75	CRS	12	21	Unpublished
Riddoch et al. [20], EYHS Portugal	1168	73	CRS	13	20	Unpublished
Total (%)	11,159	53	–	–	19	–

SRS simple random sample, *STRS* stratified random sample, *RA* random allocation as part of an intervention, *CS* convenience sample, *CRS* cluster randomized sample, *I/N* insufficient or no information

for studies with adjustment for potential confounders [27, 28, 5, 8, 29]. Effect sizes were calculated for studies that assessed participant's PA for at least 4 days [27, 28, 5, 23, 26, 20, 8], studies that obtained estimates of PA based on a 1-min epoch length [27, 28, 5, 26, 20, 22], studies that defined MVPA as 2000 counts.min^{-1} and above [26, 20], studies with valid outcome data of 75 % or more of the study sample [27, 28, 5, 26, 29], and unpublished studies [23, 26, 20]. We present pooled estimates expressed as Fisher's *z*, which represents the direction and magnitude of the relation between SPFS and PA level. A positive effect size reflects a higher level of PA among children from single-parent families, compared to children from two-parent families. Calculation of the study-specific effect sizes was based on Pearson's correlation coefficients or derivative statistics and sample sizes in three studies [8, 30, 29], *p* values and sample sizes in two studies [28, 5], and mean differences, standard deviations, and sample sizes in seven studies [20, 23, 27, 26]. Heterogeneity across the studies was evaluated with Higgins' I^2 statistics at an alpha level of 0.05.

We investigated for potential influence of bias on the pooled estimate by aspects of the study quality criteria. More specifically, we explored if our pooled estimates were influenced by the exclusion of studies with insufficient information on measurement of SPFS, studies that failed to control for potential confounders, studies with accelerometer data limited to less than 4 days, studies that used an epoch length of more than 1 min, studies based on a range of less than 2000 counts.min^{-1}, studies with less than 75 % valid outcome data, and published data. This procedure is similar to a sensitivity analysis.

The percentage of respondents from single-parent families was calculated. Coding and descriptive analysis were conducted using the statistical software Stata (version 12.1) [31]. Calculation of effect size for each individual study, pooled estimates, and estimates of heterogeneity across studies was carried out using the software Comprehensive Meta Analysis (version 2.2.064) [32].

Ethics

The manuscript does not contain clinical studies or patient data.

Results

The literature search revealed 250 published and six unpublished studies (Fig. 1). Of these, 48 studies were carefully inspected and references were obtained and assessed for inclusion. Twelve studies fulfilled the inclusion criteria of which six were unpublished (overall sample size = 11.159 children) (Table 1). Details of the 36 studies excluded and the reasons for exclusion are provided in Additional file 1. Of the 14 study authors contacted, two replied that they did not analyze their data separately by family status, as such measures were not obtained. One author no longer had access to the original data. The remaining authors did not respond.

Cross-sectional designs were used in all of the studies, except for the studies by Bradley et al. [28] and by Sallis et al. [29] who reported results from prospective cohort studies. The majority of the studies utilized some form

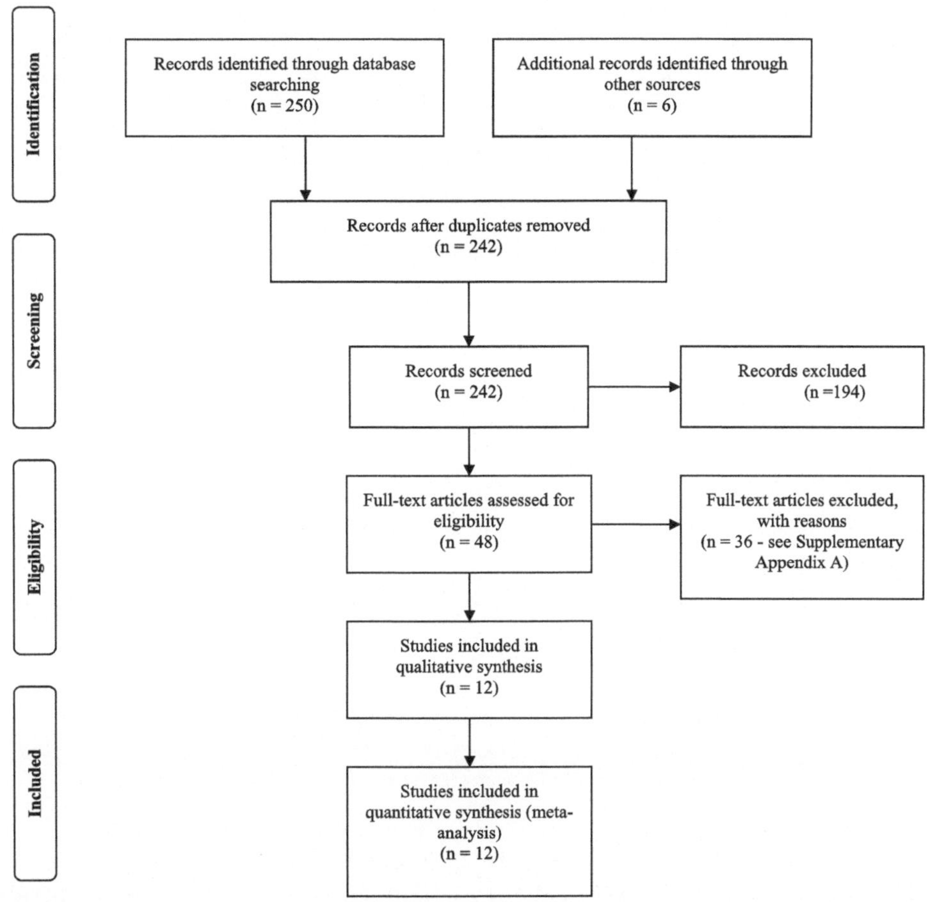

Fig. 1 PRISMA flow diagram

of random allocation of study subjects. The CoSCIS study was based on a convenience sample [22]. Sallis et al. [30] did not report the sampling strategy, and information on the sampling strategy was insufficiently reported by Bradley et al. [28]. The age of the study participants ranged from 6 to 18 years. The percentage of children from single-parent families ranged from 13 to 24 %, and two studies did not report the percentage of children from single-parent families [8, 28]. Six studies were conducted in Europe [20, 22, 26], four in North America [30, 28, 8, 29], and two in Australia [27, 5]. The studies were conducted in community or school settings with primarily Caucasian samples. Measures of reliability were reported in five studies [30, 8, 28, 22, 29].

Assessment of Risk of Bias

Overall, the quality of the studies differed considerably (Table 2). The response rate for the studies varied from 28 to 76 % (Table 1), and no study formally tested if respondents differed from non-respondents in terms of demographic factors. Seven studies provided information about how SPFS were measured [5, 8, 20] (Table 2). Estimates of PA, adjusted for potential confounding factors were provided in six studies [27, 28, 5, 30, 29, 8]. The number of days that accelerometer data were obtained varied considerably between the 12 included studies, but two studies used accelerometer data obtained for only 2 days [29, 30] (Table 3). Nine studies obtained estimates of PA based on a 1-min epoch [27, 28, 5, 26, 20, 22]. One study used counts.hour^{-1} to estimate PA [29], and two other studies by the same author did not report the epoch periods used to define PA [30, 8]. Definition of MVPA differed across studies. Four studies transformed accelerometer data to MET scores using the algorithm by Freedson et al. [33], and three studies defined MVPA as an activity occurring in the accelerometer range of 1017–3696 counts.min^{-1} [27, 28, 5]. Sallis et al. [30] used a PA level corresponding to six METS in one study and used the mean total counts as the outcome in two other studies [8, 29]. One study defined MVPA as an activity occurring of more than 1951 counts.min^{-1} [23] while the five studies from the EYHS defined MVPA as an activity occurring at 2000 or more counts.min^{-1} [26, 20] (Table 3). Valid accelerometer data was available for at least 75 % of the study sample in five studies [27, 28, 5, 29, 20].

Table 2 Assessment of study quality

Studies	Where results biased due to low response rate?	Was the exposure ascertained throughout?	Did authors adjust for confounding factors?	Was there valid outcome data for at least 75 % of the study sample?	Did authors report the number of days of PA assessment?	Did authors report the length of epoch?
Bagley et al. [27]	-	?	+	+	+	+
Bradley et al. [28]	-	?	+	+	+	+
Hesketh et al. [5]	-	+	+	+	+	+
Sallis et al. [30]	-	+	+	-	+	-
Sallis et al. [29]	-	-	+	+	+	+
Sallis et.al. [8]	?	?	+	-	+	-
Eiberg Hansen et al. [22] CoSCIS	-	?	-	-	+	+
Riddoch et al. [20], EYHS Denmark, first cohort	?	+	-	-	+	+
McMinn et al. [26], EYHS Denmark, second cohort	-	+	-	+	+	+
Riddoch et al. [20], EYHS Estonia	?	+	-	-	+	+
Riddoch et al. [20], EYHS Norway	?	+	-	-	+	+
Riddoch et al. [20], EYHS Portugal	?	+	-	-	+	+

"+" adequate information provided for assessment; "-" inadequate information provided for assessment; "?" no information provided

Effect Sizes

Pooled estimates for all 12 studies were −0.01 for boys (95 % CI −0.04–0.03, $p = 0.77$, $I^2 = 6.5$ %, $p = 0.38$) and 0.01 for girls (95 % CI −0.03–0.04, $p = 0.62$, $I^2 = 21.0$ %, $p = 0.24$), respectively, where a positive effect size (Fisher's *z*) favors single-parent status.

In an analysis of the seven studies with detailed information on measurement of SPFS, an effect size (Fisher's *z*) of −0.02 was observed among boys (95 % CI −0.06–0.02, $p = 0.35$, $I^2 = 0$ %, $p = 0.55$), and 0.00 among girls (95 % CI −0.05–0.06, $p = 0.90$, $I^2 = 45.8$ %, $p = 0.09$), respectively.

Analysis of five studies that reported estimates adjusted for potential confounders yielded an effect size of −0.02 for boys (95 % CI −0.06–0.02, $p = 0.34$, $I^2 = 9$ %, $p = 0.41$) and −0.01 for girls (95 % CI −0.05–0.03, $p = 0.51$, $I^2 = 0$ %, $p = 0.43$), respectively.

Fisher's *z* for 10 studies that obtained accelerometer data for 4 days or more was −0.01 for boys (95 % CI −0.05–0.02, $p = 0.46$, $I^2 = 0$ %, $p = 0.5$) and 0.00 for girls (95 % CI −0.03–0.04, $p = 0.85$, $I^2 = 25.8$ %, $p = 0.90$), respectively.

Effect size for nine studies that used a 1-min epoch length was −0.01 for boys (95 % CI −0.04–0.03, $p = 0.66$, $I^2 = 0$ %, $p = 0.5$) and 0.01 for girls (95 % CI −0.02–0.05, $p = 0.44$, $I^2 = 0$ %, $p = 0.44$), respectively.

Fisher's *z* for five studies that defined MVPA as 2000 counts.min^{-1} and above was 0.01 for boys (95 % CI −0.05–0.07, $p = 0.73$, $I^2 = 0$ %, $p = 0.6$) and 0.03 for girls (95 % CI −0.04–0.09, $p = 0.47$, $I^2 = 39.7$ %, $p = 0.16$), respectively.

The analysis of five studies with valid outcome data for 75 % or more of the study sample revealed an effect size of −0.00 among boys (95 % CI −0.05–0.05, $p = 0.89$, $I^2 = 12.5$ %, $p = 0.33$) and 0.00 among girls (95 % CI −0.03–0.05, $p = 0.68$, $I^2 = 0$ %, $p = 0.88$), respectively.

Six studies were unpublished. Effect size was −0.00 for boys (95 % CI −0.05–0.05, $p = 0.99$, $I^2 = 0$ %, $p = 0.6$) and 0.03 for girls (95 % CI −0.03–0.09, $p = 0.32$, $I^2 = 27.7$ %, $p = 0.23$), respectively.

As the effect size was close to zero in all analyses, and since evidence of statistically significant variability in effect size across studies was lacking, no further attempt to investigate for bias was warranted.

Discussion

The results of the present meta-analysis show no difference in the level of PA between children living in single-parent families and those living in two-parent families. Thus, the findings indicate that SPFS is not associated with children's level of PA. The overall quality of the studies was less than optimal. Most of the published studies had a low response rate, and the majority of the studies were based on small samples. As the reported percentages of children exposed to SPFS were below what is officially reported for Europe [10] and USA [11], it may suggest that respondents from single-

Table 3 Details of measurement of physical activity

Studies	Accelerometer model	Level of measurement used for calculation of effect size	Number of days (and hours) with PA assessment	Threshold, (counts.min^{-1} or counts.hour^{-1})		Cut-point used to define outcome	Percentage with valid measurements (%)
				Lower	Upper		
Bagley et.al. [27]	Manufacturing Technology Inc., Actigraph Model, AM7164-2.2C, USA	MVPA	8 days, day 2–6 included. At least four weekdays and one weekend day. At least 10 h per day	<10,000	>20,000,000	3–5.9 METS[a] counts.min^{-1} (1017–3696)	97
Bradley et al. [28]	Computer Science and Applications (CSA), Inc., Shalimar, FL	MVPA	7 days, included for 4 days if non-zero counts from 5 a.m., and 60 min zero after 9 p.m., or 30 min zero after 10 p.m., or last zero count before 12 p.m.	I/N		3+ METS[a] counts.min^{-1} (1017–3696)	75
Hesketh et al. [5]	Manufacturing Technology Inc. accelerometer, Model 7164	MVPA	6 days (24-h periods) included if complete data for at least 4 days	<10,000	>20,000,000	3+ METS[a] counts.min^{-1} (1017–3696)	89
Sallis et.al. [30]	Computer Science and Applications (CSA), Inc., Shalimar, FL model 7164	VPA	7 days complete data included if no negative counts or "no long periods with zero counts"	I/N		6+ METS[a]	I/N
Sallis et al. [29]	Caltrac accelerometer (Hemokinetics, Inc., Madison, WI)	Mean total counts	From end of school day I to beginning of school day II, next morning	I/N		counts.hour^{-1}	76
Sallis et.al. [8][b]	Caltrac accelerometer (Hemokinetics, Inc., Madison, WI)	Mean total counts	From end of school day I to beginning of school day II, next morning or during a weekend (Friday to Monday morning)[c]	I/N		I/N	5
Eiberg Hansen et al. [22], CoSCIS	MTI Actigraph (Manufacturing Technology Inc., Fort Walton Beach, Florida, USA)	MVPA	4 days, including one weekend day, included if ≥600 min/day of activity for ≥3 days, and activity between 6 a.m. and 12 p.m. for at least 10 h.	<10,000	-	>1951 counts.min^{-1}	69.7
Riddoch et al. [20], EYHS Denmark, first cohort	MTI Actigraph (Manufacturing Technology Inc., Fort Walton Beach, Florida, USA)	MVPA	5 days, including one weekend day, included if ≥600 min/day of activity for ≥3 days, and activity between 6 a.m. and 12 p.m. for at least 10 h.	<10,000	-	≥2000 counts.min^{-1}	60
McMinn et al. [26], EYHS Denmark, second cohort	MTI Actigraph (Manufacturing Technology Inc., Fort Walton Beach, Florida, USA)	MVPA	5 days, including one weekend day, included if ≥600 min/day of activity for ≥3 days, and activity between 6 a.m. and 12 p.m. for at least 10 h.	<10,000	>20,000,000	≥2000 counts.min^{-1}	85
Riddoch et al. [20], EYHS Estonia	MTI Actigraph (Manufacturing Technology Inc., Fort Walton Beach, Florida, USA)	MVPA	5 days, including one weekend day, included if ≥600 min/day of activity for ≥3 days, and activity between 6 a.m. and 12 p.m. for at least 10 h.	<10,000	-	≥2000 counts.min^{-1}	52
		MVPA		<10,000	-	≥2000 counts.min^{-1}	44

Table 3 Details of measurement of physical activity *(Continued)*

Riddoch et al. [20], EYHS Portugal	MTI Actigraph (Manufacturing Technology Inc., Fort Walton Beach, Florida, USA)		5 days, including one weekend day, included if ≥600 min/day of activity for ≥3 days, and activity between 6 a.m. and 12 p.m. for at least 10 h.				
Riddoch et al. [20], EYHS Norway	MTI Actigraph (Manufacturing Technology Inc., Fort Walton Beach, Florida, USA)	MVPA	5 days, including one weekend day, included if ≥600 min/day of activity for ≥3 days, and activity between 6 a.m. and 12 p.m. for at least 10 h.	<10,000	-	≥2000 counts.min^{-1}	66

MVPA moderate to vigorous physical activity, *VPA* vigorous physical activity, *PA* physical activity, *I/N* insufficient or no information

[a]Calculated with algorithm from Freedson et al. [33]

[b]In the study by Sallis et al. [8], parents reported information on demographic, psychological, and biological circumstances. Data was collected by questionnaires that were distributed by 3648 students from seven schools. A total of 781 returned questionnaires were found complete and available for inclusion in further analysis (21 %). From the pool of 3648 children, 400 were selected at random and invited to wear an accelerometer to monitor the level of PA for 7 days. Accelerometer data for 265 children (66.3 %) were valid and included in further analysis. Of these, complete data from questionnaire and accelerometer was found among 200 (5 %) of the originally sampled 3648 children

[c]Activity during the school day was not measured

parent families tended to participate in the studies to a lower extent than what could be expected from random sampling variability. However, none of the included studies addressed this issue. Thus, the low percentage of children from single-parent families suggests that most of the studies may be influenced by selection bias.

With regard to the outcome (accelerometer-based assessment of PA) several potential sources of bias was observed. For example, monitoring for at least 4 days has been argued as necessary to obtain reliable measurements of PA among children and adolescents [34]. In the studies included in the present analysis, monitoring varied between 1 and 8 days and the daily average level of PA estimated in studies with less than 4 days of monitoring may not reflect the participant's level of PA. Also, it has been argued that the use of a 1-min epoch length to determine the amount of time spent in different levels of PA intensity fails to capture the time children and adolescents spent in vigorous activity [35]. The majority of the included studies used a 1-min epoch length, and this may have caused underestimation of the time spent in MVPA among participants. Hence, the studies may have failed to capture differences in time spent in vigorous PA by children's family status. Interestingly, the early study by Sallis et al. [30] was confined to vigorous PA and was the only study that showed a higher level of PA among single-parent children. Definition of MVPA differed between the studies, and this reflects the ongoing debate about the most appropriate cut-point for defining intensities of accelerometer-based assessments of PA [36]. However, the level of PA was equal across SPFS in all studies but one, and the discussion about an ideal cut-point may be less relevant for results of the present analysis. A minority of the studies had valid accelerometer data for at least 75 % of the study sample. The availability of valid accelerometer data from 5 % of the sample in the study by Sallis et al. [30] is especially notable. As in that study, poor compliance of the participants to wear the accelerometers, malfunction of the devices or loss of information because of study design, may be responsible for the low availability of data. Consequently, studies with a low proportion of valid outcome data may be prone to selection bias, and as information on the family status of the participants with missing accelerometer data is rarely provided, comparability of the study results may be hampered. Thus, our results should be treated with caution.

Our results are at odds with the results of previous reviews. For example, Sallis et al. [9] concluded that single-parent status was indeterminately related to children's PA. In this respect, a clearer distinction between single-parent family structures (e.g., distinction between divorced and widowed) has been called for as failure to do so could lead to comparison across different family environments that may not be comparable [6]. Similarly, potential differences between children who experience a true SPFS and those who live in single-parent family but have dual custody/regular contact with a second parent may also influence the comparability of results. Our data did not permit us to explicitly address this issue. However, measurements of SPFS are almost always self-reported and encompass a range of family structures that are often reduced to broader categories (e.g., single/two parent) in the final analysis. The self-reported measures of family status include children with and without regular contact with a second parent. As the effect sizes between and within studies in the present meta-analysis are homogeneous, it is difficult to see how further refinement of the SPFS measurement could alter the results.

Detrimental consequences of SPFS include economic difficulties and deterioration of social networks [37]. Such consequences have been observed to exert a substantial influence on children's cognitive and emotional development and well-being later in life, through various pathways [38]. Elder [38] proposed that the key to the successful development of children exposed to adverse social conditions in childhood was their parents' ability to adequately face a difficult situation and act within the existing opportunities and constraints to counteract the child's experience of a troubled time. Others have supported this notion [39]. Thus, it is possible that single parents may successfully allocate the resources necessary to avoid restricting opportunities for children's PA and imply that the single parent try to compensate for the shortage of support by the absence of a second partner. Although these explanations are only suggestive, the findings of the present meta-analysis indicate at least that single-parent status does not inhibit children's level of PA. However, the findings do not give any indication of possible differences in patterns or intensity of PA among children, separately by family status, although such differences have been reported [4, 30, 5]. Similarly, it is possible that participation in leisure activities and membership in sports clubs may be different for children of single-parent families to those from two-parent families. These associations have not been adequately addressed in the research literature, although some tentative results do exist [40, 7]. For example, Lindquist et al. [7] observed a higher level of participation in sports activities for SPFS children but a lower level of participating in PE classes in school. These findings may be somewhat contradictory but highlight the complexity of the composition of PA among children and underscore the need for developing measurement tools that enables a detailed monitoring of the total level of PA among children, regardless of their sociocultural background.

SPFS is assumed to be a proxy for several psychosocial factors important to children's PA, with instrumental support as the most prominent [30, 9, 28, 27, 5]. It is also assumed that single-parent families differ from two-parent families in their lower level of role modeling abilities and financial capacity [41]. The results of the present analysis dismiss evidence of a differential level of PA among children from single-parent families, and the results may suggest that the assumed disadvantaged fostering milieu for PA in single-parent families is not warranted. A more subtle relation between SPFS, presence of siblings, and children's PA was suggested by Bagley et al. [27], who reported a higher level of PA for boys with an older male sibling in single-parent families and for girls growing up with siblings regardless of gender. Similarly, Duncan et al. [42], suggested that the level of PA is interdependent among siblings but not among children and parents. Children of single parents may experience less parental support for engaging in PA or lack access to observational learning situations than children of two-parent families, but may compensate for the lack of parental involvement and stimuli and seek other sources of information and role models that assist in shaping their PA level. Siblings may be one such source of information, as well as role models.

Strengths and Limitations

The inclusion of six unpublished studies strengthens the present meta-analysis by allowing a detailed inspection of variability across diverse study settings and geographical locations. Another strength was our decision to restrict the analysis to studies that used accelerometry to measure children's PA permitted a detailed evaluation of the various decisions in managing accelerometer data on PA.

Some limitations should be mentioned. The search strategy used for the present study may have been too restrictive. Firstly, only English, Danish, Swedish, and Norwegian language studies were included. Secondly, efforts to locate unpublished literature were restricted to contacting authors of published studies to request information on family status and searching four databases, although several more may exist [43]. Thirdly, assessment of risk of bias in the included studies was not blinded. However, a recent meta-analysis suggested that the effectiveness of blinding authors in bias assessment is unclear and may be redundant [44]. Fourthly, the word "accelerometry" (ACELLEROM*) may have restricted the search to studies based on PA measured with accelerometric methods, although other methods exist (e.g., doubly labeled water [45], measure of heart rate, and indirect calorimetry). It has been suggested that measurement of PA using various electronic devises may not be comparable due to variability in obtaining accurate measures of energy expenditure—the basic component of PA [1]. If so, our restricted search may have revealed studies that are comparable, at least with respect to PA. Nevertheless, the search term "accelerometry" automatically includes related terms such as "pedometer", at least in Medline [18]. A search replacing the word "accelerom"* with the MeSH term "actigraphy" revealed 15 studies, of which 10 were not previously identified but deemed irrelevant as they fell into our exclusion criteria. This suggests that the chosen search strategy was sufficient to capture relevant studies. Fifthly, we combined effect size estimates of age groups into a single estimate and this may have concealed variability in levels of PA for younger versus older children. However, we assessed the differences in PA among children aged 9 and 15 years old living in single- versus two-parent families using the data from the EYHS, and results were virtually identical to analysis with combined age groups (results not shown). Hence, our combination of estimates for age groups does not impede with the overall results. Finally, our results are obtained from studies conducted in developed countries. The countries represented may share common sociocultural characteristics that shape the SPFS–PA relationship, albeit this was not investigated. Restricting our analysis to studies that share similar sociocultural characteristics provides us with a better basis for comparing results. On the other hand, it may also restrict our ability to generalize the overall conclusions to developing countries. Hence, our results may only apply for children and families in developed countries.

Conclusions

The present meta-analysis shows that single-parent status is not associated with children's level of PA. However, the included studies are heavily biased. Hence, caution should be exercised in interpretation of the overall result. Nevertheless, no evidence exists suggesting that children of single-parent families are in special need of extraordinary measures to facilitate their level of PA.

Competing Interests

John Singhammer, Mathias Ried-Larsen, Niels Christian Møller, Peter Lund-Kristensen, Karsten Froberg, and Lars Bo Andersen declare that they have no conflict of interest.

Authors' contributions

JS and MRL searched and evaluated the literature and drafted the manuscript. NCM, PLK, KF and LBA conceptualized the design, discussed and contributed to interpretation of the data, and approved the final draft. All authors agreed to be accountable for all aspect of the work. All authors read and approved the final manuscript.

Funding

The manuscript was prepared without external funding. Data from unpublished studies were made available by RICH, (Centre of Research in Childhood Health, University of Southern Denmark).

Author details
[1]Department of Physiotherapy, VIA University College, Hedeager 2, DK8200 Aarhus, Denmark. [2]Institute of Sports Science and Clinical Biomechanics, Centre of Research in Childhood Health, University of Southern Denmark, Odense, Denmark.

References

1. Butte NF, Ekelund U, Westerterp KR. Assessing physical activity using wearable monitors: measures of physical activity. Med Sci Sports Exercise. 2012;44 Suppl 1:S5–S12. doi:10.1249/MSS.0b013e3182399c0e.
2. WHO. What is the scale of the obesity problem in your country? World Health Organization. 2006. http://www.who.int/ncd_surveillance/infobase/web/InfoBasePolicyMaker/reports/Reporter.aspx?id=1.
3. Koster A, Caserotti P, Patel KV, Matthews CE, Berrigan D, Van Domelen DR et al. Association of sedentary time with mortality independent of moderate to vigorous physical activity. PloS one. 2012;7(6). doi:10.1371/journal.pone.0037696.
4. Gorely T, Atkin AJ, Biddle SJH, Marshall SJ. Family circumstance, sedentary behaviour and physical activity in adolescents living in England: Project STIL. Int J Behav Nutr Phys Act. 2009;6(33):1–8. doi:33 10.1186/1479-5868-6-33.
5. Hesketh K, Crawford D, Salmon J. Children's television viewing and objectively measured physical activity: associations with family circumstance. Int J Behav Nutr Phys Act. 2006;3(1):36.
6. Gustafson SL, Rhodes RE. Parental correlates of physical activity in children and early adolescents. Sports Med. 2006;36(1):79–97.
7. Lindquist CH, Reynolds KD, Goran MI. Sociocultural determinants of physical activity among children. Prev Med. 1999;29(4):305–12.
8. Sallis J, Taylor W, Dowda M, Freedson P, Pate R. Correlates of vigorous physical activity for children in grades 1 through 12: comparing parent-reported and objectively measured physical activity. Pediatr Exerc Sci. 2002;14:30–44.
9. Sallis J, Prochaska J, Taylor W. A review of correlates of physical activity of children and adolescents. Medicine Sci Sports Exercise. 2000;32:963–75.
10. Population and social conditions [database on the Internet]. The European Commission. 2001. Available from: http://ec.europa.eu/eurostat/data/database. Accessed: 17.07.2014
11. Families and living arrangements [database on the Internet]. United States Census Bureau; U.S. Department of Commerce. 2012. Available from: http://www.census.gov/hhes/families/data/cps2011.html. Accessed: 2012-06-13T12:48:29.58-04:00
12. Edwardson CL, Gorely T. Parental influences on different types and intensities of physical activity in youth: a systematic review. Psychology Sport Exercise. 2010;11(6):522–35. doi:10.1016/j.psychsport.2010.05.001.
13. Van Der Horst K, Paw MJ, Twisk JW, Van Mechelen W. A brief review on correlates of physical activity and sedentariness in youth. Med Sci Sports Exerc. 2007;39(8):1241–50. doi:10.1249/mss.0b013e318059bf35.
14. Warren JM, Ekelund U, Besson H, Mezzani A, Geladas N, Vanhees L. Assessment of physical activity—a review of methodologies with reference to epidemiological research: a report of the exercise physiology section of the European Association of Cardiovascular Prevention and Rehabilitation. Eur J Cardiovasc Prev Rehabil. 2010;17(2):127–39.
15. Ekelund U. Biological determinants of physical activity; heritability, genes and early life factors. 7th European Youth Heart Study Scientific Symposium, Madeira, PT. 2012.
16. Social Science Citation Index (SSCI) [database on the Internet]. Available from: http://www.isinet.com/. Accessed: September 2011
17. American Psychological Association. Accessed: September 2011
18. United States National Library of Medicine (NLM). Accessed: September 2011
19. EBSCO. Ipswich, UK: EBSCO publishing; 2011.
20. Riddoch C, Edwards D, Page A, Froberg K, Anderssen SA, Wedderkopp N, et al. The European Youth Heart Study—cardiovascular disease risk factors in children: rationale, aims, study design, and validation of methods. J Phys Act Health. 2005;2(1):115.
21. Andersen L, Harro M, Sardinha L, Froberg K, Ekelund U, Brage S, et al. Physical activity and clustered cardiovascular risk in children: a cross-sectional study (The European Youth Heart Study). Lancet. 2006;368:299–304.
22. Eiberg Hansen S, Hasselstrøm H, Grønfeldt V, Froberg K, Andersen LB. Cardiovascular disease risk factors in 6–7-Year-old Danish children: the Copenhagen School Child Intervention Study. Prev Med. 2005;40(6):740–6. doi:10.1016/j.ypmed.2004.09.017.
23. Eiberg S, Hasselstrom H, Grønfeldt V, Froberg K, Svensson J, Andersen LB. Maximum oxygen uptake and objectively measured physical activity in Danish children 6–7 years of age: the Copenhagen School Child Intervention Study. Br J Sports Med. 2005;39(10):725–30. doi:10.1136/bjsm.2004.015230.
24. Higgins JPT, Green S. Cochrane Handbook for Systematic Reviews of Interventions. Chichester: Wiley Cochrane Series: Wiley; 2011.
25. Wells GA, Shea B, O'Connell D, Peterson J, Welch V, Losos M et al. The Newcastle-Ottawa Scale (NOS) for assessing the quality of nonrandomised studies in meta-analyses. Ottawa Hospital Research Institute/Institute de recherche de l'Hospital d'Ottawa. 2003. http://www.ohri.ca/programs/clinical_epidemiology/oxford.asp. Accessed July 17 2014.
26. McMinn AM, Van Sluijs EMF, Wedderkopp N, Froberg K, Griffin SJ. Sociocultural correlates of physical activity in children and adolescents: findings from the Danish arm of the European Youth Heart study. Pediatr Exerc Sci. 2008;20(3):319–32.
27. Bagley S, Salmon J, Crawford D. Family structure and children's television viewing and physical activity. Medicine Sci Sports Exercise. 2006;38(5):910–8.
28. Bradley R, McRitchie S, Houts R, Nader P, O'Brien M, Network tNECCR. Parenting and the decline of physical activity from age 9 to 15. Int J Behav Nutr Phys Act. 2011;8(1):33.
29. Sallis JF, Alcaraz JE, McKenzie TL, Hovell MF. Predictors of change in children's physical activity over 20 months: variations by gender and level of adiposity. Am J Prev Med. 1999;16(3):222–9. doi:10.1016/s0749-3797(98)00154-8.
30. Sallis J, Alcaraz J, McKenzie T, Hovell M, Kolody B, Nader P. Parental behavior in relation to physical activity and fitness in 9-year-old children. Am J Dis Child. 1992;146:1383–8.
31. StataCorp. Stata: Release 12.1. College Station, TX: StataCorp LP. 2012.
32. Wilson DH, Becker B, Higgins J, Shadish W, Rothstein H, Bohrenstein M, et al. Comprehensive meta analysis 2.2.064 ed. Engelwood, NJ: Biostat; 2011.
33. Freedson P, Melanson E, Sirard J. Calibration of the Computer Science and Applications, Inc. accelerometer. Med Sci Sports Exerc. 1998;30:777–81.
34. Trost SG, Pate RR, Freedson PS, Sallis JF, Taylor WC. Using objective physical activity measures with youth: how many days of monitoring are needed? Med Sci Sports Exerc. 2000;32(2):426.
35. Nilsson A, Ekelund U, Yngve A, Sjostrom M. Assessing physical activity among children with accelerometers using different time sampling intervals and placements. Pediatr Exerc Sci. 2002;14:87–96.
36. Trost SG, McIver KL, Pate RR. Conducting accelerometer-based activity assessments in field-based research. Med Sci Sports Exerc. 2005;37(11):S531–43.
37. Duncan GJ, Brooks-Gunn J. Consequences of growing up poor. New York: Russell Sage; 1999.
38. Elder G. The life course as developmental theory. Child Dev. 1998;69(1):1–12.
39. Singh-Manoux A, Marmot M. Role of socialization in explaining social inequalities in health. Soc Sci Med. 2005;60(9):2129–33.
40. Quarmby T, Dagkas S. Children's engagement in leisure time physical activity: exploring family structure as a determinant. Leis Stud. 2010;29(1):53–66.
41. Mayer S. What money can't buy: family income and children's life chances. Cambridge: Harvard University Press; 1997.
42. Duncan S, Duncan T, Strycker L, Chaumeton N. A multilevel analysis of sibling physical activity. J Sport Exercise Psychology. 2004;26(1):57–68.
43. Cooper HM, Hedges LV, Valentine JC. The handbook of research synthesis and meta-analysis. New York: Russell Sage; 2009.
44. Morissette K, Tricco Andrea C, Horsley T, Chen Maggie H, Moher D. Blinded versus unblinded assessments of risk of bias in studies included in a systematic review. Cochrane Database Syst Rev. 2011. doi:10.1002/14651858.MR000025.pub2.
45. Prentice AM. Doubly-labelled water method for measuring energy expenditure: technical recommendations for use in humans. International Atomic Energy Agency and International Dietary Energy Consultancy Group: Vienna, Austria; 1990.

11

Human tendon adaptation in response to mechanical loading: a systematic review and meta-analysis of exercise intervention studies on healthy adults

Sebastian Bohm, Falk Mersmann and Adamantios Arampatzis*

Abstract

Background: The present article systematically reviews recent literature on the *in vivo* adaptation of asymptomatic human tendons following increased chronic mechanical loading, and meta-analyzes the loading conditions, intervention outcomes, as well as methodological aspects.

Methods: The search was performed in the databases PubMed, Web of Knowledge, and Scopus as well as in the reference lists of the eligible articles. A study was included if it conducted (a) a longitudinal exercise intervention (≥8 weeks) on (b) healthy humans (18 to 50 years), (c) investigating the effects on mechanical (i.e., stiffness), material (i.e., Young's modulus) and/or morphological properties (i.e., cross-sectional area (CSA)) of tendons *in vivo*, and was reported (d) in English language. Weighted average effect sizes (SMD, random-effects) and heterogeneity (Q and I^2 statistics) of the intervention-induced changes of tendon stiffness, Young's modulus, and CSA were calculated. A subgroup analysis was conducted regarding the applied loading intensity, muscle contraction type, and intervention duration. Further, the methodological study quality and the risk of bias were assessed.

Results: The review process yielded 27 studies with 37 separate interventions on either the Achilles or patellar tendon (264 participants). SMD was 0.70 (confidence interval: 0.51, 0.88) for tendon stiffness (N=37), 0.69 (0.36, 1.03) for Young's modulus (N=17), and 0.24 (0.07, 0.42) for CSA (N=33), with significant overall intervention effects ($p<0.05$). The heterogeneity analysis (stiffness: I^2=30%; Young's modulus: I^2=57%; CSA: I^2=21%) indicated that differences in the loading conditions may affect the adaptive responses. The subgroup analysis confirmed that stiffness adaptation significantly ($p<0.05$) depends on loading intensity (I^2=0%), but not on muscle contraction type. Although not significantly different, SMD was higher for interventions with longer duration (≥12 weeks). The average score of 71±9% in methodological quality assessment indicated an appropriate quality of most studies.

Conclusions: The present meta-analysis provides elaborate statistical evidence that tendons are highly responsive to diverse loading regimens. However, the data strongly suggests that loading magnitude in particular plays a key role for tendon adaptation in contrast to muscle contraction type. Furthermore, intervention-induced changes in tendon stiffness seem to be more attributed to adaptations of the material rather than morphological properties.

* Correspondence: a.arampatzis@hu-berlin.de
Department of Training and Movement Sciences, Humboldt-Universität zu Berlin, Philippstr. 13, Haus 11, 10115 Berlin, Germany

Key points

- Tendons are highly responsive to increased mechanical loading and adapt through changes of their mechanical, material, and morphological properties.
- Changes in tendon stiffness seem to be more attributed to adaptations of the material rather than morphological properties.
- An effective training intervention for the tendon should apply a high loading intensity over a longer intervention duration (>12 weeks).

Background

Tendons transmit the force exerted by the corresponding muscle to the skeleton and, therefore, are crucial components for human locomotion [1-3]. Further, the non-rigidity of tendons allows the storage and return of strain energy during locomotion [4,5] and facilitates the muscle force potential due to the force-length-velocity relationship [6-8]. Hence, tendon properties not only affect human daily locomotion like walking/running [9] and stability performance [10], but also significantly determine athletic performances, e.g., sprinting [11,12] and jumping [8,13,14] as well as the economy of running [15-17]. Furthermore, tendons are sensitive to their mechanical environment [18-22]. Following a period of enhanced mechanical loading, tendon stiffness may increase [23-26] to maintain physiological ranges of strain during locomotion, since the ultimate tendon strain is more or less constant [27]. Two mechanisms could account for an increase of tendon stiffness: a) changes of the tendon material (i.e., increase of Young's modulus) and b) changes of the tendon morphological properties (i.e., increase of cross-sectional area) [24,28-31]. Both tendon material and morphological changes result not only from an increase of collagen synthesis but also from changes of collagen fibril morphology and levels of collagen molecular cross-linking [19,32,33]. Besides physiological adaptive responses, excessive mechanical loading (i.e., overloading) was considered as an important factor in the etiology of tendinopathy [20,34,35], which is associated with pain, focal tendon tenderness, and decreased strength and movement [32].

The development and improvement of measurement techniques in the past 15 years, especially the measurement of tendon elongation during muscle contractions by means of an ultrasound-based methodology as well as the determination of the tendon cross-sectional area (CSA) from magnetic resonance images (MRI), enabled researchers to investigate human tendon mechanical, material, and morphological properties *in vivo* and adaptive responses following chronic increased loading [2,19,36]. Kubo et al. [37] were the first who reported an increase in stiffness and Young's modulus of the patellar tendon in humans following 12 weeks of exercise-based loading. An intervention-induced region specific hypertrophy of the patellar and Achilles tendon were initially reported in 2007 by Kongsgaard et al. [24] and Arampatzis et al. [29], respectively. To date, a lot of experimental studies evidenced the adaptive potential of tendons following exercise interventions, which featured different levels of mechanical loading conditions (e.g., intensity, duration of a single loading cycle, repetitions, sets, intervention duration, and training frequency per week) [25,28,30,31,38-41]. Since some interventions reported greater adaptive tendon responses than others, the outcome of the studies seems to be affected by differences of the applied loading conditions. This means that the levels of the loading conditions may determine the material and morphological adaptive responses of tendons. Although some studies investigated the effect of different loading levels (i.e., load magnitude [24,29], loading rate [31], and load duration [31,37,42]) on tendon adaptation, the small sample sizes of 8 to 14 participants used in these studies limit the generalizability of the outcomes. A meta-analysis of relevant experimental studies that examines the interaction of the levels of loading conditions with respect to study outcome could deepen our understanding of the effectiveness of certain loading levels on tendon adaptation. Furthermore, different methodological approaches could have affected the study outcomes, thus, additionally challenging the generalization of the findings. For example, most of recent studies on tendon adaptation used a manual segmentation of magnetic resonance or ultrasonographic images to determine the tendon CSA. However, using ultrasound images instead of MRI for the manual segmentation [38,39,43,44], intervention-induced changes of the tendon CSA might have been undetected or overrated, since the reliability of this manual segmentation method was reported to be poor [45]. Considering the methodological quality (i.e., internal, statistical, external validity aspects) of each study in a systematic meta-analysis would further improve our knowledge regarding mechanical loading and tendon adaptation.

Therefore, the objectives of the present study are to systematically review recent literature reports (i.e., longitudinal study designs) on the adaptation of asymptomatic human tendons following increased mechanical loading (i.e., training intervention) *in vivo* and to meta-analyze the applied levels of loading conditions, intervention outcomes, as well as methodological aspects, which has yet to be conducted. For a complete description of the adaptive processes, we will consider tendon mechanical, material, and morphological properties. Particular attention is given to the effect of loading intensity, muscle contraction type, and intervention duration on tendon adaptive responses by performing a respective subgroup analysis. This meta-analysis may provide crucial information on how to facilitate tendon adaptation.

Methods

Search strategy

The search was performed by using the electronic bibliographic databases ISI Web of Knowledge, PubMed, and Scopus (1970 to November 2014) and by screening the reference lists of the eligible articles. The following keyword combinations (i.e., search operator AND) were separately applied in the database search (i.e., title, abstract, keywords): tendon properties adaptation, tendon stiffness adaptation, tendon function adaptation, tendon mechanical loading adaptation, tendon properties training, and tendon properties exercise.

Study selection and inclusion criteria

Two independent reviewers (S.B. and F.M.) evaluated the titles of the studies that resulted from the search and included studies when the title indicated that the following inclusion criteria were fulfilled: (a) a longitudinal exercise intervention (≥8 weeks) was conducted, (b) healthy humans (18 to 50 years) served as participants, and (c) the effects on mechanical (stiffness), material (Young's modulus), and/or morphological (CSA) properties of asymptomatic tendons *in vivo* were reported (d) in the English language. The abstracts and, thereafter, the full text of the identified studies were then examined to confirm the inclusion. If a study did not meet all criteria, the respective exclusion criterion was documented and the study was eliminated from further analysis. In the case of disagreement of the two reviewers, a third reviewer (A.A.) was consulted. Figure 1 illustrates the systematic review process of the present meta-analysis.

Methodological quality and risk of bias

A customized methodological quality scale was designed to assess the internal, statistical, and external validity of the included studies in regard to the conceptual definition (Table 1). A positive point was assigned when a specific quality criterion was fulfilled (Table 1). However, if a criterion could not be scored because it was not part of the study (e.g., mechanical but not morphological tendon properties were investigated), the criterion was excluded from the further quality assessment of the study. The quality score of each validity aspect (i.e., internal, statistical, and external) was calculated by dividing the number of items with a positive score by the total number of items (the quotient was then multiplied by 100). The scores were averaged to calculate the overall methodological quality of each study. The assessment of the risk of bias (sequence generation, allocation concealment, blinding outcome assessor, incomplete outcome data, selective outcome reporting, other sources of bias) was based on the Cochrane Risk of Bias tool [46]. The data extraction and scoring were performed by two independent observers (S.B. and F.M.), and in the case of disagreement, a third one was consulted (A.A.). A funnel plot of the tendon stiffness from all included studies was created to estimate publication bias.

Data extraction

One reviewer (S.B.) extracted the following data from the full-text articles of all included studies, and a second reviewer (F.M.) confirmed the extraction. The data were merged in a table, including the information of the source (name of the first author and year of publication), the label of the participant sample in the respective study (i.e., experimental or control group according to the inclusion criteria), the characteristics of the participants (i.e., number, gender, activity level, investigated tendon), the performed intervention with the respective loading conditions (i.e., type of training, intensity, duration of single loading cycle, repetitions, sets, intervention duration, and training frequency), and the outcome of the study for either tendon stiffness, Young's modulus, and CSA as the difference of pre and post values in percentage (i.e., ((post value − pre value)/pre value) * 100) with the corresponding significance indication. Furthermore, the part of the tendon (i.e., free tendon or tendon-aponeurosis complex) that was used for the parameter calculation was documented. In studies where both calculation approaches were used, only the values from the free tendon were included. If the stiffness or Young's modulus was calculated within several percentage intervals of the force-elongation or stress-strain relationship, the values from the highest interval were used. In case that the CSA was reported for different positions along the tendon length, the mean value and pooled standard deviation were calculated and included. If the required data (i.e., means and standard deviations of pre- and post-intervention values) were not reported in the article or presented in an inappropriate format for data extraction (e.g., graph instead of values), the corresponding authors were contacted and asked to provide the missing values. Extracting values visually from a graph was the final option. In case the relevant data were not available, the study was excluded.

Statistical analysis

In order to assess the impact of mechanical loading on tendon adaptation, the effect sizes of the intervention-induced changes (i.e., changes to baseline) of the tendon stiffness, Young's modulus, and CSA for each study were calculated. As the stiffness, Young's modulus, and CSA were not always measured using identical methodological

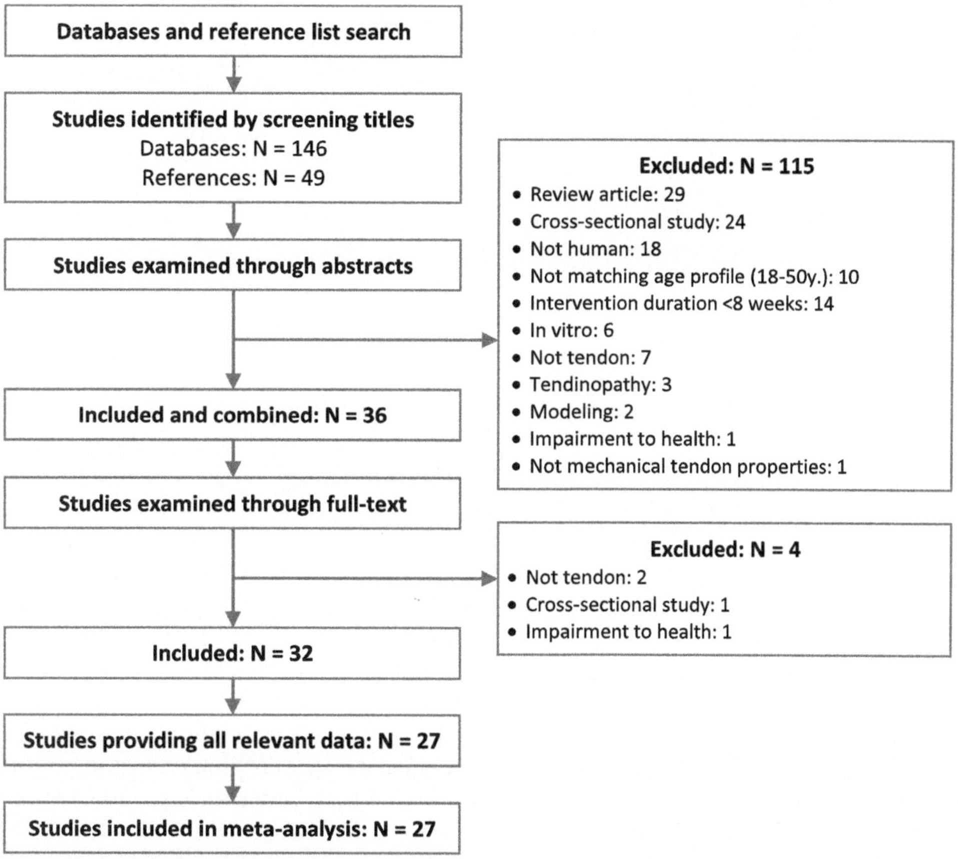

Figure 1 Flowchart of the systematic review process.

approaches, the effect size was calculated as the standardized mean difference (SMD) [47]. The SMD included further an adjustment (Hedges' adjusted *g*) for small sample bias [47]. Throughout the following manuscript, we will use the term SMD when referring to effect sizes of individual studies. The SMDs from all studies were then pooled in a meta-analysis to estimate the weighted average effect size of the tendon stiffness, Young's modulus, and CSA [47,48]. Thereto, we used a random-effects model of the generic inverse variance method, which gives more weight to larger studies (i.e., smaller standard errors) and accounts for heterogeneity of the included studies [47,49]. To analyze the presence of an overall intervention effect on the tendon stiffness, Young's modulus, and CSA, a test statistic (i.e., null hypothesis: no overall effect of the intervention) was performed [47]. A forest plot was created to illustrate the SMDs and 95% confidence intervals (CIs) of tendon stiffness, Young's modulus, and CSA for all respective studies as well as the overall effect. Further, heterogeneity between study outcomes was investigated using Q and I^2 statistics to assess if differences between outcomes are due to study diversity rather than chance [50]. A subgroup analysis was conducted on the following loading conditions: intensity (i.e., higher versus lower than 70% of maximum voluntary contraction (MVC) or one repetition maximum (RM)), muscle contraction type (i.e., isometric, eccentric, concentric-eccentric), and intervention duration (i.e., shorter and longer than 12 weeks). A second forest plot was designed to present the SMDs and CI of tendon stiffness between studies, which applied low and high loading intensities, respectively. Statistical procedures were performed by means of the software Review Manager v.5.2 [51].

Results

Literature search

The search by the defined keywords yielded 3,944 hits in the three databases. After screening all study titles and eliminating duplicates from the different databases, 146 potentially eligible studies were identified. Following the abstract examination, 35 studies remained included; however, the full text assessment showed that four more studies did not confirm all criteria and, thus, were excluded from the further analysis. The screening of the reference lists of the included studies provided a number of 49 potentially eligible studies. However, except one study, all articles did not meet the criteria or were already included. Five studies were excluded from the remaining 32 due to a lack

Table 1 Criteria of the methodological quality

	Scoring
Internal validity	
1. Study design	A positive point was assigned if the following aspects were considered:
	1. Mechanical tendon properties (stiffness)
	2. Material tendon properties (Young's modulus)
	3. Morphological tendon properties (cross-sectional area)
	4. Control group (no specific training) was included and participants were randomly assigned
2. Methods	A positive point was assigned if the following aspects were considered:
2.1 Mechanical properties	
• Object of investigation	A. Only the free tendon was assessed [79]
• Calculation of tendon force	B. Consideration of gravitational forces [80,81]
	C. Consideration of axes misalignment of dynamometer and joint [80-82]
	D. Consideration of antagonistic muscle activation [83,84]
	E. Tendon lever arm directly measured for each subject
• Measurement of tendon elongation	F. Consideration of joint angle changes during the maximal isometric contraction on the tendon elongation measurement [84,85]
	G. Using the average of multiple trials (>1) to increase the reliability of the ultrasound technique [86]
2.2 Morphological properties	A. Magnetic resonance imaging was used [45,76]
	B. Different positions along tendon length were assessed to account for potential region specific adaptations [24,29,30]
3. Cofactors	A positive point was assigned if the following aspects were considered:
	A. Influence of gender
	B. Influence of physical activity level of the participants
Statistical validity	
4. Statistical tests	A positive point was assigned if appropriate statistical tests were used
5. Power analysis	A positive point was assigned if effect sizes were calculated and reported
External validity	
6. Eligibility of sample and variable	A positive point was assigned if the intervention included:
	1. Appropriate participant sample
	2. Appropriate variables
7. Description of the exercise intervention protocol	A positive point was assigned if the following criteria were reported:
	A. Intensity of muscle contraction
	B. Duration of single stimulus
	C. Repetitions per set
	D. Number of sets
	E. Number of weeks of intervention
	F. Number of trainings per week
8. Description of the participant sample	A positive point was assigned if the following criteria were reported:
	A Age, B Gender, C Body height, D Body weight, E Activity level

of relevant information about the loading conditions [52,53] or outcome values [44,54,55]. Finally, 27 studies fulfilled all criteria and were included in the present meta-analysis (Figure 1).

Description of the included studies

All included studies assessed the effect of mechanical loading on either the patellar tendon ($N = 12$) or the Achilles tendon ($N = 15$). Nine studies applied a different loading protocol on the two legs of the participants of the exercise group, and one study investigated three different intervention groups. In the present meta-analysis, each of these interventions was treated as a separate intervention. When a study presented the data of different intervention groups, but not all of them fulfilled the inclusion criteria, only the ones that met all criteria were included. An overweighting of single studies within the meta-analysis (i.e., bias) due to this approach was, however, not expected, as the loading conditions between the separate interventions were different and independent. In fact, only this procedure allowed to include all available data for a representative meta-analysis. The articles from Foure et al. [38,56,57] reported the effect of a single intervention on different parameters of the Achilles tendon, as indicated by the same number of participants with similar anthropometrics, identical training protocol, and values of tendon CSA. The relevant parameters for the present analysis (i.e., tendon stiffness and CSA) were extracted and considered as a single intervention. Furthermore, Kubo et al. [37,42] presented the data of one intervention in two articles, as indicated by the same number of participants and anthropometrics, training protocol, and results of tendon stiffness and CSA (LC protocol exercise group in [42]). Thus, the values were only included once. In the study of Kubo et al. [58], the authors compared the results of two previous investigations [59,60] that were already included in the present meta-analysis under a new research question. These results were also not considered as a new investigation. In another article [24], the CSA pre- and post-intervention values were exclusively reported in a graph (figure four, page 116). The respective means and standard error of means were visually extracted from the graph and used in order to calculate the standard deviation and SMD.

Finally, the present meta-analysis included in total 37 interventions (participants in total $N = 264$) eligible for the research question, and their characteristics are summarized in Table 2. In all 37 interventions, the parameter tendon stiffness was used in order to quantify the training effect on the adaptive tendon responses. Thirty-three of these also examined the tendon CSA, and 17 studies further included the parameter Young's modulus. Seventeen interventions applied the mechanical stimulus on the tendon by means of isometric muscle contractions, 11 interventions used a combination of concentric and eccentric contractions or solely concentric ($N = 1$) or eccentric contractions ($N = 3$), 5 interventions performed plyometric training, 1 intervention added stretching to the resistance training, and 1 study investigated the effect of running on the tendon properties (Table 2). The loading conditions were set to different levels between studies, using high and low intensities, short and long durations of the single loading, and different numbers of repetitions and sets (Table 2). However, only three studies (i.e., eight interventions) specified the corresponding tendon strain magnitude to the muscle contraction intensity [28,29,31]. Thirty-five of the 37 interventions were performed for 8 to 14 weeks, and the participants exercised on 2 to 4 days per week. Except for four interventions [29,61,62], which included both female and male participants and one intervention including solely women [63], all other interventions were performed with men. In almost all studies, the participants were regularly physically active, but not involved in intensive sports activity. One intervention was performed with cricket players [39] and another one with runners [17]. The number of exercised participants ranged between studies from 6 to 15 with a mean of 9.8 ± 2.3.

Methodological quality and risk of bias assessment

The results of the methodological quality assessment of the included studies showed a range of achieved scores from 61% to 99% with a mean and standard deviation of 71% ± 9% (Table 3), indicating appropriate methodological qualities for most studies. Fourteen of the 27 included studies investigated mechanical, material, as well as morphological properties (i.e., stiffness, Young's modulus, and CSA), which is essential in order to clarify if a change in tendon stiffness was based on alterations of the material properties and/or tendon hypertrophy.

The risk of bias assessment indicated a low risk of bias in three interventions [24,41,61]. The judgment for the other included studies was problematic, because the randomization process, concealment of allocation, and blinding of the assessor to the data were not reported and, therefore, unclear (Table 3). The funnel plot of tendon stiffness from all included studies appeared symmetrical and, thus, indicates low risk of publication bias (Figure 2).

Meta-analysis of intervention effects

The weighted average effect size for the tendon stiffness was 0.70 (CI 0.51, 0.88), 0.69 (CI 0.36, 1.03) for tendon Young's modulus and 0.24 (CI 0.07, 0.42) for tendon CSA, indicating greater intervention effects on stiffness and Young's modulus compared to CSA (Figure 3). The overall intervention effect was significant for all three parameters ($p < 0.05$). Heterogeneity was significant for stiffness and Young's modulus ($p < 0.05$), but not for CSA ($p = 0.14$), with a moderate heterogeneity of 30% and 21% for stiffness and CSA, respectively, and a substantial heterogeneity of 57% for Young's modulus [50]. Figure 3 presents a forest plot, including the SMDs and corresponding CIs for tendon stiffness, Young's modulus, and CSA of all included interventions as well as the respective weighted average effect sizes with the overall effect test and heterogeneity analysis results.

Subgroup analysis

The subgroup analysis on the loading intensity showed that pooling interventions using muscle contraction intensities higher than 70% of MVC or RM ($N = 27$) and those using lower intensities ($N = 5$) resulted in a weighted averaged effect size of tendon stiffness of 0.90 (CI 0.71, 1.08) and 0.04 (CI −0.46, 0.53), respectively. The difference between the high and low intensity subgroup was statistically significant ($p < 0.00001$). No heterogeneity was found between the studies using high intensities ($p = 0.56$, $I^2 = 0\%$). The forest plot in Figure 4 contains the SMDs and corresponding CIs for tendon stiffness separated for interventions featuring high and low loading intensities as well as the respective weighted average effect sizes with the overall effect test and heterogeneity analysis.

When analyzing the interventions that used a high loading intensity in regard to the type of muscle contraction, the weighted averaged effect sizes of tendon stiffness showed no statistically significant ($p > 0.5$) difference between isometric ($N = 15$, SMD = 0.95, CI 0.66, 1.24), concentric-eccentric ($N = 8$, SMD = 0.82, CI 0.49, 1.15), and purely eccentric ($N = 2$, SMD = 1.04, CI 0.37, 1.72) contraction type.

The subgroup analysis of the intervention duration showed that the weighted average effect sizes of tendon stiffness were 0.91 for the interventions using longer durations (≥12 weeks: $N = 23$, CI 0.71, 1.12) and 0.81 for

Table 2 Data extraction from the included studies

Source		Participants				Intervention								Outcome							
														Stiffness			YM		CSA		
Reference	Year	Group	*N*	Sex	Activity level	Tendon	Type of training	Intensity	Duration	Reps	Sets	Weeks	Times/week	Location	%	Sig	%	Sig	Location	%	Sig
Albracht et al. [15]	2013	EP	13	m	Run	AT	Is (rep)	90% MVC	3 s	4	5	14	4	Ap (GM F)	15.8	*					
Arampatzis et al. [29]	2010	EP	11	m	Reg	AT	Is (rep)	55% MVC	1 s	20	5	14	4	Ap (GM F)	−5.2	-	−4.8	-	Free	1.3	-
		EP	11	m	Reg	AT	Is (rep)	90% MVC	1 s	12	5	14	4	Ap (GM F)	17.1	*	16.9	*	Free	0.5	-
Arampatzis et al. [28]	2007	EP	11	f, m	Reg	AT	Is (rep)	55% MVC	3 s	7	5	14	4	Ap (GM F)	7.9	-	−1.6	-	Free	4.3	-
		EP	11	f, m	Reg	AT	Is (rep)	90% MVC	3 s	4	5	14	4	Ap (GM F)	36.0	*	22.9	*	Free	9.6	*
Bohm et al. [31]	2014	EP	12	m	Reg	AT	Is (sta)	90% MVC	12 s	1	5	14	4	Ap (GM M)	24.8	*	17.7	*	Free	5.3	*
		EP	12	m	Reg	AT	Is (rep)	90% MVC	3 s	4	5	14	4	Ap (GM M)	53.9	*	45.2	*	Free	4.4	*
		EP	14	m	Reg	AT	Ply	90% MVC	Approximately 0.26 s	72	5	14	4	Ap (GM M)	28.4	-	19.6	-	Free	2.5	-
		EP	14	m	Reg	AT	Is (rep)	90% MVC	3 s	4	5	14	4	Ap (GM M)	37.3	*	36.3	*	Free	3.7	*
Carroll et al. [61]	2011	CG	7 (11)	f, m	Unt	PT	Co-Ec (rep)	74% RM	nr	2 to 3	5 to 10	12	3	Free	13.9	+	18.4	*	Free	−1.7	-
Fletcher et al. [17]	2010	EP	6	m	Run	AT	Is (sta)	80% MVC	20 s	1	4	8	3	Ap (GM F)	18.6	-					
Fouré et al. [71]	2009	EP	6	m	Exp	AT	Ply	nr	nr	150 to 280	nr	8	2	Ap (GM M)	4.1	-					
Foure et al. [38,56,57]	2010a, b,2011	EP	9	m	Reg	AT	Ply	nr	nr	200 to 600	nr	14	2.4	Ap (GM M)	26.5	*			Free	3.1	-
Foure et al. [43]	2013	EP	11	m	Reg	AT	Ec (rep)	nr	nr	200 to 600	nr	14	2.4	Ap (GM F)	16.4	-			Free	−1.5	-
Hansen et al. [62]	2003	EP	11	f, m	Unt	AT	Run	nr	30 to 50 min	1		34	2.4	Ap (GM F)	7.3	-			Free	−0.3	-
Houghton et al. [39]	2013	EP	7	nr	Cri	AT	Ply	nr	nr	4 to 10	2 to 6	8	1.9	Ap (GM M)	−8.9	-	−20	-	Free	12.9	*
Kongsgaard et al. [24]	2007	EP	12	m	Unt	PT	Co-Ec (rep)	70% RM	nr	8	10	12	3	Free	14.6	*	12.2	-	Free	3.3	nr
		EP	12	m	Unt	PT	Co-Ec (rep)	16% RM	nr	36	10	12	3	Free	−9.2	-	−4.2	-	Free	1.5	nr

Table 2 Data extraction from the included studies *(Continued)*

Kubo et al. [37,42]	2001a	EP	8	m	Reg	PT	Is (rep)	70% MVC	Rapid	50	3	12	4	Ap (VL F)	17.5	-			Free	1.4	-
	2001a,b	EP	8	m	Reg	PT	Is (sta)	70% MVC	20 s	1	4	12	4	Ap (VL F)	57.3	*	50.3	*	Free	1.4	-
Kubo et al. [25]	2002	EP	8	m	Reg	AT	Co-Ec (rep)	70% RM	nr	10	5	8	4	Ap (GM F)	31.3	*			Free	−3.3	-
		EP	8	m	Reg	AT	Co-Ec (rep) + S	70% RM	nr + 45 s	10 + 5	5 + 1	8	4 + 7 (2×/day)	Ap (GM F)	23.8	*			Free	3.4	-
Kubo et al. [63]	2003	EP2	11	f	Reg	PT	Co-Ec (rep)	BW	nr	44	1	24	6	Ap (VL F)	15.7	-					
Kubo et al. [40]	2006a	EP	9	m	nr	PT	Is (sta) [50°]	70% MVC	15 s	1	6	12	4	Ap (VL F)	9.7	-			Free	1.5	-
		EP	9	m	nr	PT	Is (sta) [100°]	70% MVC	15 s	1	6	12	4	Ap (VL F)	50.9	*			Free	1.5	-
Kubo et al. [87]	2006b	EP	8	m	Reg	PT	Is (sta)	70% MVC	15 s	1	10	12	4	Free	−0.2	-			Free	0.3	-
Kubo et al. [88]	2006c	CG	9	m	nr	PT	Co-Ec (rep)	80% RM	4 s	10	4	12	3	Free	8.5	-			Free	−0.6	-
Kubo et al. [59]	2007	EP	10	m	Unt	AT	Ply	40% RM	nr	10	5	12	4	Ap (GM M)	19.4	-			Free	3.3	-
		EP	10	m	Unt	AT	Co-Ec (rep)	80% RM	4 s	10	5	12	4	Ap (GM M)	29.7	*			Free	−1.2	-
Kubo et al. [60]	2009	EP	10	m	nr	PT	Is (sta)	70% MVC	15 s	1	10	12	4	Free	71.1	*			Free	4.0	-
		EP	10	m	nr	PT	Co-Ec (rep)	80% RM	4 s	10	5	12	4	Free	25.4	-			Free	1.3	-
Kubo et al. [52]	2010	EP	8	m	Reg	PT	Is (sta)	70% MVC	15 s	1	10	12	4	Ap (VL F)	50.9	*			Free	1.0	-
Kubo et al. [72]	2012	EP	9	m	Reg	AT	Is (sta)	80% MVC	15 s	1	15	12	4	Ap (GM M)	51.4	*			Free	2.7	-
Malliaras et al. [41]	2013	EP	9	m	Reg	PT	Co (rep)	80% RM	5 s	7 to 8	4	12	3	Free	49.9	-	52	-	Free	5.0	-
		EP	10	m	Reg	PT	Ec (rep)	80% RM	5 s	12 to 15	4	12	3	Free	39.2	-	38.6	-	Free	3.6	-
		EP	10	m	Reg	PT	Ec (rep)	80% RM (Ec)	5 s	7 to 8	4	12	3	Free	80.9	*	77.3	*	Free	5.8	-
Seynnes et al. [30]	2009	EP	15	m	Reg	PT	Co-Ec (rep)	80% RM	nr	10	4	9	3	Free	22.7	*	18.4	*	Free	3.9	*

Group (i.e., as assigned in the respective article): EP, experimental group; CG, control group. Sex: f, female; m, male. Activity level: Reg, regularly physically active and recreational sports; Unt, untrained; Exp, explosive sports (i.e., volleyball, basketball, handball); Run, runners; Cri, cricket players. Tendon: PT, patellar tendon; AT, Achilles tendon. Type of training: Is, isometric muscle contraction; Co, concentric; Ec, eccentric; Ply, plyometric; Run, running; S, stretching; rep, repetitive; sta, static. Intensity: MVC, maximum voluntary contraction; RM, one repetition maximum; BW, body weight. Outcome: YM, tendon Young's modulus; CSA, tendon cross-sectional area. Location (i.e., refers to the anatomical structure that was used for the assessment of the tendon properties): Ap, aponeurosis; GM, m. gastrocnemius medialis; VL, m. vastus lateralis; F, fiber; M, myo-tendinous junction; Free, free tendon; nr, not reported. Sig (i.e., significance): *$p < 0.05$; +$p < 0.01$; -$p > 0.05$.

Table 3 Methodological quality and risk of bias assessment of the included studies

Study	Methodological quality																				
	Internal validity																Statistical validity			External validity	
	1.1[a]	1.2[a]	1.3[a]	1.4[a]	2.1A[b]	2.1B[b]	2.1C[b]	2.1D[b]	2.1E[b]	2.1F[b]	2.1G[b]	2.2A[b]	2.2B[b]	3A[b]	3B[b]	Score [%]	4[a]	5[a]	Score [%]	6.1[a]	6.2[a]
Albracht et al., 2013 [15]	+	-	-	+	-	+	+	+	-	+	-	/	/	-	+	51	+	-	50	+	+
Arampatzis et al., 2007 [29]	+	+	+	+	-	+	+	+	-	+	-	+	+	+	-	87	+	-	50	+	+
Arampatzis et al., 2010 [28]	+	+	+	-	-	+	+	+	-	+	-	+	+	+	-	72	+	-	50	+	+
Bohm et al. [31]	+	+	+	+	-	+	+	+	+	+	+	+	+	+	+	98	+	+	100	+	+
Carroll et al., 2011 [61]	+	+	+	-	+	-	-	-	-	+	+	+	+	-	+	70	+	-	50	+	+
Fletcher et al., 2010 [17]	+	-	-	+	-	+	+	-	+	+	-	/	/	+	+	60	+	-	50	+	+
Fouré et al., 2009 [71]	+	-	-	+	-	+	-	-	-	-	-	/	/	+	+	46	+	-	50	+	+
Foure et al., 2010a,b, 2011 [38,56,57]	+	-	+	+	-	+	-	-	-	+	-	-	+	+	+	63	+	-	50	+	+
Foure et al., 2013 [43]	+	-	+	+	-	+	-	-	-	+	-	-	+	+	+	63	+	-	50	+	+
Hansen et al., 2003 [62]	+	-	+	-	-	-	-	+	+	+	-	+	+	-	+	56	+	-	50	+	+
Hougthon et al., 2013 [39]	+	+	+	+	-	+	+	+	+	+	-	-	+	+	+	84	+	+	100	+	+
Kongsgaard et al., 2007 [24]	+	+	+	-	+	+	-	+	-	+	-	+	+	+	+	74	+	-	50	+	+
Kubo et al., 2001a,b [37,42]	+	+	+	-	-	-	-	-	-	-	+	+	-	+	+	66	+	-	50	+	+
Kubo et al., 2002 [25]	+	-	+	-	-	-	-	-	-	-	+	+	-	+	+	52	+	-	50	+	+
Kubo et al., 2003 [63]	+	+	+	+	-	-	-	-	-	-	+	/	/	+	+	86	+	-	50	+	+
Kubo et al., 2006a [40]	+	-	+	-	-	-	-	+	-	+	+	+	-	+	-	49	+	-	50	+	+
Kubo et al., 2006b [87]	+	-	+	+	+	-	-	+	-	+	+	+	+	+	+	80	+	-	50	+	+
Kubo et al., 2006c [88]	+	-	+	-	+	-	-	+	-	+	-	+	+	+	-	56	+	-	50	+	+
Kubo et al., 2007 [59]	+	-	+	-	-	-	-	+	-	+	+	+	-	+	+	56	+	-	50	+	+
Kubo et al., 2009 [60]	+	-	+	-	+	-	-	+	-	+	-	+	+	+	-	56	+	-	50	+	+
Kubo et al., 2010 [52]	+	-	+	+	-	-	-	+	-	+	+	+	+	+	+	78	+	-	50	+	+
Kubo et al., 2012 [72]	+	-	+	+	-	-	-	+	-	+	+	+	+	+	-	70	+	-	50	+	+
Malliaras et al., 2013 [41]	+	+	+	+	+	-	-	+	-	+	+	-	-	+	+	80	+	-	50	+	+
Seynnes et al., 2009 [30]	+	+	+	-	+	-	-	+	+	-	-	+	+	+	+	78	+	-	50	+	+

Table 3 Methodological quality and risk of bias assessment of the included studies *(Continued)*

Study	Methodological quality													Risk of bias					
	External validity												Total score [%]	Sequence	Allocation	Blinding	Outcome	Report	Other
	7A[b]	7B[b]	7C[b]	7D[b]	7E[b]	7F[b]	8A[b]	8B[b]	8C[b]	8D[b]	8E[b]	Score [%]							
Albracht et al., 2013 [15]	+	+	+	+	+	+	-	+	+	+	+	95	65	Unclear	Unclear	Unclear	Yes	Yes	Yes
Arampatzis et al., 2007 [29]	+	+	+	+	+	+	+	+	+	+	-	95	77	Unclear	Unclear	Unclear	Yes	Yes	Yes
Arampatzis et al., 2010 [28]	+	+	+	+	+	+	+	+	+	+	-	95	72	Unclear'	Unclear'	Unclear	Yes	Yes	Yes
Bohm et al. [31]	+	+	+	+	+	+	+	+	+	+	+	100	99	Unclear	Unclear	Unclear	Yes	Yes	Yes
Carroll et al., 2011 [61]	+	-	+	+	+	+	+	+	+	+	+	96	72	Unclear'	Unclear'	Yes	Yes	Yes	Yes
Fletcher et al., 2010 [17]	+	+	+	+	+	+	+	+	+	+	+	100	70	Unclear	Unclear	Unclear	Yes	Yes	Yes
Fouré et al., 2009 [71]	-	-	+	-	+	+	+	+	+	+	+	88	61	Unclear	Unclear	Unclear	Unclear	Yes	Yes
Foure et al., 2010a,b, 2011 [38,56,57]	-	-	+	-	+	+	+	+	+	+	+	88	67	Unclear	Unclear	Unclear	Yes	Yes	Yes
Foure et al., 2013 [43]	-	-	+	-	+	+	+	+	+	+	+	88	67	Unclear	Unclear	Unclear	Yes	Yes	Yes
Hansen et al., 2003 [62]	-	+	+	+	+	+	+	+	+	+	+	96	67	Unclear'	Unclear'	Unclear	Yes	Yes	Yes
Hougthon et al., 2013 [39]	-	-	+	+	+	+	+	+	+	+	+	92	92	Unclear	Unclear	Unclear	Yes	Yes	Unclear[+]
Kongsgaard et al., 2007 [24]	+	-	+	+	+	+	+	+	+	+	+	96	73	Unclear'	Unclear'	Yes	Yes	Yes	Yes
Kubo et al., 2001a,b [37,42]	+	+	+	+	+	+	+	+	+	+	+	100	72	Unclear'	Unclear'	Unclear	Yes	Yes	Yes
Kubo et al., 2002 [25]	+	-	+	+	+	+	+	+	+	+	+	96	66	Unclear'	Unclear'	Unclear	Yes	Yes	Yes
Kubo et al., 2003 [63]	+	-	+	+	+	+	+	+	+	+	+	96	77	Unclear	Unclear	Unclear	Yes	Yes	Yes
Kubo et al., 2006a [40]	+	+	+	+	+	+	+	+	+	+	-	95	65	Unclear'	Unclear'	Unclear	Yes	Yes	Yes
Kubo et al., 2006b [87]	+	+	+	+	+	+	+	+	+	+	+	100	77	Unclear	Unclear	Unclear	Yes	Yes	Yes
Kubo et al., 2006c [88]	+	+	+	+	+	+	+	+	+	+	-	95	67	Unclear'	Unclear'	Unclear	Yes	Yes	Yes
Kubo et al., 2007 [59]	+	+	+	+	+	+	+	+	+	+	+	100	69	Unclear'	Unclear'	Unclear	Yes	Yes	Yes
Kubo et al., 2009 [60]	+	+	+	+	+	+	+	+	+	+	-	95	67	Unclear'	Unclear'	Unclear	Yes	Yes	Yes
Kubo et al., 2010 [52]	+	+	+	+	+	+	+	+	+	+	+	100	76	Unclear	Unclear	Unclear	Yes	Yes	Yes
Kubo et al., 2012 [72]	+	+	+	+	+	+	+	+	+	+	+	100	73	Unclear	Unclear	Unclear	Yes	Yes	Yes
Malliaras et al., 2013 [41]	+	+	+	+	+	+	+	+	+	+	+	100	77	Unclear	Yes	Yes	Yes	Yes	Yes
Seynnes et al., 2009 [30]	+	-	+	+	+	+	+	+	+	+	+	96	74	Unclear'	Unclear'	Unclear	Yes	Yes	Yes

Methodological quality: 1 Study design (1.1 Mechanical properties, 1.2 Material properties, 1.3 Morphological properties, 1.4 Control group), 2 Methods (2.1 Mechanical properties, 2.1A Object of investigation, 2.1B Gravitational forces, 2.1C Axes misalignment, 2.1D Antagonistic muscle activation, 2.1E Lever arm measured, 2.1F Joint angle change, 2.1G Used multiple trials, 2.2 Morphological properties, 2.2A MRI, 2.2B different positions), 3 Cofactors (3A Gender, 3B Activity level), 4 Statistical tests, 5 Power analysis, 6 Eligibility (6.1 Participants, 6.2 Variables), 7 Description exercise protocol (7A Intensity, 7B Duration single stimulus, 7C Repetitions, 7D Sets, 7E Weeks, 7F Times per week), 8 Description participants (8A Gender, 8B Age, 8C Body height, 8D Body weight, 8E Activity level). The single criteria were rated (+, point; -, no point; /, not included) and used to calculate the quality score for each category (i.e., internal, statistical, and external validity). The average of the three scores gives the total score. [a]A full point was assigned to each sub-category for the calculation of the score in the respective validity section (assigned points/possible points * 100). [b]The sub-categories of the respective block were pooled to a single point (assigned points/possible points). Risk of bias [46]: Sequence, adequate sequence generation; Allocation, allocation concealment; Blinding, blinding outcome assessor; Outcome, incomplete outcome data; Report, selective outcome reporting; Other, other sources of bias. Judgments: Yes, low risk of bias; Unclear, insufficient information reported (', only one group; [+], significant difference of baseline tendon cross-sectional area values between the control and training group). The three studies of Foure et al. [38,56,57] and the two studies of Kubo et al. [37,42] were merged as one, since the results of one intervention were reported in different publications.

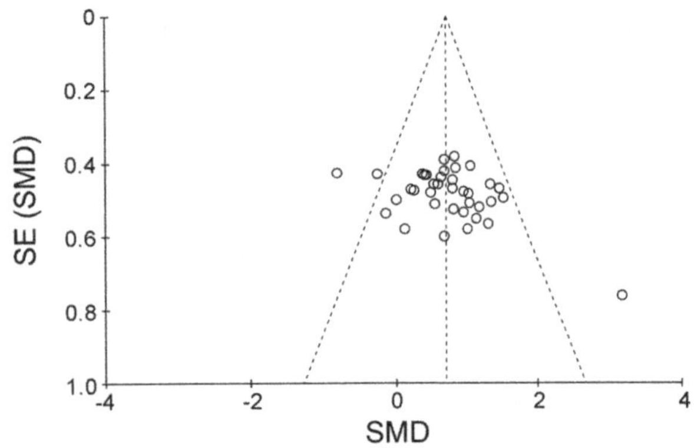

Figure 2 Funnel plot of standardized mean differences (SMDs) against standard error of the mean (SE). Values represent the tendon stiffness from all studies included in the meta-analysis.

the shorter ones (8 to 12 weeks: $N = 4$, CI 0.33, 1.29). No statistical significant difference was found between the two durations ($p = 0.7$).

Discussion

The present meta-analysis assessed the effect of chronic mechanical loading on the adaptive responses of tendon mechanical (stiffness), material (Young's modulus), and morphological (CSA) properties reported in the recent literature. Twenty-seven studies, which provided an overall number of 37 separate exercise interventions (participants in total $N = 264$), were included in the analysis. The weighted averaged effect size of the intervention-induced adaptations was 0.70 for tendon stiffness ($N = 37$), 0.69 for Young's modulus ($N = 17$), and 0.24 for CSA ($N = 33$), indicating a moderate to large effect for the first two parameters and a small to moderate effect for the latter. The overall intervention effect for stiffness, Young's modulus, and CSA was significant, regardless of the variety of applied loading regimens. However, the significant heterogeneity of stiffness and Young's modulus between the included interventions indicated that the different levels of the loading conditions might have affected the adaptive responses. The subgroup analysis revealed that high loading intensities are more effective compared to low intensities to induce adaptive responses whereas the type muscle contraction seems irrelevant. This meta-analysis gives further evidence for the plasticity of human tendon mechanical, material, and morphological properties *in vivo* in response to chronic loading of various types. Moreover, the analysis showed that the adaptive response of the tendon to intervention-induced chronic mechanical loading might be more pronounced for the material compared to morphological properties.

The averaged effect size of the intervention-based changes of tendon stiffness was 0.70, featuring a significant overall effect of all included exercise interventions. Out of the 37 interventions that measured tendon stiffness, 26 showed SMDs above 0.5 (i.e., medium to large effects [64]). Therefore, the present meta-analysis emphasizes the adaptive potential of tendons to increased mechanical loading, which was quite consistently shown despite the marked variety of loading protocols. However, the significant heterogeneity of tendon stiffness changes between studies indicated that especially the different levels of the applied loading conditions (e.g., intensity, duration of single loading cycle, repetitions, sets, intervention duration, and training frequency per week) and general exercise conditions (e.g., type of muscle contraction (isometric, concentric, or eccentric) applied repetitively or statically, differences in joint angles that affect the tendon lever arm length and, thus, acting stress on the tendon) may considerably affect tendon adaptive responses. For example, Arampatzis et al. [28,29], Kongsgaard et al. [24], and Malliaras et al. [41] investigated the effect of the magnitude of the mechanical load by means of low and high muscle contraction intensities. The studies reported a significant increase of tendon stiffness solely following the training using the high contraction intensities (i.e., 90% MVC, 70% RM, 80% eccentric RM, respectively). The conducted subgroup analysis confirmed the importance of high tendon loading intensities for tendon adaptation. Analyzing the interventions that used muscle contraction intensities higher than 70% of MVC or RM and those using lower intensities revealed significantly different weighted averaged effect sizes of tendon stiffness of 0.90 and 0.04, respectively. No heterogeneity ($I^2 = 0\%$) between studies using high intensities was found. Furthermore, considering the high contraction intensity studies, the analysis further indicates that the effect of the type of muscle contraction was only minor (Table 2). The subgroups of either isometric, concentric-eccentric, or purely eccentric contraction type showed comparable (statistically insignificant) weighted averaged effect sizes of 0.95, 0.82, and 1.04, respectively. Therefore, we can argue that the level of tendon loading (in terms of muscle contraction intensity) determines the effect on tendon adaptation independent of the muscle contraction type, which may explain the lack of differences between the interventions using different muscle contraction types. This assumption is in accordance to reports from earlier *in vitro* studies, suggesting that loading intensity-related tendon cell deformation is an important stimulus that affects catabolic and/or anabolic cellular and molecular adaptive responses [65,66]. With increasing strain, a loss of collagen crimp and an increase in fiber recruitment was observed [67,68], which very likely results in an increased number of cells being deformed [69] inducing adaptive processes in an intensity-dependent manner [65,66,70].

Study	Stiffness				Young's modulus				CSA			
	SMD	-CI	+CI	W	SMD	-CI	+CI	W	SMD	-CI	+CI	W
Albracht et al., 2013 [15]	0.82	0.02	1.63	3.3%								
Arampatzis et al., 2007 [29]	0.36	-0.49	1.20	3.1%	-0.05	-0.88	0.79	6.4%	0.23	-0.61	1.07	3.3%
	1.52	0.55	2.49	3.0%	0.75	-0.12	1.62	6.3%	0.64	-0.22	1.50	3.3%
Arampatzis et al., 2010 [28]	-0.25	-1.09	0.59	3.1%	-0.19	-1.03	0.64	6.4%	0.08	-0.75	0.92	3.3%
	0.79	-0.09	1.66	2.6%	0.56	-0.30	1.41	6.2%	0.00	-0.84	0.84	3.2%
Bohm et al., [31]	0,66	-0,17	1,49	3.2%	0,55	-0,25	1,35	6.6%	0,36	-0,44	1,17	3.5%
	1,46	0,54	2,38	2.8%	1,28	0,41	2,16	6.2%	0,34	-0,47	1,15	3.5%
	0,67	-0,09	1,44	3.5%	0,54	-0,22	1,29	6.9%	0,14	-0,60	0,88	4.0%
	1,04	0,25	1,84	3.4%	1,04	0,25	1,84	6.6%	0,23	-0,52	0,97	4.0%
Carroll et al., 2011 [61]	0.99	-0.14	2.13	2.0%	1.42	0.20	2.64	4.4%	-0.19	-1.03	0.65	3.3%
Fletcher et al., 2010 [17]	0.66	-0.52	1.84	1.9%								
Fouré et al., 2009 [71]	0.12	-1.01	1.26	2.0%								
Foure et al., 2010a,b, 2011 [38,56,57]	0.48	-0.46	1.42	2.7%					0.08	-0.85	1.00	2.9%
Foure et al., 2013 [43]	0.39	-0.45	1.24	3.1%					-0.11	-0.95	0.73	3.3%
Hansen et al., 2003 [62]	0.63	-0.23	1.49	3.0%					0.00	-0.84	0.84	3.3%
Hougthon et al., 2013 [39]	-0.15	-1.20	0.90	2.3%	-0.36	-1.42	0.70	5.1%	1.12	-0.04	2.28	2.0%
Kongsgaard et al., 2007 [24]	1.33	0.43	2.22	2.9%	1.05	0.19	1.92	6.2%	0.33	-0.48	1.13	3.5%
	-0.8	-1.64	0.03	3.2%	-0.29	-1.09	0.52	6.6%	0.46	-0.36	1.27	3.6%
Kubo et al., 2001a,b [37,42]	0.54	-0.47	1.54	2.5%					0.16	-0.82	1.14	2.6%
	1.31	0.20	2.42	2.1%	4.45	2.42	6.47	2.2%	0.15	-0.84	1.13	2.6%
Kubo et al., 2002 [25]	0.8	-0.23	1.83	2.4%					-0.22	-1.21	0.76	2.6%
	0.94	-0.11	1.99	2.3%					0.21	-0.78	1.19	2.6%
Kubo et al., 2003 [63]	0.42	-0.43	1.27	3.1%								
Kubo et al., 2006a [40]	0.25	-0.68	1.17	2.7%					0.14	-0.79	1.06	2.9%
	1.17	0.15	2.18	2.4%					0.19	-0.74	1.12	2.8%
Kubo et al., 2006b [87]	-0.01	-0.99	0.97	2.5%					0.00	-0.98	0.98	2.6%
Kubo et al., 2006c [88]	0.2	-0.73	1.13	2.7%					0.00	-0.92	0.92	2.9%
Kubo et al., 2007 [59]	0.51	-0.38	1.41	2.9%					0.21	-0.67	1.09	3.1%
	1.01	0.07	1.96	2.7%					-0.12	-1.00	0.76	3.1%
Kubo et al., 2009 [60]	0.94	0.01	1.88	2.7%					0.25	-0.63	1.14	3.1%
	0.58	-0.32	1.48	2.9%					0.13	-0.75	1.01	3.1%
Kubo et al., 2010 [52]	1.12	0.04	2.20	2.2%					0.05	-0.93	1.03	2.6%
Kubo et al., 2012 [72]	3.17	1.68	4.66	1.3%					0.23	-0.70	1.16	2.8%
Malliaras et al., 2013 [41]	1.03	0.03	2.03	2.5%	1.22	0.19	2.24	5.3%	0.62	-0.33	1.57	2.7%
	0.78	-0.13	1.70	2.8%	0.75	-0.17	1.66	5.9%	0.32	-0.56	1.21	3.1%
	1.35	0.36	2.34	2.5%	1.25	0.28	2.23	5.6%	0.35	-0.53	1.24	3.1%
Seynnes et al., 2009 [30]	0.81	0.06	1.56	3.6%	0.57	-0.16	1.31	7.1%	3.89	2.62	5.17	1.7%
Weighted average effect size	0.70	0.51	0.88		0.69	0.36	1.03		0.24	0.07	0.42	
Test for overall effect	P < 0.00001				P < 0.0001				P = 0.006			
Heterogeneity	P = 0.05	I^2= 30%			P = 0.002	I^2= 57%			P = 0.14	I^2= 21%		

Forest plot

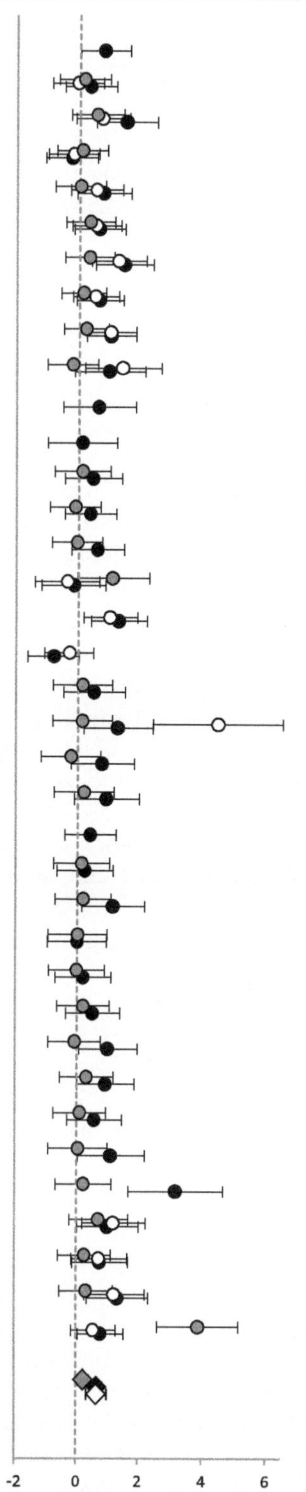

Figure 3 Forest plot for the meta-analysis of the effect of mechanical loading on tendon properties. Illustrated are the exercise intervention-induced changes on tendon stiffness (black), Young's modulus (white), and cross-sectional area (CSA, gray), respectively, featuring the single-study effect sizes (SMD, circles), the corresponding confidence intervals (CIs, error bars), and study weight in the overall comparison (W) as well as the respective weighted average effect sizes (random-effects model, diamonds) with the overall effect test and heterogeneity analysis.

However, several of the included studies evidenced that besides the magnitude of tendon loading additional loading and exercise conditions may affect tendon adaptation, e.g., loading frequency [28], loading rate [31], joint angle [40], loading duration [31,37,42], and repetitive vs. static loading [31,60].

Furthermore, the effect of plyometric training on tendon properties seems yet ambiguous, since the five plyometric training interventions [31,38,56,57,59,71] included in the present meta-analysis reported controversial results. The changes in tendon stiffness ranged from +28% [31] to −9% [39]. However, only the 27% increase reported by Foure et al. [38,56,57] reached statistical significance. The different jumping exercises, uncontrolled [38,39,43,56,71] or comparably low (40% RM [59]) tendon load magnitude, and dissimilar intervention durations (8 to 14 weeks) might be the reason for the inhomogeneous findings. Comparing dynamic (concentric-eccentric) and isometric training with plyometric training, Kubo et al. [59] and Bohm et al. [31] reported a statistically significant increase of Achilles tendon stiffness solely following the dynamic and isometric but not after the plyometric training. Bohm et al. [31] suggested that the short loading duration during jumping constrains the transduction of the mechanical stimulus to the cellular level due to the viscosity of the tendinous tissue and, therefore, may not be optimal to facilitate adaptive responses of the tendon.

In regard to the duration of the exercise intervention, several of the included studies featuring a duration of 8 weeks found significant adaptations of tendon stiffness [17,25,30], indicating that tendons already respond to increased mechanical loading within 2 months. Pooling the interventions featuring a high intensity with respect to the intervention duration in the subgroup analysis, the weighted average effect sizes of tendon stiffness were 0.91 for the interventions ($N = 23$) using longer durations (≥12 weeks) and 0.81 ($N = 4$) for the shorter ones (8 to 12 weeks) without a statistically significant difference. The present analysis showed that shorter intervention durations (8 to 12 weeks) may induce tendon adaptive responses; however, longer durations (≥12 weeks) seem to be more efficient, and their effect has been clearly demonstrated in many studies. For example, Kubo et al. [72,73] showed that within the time-course of training, Achilles and patellar tendon stiffness did not increase significantly after 2 months but reached statistical significance at the end of the 3-month training period.

The present meta-analysis solely included data of Achilles and patellar tendons. However, as to be expected, similar loading protocols on different types of tendons induced similar adaptive responses [58]. Therefore, evidence-based interventions that facilitate tendon adaptation should be applicable to various tendons and prove valuable in regard to athletic training as well as the therapy and prevention of tendon injuries.

Increases in tendon stiffness may be a result of either change in tendon material properties (i.e., Young's modulus) and/or tendon morphological properties (i.e., cross-sectional area and tendon rest length). Several studies reported increases in tendon CSA following training interventions [24,28-31]. However, it is feasible that no such reports exist for an exercise-induced change of tendon rest length, which hence can be excluded from being a relevant adaptive mechanism in response to increased mechanical loading. Regardless of the differences between the applied loading regimens, the averaged effect size for Young's modulus ($N = 17$) was 0.69 and for CSA 0.24 ($N = 33$). The overall intervention effect was significant for both Young's modulus and CSA, and the heterogeneity between studies was significant for Young's modulus and moderate for CSA. As averaged effect size of stiffness and Young's modulus were very similar and comparably higher as the CSA effect size, we can argue that the increase in stiffness may be primarily attributed to alterations of the material properties rather than morphological properties. Changes of the material properties were mentioned to be an early mechanism for increased stiffness, whereas tendon hypertrophy could be a long-term effect of mechanical loading [19,32]. Several studies included in the present meta-analysis found an increase in tendon Young's modulus following the exercise interventions without changes in the tendon CSA [26,28,42], supporting the assumption that material properties demonstrate greater plasticity and change more instantaneous in response to enhanced chronic mechanical loading. Taking into account that the average duration of all included interventions was 12.9 ± 4.5 weeks (two studies with longer durations than 14 weeks: running training [62] and low load resistance bodyweight training [63]), the reason for the small averaged effect size of CSA in contrast to the larger effects of Young's modulus may be the relatively short intervention durations. Yet, tendon hypertrophy could be more pronounced following longer periods of loading (i.e., habitual loading) compared to durations commonly used in exercise interventions.

Besides physiological adaptive responses of the tendon to increased mechanical loading in terms of a functional relevant improvement, excessive mechanical loading (i.e., overloading) was considered an important factor in the etiology of tendinopathy [20,34,35], which is characterized by activity-related pain, focal tendon tenderness, and decreased strength and flexibility [32]. It was suggested that repetitive strains, though below the failure threshold of the tendon, cause tendon micro-injuries and subsequently tendon inflammation, which may contribute to the development of tendon degeneration [22]. None of the

Study or Subgroup	Stiffness SMD	-CI	+CI	W
High intensity (N=27)				
Albracht et al., 2013 [15]	0.82	0.02	1.63	5.1%
Arampatzis et al., 2007 [29]	1.52	0.55	2.49	4.3%
Arampatzis et al., 2010 [28]	0.79	-0.09	1.66	3.5%
Bohm et al., [31]	0,66	-0,17	1,49	4.8%
	1,46	0,54	2,38	3.9%
	0,67	-0,09	1,44	5.6%
	1,04	0,25	1,84	5.2%
Carroll et al., 2011 [61]	0.99	-0.14	2.13	2.6%
Fletcher et al., 2010 [17]	0.66	-0.52	1.84	2.4%
Kongsgaard et al., 2007 [24]	1.33	0.43	2.22	4.1%
Kubo et al., 2001a,b [37,42]	0.54	-0.47	1.54	3.3%
	1.31	0.20	2.42	2.7%
Kubo et al., 2002 [25]	0.8	-0.23	1.83	3.1%
	0.94	-0.11	1.99	3.0%
Kubo et al., 2006a [40]	0.25	-0.68	1.17	3.8%
	1.17	0.15	2.18	3.2%
Kubo et al., 2006b [87]	-0.01	-0.99	0.97	3.4%
Kubo et al., 2006c [88]	0.2	-0.73	1.13	3.8%
Kubo et al., 2007 [59]	1.01	0.07	1.96	3.7%
Kubo et al., 2009 [60]	0.94	0.01	1.88	3.9%
	0.58	-0.32	1.48	4.1%
Kubo et al., 2010 [52]	1.12	0.04	2.20	2.8%
Kubo et al., 2012 [72]	3.17	1.68	4.66	1.5%
Malliaras et al., 2013 [41]	1.03	0.03	2.03	3.3%
	0.78	-0.13	1.70	3.9%
	1.35	0.36	2.34	3.3%
Seynnes et al., 2009 [30]	0.81	0.06	1.56	5.9%
Weighted average effect size	0.90	0.71	1.08	
Test for overall effect	P < 0.00001			
Heterogeneity	P = 0.56	I^2 = 0%		
Low intensity (N=5)				
Arampatzis et al., 2007 [29]	0.36	-0.49	1.20	20.3%
Arampatzis et al., 2010 [28]	-0.25	-1.09	0.59	20.2%
Kongsgaard et al., 2007 [24]	-0.80	-1.64	0.03	20.4%
Kubo et al., 2003 [63]	0.42	-0.43	1.27	20.1%
Kubo et al., 2007 [59]	0.51	-0.38	1.41	18.9%
Weighted average effect size	0.04	-0.46	0.53	
Test for overall effect	P = 0.88			
Heterogeneity	P = 0.15	I^2= 41%		

Forest plot

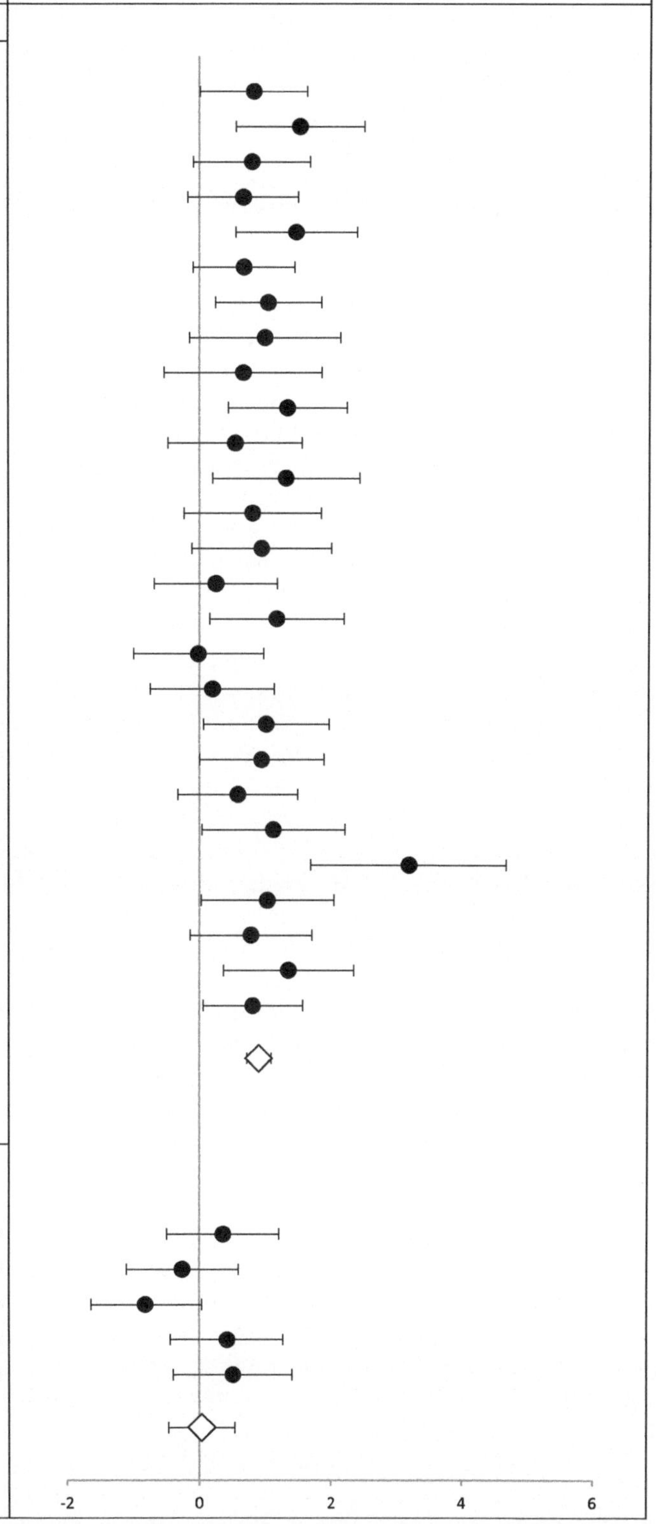

Figure 4 Forest plot for the meta-analysis of the effect of mechanical loading on tendon properties. Illustrated are the exercise intervention-induced changes on tendon stiffness (black), Young's modulus (white), and cross-sectional area (CSA, gray), respectively, featuring the single-study effect sizes (SMD, circles), the corresponding confidence intervals (CIs, error bars), and study weight in the overall comparison (W) as well as the respective weighted average effect sizes (random-effects model, diamonds) with the overall effect test and heterogeneity analysis.

included interventions reported a significant dropout of participants due to clinical symptoms of overloading. Nevertheless, adequate regeneration times and slower adaptation rates of tendon compared to muscle [72-74] should be considered in an exercise intervention to avoid episodes of high tendon strain and stress [75] that may cause maladaptation and tendon damage.

The appropriate investigation of tendon properties needs to include numerous methodological considerations. The total methodological quality score used in the present meta-analysis ranged from 61% to 99% with a mean of 71% ± 9%, indicating adequate to high methodological qualities for most studies and, thus, study validity. However, several aspects of the internal study validity (i.e., study design, methods, and cofactors) were not considered in every study. First, only 17 of the 37 included interventions reported the values of stiffness, Young's modulus, and CSA and, therewith, provided a complete examination of the adaptive processes of the mechanical, material, and morphological tendon properties and their interaction. Only about half (i.e., 19) of the interventions included a control group. To determine the tendon CSA, four studies (six interventions) used ultrasonographic images instead of MRI [76] for the manual segmentation, although the reliability for this method was reported to be poor [45]. However, advancements in the analysis of ultrasound signals (e.g., ultrasound tissue characterization) for the assessment of tendon dimensions are promising [77,78] and may be attractive for the detection of intervention-induced increases of tendon CSA in future studies. With regard to the measurement and calculation of the tendon force, tendon elongation, and CSA, not a single study considered all relevant methodological aspects (e.g., accounting for gravitational forces, axes misalignment of joint and dynamometer, averaging multiple trials to reliably assess tendon elongation, measuring the tendon moment arm directly), which affects the validity of the applied method. In consequence, the score for the internal validity was in average only 66% ± 15% (range: 49% to 98%). Considering the statistical validity, all studies applied appropriate statistical tests, but only two studies [31,39] calculated the effect size to estimate the effect of the intervention-induced tendon adaptations. Furthermore, there was a clear deficit in controlling and reporting all relevant loading conditions (e.g., intensity, duration of single loading cycle) [38,39,43,56,71], compromising the comparability of the results between interventions and their interpretations in regard to potential causalities. Nevertheless, a mean external validity score of 96 ± 4% (range 88% to 100%) indicated a high external validity of all included studies. Although already considered in most of the included studies, future investigations on tendon adaptation should account for these methodological quality criteria to ensure high study validity. The risk of bias assessment was difficult, since important information were not reported in most articles. In particular, details of the randomization process, concealment of allocation, and/or blinding of the assessor to the outcome data were missing in 34 of the 37 interventions, and therefore, the risk of bias judgment was inadequate for most included interventions. Only three studies [24,41,61] provided the necessary information, and the assessment indicated a low risk of bias. However, the judgment of the other domains (i.e., incomplete outcome data, selective outcome reporting, and other sources of bias) indicated a low risk of bias for almost every included study. Future investigations should account for an appropriate consideration and/or presentation of these aspects to allow for risk of bias estimation. Although the risk of bias assessment could not be performed adequately due to a lack of information, the overall assessment together with the methodological quality scale suggests an appropriate validity of the included studies. Furthermore, the funnel plot indicated a low risk of publication bias. Therefore, the outcome of the present meta-analysis provides profound evidence.

The current review and meta-analysis may feature some limitations in regard to the sample sizes, recruited participants, and durations of the included interventions. All included studies were performed on small sample sizes (6 to 15 participants), most likely due to the great study effort, and thus, conclusions with regard to a greater population based on solely one intervention should be drawn carefully. However, the present meta-analysis on recent literature confirmed the effects of chronic loading on the adaptation of mechanical, material, and morphological tendon properties. To a greater part, the included participants were male (237 of 264) and involved in recreational activity (approximately 164 of 264), which could have biased the generalizability of the study outcomes to a greater mixed-gender population with a different activity profile. Furthermore, the duration of 35 of the 37 included interventions was short term (≤14 weeks). However, longer durations may affect the adaptive responses of the separate tendon properties (material and morphological) in a different way. Moreover, the present meta-analysis only considered studies in the English language.

Conclusions

In conclusion, the present meta-analysis on the effect of chronic mechanical loading on human tendon adaptation *in vivo* included 27 studies featuring 37 separate exercise interventions. The meta-analysis showed that tendons are highly responsive to increased mechanical loading and adapt through changes of their mechanical, material, and morphological properties. Intervention-induced changes in tendon stiffness seem to be more attributed to adaptations of the material rather than morphological properties. Based on the results of the present meta-analysis, we can conclude that high magnitude loading (i.e., muscle contraction intensity) is most effective to elicit tendon adaptation and that longer intervention durations (>12 weeks) are beneficial compared to shorter ones. The effect of muscle contraction type (isometric, concentric-eccentric, or isometric) seems insignificant; however, the review suggests that plyometric training may not be optimal to facilitate tendon adaptation.

Competing interests

The authors declare that they have no competing interests.

Authors' contributions

SB conceived, designed and executed the systematic review and meta-analysis, contacted authors, interpreted the findings, and drafted and revised the article; FM executed the systematic review, interpreted the findings, and drafted and revised the article; AA conceived and designed the systematic review and meta-analysis, interpreted the findings, and drafted and revised the article. All authors read and approved the final manuscript.

Acknowledgements

No financial support was received for the conduct of this study or preparation of this manuscript.

References

1. Elliott DH. Structure and function of mammalian tendon. Biol Rev. 1965;40:392–421.
2. Magnusson SP, Narici MV, Maganaris CN, Kjaer M. Human tendon behaviour and adaptation, in vivo. J Physiol. 2008;586:71–81.
3. McNeill AR. Tendon elasticity and muscle function. Comp Biochem Physiol A Mol Integr Physiol. 2002;133:1001–11.
4. Alexander R. Energy-saving mechanisms in walking and running. J Exp Biol. 1991;160:55–69.
5. Fukunaga T, Kubo K, Kawakami Y, Fukashiro S, Kanehisa H, Maganaris CN. In vivo behaviour of human muscle tendon during walking. Proc R Soc B Biol Sci. 2001;268:229–33.
6. Ettema GJ, Huijing PA, van Ingen Schenau GJ, de Haan A. Effects of prestretch at the onset of stimulation on mechanical work output of rat medial gastrocnemius muscle-tendon complex. J Exp Biol. 1990;152:333–51.
7. Ettema GJ, van Soest AJ, Huijing PA. The role of series elastic structures in prestretch-induced work enhancement during isotonic and isokinetic contractions. J Exp Biol. 1990;154:121–36.
8. Kawakami Y, Muraoka T, Ito S, Kanehisa H, Fukunaga T. In vivo muscle fibre behaviour during counter-movement exercise in humans reveals a significant role for tendon elasticity. J Physiol Lond. 2002;540:635–46.
9. Lichtwark GA, Bougoulias K, Wilson AM. Muscle fascicle and series elastic element length changes along the length of the human gastrocnemius during walking and running. J Biomech. 2007;40:157–64.
10. Karamanidis K, Arampatzis A, Mademli L. Age-related deficit in dynamic stability control after forward falls is affected by muscle strength and tendon stiffness. J Electromyogr Kinesiol. 2008;18:980–9.
11. Kubo K, Ikebukuro T, Yata H, Tomita M, Okada M. Morphological and mechanical properties of muscle and tendon in highly trained sprinters. J Appl Biomech. 2011;27:336–44.
12. Stafilidis S, Arampatzis A. Muscle – tendon unit mechanical and morphological properties and sprint performance. J Sports Sci. 2007;25:1035–46.
13. Ishikawa M, Niemela E, Komi PV. Interaction between fascicle and tendinous tissues in short-contact stretch-shortening cycle exercise with varying eccentric intensities. J Appl Physiol. 2005;99:217–23.
14. Lichtwark GA, Wilson AM. In vivo mechanical properties of the human Achilles tendon during one-legged hopping. J Exp Biol. 2005;208:4715–25.
15. Albracht K, Arampatzis A. Exercise-induced changes in triceps surae tendon stiffness and muscle strength affect running economy in humans. Eur J Appl Physiol. 2013;113:1605–15.
16. Arampatzis A, De Monte G, Karamanidis K, Morey-Klapsing G, Stafilidis S, Brueggemann G-P. Influence of the muscle-tendon unit's mechanical and morphological properties on running economy. J Exp Biol. 2006;209:3345–57.
17. Fletcher JR, Esau SP, MacIntosh BR. Changes in tendon stiffness and running economy in highly trained distance runners. Eur J Appl Physiol. 2010;110:1037–46.
18. Galloway MT, Lalley AL, Shearn JT. The role of mechanical loading in tendon development, maintenance, injury, and repair. J Bone Joint Surg. 2013;95:1620–8.
19. Heinemeier KM, Kjaer M. In vivo investigation of tendon responses to mechanical loading. J Musculoskelet Neuronal Interact. 2011;11:115–23.
20. Kjaer M. Role of extracellular matrix in adaptation of tendon and skeletal muscle to mechanical loading. Physiol Rev. 2004;84:649–98.
21. Lavagnino M, Arnoczky SP. In vitro alterations in cytoskeletal tensional homeostasis control gene expression in tendon cells. J Orthop Res. 2005;23:1211–8.
22. Wang JH-C. Mechanobiology of tendon. J Biomech. 2006;39:1563–82.
23. Arampatzis A, Karamanidis K, Morey-Klapsing G, De Monte G, Stafilidis S. Mechanical properties of the triceps surae tendon and aponeurosis in relation to intensity of sport activity. J Biomech. 2007;40:1946–52.
24. Kongsgaard M, Reitelseder S, Pedersen TG, Holm L, Aagaard P, Kjaer M. Region specific patellar tendon hypertrophy in humans following resistance training. Acta Physiol. 2007;191:111–21.
25. Kubo K, Kanehisa H, Fukunaga T. Effects of resistance and stretching training programmes on the viscoelastic properties of human tendon structures in vivo. J Physiol. 2002;538:219–26.
26. Reeves ND, Maganaris CN, Narici MV. Effect of strength training on human patella tendon mechanical properties of older individuals. J Physiol Lond. 2003;548:971–81.
27. LaCroix AS, Duenwald-Kuehl SE, Lakes RS, Vanderby Jr R. Relationship between tendon stiffness and failure: a metaanalysis. J Appl Physiol (Bethesda Md: 1985). 2013;115:43–51.
28. Arampatzis A, Peper A, Bierbaum S, Albracht K. Plasticity of human Achilles tendon mechanical and morphological properties in response to cyclic strain. J Biomech. 2010;43:3073–9.
29. Arampatzis A, Karamanidis K, Albracht K. Adaptational responses of the human Achilles tendon by modulation of the applied cyclic strain magnitude. J Exp Biol. 2007;210:2743–53.
30. Seynnes OR, Erskine RM, Maganaris CN, Longo S, Simoneau EM, Grosset JF. Training-induced changes in structural and mechanical properties of the patellar tendon are related to muscle hypertrophy but not to strength gains. J Appl Physiol (Bethesda, Md: 1985). 2009;107:523–30.
31. Bohm S, Mersmann F, Tettke M, Kraft M, Arampatzis A. Human Achilles tendon plasticity in response to cyclic strain: effect of rate and duration. J. Exp. Biol. 2014. doi:10.1242/jeb.112268.
32. Kjaer M, Langberg H, Heinemeier K, Bayer ML, Hansen M, Holm L. From mechanical loading to collagen synthesis, structural changes and function in human tendon. Scand J Med Sci Sports. 2009;19:500–10.
33. Miller BF, Olesen JL, Hansen M, Døssing S, Crameri RM, Welling RJ. Coordinated collagen and muscle protein synthesis in human patella tendon and quadriceps muscle after exercise. J Physiol. 2005;567:1021–33.
34. Wang JH-C, Guo O, Li B. Tendon biomechanics and mechanobiology—a minireview of basic concepts and recent advancements. J Hand Ther. 2012;25:133–41.
35. Magnan B, Bondi M, Pierantoni S, Samaila E. The pathogenesis of Achilles tendinopathy: a systematic review. Foot Ankle Surg. 2014;20:154–9.
36. Arampatzis A, Karamanidis K, Mademli L, Albracht K. Plasticity of the human tendon to short- and long-term mechanical loading. Exerc Sport Sci Rev. 2009;37:66–72.
37. Kubo K, Kanehisa H, Ito M, Fukunaga T. Effects of isometric training on the elasticity of human tendon structures in vivo. J Appl Physiol. 2001;91:26–32.
38. Foure A, Nordez A, Cornu C. Effects of plyometric training on plantar flexor mechanical properties. Comput Methods Biomech Biomed Engin. 2010;13:57–9.

39. Houghton LA, Dawson BT, Rubenson J. Effects of plyometric training on Achilles tendon properties and shuttle running during a simulated cricket batting innings. J Strength Cond Res. 2013;27:1036–46.
40. Kubo K, Ohgo K, Takeishi R, Yoshinaga K, Tsunoda N, Kanehisa H. Effects of isometric training at different knee angles on the muscle-tendon complex in vivo. Scand J Med Sci Sports. 2006;16:159–67.
41. Malliaras P, Kamal B, Nowell A, Farley T, Dhamu H, Simpson V. Patellar tendon adaptation in relation to load-intensity and contraction type. J Biomech. 2013;46:1893–9.
42. Kubo K, Kanehisa H, Fukunaga T. Effects of different duration isometric contractions on tendon elasticity in human quadriceps muscles. J Physiol. 2001;536:649–55.
43. Foure A, Nordez A, Cornu C. Effects of eccentric training on mechanical properties of the plantar flexor muscle-tendon complex. J Appl Physiol. 2013;114:523–37.
44. Urlando A, Hawkins D. Achilles tendon adaptation during strength training in young adults. Med Sci Sports Exerc. 2007;39:1147–52.
45. Ekizos A, Papatzika F, Charcharis G, Bohm S, Mersmann F, Arampatzis A. Ultrasound does not provide reliable results for the measurement of the patellar tendon cross sectional area. J Electromyogr Kinesiol Off J Int Soc Electrophysiol Kinesiol. 2013;23:1278–82.
46. Higgins JPT, Green S (editors). Cochrane Handbook for Systematic Reviews of Interventions Version 5.1.0 [updated March 2011]. The Cochrane Collaboration, 2011. Available from www.cochrane-handbook.org.
47. Deeks JJ, Higgins JPT, Altman DG (editors). Chapter 9: Analysing data and undertaking meta-analyses. In: Higgins JPT, Green S (editors). Cochrane Handbook for Systematic Reviews of Interventions Version 5.1.0 (updated March 2011). The Cochrane Collaboration, 2011. Available from www.cochrane-handbook.org.
48. Cooper H. Research synthesis and meta-analysis: a step-by-step approach. 4th ed. Thousand Oaks. Sage Publications, Inc; 2010.
49. Deeks JJ, Altman DG, Bradburn MJ. Statistical methods for examining heterogeneity and combining results from several studies in meta-analysis. In: Egger M, Smith GD, Altman DG, editors. Systematic reviews in healthcare. BMJ Publishing Group; Chichester: UK, 2001. p. 285–312.
50. Higgins JPT, Thompson SG, Deeks JJ, Altman DG. Measuring inconsistency in meta-analyses. BMJ. 2003;327:557–60.
51. The Cochrane Collaboration. Review Manager (RevMan). Copenhagen: The Nordic Cochrane Centre; 2012.
52. Kubo K, Tabata T, Ikebukuro T, Igarashi K, Tsunoda N. A longitudinal assessment of running economy and tendon properties in long-distance runners. J Strength Cond Res Natl Strength Cond Assoc. 2010;24:1724–31.
53. Milgrom Y, Milgrom C, Altaras T, Globus O, Zeltzer E, Finestone AS. Achilles tendons hypertrophy in response to high loading training. Foot Ankle Int. 2014. doi:10.1177/1071100714550651.
54. Bloomquist K, Langberg H, Karlsen S, Madsgaard S, Boesen M, Raastad T. Effect of range of motion in heavy load squatting on muscle and tendon adaptations. Eur J Appl Physiol. 2013;113:2133–42.
55. Farup J, Rahbek SK, Vendelbo MH, Matzon A, Hindhede J, Bejder A. Whey protein hydrolysate augments tendon and muscle hypertrophy independent of resistance exercise contraction mode. Scand J Med Sci Sports. 2014;24:788–98.
56. Foure A, Nordez A, Cornu C. Plyometric training effects on Achilles tendon stiffness and dissipative properties. J Appl Physiol. 2010;109:849–54.
57. Foure A, Nordez A, McNair P, Cornu C. Effects of plyometric training on both active and passive parts of the plantarflexors series elastic component stiffness of muscle-tendon complex. Eur J Appl Physiol. 2011;111:539–48.
58. Kubo K, Ikebukuro T, Yata H, Tsunoda N, Kanehisa H. Effects of training on muscle and tendon in knee extensors and plantar flexors in vivo. J Appl Biomech. 2010;26:316–23.
59. Kubo K, Morimoto M, Komuro T, Yata H, Tsunoda N, Kanehisa H. Effects of plyometric and weight training on muscle-tendon complex and jump performance. Med Sci Sports Exerc. 2007;39:1801–10.
60. Kubo K, Ikebukuro T, Yaeshima K, Yata H, Tsunoda N, Kanehisa H. Effects of static and dynamic training on the stiffness and blood volume of tendon in vivo. J Appl Physiol (Bethesda Md: 1985). 2009;106:412–7.
61. Carroll CC, Dickinson JM, LeMoine JK, Haus JM, Weinheimer EM, Hollon CJ. Influence of acetaminophen and ibuprofen on in vivo patellar tendon adaptations to knee extensor resistance exercise in older adults. J Appl Physiol (Bethesda Md: 1985). 2011;111:508–15.
62. Hansen P, Aagaard P, Kjaer M, Larsson B, Magnusson SP. Effect of habitual running on human Achilles tendon load-deformation properties and cross-sectional area. J Appl Physiol. 2003;95:2375–80.
63. Kubo K, Kanehisa H, Miyatani M, Tachi M, Fukunaga T. Effect of low-load resistance training on the tendon properties in middle-aged and elderly women. Acta Physiol Scand. 2003;178:25–32.
64. Cohen J. Statistical power analysis for the behavioral sciences. Psychology Press; Hillsdale, New Jersey: US, 1988.
65. Arnoczky SP, Tian T, Lavagnino M, Gardner K. Ex vivo static tensile loading inhibits MMP-1 expression in rat tail tendon cells through a cytoskeletally based mechanotransduction mechanism. J Orthop Res Off Publ Orthop Res Soc. 2004;22:328–33.
66. Lavagnino M, Arnoczky SP, Tian T, Vaupel Z. Effect of amplitude and frequency of cyclic tensile strain on the inhibition of MMP-1 mRNA expression in tendon cells: an in vitro study. Connect Tissue Res. 2003;44:181–7.
67. Hansen KA, Weiss JA, Barton JK. Recruitment of tendon crimp with applied tensile strain. J Biomech Eng Trans Asme. 2002;124:72–7.
68. Schatzmann L, Brunner P, Stäubli HU. Effect of cyclic preconditioning on the tensile properties of human quadriceps tendons and patellar ligaments. Knee Surg Sports Traumatol Arthrosc Off J ESSKA. 1998;6 Suppl 1:S56–61.
69. Arnoczky SP, Tian T, Lavagnino M, Gardner K, Schuler P, Morse P. Activation of stress-activated protein kinases (SAPK) in tendon cells following cyclic strain: the effects of strain frequency, strain magnitude, and cytosolic calcium. J Orthop Res Off Publ Orthop Res Soc. 2002;20:947–52.
70. Lavagnino M, Arnoczky SP, Kepich E, Caballero O, Haut RC. A finite element model predicts the mechanotransduction response of tendon cells to cyclic tensile loading. Biomech Model Mechanobiol. 2008;7:405–16.
71. Fouré A, Nordez A, Guette M, Cornu C. Effects of plyometric training on passive stiffness of gastrocnemii and the musculo-articular complex of the ankle joint. Scand J Med Sci Sports. 2009;19:811–8.
72. Kubo K, Ikebukuro T, Maki A, Yata H, Tsunoda N. Time course of changes in the human Achilles tendon properties and metabolism during training and detraining in vivo. Eur J Appl Physiol. 2012;112:2679–91.
73. Kubo K, Ikebukuro T, Yata H, Tsunoda N, Kanehisa H. Time course of changes in muscle and tendon properties during strength training and detraining. J Strength Cond Res. 2010;24:322–31.
74. de Boer MD, Maganaris CN, Seynnes OR, Rennie MJ, Narici MV. Time course of muscular, neural and tendinous adaptations to 23 day unilateral lower-limb suspension in young men. J Physiol. 2007;583:1079–91.
75. Mersmann F, Bohm S, Schroll A, Boeth H, Duda G, Arampatzis A. Evidence of imbalanced adaptation between muscle and tendon in adolescent athletes. Scand J Med Sci Sports. 2014;24:e283–9.
76. Couppé C, Svensson RB, Sødring-Elbrønd V, Hansen P, Kjaer M, Magnusson SP. Accuracy of MRI technique in measuring tendon cross-sectional area. Clin Physiol Funct Imaging. 2014;34:237–41.
77. Noble JA. Ultrasound image segmentation and tissue characterization. Proc Inst Mech Eng Part H-J Eng Med. 2010;224:307–16.
78. Van Schie HTM, de Vos RJ, de Jonge S, Bakker EM, Heijboer MP, Verhaar JA. Ultrasonographic tissue characterisation of human Achilles tendons: quantification of tendon structure through a novel non-invasive approach. Br J Sports Med. 2010;44:1153–9.
79. Kongsgaard M, Nielsen CH, Hegnsvad S, Aagaard P, Magnusson SP. Mechanical properties of the human Achilles tendon, in vivo. Clin Biomech. 2011;26:772–7.
80. Arampatzis A, Morey-Klapsing G, Karamanidis K, DeMonte G, Stafilidis S, Brüggemann G-P. Differences between measured and resultant joint moments during isometric contractions at the ankle joint. J Biomech. 2005;38:885–92.
81. Arampatzis A, Karamanidis K, De Monte G, Stafilidis S, Morey-Klapsing G, Brüggemann G-P. Differences between measured and resultant joint moments during voluntary and artificially elicited isometric knee extension contractions. Clin Biomech (Bristol, Avon). 2004;19:277–83.
82. Arampatzis A, Stafilidis S, DeMonte G, Karamanidis K, Morey-Klapsing G, Brüggemann GP. Strain and elongation of the human gastrocnemius tendon and aponeurosis during maximal plantarflexion effort. J Biomech. 2005;38:833–41.
83. Mademli L, Arampatzis A, Morey-Klapsing G, Brüggemann G-P. Effect of ankle joint position and electrode placement on the estimation of the antagonistic moment during maximal plantarflexion. J Electromyogr Kinesiol. 2004;14:591–7.
84. Magnusson SP, Aagaard P, Dyhre-Poulsen P, Kjaer M. Load-displacement properties of the human triceps surae aponeurosis in vivo. J Physiol. 2001;531:277–88.

85. Arampatzis A, Monte GD, Karamanidis K. Effect of joint rotation correction when measuring elongation of the gastrocnemius medialis tendon and aponeurosis. J Electromyogr Kinesiol Off J Int Soc Electrophysiol Kinesiol. 2008;18:503–8.
86. Schulze F, Mersmann F, Bohm S, Arampatzis A. A wide number of trials is required to achieve acceptable reliability for measurement patellar tendon elongation in vivo. Gait Posture. 2012;35:334–8.
87. Kubo K, Yata H, Kanehisa H, Fukunaga T. Effects of isometric squat training on the tendon stiffness and jump performance. Eur J Appl Physiol. 2006;96:305–14.
88. Kubo K, Komuro T, Ishiguro N, Tsunoda N, Sato Y, Ishii N. Effects of low-load resistance training with vascular occlusion on the mechanical properties of muscle and tendon. J Appl Biomech. 2006;22:112–9.

12

The Impact of Gastrointestinal Symptoms and Dermatological Injuries on Nutritional Intake and Hydration Status During Ultramarathon Events

Ricardo J. S. Costa[1*], Rhiannon Snipe[1], Vera Camões-Costa[1], Volker Scheer[2] and Andrew Murray[3]

Abstract

Background: Debilitating gastrointestinal symptoms (GIS) and dermatological injuries (DI) are common during and after endurance events and have been linked to performance decrements, event withdrawal, and issues requiring medical attention. The study aimed to determine whether GIS and DI affect food and fluid intake, and nutritional and hydration status, of ultramarathon runners during multi-stage (MSUM) and 24-h continuous (24 h) ultramarathons.

Methods: Ad libitum food and fluid intakes of ultramarathon runners (MSUM $n = 54$; 24 h $n = 22$) were recorded throughout both events and analysed by dietary analysis software. Body mass and urinary ketones were determined, and blood samples were taken, before and immediately after running. A medical log was used to monitor symptoms and injuries throughout both events.

Results: GIS were reported by 85 and 73 % of ultramarathon runners throughout MSUM and 24 h, respectively. GIS during MSUM were associated with reduced total daily, during, and post-stage energy and macronutrient intakes ($p < 0.05$), whereas GIS during 24 h did not alter nutritional variables. Throughout the MSUM 89 % of ultramarathon runners reported DI. DI during MSUM were associated with reduced carbohydrate ($p < 0.05$) intake during running and protein intake post-stage ($p < 0.05$). DI during 24 h were low; thus, comparative analyses were not possible. Daily, during running, and post-stage energy, macronutrient and water intake variables were observed to be lower with severity of GIS and DI ($p < 0.05$) throughout the MSUM only.

Conclusions: GIS during the MSUM, but not the 24 h, compromised nutritional intake. DI presence and severity also compromised nutrient intake during running and recovery in the MSUM.

Key Points

- Gastrointestinal symptoms (GIS) were a common feature in both the MSUM and 24 h; however, dermatological injuries (DI) were high during the MSUM, but relatively low during the 24 h.
- Incidence and severity of GIS appeared to be associated with greater disturbances to daily energy balance, reduced daily macronutrient intake, and reduced nutritional intake during running and recovery throughout the MSUM, but not the 24 h.
- Incidence and severity of DI appeared to be associated with reduced nutritional intake during running and recovery throughout the MSUM.

* Correspondence: ricardo.costa@monash.edu
[1]Department of Nutrition & Dietetics, Monash University, Notting Hill, Victoria, Australia
Full list of author information is available at the end of the article

Background

Ultramarathon running events (>42.195 km) have increased in popularity over the past decade [1] and are predicted for future growth within recreational endurance sports participation. Despite popularity, research into the demands of such an extreme sport is scarce in comparison to shorter endurance running events (e.g. marathon and sub-marathon) [2]. Participation in ultra-endurance events often requires competitors to perform loaded prolonged physical exertion, sleep rough on consecutive days, and manage food and fluid provisions throughout competition to maintain performance and avoid adverse health outcomes [3, 4]. Such diverse challenges demonstrates the uniqueness of extreme endurance sports and highlights areas for potential performance decrements and health issues to exacerbate.

Extreme energy deficits are a common feature of continuous and multi-stage ultramarathon running events and have been associated with poor recovery quality and sustained fatigue [5, 6]. Development of unintentional symptoms (e.g. gastrointestinal) and injury (e.g. dermatological) may limit total food and fluid intake during consecutive days of exertional stress with and without the additional impact of environmental extremes [3, 7]. Moreover, sub-optimal nutrition and hydration during periods of extreme exertion is clinically relevant, having been implicated in exacerbating exercise-induced immunodepression, impaired repair and healing, cytokine dysfunction associated with chronic fatigue, rapid onset microcytic anaemia, exercise-induced rhabdomyolysis, and exertional heat illnesses [3, 8–13].

Gastrointestinal symptoms (GIS) are a common feature of endurance sports and appear to be more pronounced in running compared to other exercise modes [14] and greater in a dehydrated state compared with a euhydrated state [15]. Indeed, 93 % of a participant cohort reported GIS during a long distance triathlon event, with upper-GIS (e.g. belching, bloating, and vomiting) and nausea reported to predominate [16]; whereas 60 % of ultramarathon runners during a continuous 161-km ultramarathon reported upper- (e.g. vomiting) and lower (e.g. abdominal cramps and diarrhoea)-GIS, with 89 % of participants with symptoms also reporting nausea [17]. Gastrointestinal symptoms (e.g. nausea and vomiting) have also been reported to be a key contributing factor in performance decrements and event withdrawal during ultramarathon running competition [18, 19].

The causes of GIS during prolonged exertion are multi-factorial in origin. Splanchnic hypoperfusion, ischaemia, alterations to intestinal motility, and mechanical trauma appear to play a key role [15, 20, 21]. When exertion is performed in hot environmental conditions (>30 °C), enhanced thermoregulatory strain, increased body water losses, and accompanying hypovolaemia promote further splanchnic hypoperfusion, ischaemia, and disruption of intestinal epithelial integrity [22–24]. Such perturbations have been linked to increased epithelial permeability of bacterial endotoxins, originating from the intestinal microbiota, leading to endotoxaemia and subsequent responsive cytokinaemia [25, 26], in which nausea is a common feature. Moreover, nausea and (or) vomiting has also been reported during episodes of heat illness [27], asymptomatic and symptomatic exercise-associated hyponatremia (with or without encephalopathy) [28, 29], and may occur if ultramarathon runners attempt to meet high energy and water demands through constant forced feeding and stimulation of the ileal brake [30].

Dermatological injuries (DI) (e.g. blisters, subungual haematoma, chafing, abrasions, and sunburn) are also a common feature of endurance sports [4, 31–33]. Dermatological injuries account for the greatest number of medical interventions and event withdrawals during multi-stage ultramarathon events [7, 33, 34] and the prime factor to adversely affect performance in continuous ultramarathon competition [18, 35]. The main causes of such injuries are excessive frictional forces and surface exposure, which are exacerbated by heat, poorly-fitted clothing and equipment, carrying load, and individual characteristics (i.e. skin surface roughness) [33, 36]. An anecdotal observational case scenario from the seven-stages 245 km 2008 Marathon des Sables indicated that all members ($n = 6$) of tent 96 developed foot injuries by stage 2, with injury numbers and severity increasing thereafter. All members reported investing a substantial amount of time with injury care and pain management (i.e. 2–3 h during recovery; including self-management, awaiting and receiving medical attention), deterring focus and priority away from scheduled feeding regimes, and potentially creating a barrier towards meeting high nutritional and hydration requirement, which can substantially effect running performance.

To date, the impact of GIS and DI on nutritional intake and hydration status during continuous ultramarathon events longer than 161 km, and multi-stage ultramarathon events, has not been thoroughly investigated. The purpose of this study was to determine whether GIS or DI affects food and fluid intake, and nutrition and hydration status, of ultramarathon runners during a multi-stage ultramarathon and a 24-h continuous ultramarathon.

Methods

Ultramarathon Events and Participants

The multi-stage ultramarathon (MSUM) component of the study was conducted during the 2010 and 2011 Al Andalus Ultimate Trail (*www.alandalus-ut.com*), held during the second week of July, in the region of Loja, Spain (Table 1). The 24-h continuous ultramarathon (24 h) component of the study was conducted during the 2011 and 2012 Glenmore24 Trail Race (*http://runyabam.com/glenmore-24/*), held during the first week of September, in the Cairngorms National Park, Scottish Highlands, UK.

After ethical approval from the University Ethics Committee that conforms with the Helsinki declaration for human research ethics, 74 out of 134 ultramarathon

Table 1 Participant and event characteristics of the multi-stage (MSUM) and 24-h continuous (24 h) ultramarathons

	MSUM	24 h
Participant characteristics		
Total (*n*)	54	22
Male	33	16
Female	21	6
Age (year)	40 ± 8	40 ± 7
Height (m)	171 ± 15	177 ± 8
Body mass (kg)	70 ± 11	78 ± 11
Number of previous ultramarathon events	5 ± 7	16 ± 13
Ultramarathon characteristics		
Distance (km)	total 225	range 122 to 208
Ambient temperature (°C)	range 32 to 40	range 0 to 20
Relative humidity (% range)	range 32 to 40	range 54 to 82
Altitude (m)	range 473 to 1443	range 39 to 645
Course description	Off-road trails and paths, steep and narrow mountain passes, and occasional road	Off-road terrains, including trails, paths, and grasslands

Mean ± SD (otherwise specified)

runners entered in the MSUM event, and 25 out of 48 ultramarathon runners entered in the 24 h event provided informed consent to participate in the study. However, complete gastrointestinal and dermatological profiles and nutritional and hydration variables were obtained in $n = 54$ and $n = 22$ for the MSUM and 24 h events, respectively (Table 1). Only participants who presented complete gastrointestinal and dermatological profiles and nutritional and hydration variables were used in comparative data analysis.

Study Design and Data Collection

Both ultramarathons were self-sufficient, whereby participants planned and provided their own ad libitum foods and fluids along the duration of the events. Only plain water was provided by the race organisers. Aid stations along the running course were situated approximately 10 and 3 km apart for the MSUM and 24 h, respectively. For the MSUM, estimated total daily energy expenditure was calculated through predictive equations [37] and verified through SenseWear (7.0, BodyMedia Inc., Pittsburgh, PA, USA) in a sub-sample of ultramarathon runners using convenience sampling (22 verifications, coefficient of variation 5.6 %), as previously used to guide sports dietetic support during MSUM competition [38]. For the 24 h, estimated total energy expenditure was determined by SenseWear in all participants. The triaxial accelerometry, which also included measurements of heat flux, skin temperature, and galvanic skin responses, was attached firmly to the upper arm of the participants, over the mid-point of the triceps muscle, during the measurement period. Data were processed using proprietary algorithms available in the software (version 7.0, algorithm version 2.2.4).

Before the start of each event (and each stage of the MSUM), participants were asked to provide a mid-flow urine sample into 30 ml universal tubes, followed by body mass and height measurements. Participants were then required to sit for 10 min before blood sampling. Whole blood samples were collected by venepuncture without venostasis from an antecubital vein using a 21G butterfly syringe into one lithium heparin (6 ml, 1.5 IU/ml heparin; Becton Dickinson, Oxford, UK) and one K_3EDTA (6 ml, 1.6 mg/ml of K_3EDTA; Becton Dickinson, Oxford, UK) vacutainer tube. Blood samples were immediately centrifuged and plasma aliquoted into eppendorfs and stored frozen initially at −20 °C during the ultramarathon events in a sterile field laboratory setup, prior to transferring to −80 °C storage after completion of the experimental procedure. Immediately after event completion (and each stage of the MSUM), blood samples were collected, followed by a mid-flow urine sample at the earliest convenience.

At the end of each competition day on stages 1 to 4 in the MSUM, and within the hour after event completion in the 24 h, trained researchers conducted a standardised interview on participants and support crews to ascertain all foods and fluids ingested, symptoms, and injuries. To improve dietary recording accuracy, before competition, participants and their support crews were educated and instructed to record in detail all foods and fluids ingested during the competition period (i.e. pre, during, immediately post (within 1 h of cessation), and rest periods, as per MSUM and 24 h relevance) in real time. Additionally, participants and support crews were instructed to keep food and beverage packaging of all foods and fluids consumed, which were collected by researchers.

Gastrointestinal symptoms and DI were explored through a symptomology tool and a medical log with physician verification. A Likert-type rating scale was used to quantify GIS, whereby symptoms were classified as indicated by ≥50 mm on a standard 100 mm visual analogue scale, with 0 mm indicative of no symptoms to 100 mm indicative of extreme symptoms resulting in event withdrawal. Severity of GIS was classified as low, moderate, and high based on the incidence of GIS reported (1 GIS, 2–3 GIS, and ≥4 GIS; respectively).

Dermatological injuries were classified through visual identification. Severity of DI was also classified as low, moderate, and high based on the reported incidence of DI, the level of self-management and (or) medical intervention by the medical crew the injury received, associated pain severity (0 = no pain, 1 = minimal pain, 2 = mild pain, 3 = moderate pain, 4 = severe pain, and 5 = elimination from event), and evidence of established and progressive infection and inflammation through physician verification. Additionally, to determine carbohydrate adequacy, urine reagent strips (10SG urinalysis strips, Siemans Healthcare Diagnostic, NY, USA) were used to identify urinary ketones (i.e. acetoacetic acid) in pre- and post-running urine samples [12].

Dietary Analysis

Food and fluid ingestion records from both ultramarathon events were used to calculate energy, nutrient, and water intake variables through Dietplan6 dietary analysis software (v.6.60, Forestfield Software, Horsham, West Sussex, UK). To improve the validity of the dietary analysis, all the nutritional information gathered from food and beverage packages were entered into the dietary analysis software program. In addition, to improve the reliability of the dietary analysis, all the completed dietary interview logs were blindly analysed by a second-trained researcher.

Assessment of Hydration Status

Pre- and post-running plasma osmolality (P_{Osmol}) was determined from 50 μl lithium heparin plasma samples in duplicate by freezepoint osmometry (Osmomat 030, Gonotec, Germany), as recommended previously [39]. Whole blood K_3EDTA samples were used to determine haemoglobin concentration and haematocrit through a cell counter (Coulter ACT Diff, Beckham Coulter, USA), which were subsequently used to estimate changes in plasma volume (P_V) relative to pre-competition values [40].

Data Analysis

Data in the text, tables, and figures are presented as mean value ± standard deviation (SD), unless otherwise specified. Considering the potential influence of individual body mass differences on dietary intake variables, data analysis was performed on total values and adjusted for body mass [5, 6, 41]. Diagnostic checks (Shapiro–Wilks test of normality and Levene's homogeneity of variance test) were performed before applying parametric statistics (SPSS v.22, IL, US). One-way ANOVA (or Kruskal–Wallis one-way) was applied to determine stage differences in GIS and DI incidence and impact of severity of symptoms and injuries on dependant variables. Significant main effects were analysed using post hoc Tukey's HSD test. Independent-sample *t* test (or Mann–Whitney *U* test) was applied to determine dependant variable differences between groups (GIS and DI), including sub-group comparisons (running speed (slow ultramarathon runners: average speed <8 km/h and fast ultramarathon runners: average speed ≥8 km/h) and sexes). Significance was accepted at $p < 0.05$.

Results

Gastrointestinal Symptoms

Gastrointestinal symptoms were a common feature during the MSUM, with 85 % of the study cohort presenting at least one GIS along the event (Fig. 1a). No statistically significant differences in GIS incidence or severity were observed between stages. No significant difference in GIS were observed between sexes. However, male ultramarathon runners reported greater occurrence ($p = 0.04$) of diarrhoea along the MSUM. Despite the presence of GIS being associated with a slower time to completion (28 h 43 min ± 4 h 32 min; 7.9 ± 1.3 km/h) compare with no-GIS (25 h 52 min ± 4 h 12 min; 8.9 ± 1.3 km/h), no significant difference in GIS was observed for running speed.

Gastrointestinal symptoms were a common feature during the 24 h, with 73 % of the study cohort presenting at least one GIS during the event (Fig. 1b). No significant differences in GIS were observed between sexes. Gastrointestinal symptoms were greater in fast (2.5-fold) compared with slow ultramarathon runners ($p < 0.01$). Fast ultramarathon runners reported greater occurrence of urge to vomit ($p = 0.04$), vomiting ($p = 0.04$), belching ($p = 0.04$), and diarrhoea ($p = 0.04$) compared with slow ultramarathon runners. On the contrary to the MSUM, the presence of GIS was not associated with a lower distance covered over the 24 h (166 ± 28 km; 6.9 ± 1.2 km/h) compare with no-GIS (139 ± 15 km; 5.8 ± 0.6 km/h).

Dermatological Injuries

Throughout the MSUM, 89 % of participants presented at least one DI, irrespective of severity. However, 76 % of participants required self-management and (or) sought (and received) medical intervention for DI. The incidence ($p < 0.01$) and severity ($p < 0.01$) of DI significantly increased as the MSUM progressed. No significant difference in DI incidence was observed between sexes and running speed. However, the presence of DI were associated within a slower time to completion (29 h 03 min ± 4 h 39 min; 7.8 ± 1.3 km/h) compare with no-DI (26 h 38 min ± 4h39min; 8.7 ± 1.3 km/h). Dermatological injuries that required self-management and (or) medical attention during the 24 h was low (14 %); thus, comparative analyses on intake and status variables were not possible (Fig. 2).

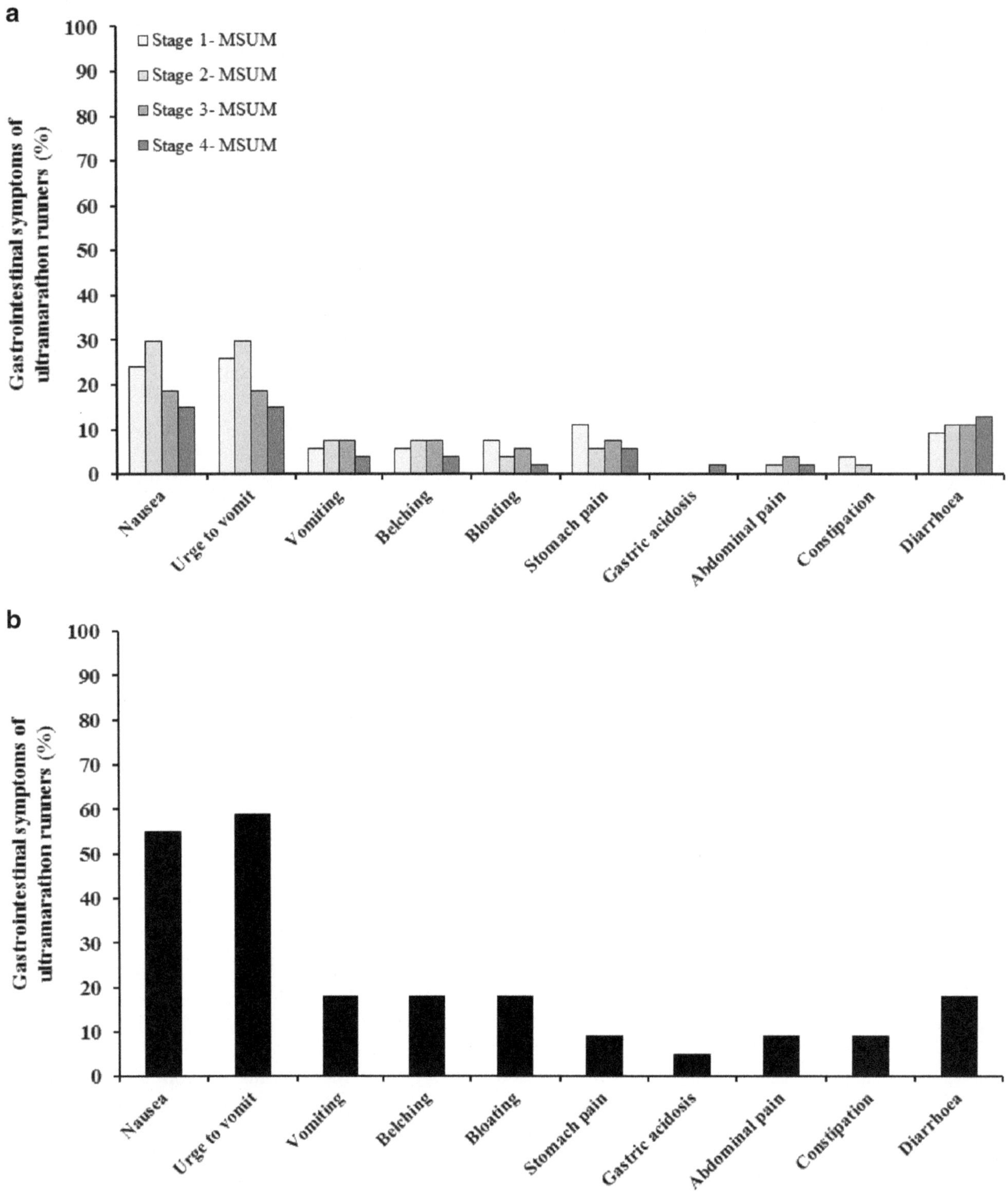

Fig. 1 Gastrointestinal symptoms of ultramarathon runners during a multi-stage ultramarathon (**a**) and a 24-h continuous ultramarathon (**b**) (MSUM $n = 54$ and 24 h $n = 22$)

Hydration Status

No statistically significant difference in pre- and post-stage P_{Osmol} (coefficient of variation: 3.5 %) was observed between participants presenting GIS and no-GIS in the MSUM (overall mean 286 ± 8 mOsmol/kg) and the 24 h (overall mean 286 ± 11 mOsmol/kg) and

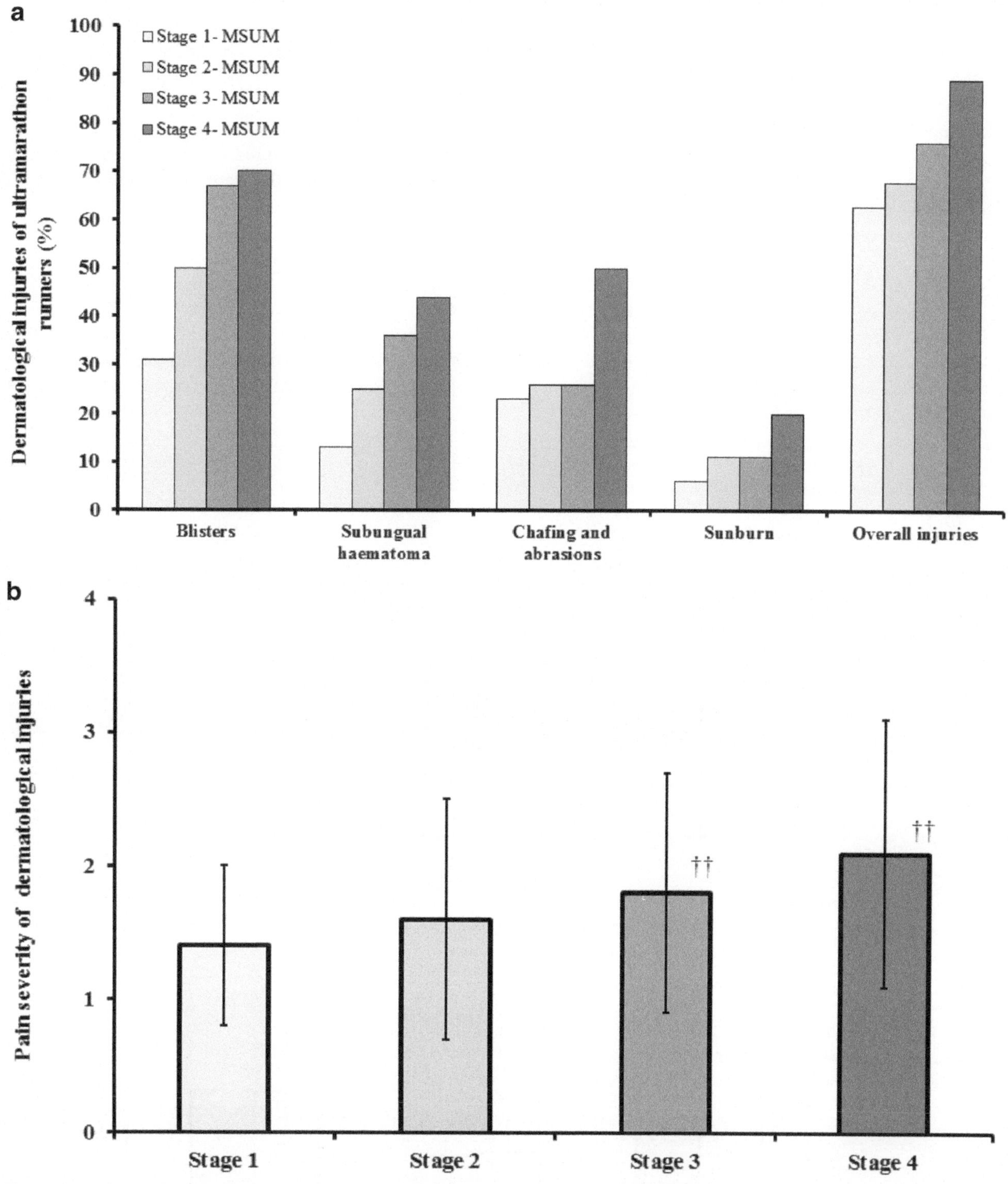

Fig. 2 Dermatological injuries (**a**) and pain severity of dermatological injuries (**b**) of ultramarathon runners during a multi-stage ultramarathon. Pain severity scale: 0 = no pain, 1 = minimal pain, 2 = mild pain, 3 = moderate pain, 4 = severe pain, and 5 = elimination from event. Mean ± SD ($n = 54$): $^{\dagger\dagger}p < 0.01$ vs. Stage 1

between participants presenting DI and no-DI in the MSUM (overall mean: 287 ± 7 mOsmol/kg). Similarly, no statistically significant difference in P_V change was observed between participants presenting GIS and no-GIS in the MSUM (peak value 21 ± 12 %) and the 24 h (peak value 9 ± 11 %) and between participants presenting DI and no-DI in the MSUM.

Energy Balance

Gastrointestinal symptoms during the MSUM were associated with a lower daily energy intake (total $p < 0.01$ and adjusted $p = 0.03$) and greater energy deficit (78 %; $p = 0.04$) compared with no-GIS (Fig. 3a). The severity of GIS did not further disturb energy balance along the MSUM. No significant differences in energy intake (total and adjusted), energy expenditure, and energy deficit were observed between GIS and no-GIS in the 24 h (Fig. 3b). Gastrointestinal symptoms along the MSUM were also associated with a reduction in energy intake during running compared with no-GIS (Table 2). Furthermore, greater GIS severity along the MSUM was associated with a lower energy (total (−1.5 MJ) $p = 0.01$ and adjusted $p = 0.01$) intake during running. Additionally, GIS along the MSUM were associated with a lower energy intake during the recovery period (Table 2); however, severity of GIS did not significantly exacerbate the reduction.

The presence and severity of DI along the MSUM did not result in significant differences of daily energy balance variables compared with no-DI. Incidence of DI did not significantly impact on energy intake during running (Table 3); however, greater severity of DI along the

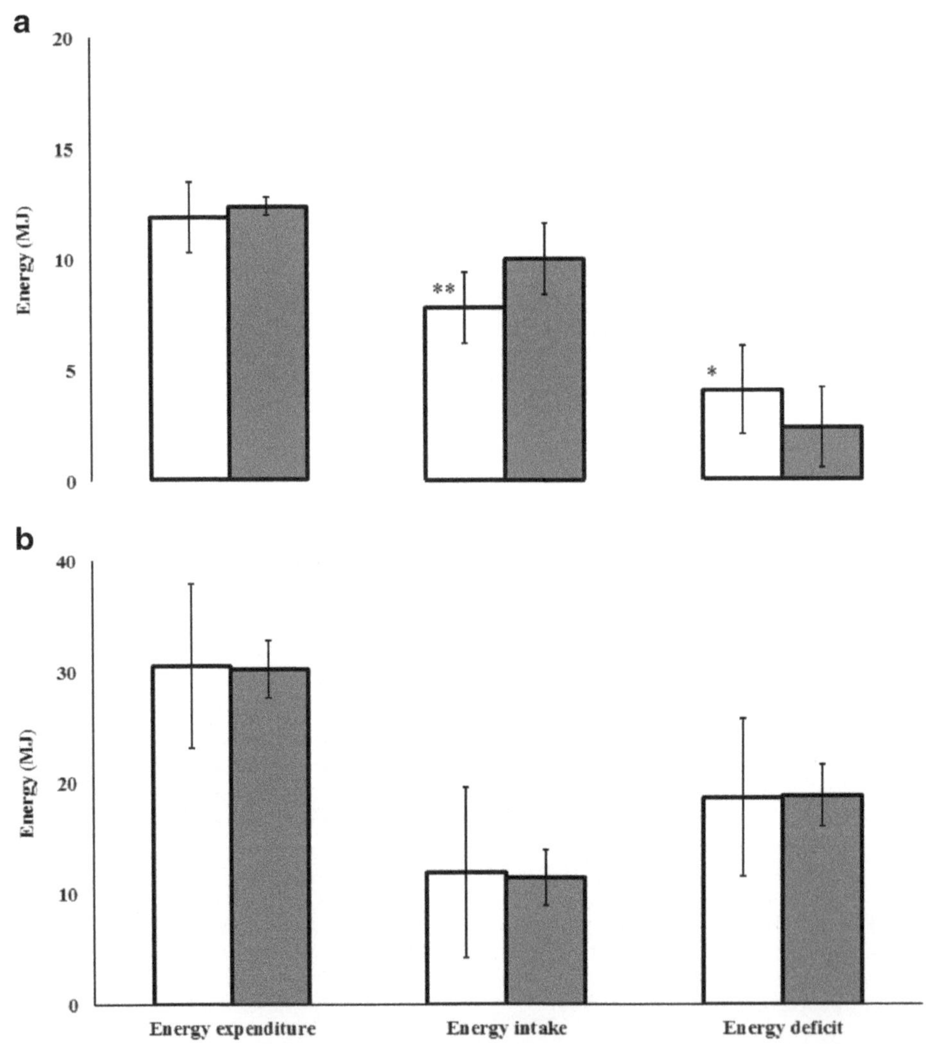

Fig. 3 Energy expenditure, intake, and deficit of ultramarathon runners presenting (*white*) and not presenting (*grey*) gastrointestinal symptoms during a multi-stage ultramarathon (**a**) and a 24-h continuous ultramarathon (**b**). Mean ± SD (MSUM $n = 54$ and 24 h $n = 22$): $^{**}p < 0.01$ and $^{*}p < 0.05$ vs. no-GIS

Table 2 During running and post-stage recovery energy, macronutrient, and water (through foods and fluids) intake of ultramarathon runners presenting (GIS) and not presenting (no-GIS) gastrointestinal symptoms during a multi-stage ultramarathon (MSUM)

	During			Post-stage recovery		
	GIS	no-GIS	*p* value	GIS	no-GIS	*p* value
Energy (MJ)						
Total	3.1 ± 2.0	4.0 ± 1.5	<0.05	2.4 ± 1.1	3.4 ± 1.4	<0.01
Adjusted[a]	0.046 ± 0.003	0.052 ± 0.002	0.36	0.036 ± 0.002	0.043 ± 0.002	0.07
Protein (g)						
Total	13 ± 28	13 ± 9	0.91	14 ± 14	23 ± 13	<0.01
Adjusted[a]	0.2 ± 0.4	0.2 ± 0.1	0.89	0.2 ± 0.2	0.3 ± 0.2	<0.05
Carbohydrate (g)						
Total	137 ± 75	175 ± 69	<0.05	108 ± 50	141 ± 87	0.07
Adjusted[a]	2.0 ± 0.9	2.3 ± 1.0	0.14	1.6 ± 0.8	1.6 ± 0.7	0.77
Poly (%)[b]	19 ± 16	26 ± 15	0.10	18 ± 21	10 ± 16	0.49
Oligo/di/mono (%)[b]	81 ± 16	74 ± 15	0.06	82 ± 21	90 ± 16	0.07
Fibre	3 ± 5	6 ± 4	<0.01	3 ± 3	3 ± 3	0.96
Fat (g)						
Total	15 ± 16	21 ± 15	0.06	10 ± 11	18 ± 13	<0.01
Adjusted[a]	0.2 ± 0.2	0.3 ± 0.2	0.34	0.2 ± 0.2	0.2 ± 0.2	<0.05
Water						
Total (L)	4.4 ± 1.5	3.9 ± 1.7	0.13	1.1 ± 0.6	1.5 ± 0.9	0.17
Adjusted (ml)[a]	65 ± 23	51 ± 22	<0.01	18 ± 10	20 ± 14	0.52

Mean ± SD ($n = 54$). The overall mean inter-observer coefficient of variation for energy, macronutrient, and water variables analysed were 1.3, 2.3, and 0.7 %, respectively
[a]Adjusted for body mass
[b]Saccharides

MSUM was associated with a lower energy (total (−1.2 MJ) $p = 0.02$ and adjusted $p = 0.01$) during running. Incidence and severity of DI did not significantly impact on energy intake in the post-stage recovery period (Table 3).

No acetoacetic acid was identified in pre-stage urine samples throughout the MSUM and pre-event urine samples in the 24 h. Acetoacetic acid (concentration range 1.5 to 8.0 mmol/l) in post-stage urine samples was evident in 46 % of participants at some point along the MSUM and 90 % of participants in the 24 h. No significant differences in pre- and post-stage acetoacetic acid concentration were observed between GIS and no-GIS and DI and no-DI along the MSUM. No significant differences in pre- and post-event acetoacetic acid concentration were observed between GIS and no-GIS in the 24 h.

Macronutrient and Water Intake (Gastrointestinal Symptoms vs. No-Gastrointestinal Symptoms)

The presence of GIS during the MSUM was associated with a significant reduction in daily carbohydrate and fat intakes, compared with no-GIS (Table 4). Conversely, higher daily water intake was observed in participants reporting GIS (vs. no-GIS). The severity of GIS along the MSUM did not result in substantial differences of daily macronutrient intake. However, greater GIS severity did result in lower daily water intake (total (−851 ml/day) $p = 0.04$ and adjusted $p < 0.01$).

Incidence and severity of GIS during the 24 h did not alter macronutrient and water intake variables (total and adjusted) during running (Table 5); whereas GIS along the MSUM were associated with significant reductions in carbohydrate and fat intakes during running compared with no-GIS (Table 2). Rate of carbohydrate intake during running was also significantly lower (−8 g/h) in participants reporting GIS ($p < 0.01$ vs. no-GIS) (Fig. 4). Conversely, higher water intake during running was observed in participants reporting GIS (vs. no-GIS). Furthermore, greater GIS severity along the MSUM was associated with significantly lower protein (total (−19 g) $p = 0.01$ and adjusted $p = 0.01$), fat (total (−11 g) $p = 0.03$ and adjusted $p = 0.01$), and water (total (−902 ml) $p = 0.01$, adjusted $p < 0.01$, and rate per hour (−122 ml/h) $p = 0.01$) intakes during running.

Table 3 During running and post-stage recovery energy, macronutrient, and water (through foods and fluids) intake of ultramarathon runners presenting (DI) and not presenting (no-DI) dermatological injuries during a multi-stage ultramarathon (MSUM)

	During			Post-stage recovery		
	DI	no-DI	*p* value	DI	no-DI	*p* value
Energy (MJ)						
Total	3.2 ± 2.2	3.2 ± 1.3	0.99	2.4 ± 1.2	2.6 ± 1.1	0.31
Adjusted[a]	.046 ± .031	.048 ± .021	0.63	.036 ± .018	0.040 ± 0.017	0.15
Protein (g)						
Total	13 ± 29	13 ± 12	0.93	14 ± 14	18 ± 15	0.07
Adjusted[a]	0.2 ± 0.4	0.2 ± 0.2	0.79	0.2 ± 0.2	0.3 ± 0.2	<0.05
Carbohydrate (g)						
Total	138 ± 77	151 ± 66	0.29	107 ± 51	115 ± 48	0.34
Adjusted[a]	1.9 ± 0.9	2.3 ± 1.0	<0.05	1.6 ± 0.8	1.7 ± 0.7	0.27
Poly (%)[b]	20 ± 17	19 ± 14	0.59	16 ± 19	20 ± 23	0.78
Oligo/di/mono (%)[b]	80 ± 17	81 ± 14	0.10	84 ± 19	80 ± 23	0.21
Fibre	4 ± 5	3 ± 2	0.11	3 ± 3	3 ± 5	0.75
Fat (g)						
Total	16 ± 18	14 ± 10	0.38	11 ± 11	13 ± 12	0.19
Adjusted[a]	0.2 ± 0.3	0.2 ± 0.1	0.76	0.2 ± 0.2	0.2 ± 0.2	0.25
Water						
Total (L)	4.5 ± 1.6	4.1 ± 1.1	0.05	1.1 ± 0.7	1.2 ± 0.6	0.75
Adjusted (ml)[a]	65 ± 24	61 ± 19	0.31	18 ± 11	18 ± 9	0.96

Mean ± SD ($n = 54$). The overall mean inter-observer coefficient of variation for energy, macronutrient, and water variables analysed were 1.3, 2.3, and 0.7 %, respectively
[a]Adjusted for body mass
[b]Saccharides

Table 4 Daily macronutrient and water (through foods and fluids) intake of ultramarathon runners presenting and not presenting (no-) gastrointestinal symptoms (GIS) and dermatological injuries (DI) during a multi-stage ultramarathon

	GIS	no-GIS	*p* value	DI	no-DI	*p* value
Protein (g)						
Total	104 ± 39	114 ± 28	0.20	106 ± 39	103 ± 38	0.68
Adjusted	1.5 ± 0.6	1.4 ± 0.3	0.46	1.5 ± 0.5	1.6 ± 0.6	0.61
Carbohydrate (g)						
Total	506 ± 137	635 ± 124	<0.01	516 ± 138	535 ± 151	0.39
Adjusted[a]	7.4 ± 2.0	7.9 ± 1.5	0.25	7.4 ± 1.8	7.8 ± 2.3	0.17
Poly (%)[b]	41 ± 11	35 ± 10	0.13	40 ± 11	39 ± 11	0.70
Oligo/di/mono (%)[b]	59 ± 11	65 ± 10	<0.01	60 ± 11	61 ± 11	0.37
Fibre	17 ± 9	29 ± 12	<0.01	18 ± 9	20 ± 12	0.35
Fat (g)						
Total	90 ± 36	126 ± 57	<0.01	95 ± 42	89 ± 36	0.33
Adjusted[a]	1.3 ± 0.6	1.6 ± 0.7	<0.05	1.4 ± 0.6	1.3 ± 0.5	0.62
Water						
Total (L)	7.8 ± 2.0	7.1 ± 2.2	0.09	7.9 ± 1.9	7.1 ± 2.1	<0.05
Adjusted (ml)[a]	117 ± 32	93 ± 31	<0.01	116 ± 31	109 ± 37	0.20

Mean ± SD ($n = 54$). The overall mean inter-observer coefficient of variation for energy, macronutrient, and water variables analysed were 1.3, 2.3, and 0.7 %, respectively
[a]Adjusted for body mass
[b]Saccharides

Table 5 Macronutrient and water (through foods and fluids) intake of ultramarathon runners presenting and not presenting (no-) gastrointestinal symptoms (GIS) during a 24-h continuous ultramarathon

	GIS	no-GIS	*p* value
Protein (g)			
Total	79 ± 31	109 ± 49	0.12
Adjusted[a]	1.3 ± 0.4	1.3 ± 0.5	0.46
Carbohydrate (g)			
Total	937 ± 683	759 ± 184	0.54
Adjusted[a]	12.4 ± 8.7	8.7 ± 1.7	0.29
Poly (%)[b]	31 ± 10	33 ± 18	0.60
Oligo/di/mono (%)[b]	69 ± 10	67 ± 18	0.56
Fibre	23 ± 10	22 ± 15	0.82
Fat (g)			
Total	104 ± 53	143 ± 47	0.15
Adjusted[a]	1.1 ± 0.7	1.7 ± 0.6	0.51
Water			
Total (L)	9.1 ± 4.2	9.1 ± 3.8	0.98
Adjusted (ml)[a]	125 ± 54	105 ± 44	0.45

Mean ± SD ($n = 22$). The overall mean inter-observer coefficient of variation for energy, macronutrient, and water variables analysed were 0.8, 1.4, and 0.5 %, respectively
[a]Adjusted for body mass
[b]Saccharides

Gastrointestinal symptoms along the MSUM were associated with a reduced recovery nutrition profile, whereby significantly lower total protein, carbohydrate, and fat intakes were observed during the post-stage recovery period compared with no-GIS (Table 2). The severity of GIS along the MSUM did not however result in significant differences of macronutrient and water intake variables in the post-stage recovery period.

Macronutrient and Water Intake (Dermatological Injuries vs. No-Dermatological Injuries)

Dermatological injuries along the MSUM did not result in substantial differences of daily macronutrient intakes compared with no-DI (Table 4). However, the presence of DI was associated with significantly higher daily water intake. Greater severity of DI along the MSUM was associated with significantly lower daily fat intake (total $p = 0.01$).

Dermatological injuries along the MSUM were associated with significant reductions in total protein and rate of carbohydrate (−4 g/h; $p = 0.05$; Fig. 4) intake during running compared with no-DI (Table 3). Conversely, higher water intake during running was observed in participants reporting DI (vs. no-DI). Greater severity of DI along the MSUM was associated with significantly lower carbohydrate (total (−40 g) $p = 0.03$ and rate per hour (−6 g/h) $p = 0.02$) intake and rate of water intake per hour (−105 ml/h; $p = 0.02$) during running.

The presence of DI along the MSUM did not significantly reduced recovery nutrition profile (Table 3). However, greater severity of DI along the MSUM was associated with significant reductions in the recovery nutrition profile, whereby lower protein (0.1 g/kg; adjusted $p = 0.02$) and water (total (−270 ml) $p = 0.04$ and adjusted $p = 0.02$) intakes were observed with increased severity.

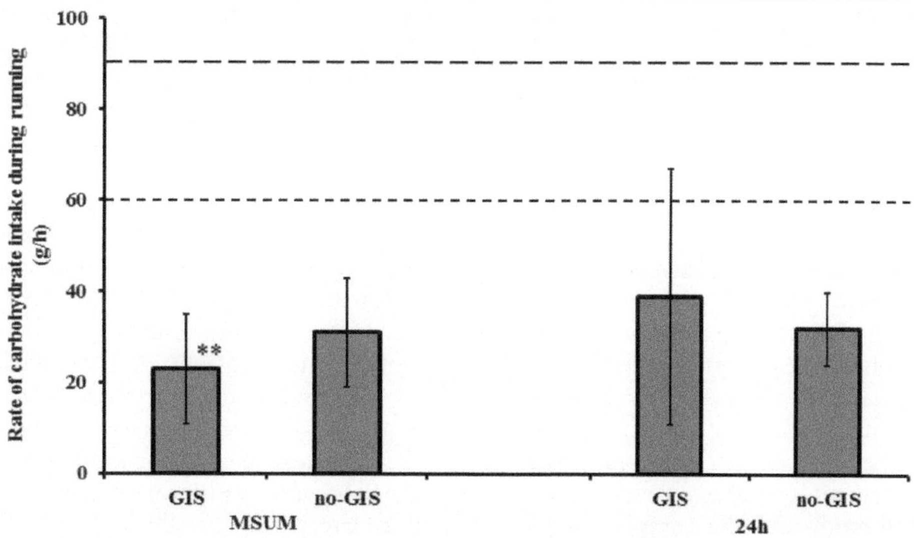

Fig. 4 Rate of carbohydrate intake during running of ultramarathon runners presenting (*GIS*) and not presenting (no-GIS) gastrointestinal symptoms during a multi-stage ultramarathon (MSUM) and a 24-h continuous ultramarathon (24 h). Values compared to carbohydrate intake recommendation for glucose (*short broken line*) and glucose-fructose (*long broken line*) [43]. Mean ± SD (MSUM $n = 54$ and 24 h $n = 22$): $^{**}p < 0.01$ vs. no-GIS

Discussion

The current study aimed to determine whether GIS or DI affects food and fluid intake, and nutrition and hydration status, of ultramarathon runners during multi-stage and 24-h ultra-marathons. Gastrointestinal symptoms were a common feature in both the MSUM and 24 h; however, reported incidence of DI requiring self-management and (or) medical intervention were high during the MSUM, but relatively low during the 24 h. The presence of GIS appeared to be associated with greater disturbances to daily energy balance, reduced daily macronutrient intake, and reduced nutritional intake during running and recovery throughout the MSUM. Similarly, the presence of DI appeared to be associated with reduced nutritional intake during running and recovery throughout the MSUM. Increasing severity of GIS and DI along the MSUM was associated with further reductions in energy, macronutrient, and fluid intakes. Gastrointestinal symptom incidence and severity did not alter energy, macronutrient, and fluid intakes during the 24 h. From a performance perspective and considering previous research has identified performance issues with GIS and DI [18], these clinical manifestation resulted in a longer time to complete the MSUM, but not distance covered in the 24 h, despite not reaching significance possibly due to large individual variations within group comparisons.

In both events, upper-GIS and nausea were the most commonly reported symptoms, with lower-GIS (i.e. predominantly diarrhoea) incidence being reported to a lesser extent. These results are in accordance with previous field observations, whereby 89 % of ultramarathon runners presenting gastrointestinal distress during a 161-km ultramarathon also reported nausea, whilst abdominal cramping (44 %) and diarrhoea (44 %) were reported to a lesser extent [17, 18]. Such observations are however contrary to previously reported indications that lower-GIS are the predominant GIS during running [14]. Moreover, incidence of GIS were greater than those previously reports during long distance triathlon events, marathon, and ultramarathon running [14, 17]. This finding is not surprising, considering the greater exertional and thermoregulatory strain compared with previous studies. It is unfortunate that on this occasion, the timing or distance at which symptoms occurred was not determined. If ultramarathon runners presented symptom later, after running onset, it would be expected to have lesser impact on nutritional intake than if symptoms were presented earlier. Considering the field setting of the study and the competitive nature of the events, the current study design per se did not allow symptom data to be collected during the actual competitive segment of each event. However, recent preliminary data from controlled laboratory trials has indicated GIS significantly increasing by 30 min (equivalent to 5.0-km distance point) and remained elevated thereafter, during a 3 h running protocol in thermoneutral condition (23.3 °C, 51 % RH) whereby participants consumed 30 g carbohydrate (2:1 glucose to fructose ratio) every 20 min [42, 43].

Taking into account that (a) no significant difference in GIS incidence and severity was seen between stages in the MSUM, (b) participants reported symptoms 'coming and going' along the consecutive days of competition, and (c) the variety of symptoms reported in both events; the precise causal mechanism/s for the high GIS incidence is not clear, but appears to be multi-factorial in origin. Exertion induced splanchnic hypoperfusion, ischemia, mechanical trauma, neuroendocrine stimulation, altered gastrointestinal motility, malabsorption, and altered epithelial permeability have all been directly or indirectly implicated [15, 20–26, 44]. It is however likely that the exertional heat stress exposure along the MSUM substantially contributed to the high GIS rates, since greater perturbations to gastrointestinal integrity (i.e. splanchnic hypoperfusion, splanchnic ischemia, and increase epithelial permeability) have been observed in heat stress experimental models (>30 °C ambient temperature) compared with thermoneutral conditions [21, 24, 45]. Indeed, lower perceptive tolerance rating to heat has been associated with greater reports of GIS in ultramarathon runners [5]. Moreover, daily and during running water intakes (through foods and fluids) were observed to be greater in ultramarathon runners reporting GIS. Since over-drinking behaviours and asymptomatic hyponatraemia were evident in the current MSUM event [41], it is possible that fluid intake strategies of ultramarathon runners may have also contribute to GIS [27–29], especially upper-GIS (e.g. gastric fluid load above individual tolerance), nausea, and vomiting (e.g. hyponatraemia). Gastrointestinal symptoms along the 24 h were likely to have been induced by the extreme duration of exertional stress, with or without feeding tolerance (i.e. forced feeding of scheduled dietary strategy) [15, 46, 47]. Similar to the 24 h findings, total carbohydrate intake rates have been reported to be positively correlated with nausea and GIS, but resulted in faster finishing times in long distance triathlon events [14]. Systemic endotoxaemic and cytokinaemic responses were observed in the current MSUM and 24 h events [25, 26]. Such responses have also been linked to GIS; therefore, exertional or exertional heat stress induced intestinal bacteria translocation and subsequent systemic inflammatory responses cannot be discounted as GIS promoters during ultramarathon events. On this occasion, during both the MSUM and 24 h, the type of carbohydrates consumed (i.e. quantity of highly resistant and fermentable carbohydrates associated with GIS [48]) did not differ between GIS and no-GIS. This suggests that gastrointestinal mechanisms and intake volumes are potentially responsible for GIS and not necessarily food and fluid choices. It is worth noting that excessive carbohydrate intakes during exercise above individually tolerated levels may directly contribute to the high occurrence of upper-GIS through neural and humoral-driven pathways stimulating the ileal break [30]. It is thus evident that GIS during ultramarathon running is multi-factorial. Conducting a series of controlled laboratory experiments to assess exertional stress (with and without heat stress) on gastrointestinal integrity and functional markers, and links to symptoms, would shed light on the key aetiological pathways of exertional induced upper- and lower-GIS.

Considering the already compromised nutrition status of ultramarathon runners during MSUM and 24 h events [5, 6], GIS further compromised the ability to consume energy, macronutrients, and fluid along the MSUM, but not during the 24 h. Indeed, compared with no-GIS, incidence of GIS were associated with (1) lower daily energy, carbohydrate, and fat intakes; (2) lower energy and carbohydrate intakes during running; and (3) poorer recovery nutrition throughout the MSUM. The severity of GIS appeared not to impact on total daily energy and macronutrient intakes, but high severity did result in a lower total daily water intake. The severity of GIS also appeared not to impact on recovery nutrition, but high severity did result in lower energy, protein, fat, and water intakes during running. Thus, the debatable question is whether symptoms per se limited the ability to consume foods and fluids or whether additional nutrient availability in the gastrointestinal tract prevented or suppressed symptoms. It has previously been shown that carbohydrate ingestion before and during exertion attenuated the reductions in post-exercise superior mesenteric artery and portal vein blood flow by Doppler method [49, 50]. This suggests that nutrient presence in the gastrointestinal tract may be protective against exertion induced splanchnic hypoperfusion and subsequent associated damage and symptoms [51].

The current study was the first to comprehensively assess DI during various ultramarathon events and its impact on nutritional intake and status. Dermatological injuries that warranted self-management and (or) medical intervention were a common feature during the MSUM; but relatively low incidence was observed in the 24 h. The discrepancy between the MSUM and 24 h is likely due to MSUM participants having sufficient time to manage DI, whilst stopping during the 24 h event would cost the participant valuable time. It is speculated that incidence of DI were likely to be substantially higher in the 24 h, but participants did not choose to investigate damage during the event. Nevertheless, incidence and severity of DI increased as the MSUM progressed. Foot injury (e.g. blisters) was the most common DI reported, with severity of foot injury associated with infection, local inflammation, and pain. Participants reported investing time and effort into self-management or seeking and receiving medical attention for injuries. This was especially apparent from Stage 3 onwards, in which medical crews reported observing concerning levels of infection and inflammation surrounding blisters in several participants.

Dermatological injuries were associated with a lower rate of carbohydrate intake during running, but the incidence of DI did not promote any additional decrements in other nutritional and hydration status variables per se compared with no-DI. However, as the severity of DI increased, lower energy, carbohydrate, and water intakes during running and lower protein and water intakes as part of recovery nutrition were observed. It thus appears, the greater the number of DI and subsequent progressive presentation of infection, inflammation, and pain, the more attention is focused towards the management and treatment of injuries, whilst nutrition was deprioritised.

From a performance and clinical perspective, carbohydrate energy substrate plays a crucial role in exercise performance [43, 52], fatigue attenuation [12], and immune competence [53] during periods of exertional stress. Sub-optimal daily and during exercise carbohydrate intake has been linked with hormonal (e.g. cortisol) and immune (e.g. cytokine profile and innate immune responses) dysfunction, potentially leading to states of chronic fatigue and depressed immunity [11, 12, 53, 54]. Additionally, carbohydrate, protein, and water play a fundamental role in recovery processes, with poor recovery nutrition being linked to reduced glycogen and tissue protein synthesis, hypohydration, and immunodepression [8, 9, 43, 53, 55, 56]. Indeed, positive correlations have been observed between energy and carbohydrate intakes with perceived recovery quality during a multi-stage ultramarathon event [5]. It is thus concerning that incidence and severity of both GIS and DI promoted further reductions in daily, during exercise, and recovery nutrition.

Conclusions

High rates of GIS were reported in both events; however, incidence and severity of GIS only negatively altered nutritional intake during MSUM. Dermatological injury incidence and severity reduced nutrient intake during running and recovery in the MSUM. Considering the already compromised nutritional status of ultramarathon runners during multi-stage events, these findings demonstrate that GIS and DI further compromises intake. Effective GIS and DI prevention and management strategies should be investigated, especially in respect to consecutive days of exertional stress.

Abbreviations

24 h: 24-h ultramarathon; DI: dermatological injuries; GIS: gastrointestinal symptoms; MSUM: multi-stage ultramarathon; P_{Osmol}: plasma osmolality; P_V: plasma volume; SD: standard deviation.

Competing Interests

The authors declare that they have no competing interests.

Authors' Contributions

The authors' contributions are as follows: RC was the chief investigator of this research. RC, VS, and AM were responsible for the original research idea and contributed to the development of the experimental design. RC, RS, and VC contributed to the analysis of the raw data. All authors contributed to the various aspects of data collection and sample analysis and the preparation review of the manuscript. All authors read and approved the final manuscript.

Authors' Information

RC is a lecturer, researcher, and practitioner in sport dietetics. RS is a PhD candidate and sports dietetic practitioner. VC is a teaching and research associate and psychology practitioner. VS and AM are sports medicine practitioners.

Acknowledgements

Firstly, the authors would like to thank all the ultramarathon runners that volunteered to participate in this study. The authors acknowledge the Al Andalus Ultimate Trail (www.alandalus-ut.com) and Glenmore24 Trail Race (http://runyabam.com/glenmore-24/) race directors for assisting and supporting various aspects of this study. The authors also acknowledge the members of Coventry University Sport & Exercise Nutritional Support & Research Team and collaborators for their support during the process of the sample and data collection. Finally, the authors would like to especially thank David Allen, David Wylie, Julian Evans, Karl Platt, and Simon Thomson from tent 96 of the 2008 Marathon des Sables for their valuable personal experience contribution. The study was funded by Coventry University Sport & Exercise Science Applied Research Group and the Department of Health Professionals. Funded contributions were also provided by the Coventry University as part of Dr. Ricardo Costa's Applied Research Fellowship.
All authors declare no conflict of interest.

Author details

[1]Department of Nutrition & Dietetics, Monash University, Notting Hill, Victoria, Australia. [2]British Forces Germany Health Services, Paderborn, Germany. [3]Centre of Sports & Exercise, Edinburgh University, Edinburgh, UK.

References

1. Knoth C, Knechtle B, Rust CA, Rosemann R, Lepers R. Participation and performance trends in multi-stage ultra-marathon- the 'Marathon des Sables' 2003–2012. Extreme Physiol Med. 2012;1:1–11.
2. Murray A, Costa RJS. Born to run. Studying the limits of human performance. BMC Med. 2012;10(76):1–3.
3. Hoffman MD, Pasternak A, Rogers IR, Khodaee M, Hill JC, Townes DA, et al. Medical services at ultra-endurance food races in remote environments: medical issues and consensus guidelines. Sports Med. 2014;44(8):105–1069.
4. Krabak BJ, Waite B, Lipman G. Evaluation and treatment of injury and illness in the ultramarathon athlete. Phys Med Rehabil Clin N Am. 2014;25(4):845–63.
5. Costa RJS, Swancott A, Gill SK, Hankey J, Scheer V, Murray A, et al. Compromised energy and nutritional intake of ultra-endurance runners during a multi-stage ultra-marathon conducted in a hot ambient environment. Int J Sports Sci. 2013;3:51–61.
6. Costa RJS, Gill SK, Hankey J, Wright A, Marczak S. Perturbed energy balance and hydration status in ultra-endurance runners during a 24 h ultra-marathon. Br J Nutri. 2014;112:428–37.
7. Scheer BV, Murray A. Al Andalus Ultra Trail: an observation of medical interventions during a 219km, 5 day ultramarathon stage race. Clin J Sport Med. 2011;21:444–6.
8. Costa RJS, Oliver SJ, Laing SJ, Walters R, Bilzon JLJ, Walsh NP. Influence of timing of postexercise carbohydrate-protein ingestion on selected immune indices. Int J Sport Nutr Exerc Metab. 2009;19(4):366–284.
9. Costa RJS, Walters R, Bilzon JLJ, Walsh NP. Effects of immediate post-exercise carbohydrate ingestion with and without protein on neutrophil degranulation. Int J Sport Nutr Exerc Metab. 2011;21(3):205–13.
10. Dempster S, Britton R, Murray A, Costa RJS. Case study: nutrition and hydration status during 4254 km of running over 78 consecutive days. Int J Sport Nutr Exerc Metab. 2013;23(5):533–41.
11. Robson-Ansley P, Barwood M, Canavan J, Hack S, Eglin C, Davey S, et al. The effect of repeated endurance exercise on IL-6 and sIL-6R and their relationship with sensations of fatigue at rest. Cytokine. 2009;45:111–6.
12. Robson-Ansley PJ, Gleeson M, Ansley L. Fatigue management in the preparation of Olympic athletes. J Sports Sci. 2009;27:1409–20.
13. Walsh NP, Gleeson M, Shephard RJ, Gleeson M, Woods JA, Bishop NC, et al. Position statement. Part one: immune function and exercise. Exerc Immunol Rev. 2011;17:6–63.
14. Pfeiffer B, Stellingwerff T, Hodgson AB, Randell R, Pöttgen K, Res P, et al. Nutritional intake and gastrointestinal problems during competitive endurance events. Med Sci Sports Exerc. 2012;44:344–51.
15. Rehrer NJ, McLaughlin J, Wasse LK. Importance of gastrointestinal function to athletic performance and health. In: Maughan R editor. The encyclopaedia of sports medicine, an IOC medical commission publication: Sports Nutrition. Wiley-Blackwell, Hoboken, New Jersey, United States.; 2014. p. 526–38.
16. Jeukendrup AE, Vet-Joop K, Sturk A, Stegen JH, Senden J, Saris WH, et al. Relationship between gastro-intestinal complaints and endotoxaemia, cytokine release and the acute-phase reaction during and after a long-distance triathlon in highly trained men. Clin Sci. 2000;98:47–55.
17. Stuempfle KJ, Hoffman MD, Hew-Butler T. Association of gastrointestinal distress in ultramarathoners with race diet. Int J Sport Nutr Exerc Metab. 2013;23:103–9.
18. Hoffman MD, Fogard K. Factors related to successful completion of a 161-km ultramarathon. Int J Sports Physiol Perform. 2011;6(1):25–37.
19. Stuempfle KJ, Hoffman MD. Gastrointestinal distress is common during a 161-km ultramarathon. J Sports Sci. 2015;33(17):1814–21.
20. ter Steege RW, Kolkman JJ. The pathophysiology and management of gastrointestinal symptoms during physical exercise, and the role of splanchnic blood flow. Aliment Pharmacol Ther. 2012;35:516–28.
21. van Wijck K, Lenaerts K, Grootjans J, Wijnands KA, Poeze M, van Loon LJ, et al. Physiology and pathophysiology of splanchnic hypoperfusion and intestinal injury during exercise: strategies for evaluation and preventions. Am J Physiol. 2012;303:G155–68.
22. Lambert GP. Stress-induced gastrointestinal barrier dysfunction and its inflammatory effects. J Anim Sci. 2009;87:E101–8.
23. O'Connor FG, Casa DJ, Bergeron MF, Carter R, Deuster P, Heled Y, et al. American College of Sports Medicine round table on exertional heat stroke. Return to duty/return to play: conference proceedings. Curr Sports Med Rep. 2010;9:314–21.
24. Yeh YJ, Law LY, Lim CL. Gastrointestinal response and endotoxemia during intense exercise in hot and cool environments. Eur J Appl Physiol. 2013; 113(6):1575–83.
25. Gill SK, Hankey J, Wright A, Marczak S, Hemming K, Allerton DM, et al. The impact of a 24-hour ultra-marathon on circulatory endotoxin and cytokine profile. Int J Sports Med. 2015;36(8):688–95.
26. Gill SK, Teixeira A, Rama L, Rosado F, Hankey J, Scheer V, et al. Circulatory endotoxin concentration and cytokine profile in response to exertional-heat stress during a multi-stage ultra-marathon competition. Exerc Immunol Rev. 2015;21:114–28.
27. Backer HD, Shopes E, Collins SL, Barkan H. Exertional heat illness and hyponatremia in hikers. Am J Emerg Med. 1999;17(6):532–9.
28. Hew-Butler T, Rosner MH, Fowkes-Godek S, Dugas JP, Hoffman MD, Lewis DP, et al. Statement of the third international exercise-associated hyponatremia consensus development conference, Carlsbad, California, 2015. Clin J Sport Med. 2015;25(4):303–20.
29. Siegel AJ, d'Hemecourt P, Adner MM, Shirey T, Brown JL, Lewandrowski KB. Exertional dysnatremia in collapsed marathon runners: a critical role for point-of-care testing to guide appropriate therapy. Am J Clin Pathol. 2009; 132(3):336–40.
30. Shin HS, Ingram JR, McGill, Poppitt SD. Lipids, CHOs, proteins: can all macronutrients put a 'brake' on eating? Physiol Behav. 2013;120:114–23.

31. Lipman GS, Scheer BV. Blisters: the enemy of the feet. Wilderness Environ Med. 2015;26(2):275–6.
32. Lipman GS, Ellis MA, Lewis EJ, Waite BL, Lissoway J, Chan GK, et al. A prospective randomized blister prevention trial assessing paper tape in endurance distances (Pre-TAPED). Wilderness Environ Med. 2014;25(4):457–61.
33. Scheer BV, Reljic D, Murray A, Costa RJS. The enemy of the foot: blisters in ultra-endurance runners. J Am Podiatr Med Assoc. 2014;104(5):473–8.
34. Krabak BJ, Waite B, Schiff MA. Study of injury and illness rates in multiday ultramarathon runners. Med Sci Sport Exerc. 2011;43(12):2314–20.
35. Schwabe K, Schwellnus MP, Derman W, Swanevelder S, Jordaan E. Less experience and running pace are potential risk factors for medical complications during a 56 km road running race: a prospective study in 26 354 race starters-SAFER study II. Br J Sports Med. 2014;48(11):905–11.
36. American Dietetic Association, Dietitians of Canada, American College of Sports Medicine, Rodriguez NR, Di Marco NM, Langley S. American College of Sports Medicine position stand. Nutrition and athletic performance. Med Sci Sports Exerc. 2009;41(3):709–31.
37. American Dietetic Association, Dietitians of Canada, American College of Sports Medicine, Rodriguez NR, Di Marco NM, Langley S. American College of Sports Medicine position stand. Nutrition and athletic performance. Med Sci Sports Exerc. 2009;41(3):709–31.
38. Britton R, Dempster S, Moore JP, Costa RJS. The use of triaxial accelerometry to support dietary intervention during a multi-stage mountain ultra-marathon: a case study approach. J Sport Sci. 2011;29 Suppl 2:S132.
39. Seifarth CC, Miertschischk J, Hahn EG, Hensen J. Measurement of serum and plasma osmolality in healthy young humans—influence of time and storage conditions. Clin Chem Lab Med. 2004;42:927–32.
40. Costa RJS, Crockford MJ, Moore JP, Walsh NP. Heat acclimation responses of an ultra-endurance running group preparing for hot desert based competition. Eur J Sport Sci. 2014;14(S1):S131–41.
41. Costa RJS, Teixiera A, Rama L, Swancott AJ, Hardy LD, Lee B, et al. Water and sodium intake habits and status of ultra-endurance runners during a multi-stage ultra-marathon conducted in a hot ambient environment: an observational study. Nutri J. 2013;12(13):1–16.
42. Miall A, Khoo A, Rauch C, Gibson P, Costa RJS. Repetitive gut challenge reduces gastrointestinal symptoms and malabsorption of carbohydrates during exertional stress. J Nutr Intermediary Metab. 2014;1:31–2.
43. Burke LM, Hawley JA, Wong SHS, Jeukendrup AE. Carbohydrates for training and competition. J Sports Sci. 2011;29 Suppl 1:S17–27.
44. Peters HP, Akkermans LM, Bol E, Mosterd WL. Gastrointestinal symptoms during exercise. The effect of fluid supplementation. Sports Med. 1995;20(2):65–76.
45. Selkirk GA, McLellan TM, Wright HE, Rhind SG. Mild endotoxemia, NF-kB translocation, and cytokine increase during exertional heat stress in trained and untrained individuals. Am J Physiol Regul Integr Comp Physiol. 2008;295:611–23.
46. Van Nieuwenhoven MA, Brummer RM, Brouns F. Gastrointestinal function during exercise: comparison of water, sports drink, and sports drink with caffeine. J Appl Physiol. 2000;89(3):1079–85.
47. Peters HP, Schep G, Koster DJ, Douwes AC, de Vries WR. Hydrogen breath test as a simple noninvasive method for evaluation of carbohydrate malabsorption during exercise. Eur J Appl Physiol Occup Physiol. 1994;68(5):435–40.
48. Halmos EP, Christophersen CT, Bird AR, Shepherd SJ, Gibson PR, Muir JG. Diets that differ in their FODMAP content alter the colonic luminal microenvironment. Gut. 2015;64:93–100.
49. Qamar MI, Read AE. Effects of exercise on mesenteric blood flow in man. Gut. 1987;28(5):583–7.
50. Rehrer NJ, Goes E, DuGardeyn C, Reynaert H, DeMeirleir K. Effect of carbohydrate on portal vein blood flow during exercise. Int J Sports Med. 2005;26(3):171–6.
51. Matheson PJ, Wilson MA, Garrison RN. Regulation of intestinal blood flow. J Surg Res. 2000;93(1):182–96.
52. Stellingwerff T, Cox GR. Systematic review: carbohydrate supplementation on exercise performance or capacity of varying durations. Appl Physiol Nutr Metab. 2014;39:1–14.
53. Walsh NP, Gleeson M, Pyne DB, Nieman DC, Dhabhar FS, Shephard RJ, et al. Position statement. Part two: maintaining immune health. Exerc Immunol Rev. 2011;17:64–103.
54. Costa RJS, Jones GE, Lamb KL, Coleman R, Williams JH. The effects of a high carbohydrate diet on cortisol and salivary immunoglobulin A (s-IgA) during a period of increase exercise workload amongst Olympic and Ironman triathletes. Int J Sports Med. 2005;26(10):880–5.
55. Beelen M, Burke LM, Gibala MJ, van Loon LJC. Nutritional strategies to promote postexercise recovery. Int J Sport Nutri Exerc Metab. 2010;20:515–32.
56. American College of Sports Medicine, Sawka MN, Burke LM, Eichner ER, Maughan RJ, Montain SJ, et al. American College of Sports Medicine position stand. Exercise and fluid replacement. Med Sci Sports Exerc. 2007;39:377–90.

13

Image-Guided Hyaluronic Acid Injection and Knee Bracing Significantly Improve Clinical Outcomes for High-Grade Osteoarthritis

Terry K. Morgan[1*], Emilie Jensen[1], Jeong Lim[2] and Russell Riggs[3]

Abstract

Background: Intra-articular hyaluronic acid (HA) injection is an intermediate option between analgesics and knee joint replacement in patients with osteoarthritis (OA). Our objective was to test whether image-guided HA injections may improve knee OA outcomes after 6 months of treatment independent of potential covariates.

Methods: This is a retrospective case series with multivariate outcome-based analysis of 207 consecutive adult patients with mild to severe knee OA treated at a single out-patient clinic employing fluoroscopy-guided HA injections. We employed a customized pain (scored 0–10) and function (scored 0–120) questionnaire based on the Likert scale to compare baseline scores with 6-month outcomes. Linear and logistic (based on >9-point score improvement) regression analysis was used to adjust for potential covariates, including grade of disease, patient age, gender, body mass index, smoking history, medical history (e.g., diabetes or heart disease), use of daily pain medications, fish oil supplementation, knee bracing, and physical therapy.

Results: Significant covariates included OA grade, knee bracing, and analgesic use. Most of the study subjects were women (124/207, 60 %) and obese (113/207, 55 %). Clinically significant improvements in index scores (>9 points) at 6 months were observed in more than 50 % of cases post-image-guided HA injection. Regression analysis revealed a complimentary affect with knee bracing, especially in severe grade 4 disease (odds ratio 5.5 [1.14–27.0], $P < 0.05$). Daily analgesic use reflected a poor clinical response to treatment.

Conclusions: Our data suggest image-guided HA injections coupled with knee bracing may benefit patients with moderate to severe knee osteoarthritis.

Key Points:

- Image-guided hyaluronic acid injections significantly improve clinical outcomes at 6 months for mild, moderate, and severe knee osteoarthritis.
- Knee bracing is a significant covariate for clinical improvement in severe grade 4 disease.
- Daily analgesic use is associated with high-grade disease and less clinical improvement.

Keywords: Knee osteoarthritis; Hyaluronic acid; Intra-articular injection; Fluoroscopy

* Correspondence: morgante@ohsu.edu
[1]Department of Pathology, Oregon Health & Science University, 3181 SW Sam Jackson, Mail Code L-471, Portland, OR 97239, USA
Full list of author information is available at the end of the article

Background

Osteoarthritis (OA) of the knee is a leading cause of adult disability [1], affecting approximately 10–15 % of Americans over the age of 60 years [2]. The estimated cost to the United States economy is over $100 billion per year [3, 4], and the prevalence of the disease is expected to increase over the next decade due to obesity and aging of the population.

A wide variety of treatment options are available [5], including weight loss, knee bracing, physical therapy, analgesics, intra-articular injections (e.g., hyaluronic acid [HA], methylprednisolone), and surgery (e.g., debridement or joint replacement). Non-surgical conservative approaches such as HA injection provide an intermediate approach between analgesics and joint replacement with the objective of decreasing pain, improving function, and delaying the need for joint replacement. Recent meta-analyses provide conflicting opinions about the efficacy of HA injections [6–8], which may affect providers' willingness to recommend this type of treatment. However, we suspect many patients may potentially benefit from image-guided injections [9, 10] after controlling for covariates.

We hypothesized that image-guided intra-articular HA injections improve 6-month clinical outcomes in adults with mild to severe knee OA. Moreover, supplemental knee bracing and analgesic support may improve outcomes compared with image-guided HA injection alone.

Methods

Study Design

This is a retrospective case series with multivariate outcome-based analysis using an Oregon Health & Science University Institutional Review Board approved protocol to extract clinical chart data from 207 adult patients (25–105 years old) with mild (grade 2), moderate (grade 3), or severe (grade 4) knee OA treated at a single out-patient clinic in 2013. All study subjects were Caucasian with 6 months of clinical follow-up after a series of three fluoroscopy-guided (1.0 ml of IsoVue contrast injected into the knee with a 21-gauge needle) HA (*Euflexxa*, 1 % Sodium Hyaluronate, Ferring Pharm. Inc. Parsippany, NJ) injections administered 1 week apart by an experienced physician (RR). Clinical data were extracted from uniform patient questionnaires using a customized pain (scored 0–10) and function (scored 0–120) assessment based on the Likert scale [7, 11]. Physical examination and clinical history were screened for potential covariates, including the grade of osteoarthritis, which was defined by the Kellgren-Lawrence criteria [12]: grade 2 (mild) had definite joint space narrowing and osteophytic lipping, grade 3 (moderate) also showed sclerosis and possible bone contour deformity, and grade 4 (severe) had severe sclerosis, joint narrowing, large osteophytes, and bone contour deformities. Patient age, gender, body mass index, smoking history, significant medical history (e.g., diabetes or heart disease), subjective reporting of over-the-counter daily analgesics (e.g., NSAIDs), daily fish oil supplements, and duration of disease were also documented. More than half of the study subjects (110/207) were fitted with a non-customized single-hinged medial off-loading knee brace (V/Q OrthoCare, Vista, CA) after HA injection for the duration of the 6-month interval available for outcome metrics. Knee bracing was recommended to patients with limitations in activity defined by the ability to ambulate up and down a flight of stairs ±knee brace. Physical therapy was recommended for all study subjects. Of these, 100 study subjects regularly participated in knee-centric physical therapy (8–10 sessions over 6-month study period). Patients completed follow-up questionnaires and had a physical examination at 2 and 6 months post-image-guided HA injection. This archived patient chart data was extracted into a coded file without patient identifiers (e.g., name, birthdate) for statistical analysis. Extraction quality assurance was verified by 10 % independent review (20/207 cases).

Statistical Analyses

All statistical analyses were performed using SAS (version 9.4, SAS Institute, Cary, NC). Patient demographics, potential covariates, and outcome metrics were examined by univariate analysis using the Student *t*-test. Potential covariates (e.g., knee bracing, analgesics) were analyzed as binary variables (yes or no). In the cases with bilateral knee involvement, the highest OA grade knee was employed for analysis. The primary outcome metric was pain and function outcomes at 2 and 6 months compared with baseline (before first HA injection) for linear regression analysis, and "clinically significant" improvement was defined as >9-point decrease in score for logistic regression analysis. Subjective pain index (0–10) was a secondary outcome analyzed by linear regression.

Results

Multivariate regression analysis demonstrated that knee osteoarthritis grade was the most significant covariate affecting clinical outcomes at 2 months ($P < 0.0001$) and 6 months ($P < 0.0001$) post-image-guided HA injection. Therefore, all analyses were reported separately for each OA grade: mild (grade 2), moderate (grade 3), and severe (grade 4) disease (Table 1). As expected, univariate analysis showed that increasing severity of knee OA was related to increasing subject age and body mass index. Most of the study subjects were obese with BMIs ≥30.0 (113/207, 55 %) and most were women (124/207, 60 %). Univariate analysis did not show a relationship between OA grade and smoking, daily analgesic use, or physical

Table 1 Patient demographics and outcomes treated by image-guided hyaluronic acid injection

	OA grade 2 (*n* = 58)	OA grade 3 (*n* = 98)	OA grade 4 (*n* = 51)	*P* value X^2 or ANOVA
Age (mean, SD)	56.3 ± 12.4	64.0 ± 11.3	69.8 ± 12.2	*P* < 0.0001
Male gender (*n*, [%])	20 (35 %)	41 (42 %)	21 (42 %)	*P* = 0.62
Body mass index (mean, SD)	29.6 ± 6.5	31.2 ± 6.5	34.6 ± 9.3	*P* < 0.01
Never smoked (*n*, [%])	49 (85 %)	86 (88 %)	42 (82 %)	*P* = 0.29
Physical therapy (*n*, [%])	27 (47 %)	44 (45 %)	20 (39 %)	*P* = 0.72
Daily analgesics (*n*, [%])	23 (40 %)	41 (42 %)	26 (51 %)	*P* = 0.39
Knee bracing (*n*, [%])	20 (35 %)	60 (61 %)	31 (61 %)	*P* < 0.01
Fish oil (*n*, [%])	43 (74 %)	64 (65 %)	43 (84 %)	*P* = 0.05
Function index baseline (mean, SD)	34.7 ± 16.1	46.0 ± 15.4	48.1 ± 13.3	*P* < 0.0001
Index at 6 months (mean, SD)	27.2 ± 15.9	26.3 ± 14.9	36.4 ± 17.7	*P* < 0.01
Mean improvement (±SD)	6.7 ± 19.0	19.3 ± 16.8	12.5 ± 14.6	*P* < 0.001
Percentage improvement (±SD)	19 % ± 32 %	40 % ± 32 %	26 % ± 31 %	*P* < 0.001
>9-point improvement (*n*, [%])	32 (55 %)	67 (68 %)	26 (51 %)	*P* = 0.07
Average pain baseline (mean, SD)	5.5 ± 2.5	6.2 ± 2.1	7.1 ± 2.1	*P* < 0.01
Pain at 6 months (mean, SD)	3.9 ± 2.0	3.8 ± 2.1	5.2 ± 2.5	*P* < 0.01
Mean improvement (mean, SD)	1.66 ± 2.1	2.74 ± 2.5	2.3 ± 2.8	*P* = 0.05
Percentage improvement (±SD)	21 % ± 38 %	40 % ± 37 %	25 % ± 47 %	*P* = 0.04

Univariate analysis of patient demographics and treatment outcomes relative to knee osteoarthritis (OA) severity (grades 2–4). Data are presented as the mean ± standard deviation (SD) or percent (%) within OA grade

therapy. Moderate to severe OA were more likely to be fitted with a knee brace. Surprisingly, the greatest frequency of improvement was seen in more severe disease (68 % of study subjects), which also showed the most improvement in pain index (40 % compared with 21 % in mild disease).

Regression analysis revealed that knee bracing provided a positive complimentary effect to HA injection in severe OA cases (Table 2) to improve outcomes with an odds ratio of 5.5 (1.14–27.0) and *P* value <0.05. Analgesic use reflected a poor clinical response to treatment, rather than positive additive effect as first postulated. Physical therapy significantly decreased subjective pain index for mild OA ($P < 0.01$), but it had no effect on moderate or severe disease. Outcomes at 2 months were not significantly different than 6-month outcomes in this case series (data not shown) with the exception that bracing appeared to positively affect outcomes in moderate cases at 2 months (odds ratio 2.17 [0.86–5.48], *P* value 0.02), which remained a positive effect at 6 months, but the effect was not statistically significant (Table 2). Mild OA did not respond to knee bracing at either 2 or 6 months of evaluation, although logistic regression suggested a positive trend ($P = 0.19$).

Table 2 Regression analysis of significant covariates for clinical improvement

	OA grade 2 (*n* = 58)		OA grade 3 (*n* = 98)		OA grade 4 (*n* = 51)	
Function index linear regression	Parameter estimate	*P* value	Parameter estimate	*P* value	Parameter estimate	*P* value
Knee bracing	+2.69	0.67	+2.56	0.51	+10.81	0.04
Daily analgesics	−5.58	0.38	−8.6	0.03	−13.94	0.003
Logistic regression (>9-point improvement)	Odds ratio [95 % C.I.]	*P* value	Odds ratio [95 % C.I.]	*P* value	Odds ratio [95 % C.I.]	*P* value
Knee bracing	2.4 [0.66–8.81]	0.19	1.22 [0.45–2.22]	0.70	5.54 [1.14–27.0]	0.03
Daily analgesics	0.12 [0.03–0.53]	0.005	0.55 [0.18–1.63]	0.28	0.12 [0.03–0.61]	0.009
Average pain index linear regression	Parameter estimate	*P* value	Parameter estimate	*P* value	Parameter estimate	*P* value
Knee bracing	+0.94	0.25	+0.30	0.67	+1.81	0.10
Daily analgesics	−0.59	0.46	−1.06	0.14	−2.15	0.03
Physical therapy	+2.11	0.004	−0.25	0.73	−1.30	0.22

In addition to intra-articular HA injection, knee bracing significantly improved clinical outcomes with positive (+) effect on clinical indices at 6 months in severe (grade 4) osteoarthritis (OA) analyzed by both linear and logistic regression. In contrast, daily analgesic use was a sign of poor clinical response to treatment with worsening scores (−)

Discussion

Intra-articular HA knee injections are commonly performed by orthopedic surgeons [13] and increasingly by primary care physicians [5]. Although recent meta-analyses provide conflicting opinions about the efficacy of HA injections [6–8], it should be no surprise that image-guided injections may yield significantly better results [9, 10]. Our retrospective analysis of fluoroscopy-guided HA knee injections supports this conclusion. Moreover, our multivariate regression analysis reveals OA grade and bracing may significantly affect clinical outcomes.

Most of the image-guidance literature centers on corticosteroid injections. For example, Jones et al. [10] reported that ultrasound guidance yielded clinically significant improvement in 28/54 (52 %) of their study subjects, while only 7/30 (23 %) showed improvement without imaging. They attributed this discrepancy to incorrectly placed injections, which missed the joint space. Indeed, meta-analyses have shown that image-guided intra-articular knee injections yield ~97 % accuracy for needle placement compared with ~81 % accuracy without imaging [9], which of course means better efficacy and increased cost-effectiveness [14, 15].

An important limitation of our retrospective case series is the fact that all the study subjects received image-guided injections. They were not randomized into guided and non-guided HA injections for comparison. However, our data suggest future studies should test whether guidance together with knee bracing improves short-term and long-term outcomes when treating knee OA with HA. This is especially important for severe disease, which is a group most likely to require joint replacement and may benefit most from combined HA injection and knee bracing.

Analgesic use showed no positive effects in our data, and the literature suggests they have little clinical effect [16]. Notably, daily analgesic use was not prescribed in our study. Patients who reported daily analgesic use were more likely to have high-grade disease, less likely to show a functional improvement by 6 months, and less likely to report a reduction in the subjective pain index relative to baseline. We therefore suspect these patients may be more likely to be long-term non-responders to HA injection and knee bracing. This data also suggest the mechanism of action of HA injections may not be solely anti-inflammatory.

The biological actions of HA viscosupplementation are only beginning to be understood. For example, HA may increase synovial fluid viscosity [17] and regulate a number of cytokines involved in both anti-inflammatory activity and extracellular matrix restorative mechanisms. Recent studies exploring the effects of HA on activated CD4 positive T cells in synovial fluid [18] and reduction of joint tissue catabolism [19] are intriguing. Both mechanisms suggest that in some patients HA may have more long-term positive effects than only short-term improvements in pain and patient function. Long-term outcome data were not available for our analysis, but they are needed to test whether image-guided HA injections with knee bracing may delay joint replacement. Over 75 % of OA patients with joint space narrowing progress to total knee replacement within 18 years of diagnosis [20]. Delaying joint replacement is therefore very important because the lifespan of the device is 10–15 years. In an obese aging population, cost-effective interventions like HA injection and knee bracing make sense.

Conclusions

Our data suggest image-guided HA injections coupled with knee bracing may benefit patients with moderate to severe knee osteoarthritis. With the current rates of obesity and the advanced aging of the population, it is reasonable to speculate that many more patients will require revision surgery if alternative intervention methods like viscosupplementation are not effective. A randomized prospective trial to thoroughly evaluate the short-term and long-term impact of image-guided HA injection with and without knee bracing is needed.

Abbreviations

BMI: body mass index; HA: Hyaluronic acid; OA: Osteoarthritis.

Competing interests

Dr. Russell Riggs is the owner and medical director of the *Reflex Clinic*. Although he participated in the original documentation of patient data during treatment, these clinical charts were not intended for publication. Dr. Riggs did not participate in retrospective data extraction from the *Reflex Clinic* clinical records or data analysis performed at Oregon Health & Science University. However, this study was funded by the *Reflex Clinic* to support independent coded data extraction by the Morgan laboratory and statistical analysis.

Emilie Jensen and Drs. Morgan and Lim declare they have no competing interests.

Authors' contributions

TKM was principal investigator and managed all aspects of study design, data collection, and analysis. EJ was a summer intern at the Morgan laboratory and collected coded data from the Reflex Clinic archives for analysis. JL analyzed the data. RR provided access to his clinic's data, necessary funding, and the clinical methods described in the manuscript. All authors participated in the drafting of this manuscript and have given final approval for publication.

Author details

[1]Department of Pathology, Oregon Health & Science University, 3181 SW Sam Jackson, Mail Code L-471, Portland, OR 97239, USA. [2]Department of Public Health & Preventative Medicine, Oregon Health & Science University, Portland, OR, USA. [3]Reflex Clinic, Portland, OR, USA.

References

1. Peat G, McCarney R, Croft P. Knee pain and osteoarthritis in older adults: a review of community burden and current use of primary health care. Ann Rheum Dis. 2001;60(2):91–7.

2. Dillon C, Rasch E, Gu Q, Hirsch R. Prevalence of knee osteoarthritis in the United States: arthritis data from the Third National Health and Nutrition Examination Survey 1991–94. J Rheumatol. 2006;33(11):2271–9.
3. Buckwalter J, Saltzman C, Brown T. The impact of osteoarthritis: implications for research. Clin Orthop Relat Res. 2004;427(Suppl):S6–15.
4. Jackson D, Simon T, Aberman H. Symptomatic articular cartilage degeneration: the impact in the new millennium. Clin Orthop Relat Res. 2001;391(Suppl):S14–25.
5. Crawford D, Miller L, Block J. Conservative management of symptomatic knee osteoarthritis: a flawed strategy? Ortho Rev (Pavia). 2013;5(1), e2.
6. Bannuru R, Natov N, Dasi U, Schmid C, McAlindon T. Therapeutic trajectory following intra-articular hyaluronic acid injection in knee osteoarthritis—meta-analysis. Osteoarthr Cartil. 2011;19(6):611–9.
7. Leighton R, Akermark C, Therrien R, Richardson J, Andersson M, Todman M, et al. NASHA hyaluronic acid vs methylprednisone for knee osteoarthritis: a prospective, multicenter, randomized, non-inferiority trial. Osteoarthr Cartil. 2014;22:17–25.
8. Rutjes A, Juni P, da Costa B, Trelle S, Nuesch E, Reichenbach S. Viscosupplementation for osteoarthritis of the knee. Ann Intern Med. 2012;157(3):180–91.
9. Berkoff D, Miller L, Block J. Clinical utility of ultrasound-guidance for intra-articular knee injections: a review. Clin Interv Aging. 2012;7:89–95.
10. Jones A, Regan M, Ledingham J, Pattrick M, Manhire A, Doherty M. Importance of placement of intra-articular steroid injections. BMJ. 1993;307(6915):1329–30.
11. Bellamy N, Buchanan W, Goldsmith C, Campbell J, Stitt L. Validation study of WOMAC: a health status instrument for measuring clinically important patient relevant outcomes to antirheumatic drug therapy in patients with osteoarthritis of the hip or knee. J Rheumatol. 1988;15(12):1833–40.
12. Kellgren J, Lawrence J. Radiographic assessment of osteoarthritis. Ann Rheum Dis. 1957;16(4):494–502.
13. Yiasemidou M, Munir U, Glassman D, Teanby D. Efficacy and safety of biweekly viscosupplementation regimen for knee osteoarthritis. J Knee Surg. 2015. doi:10.1055/s-0034-1394300.
14. Hatoum H, Fierlinger A, Lin S, Altman R. Cost-effectiveness analysis of intra-articular injections of a high molecular weight bioengineered hyaluronic acid for the treatment of osteoarthritis knee pain. J Med Econ. 2014;17(5):326–37.
15. Sibbitt W, Brand P, Kettwich L, Chavez-Zhiang N, Delea S, Bankhurst A. A randomized controlled trial evaluating the cost-effectiveness of sonographic guidance for intra-articular injection of the osteoarthritic knee. J Clin Rheumatol. 2011;17(8):409–15.
16. Scott D, Berry H, Capell H. The long-term effects of non-steroidal anti-inflammatory drugs in osteoarthritis of the knee: a randomized placebo-controlled trial. Rheumatology (Oxford). 2000;39(10):1095–101.
17. Zhou PH, Liu SQ, Peng H. The effect of hyaluronic acid on IL-1beta-induced chondrocyte apoptosis in a rat model of osteoarthritis. J Orthop Res. 2008;26(12):1643–8.
18. Lurati A, Laria A, Mazzocchi D, Re K, Marrazza M, Scarpellini M. Effects of hyaluronic acid (HA) viscosupplementation on peripheral Th cells in knee and hip osteoarthritis. Osteoarthr Cartil. 2015;23(1):88–93.
19. Sundman E, Cole B, Karas V, Valle C, Tetreault M, Mohammed H, et al. The anti-inflammatory and matrix restorative mechanisms of platelet-rich plasma in osteoarthritis. Am J Sports Med. 2014;42(1):35–41.
20. Wolfe F, Lane N. The long term outcome of osteoarthritis: rates and predictors of joint space narrowing in symptomatic patients with knee osteoarthritis. J Rheumatol. 2002;29(1):139–46.

14

Ultra-Marathon Athletes at Risk for the Female Athlete Triad

Lindy-Lee Folscher[1*], Catharina C Grant[1], Lizelle Fletcher[2] and Dina Christina Janse van Rensberg[1]

Abstract

Background: Worldwide female participation in ultra-endurance events may place them at risk for the female athlete triad (FAT). The study objectives were to establish triad knowledge, occurrence of disordered eating and triad risk amongst participants of the 2014 89-km Comrades Marathon event.

Methods: A survey utilising the Low Energy Availability in Females questionnaire (LEAF-Q) and Female Athlete Screening Tool (FAST) questionnaire was conducted on female participants in order to determine the risk. In addition, seven questions pertaining to the triad were asked in order to determine the athlete's knowledge of the triad. Athletes were requested to complete the anonymous questionnaire after written informed consent was obtained while waiting in the event registration queues. Statistical analyses included Pearson product–moment correlations, chi-square tests and cross-tabulations to evaluate associations of interest.

Results: Knowledge of the triad was poor with 92.5 % of participants having not heard of the triad before and most of those who had, gained their knowledge from school or university. Only three athletes were able to name all 3 components of the triad. Amenorrhoea was the most commonly recalled component while five participants were able to name the component of low bone mineral density. Of the 306 athletes included in the study, 44.1 % were found to be at risk for the female athlete triad. One-third of participants demonstrated disordered eating behaviours with nearly half reporting restrictive eating behaviours. There is a significant association between athletes at risk for the triad according to the LEAF-Q and those with disordered eating ($\chi^2(1) = 8.411$, $p = 0.014$) but no association (or interaction) between triad knowledge and category (at risk/not at risk) of LEAF-Q score ($\chi^2(1) = 0.004$, $p = 0.949$). More athletes in the groups with clinical and sub-clinical eating disorders are at risk for the triad than expected under the null hypothesis for no association.

Conclusions: Only 7.5 % of the female Comrades Marathon runners knew about the triad despite 44.1 % being at a high risk for the triad. Therefore, education and regular screening programmes targeting these athletes are overdue. Postmenopausal athletes are at particularly high risk for large losses in bone mass if they experience chronic energy deficiency and hence require special focus.

MESH terms: Female athlete triad; Ultra-marathon runners; Risk of female athlete triad; Knowledge of female athlete triad

Key points

- Knowledge of the triad is very poor amongst South African ultra-marathon runners.
- There are many misconceptions about menstrual function and exercise training amongst these endurance athletes.
- High rates (32 %) of disordered eating exist amongst female Comrades Marathon runners.
- 44.1 % of Comrades Marathon runners are at risk for the triad.

* Correspondence: folscherl@gmail.com
[1]Section Sports Medicine, Faculty of Health Sciences, University of Pretoria, Hatfield, Pretoria 0002, South Africa
Full list of author information is available at the end of the article

Background

Female sports participation and ultra-marathon running has increased exponentially worldwide over the past three decades [1, 2]. This is reflected by female finishers of the annual 89-km Comrades Marathon run between Pietermaritzburg and Durban, South Africa which increased from 33 in 1980 to 2429 in 2014 [3]. Sport participation benefits weight management, chronic disease, high risk behaviour reduction, improved mental health, enhanced self-esteem and academic performance [4]. Unfortunately, intense training poses risks for female endurance athletes [5].

The female athlete triad (FAT) is a syndrome involving an interplay between low energy availability, menstrual dysfunction and altered bone mineral density [6]. Endurance runners are at increased risk posed by high energy demands of their training regimen and a potential desire for leanness for improved performance [7, 8]. Studies of collegiate and young adult endurance runners demonstrated higher prevalence of low bone mineral density (39.8 vs 10 %) amongst elite and recreational runners compared to non-runners [9].

Adequate dietary intake supplies energy for numerous physiological processes. This requires excess energy after exercise energy expenditure. If excessive exercise or dietary restriction reduces available energy below 30 $kcal.kg^{-1}$ of fat free mass per day, physiological processes are compromised with suppression of reproductive function and new bone formation and consequent infertility, osteoporosis and stress fractures [5, 6, 10]. Adequate nutrients are also essential to maintain muscle mass, repair exercise-induced tissue damage and recover from illness and injury. Hence, energy deficiency results in injuries and poor recovery from intense training [10].

Low energy availability from excessive exercise expenditure, poor nutritional habits or eating disorders is the central pathological process of the triad [8, 11]. The Female Athlete Triad Screening Tool (FAST) was designed and validated to identify females at risk for disordered eating. The validated Low Energy Availability in Females questionnaire (LEAF-Q) determines triad risk by assessing injury history and gastrointestinal and menstrual function [12, 13].

Previous prevalence studies have investigated adolescents and collegiate cross country and recreational distance runners (5–20 km), demonstrating rates of at least one triad component between 16 and 78 % [14, 15]. Prevalence data amongst ultra-marathon athletes is limited. Study results from the Two Oceans Ultra-marathon athletes found disordered eating in 14.7 % of those interviewed [16]. The self-loathing subscale used utilised only four questions and more comprehensive screening may have uncovered higher rates. Additional prevalence data is also required amongst recreational athletes [15].

Treatment of the triad is complex due to psychological and performance-related aspects therefore prevention should be prioritised and requires education of athletes and coaches, which is often sorely lacking. An Australian study demonstrated that only 10 % of 18–40-year-old exercisers interviewed were able to name all triad components [8]. No studies were found on triad knowledge amongst South African female ultra-marathon runners.

The Comrades Marathon, considered "the holy grail" of road running amongst South Africans, requires consistent weekly training of 80–200 km during the 6 months preceding the event, which places these athletes at risk for low energy availability and its health consequences. The primary objective of this study was to establish knowledge of the triad amongst these athletes and then determine their level of risk.

Methods

A cross-sectional, descriptive study utilising a questionnaire survey was conducted after ethical approval (159\2014) from the Faculty of Health Sciences, University of Pretoria, Ethics Committee. All study procedures followed were in accordance with the Helsinki Declaration of 1975, as revised in 2013. Registered female participants for the 2014 Comrades Marathon were invited to be study participants during race registration at the International Conference Centre, Durban, KwaZulu-Natal, South Africa. Participants provided written informed consent prior to questionnaire completion and no participation incentives were offered.

Data Collection

Females waiting in the registration queue were arbitrarily approached and asked to complete an anonymous questionnaire after reading the information and consent form. Three-hundred and seventy-one athletes were approached and 351 agreed to participate. Forty-five incomplete questionnaires were excluded from analysis. Three-hundred and six completed questionnaires, of which 42 were from international runners, were included in the sample representing 12.6 % of the 2429 females who completed the 2014 event. Research assistants were available to clarify any questions while participants completed the paper-based questionnaires. On completion, questionnaires were collected and placed in a sealed box. Questionnaires were marked and scored by the principle investigator according to the scoring tool for the LEAF-Q and FAST questionnaires.

Questionnaire Data

Questionnaire data included age, self-reported weight and height, training mileage, average training pace, number of Comrades Marathons completed and fastest finishing time. Participants were asked about their familiarity with the FAT, and if so, the source of their knowledge. In order to identify athletes at risk for the triad and disordered eating behaviours, the LEAF-Q and FAST were incorporated into the questionnaire. The FAST, developed to identify disordered eating behaviours in athletes, is reliable with a high internal consistency (Cronbach's α = 0.87). Higher FAST scores are associated with eating disorders as identified by the Eating Disorder Examination Questionnaire (0.60, $p < 0.05$) and Eating Disorder Inventory (0.89, $p < 0.001$) [13]. The 25 item LEAF-Q was developed to identify athletes at risk for low energy availability by utilising subsets of gastrointestinal symptoms, injury frequency and menstrual dysfunction. The LEAF-Q was validated in endurance athletes (Cronbach's $\alpha \geq 0.71$) with scores ≥8 producing a sensitivity of 78 % and specificity of 90 % to correctly classify energy availability and/or reproductive function and/or bone health [12].

Statistical Analysis

Data from completed questionnaires were analysed using IBM Statistics SPSS 22. Descriptive statistics were calculated and Pearson product–moment correlations and chi-square tests were used to assess associations of interest.

Results

Participant Characteristics

Comrades Marathon 2014 participants are older athletes with a range of ultra-marathon experience, performance and training load as shown in Table 1.

Demographic Data

Knowledge of the Female Athlete Triad

Most participants had never heard of the triad before (Table 2) and most of those who had, gained their knowledge from school or university. Only three athletes were able to name all three components of the triad. Amenorrhoea was the most commonly recalled component while five participants were able to name the component of low bone mineral density.

Table 1 Demographic data, training load, running experience and performance

	Mean	Standard deviation	Median	[Min; max]
Age (years)	39.45	7.97	40.00	[21;65]
Weight (kg)	59.15	6.97	59.00	[42;83]
Height (m)	1.65	0.08	1.65	[1.3;1.85]
Number of Comrades Marathons completed	2.24	3.03	1.00	[0;22]
Fastest Comrades Marathon (89 km) time (hr:min)	10:05	1:34	10:35	[7:02;12:00]
Average training during peak training (h/week)	8.66	3.14	8.00	[1.5;20]
Average training pace (min/km)	5.55	0.70	6.00	[4.20;9.00]
Fastest standard marathon (42 km) time in last 6 months (hr:min)	4:06	0:64	4:19	[2:42;5:59]

Table 2 Knowledge of the female athlete triad amongst female participants in the 2014 Comrades Marathon

Question	Frequency	Percentage (%)
1. Familiarity with triad	23	7.5
2. No previous knowledge	283	92.5
3. If yes, where did you hear about it?		
Sports magazine	2	0.65
Running book	2	0.65
University/school	13	4.2
Internet	3	1.0
Coach	1	0.35
Race expo	2	0.65
Not applicable	283	92.5
4. Ability to name components		
Unable to name any	286	93.5
Of the 20 participants attempting to name components:		
Able to name only one	6	2.0
Able to name two	7	2.2
Able to name all three	3	1.0
Incorrect	4	1.3

Knowledge of the Health Implications for the Female Athlete Triad

Of the 23 participants who had heard of the triad before only 12 could name 2 negative health consequences. Seven could correctly name 1 and 4 were unable to name any. The most commonly mentioned negative consequence was osteoporosis.

Self-Assessed Risk for the Triad

Only 2.3 % of participants thought they were at risk for the triad. The overwhelming majority (83.3 %) were uncertain whether they were at risk and 14.4 % believed that they were not.

Beliefs About Female Menstrual Function with Training

There was an even split (48.4 %, respectively) between participants who believed it normal to cease menstruation with heavy training and those who did not, while the remainder (3.2 %) expressed uncertainty. Even though many participants stated that amenorrhoea was a normal consequence of heavy training, the majority (83.3 %) believed it to be unhealthy.

Key Components of the LEAF Questionnaire

Table 3 highlights some key LEAF-Q responses. Many athletes reported injuries, the most common being muscular strain/tears and iliotibial band friction syndrome. Menstrual changes were common with increased exercise with one-fifth of those capable of menstruation reporting amenorrhoea with heavy training loads. Gastrointestinal disturbances were less frequent than menstrual disturbances and injuries.

LEAF-Q Scores

Nearly half (44.1 %) of participants are classified as being at risk for the triad according to their LEAF-Q scores.

FAST Questionnaire Scores

Table 4 shows that according to FAST questionnaire responses, almost one-third of participants are at risk for low energy availability related to their eating behaviours. The majority of participants believed their running performance was related to their weight with 60.5 % expecting performance improvements with weight reduction and 67.4 % worrying that weight gain would impair their performance. Restrictive eating was reported by nearly half of participants with 47.7 % controlling fat and calorie intake and 44.5 % limiting carbohydrate intake. Many participants reported using exercise for weight management with 50.3 % reporting that they trained intensely in order to avoid weight gain and 71.8 % stating that they would worry about weight gain if unable to exercise or injured and therefore restrict their calorie intake. A large percentage (68.3 %) considered sport participation as important for their self-esteem.

Correlative Analysis

Table 5 shows that higher LEAF-Q scores correlate negatively with faster race performance, while higher FAST scores correlate positively with LEAF-Q scores, weight and BMI.

Cross-tabulation

The cross-tabulation of FAST and LEAF-Q categories (Table 6) demonstrates more athletes at risk for the triad in the groups with clinical and sub-clinical eating disorders than expected under the null hypothesis of no association (count vs. expected count).

Cross-tabulation of triad knowledge (Yes/No) by LEAF-Q score (Not at risk/At risk) demonstrated no association between triad knowledge and LEAF-Q score category ($\chi^2(1) = 0.004$, $p = 0.949$).

Discussion

Ultra-endurance sport attracts older athletes due to age restrictions on participation and possibly the fact that many long distance athletes compete in shorter distances before attempting ultra-endurance events. The mean age of athletes studied was 39 years. Marathon finishing times of participants demonstrated that both elite runners and recreational athletes were included in the sample,

Table 3 Responses to key components of LEAF-Q as reported by female participants of the 2014 Comrades Marathon

LEAF questionnaire component	Frequency	Percent
1. Injury history		
Number of days lost from participation due to injury in past year:		
0	120	39.2
1–7	91	29.7
8–14	39	12.8
15–21	24	7.8
≥22	32	10.5
Most common injuries reported:		
(Respondents could choose more than one)		
Muscular strain/tear	38	11.8
Iliotibial band friction syndrome (ITB)	36	11.2
Knee injury	24	7.4
Hamstring injury	18	5.6
Achilles tendonitis/ankle injury	14	4.3
Plantar fasciitis/foot injury	14	4.3
Stress fractures	11	3.4
2. Menstrual function		
Exercise-related menstrual changes:		
Bleed less	79	72.5
Menstruation stops	22	20.2
Increased bleeding	8	7.3
Number of periods in the last year (if still menstruating)		
≥9	184	60.2
5–8	20	6.6
0–2	2	0.7
Secondary amenorrhoea	71	23.2
Current and not menopausal		
Postmenopausal	14	4.6
Hysterectomy	30	9.8
3. Gastrointestinal disturbances		
Abdominal bloated/gaseous when not having periods:		
Daily–weekly	55	14.7
Seldom	76	24.8
Rarely or never	185	60.5
Cramps/stomach ache not related to your menstruation:		
Daily–weekly	42	13.8
Seldom	57	18.6
Rarely or never	207	67.6

Table 4 Number of female athletes with disordered eating according to FAST questionnaire results

	Frequency	Percent	Mean FAST score	SD
No eating disorder	208	68.0	61.79	9.59
Subclinical eating disorder	82	26.8	82.70	4.68
Clinical eating disorder	16	5.2	100.13	6.04

increasing the likelihood of results being representative of the female ultra-marathon running community.

A disturbingly small percentage (7.5 %) of participants knew about the triad. The majority (80 %) of these were international runners from Europe, USA or Australia. The most knowledgeable athletes had obtained their knowledge at school or university. It is likely that these are younger athletes with recent education which has been influenced by the Female Athlete Triad Coalition and other regulatory bodies' drive for pre-participation evaluation and education [11, 17]. This lack of knowledge is concerning since endurance athletes are at increased risk due to the high volume training associated with ultra-marathon preparation and possible inadvertent low energy availability [18]. Only 1 % of participants could name all three triad components which is lower than the 10 % reported by Australian women [8]. Knowledge of negative health implications of the triad was equally poor with only 3.9 and 2.3 % able to name one and two negative consequences, respectively. Similar rates were found in an American study in which more than 90 % of female high school track athletes were unable to link menstrual irregularity with negative bone consequences [17].

Very few participants believed they were at risk for the triad, possibly since 83.3 % were unsure what the triad was. The 44 participants who explicitly stated that they were not at risk demonstrate blissful ignorance and are therefore unlikely to pursue further understanding of the triad. It could be argued that simply engaging in endurance training places female athletes at risk, which may be mitigated by education on nutritional intake and careful dietary monitoring. However, female endurance athletes often seek to reduce body weight without seeking professional guidance, resulting in chronic energy deficiency [19].

Table 5 Summary of bivariate correlations

Variables	Pearson coefficient	p for H_0: $\rho = 0$
LEAF-Q score and Comrades performance	−0.159	0.029
FAST score and LEAF-Q score	0.244	<0.001
FAST score and weight	0.198	0.001
FAST score and BMI	0.186	0.001

The fact that 48.4 % of participants believed amenorrhoea to be normal with heavy training is concerning and higher than the 35 % reported by Australian women [8]. These athletes are unlikely to seek medical attention for amenorrhoea, resulting in a missed opportunity for early intervention. In addition, this belief may cause athletes to use amenorrhoea as an indicator of hard training, driving them towards this "marker" of adequate training. Amenorrhoea may also be considered "convenient" by athletes since they are relieved of the discomfort caused by menstruation. Conversely, low energy might initially result in subclinical menstrual disorders still placing athletes at risk since these disorders go undetected when athletes use amenorrhoea as a "red flag" for excessive training [20, 21].

Fifty percent of women capable of normal menstrual cycles reported changes with increasing exercise, similar to other studies that reported 43–78 % of athletes with menstrual dysfunction, exacerbated by increasing training [16, 21, 22]. Menstrual dysfunction is a useful triad screening tool but was not applicable to many older athletes due to Mirena® use, postmenopausal status or previous hysterectomy [11, 21, 23]. Postmenopausal females are already in a hypo-estrogenic state and at risk for osteoporosis. Energy deficits with resultant oestrogen deficiency leads to abnormal bone remodelling placing energy deficient postmenopausal athletes at risk [21]. Protective effects of weight-bearing exercise on postmenopausal bone loss may be lost with high training volumes and therefore more research may be required on these vulnerable athletes [24].

If triad knowledge is so poor amongst this group of athletes, they probably have inadequate nutritional knowledge to prevent inadvertent energy deficiency. Previous studies revealed that female endurance athletes often consume an incorrect macronutrient balance causing calorie deficiencies [25, 26]. One-third of athletes were categorised as having disordered eating by FAST scores—higher than the 14.7 % reported by Micklesfield et al. in Two Oceans athletes but similar to rates reported by Cobb et al. (25.5 %) amongst competitive distance runners [16, 23]. The majority of these athletes demonstrate a subclinical eating disorder with only 5.2 % meeting clinical eating disorder criteria, only marginally higher than general population rates (2–4 %) [27]. There were more athletes than expected with disordered eating behaviours in athletes at risk according to LEAF-Q scores confirming the interaction between disordered eating and triad risk. Since disordered eating is associated with low bone mineral density in competitive female distance runners without menstrual irregularity, screening of these athletes is advisable [23]. Dietary restraint is the disordered eating behaviour most closely associated with bone mineral loss and is therefore an important risk factor [28]. Nutritional trends amongst

Table 6 Cross-tabulation of FAST and LEAF-Q score categories

FAST score category:		Not at risk for triad according to LEAF-Q score	At risk for triad according to LEAF-Q score	Total
No eating disorder	Count	125	83	208
	Expected count	116.2	91.8	
	Column %	73.1 %	61.5 %	68 % of 306
Subclinical eating disorder	Count	42	40	82
	Expected count	45.8	36.2	
	Column %	24.6 %	29.6 %	26.8 % of 306
Clinical eating disorder	Count	4	12	16
	Expected count	8.9	7.1	
	Column %	2.3 %	8.9 %	5.2 % of 306

Pearson chi-square = 8.411; degrees of freedom = 2; $p = 0.015$

athletes have drastically changed in recent years following publicised low carbohydrate/high fat diets. Nearly 45 % of participants reported carbohydrate restriction. This is likely due to proposed benefits of improved body composition and performance without adequate input from a dietician thereby placing themselves at greater risk for calorie deficits. While low carbohydrate/high fat diets assist in weight loss, performance benefits for endurance athletes as well as the long-term health implications of such diets may be questioned. In addition to this, appetite often declines with intensive training and cannot be used as an indicator of energy requirements for endurance athletes [19]. Therefore, nutritional assessment and support may be beneficial for this group.

Weight control may be the motivation for or consequence of endurance exercise. Half of participants reported weight management as a motivation for training and 68 % expressed performance-related weight beliefs. Gibbs et al. demonstrated an association between a high drive for thinness amongst exercising women and energy deficiency, highlighting the need to screen athletes for energy and menstrual status if direct measurement is not feasible [29]. The high proportion demonstrating "weight consciousness" highlights the urgent need for screening of these athletes to detect compulsive attitudes towards exercise as well as eating psychopathology which is directly linked to the triad and stress fracture risk [22].

Self-reported injury rates were fairly high with 59.1 % of participants reporting injuries in the preceding year. This injury rate is similar to other studies which report injury rates as high as 79.3 %. Typical injuries occur in the lower extremities and increase with increased training distance, participation in longer distance events and training on hard surfaces (mainly concrete). These factors are all relevant to this group studied [30–32]. The majority of reported injuries were overuse injuries in keeping with other studies on athletes with high training loads [31, 33].

LEAF-Q scores classified 44.1 % of participants at risk for the triad with a correlation between faster race performance and higher triad risk. Faster race performance, higher training volume and intensity have a strong association with bone stress injury and triad risk [18].

With the above in mind, prevention is considered "the ultimate treatment strategy" [5, 17]. Screening and educational interventions are the most effective preventative strategy amongst endurance athletes [6, 7, 11]. Education should include healthcare professionals managing athlete injuries/illnesses, club coaches, family and friends of athletes [5]. Unfortunately, knowledge of the triad is also poor amongst health-care professionals with only 48 % of USA physicians, 43 % of physical therapists, 32 % of athletic trainers and 8 % of coaches able to name all three components [34]. It is unlikely that the situation is any different amongst healthcare professionals treating these participants therefore education about the triad should be extended to include these professionals. In addition, governing bodies should ensure effective implementation of educational programmes [5]. Athletics South Africa (ASA), the governing body of running in South Africa, should become activists for the education of female athletes. Pre-participation medical screening questionnaires are required by organisers before entry into certain events and cover mainly chronic illness and medical/injury history. It is recommended that triad screening questions be included in these questionnaires.

Strengths of the Study

All female athletes in the registration queue during sampling were requested to participate in the study to avoid selection bias from research assistants singling out "thin" athletes. South African runners as well as 42 international runners were asked to participate in order to get representation of the global female running community. Questions were simple and easy to understand.

Limitations

The study is limited to female participants in the 2014 South African Comrades Marathon. The data is self-reported and therefore dependent on the understanding of the questions and honesty of completion. The 45 incomplete questionnaires were excluded from analysis. It was assumed that these were incomplete due to time constraints. It may however be that some questions were too sensitive, especially those about eating behaviours. It is therefore possible that occurrence rates of participants with clinical or subclinical eating disorders are underreported.

Conclusions

This study highlights a group of athletes at high risk for the triad and calls for urgent educational interventions and regular screening for this group of athletes. Pre-participation screening should become mandatory and should be performed by race organisers or athletic governing bodies [17, 35]. This study population includes some older athletes entering menopausal years who are at particularly high risk for large losses in bone mass if exposed to chronic energy deficiency due to endurance exercise. More research may be required on this group of athletes.

What is Already Known:

- The female athlete triad consists of an interaction between low energy availability, hormonal dysfunction with resultant menstrual disturbances and altered bone mineral density
- While ultra-marathon running is protective against chronic illness, runners are at risk for the negative health consequences of female athlete triad
- Disordered eating places athletes at risk for the triad particularly if engaged in high volume/high intensity training

Competing Interests

L-LF, CCG, LF and DCJvR declare that they have no conflict of interest.

Authors' Contributions

L-LF conceived and designed the study as well as conducted data collection and wrote the paper. LF assisted in data interpretation, statistical analysis and revision of the report. CCG provided technical advice, supervision and revision of the report. DCJvR provided support with literature search and revision of the report. All authors read and approved the final manuscript.

Acknowledgements

The authors would like to thank Douglas Grantham, Lisa Grantham and Melanie Mandy for assistance in data collection, Danny Folscher for co-ordination of questionnaire collection and the female participants who took the time to complete the questionnaire. Thanks also to Joyce Jordaan for assistance with data capturing and analysis.

Funding

No financial support was received for the conduct of this study or preparation of this manuscript.

Author details

[1]Section Sports Medicine, Faculty of Health Sciences, University of Pretoria, Hatfield, Pretoria 0002, South Africa. [2]Department of Statistics, University of Pretoria, Hatfield, Pretoria 0002, South Africa.

References

1. Andersen JJ. [cited 2015 23 June]; Available from: http://runrepeat.com/research-marathon-performance-across-nations.
2. Running USA. [cited 2014 28 February]; Available from: http://www.runningusa.org/statistics.
3. Comrades Marathon Association. [cited 2014 10 October]; Available from: http://www.comrades.com.
4. Khodaee M, Ansari M. Common ultramarathon injuries and illnesses: race day management. Curr Sports Med Rep. 2012;11:290–7.
5. Temme KE, Hoch AZ. Recognition and rehabilitation of the female athlete triad/tetrad: a multidisciplinary approach. Curr Sports Med Rep. 2013;12(3):190–9.
6. Deimel JF, Dunlan BJ. The female athlete triad. Clin Sports Med. 2012;31:247–54.
7. Nazem TG, Ackerman KE. The female athlete triad. Sports Health. 2012;4(4):302–11.
8. Miller SM, Kukuljan S, Turner AI, van der Pligt P, Ducher G. Energy deficiency, menstrual disturbances and low bone mass: what do exercising Australian women know about the female athlete triad? Int J Sport Nutr Exerc Metab. 2012;22:131–8.
9. Torstveit MK, Sundgot-Borgen J. The female athlete triad exists in both elite athletes and controls. Med Sci Sports Exerc. 2005;37(9):1449–59.
10. Manore MM, Kam LC, Loucks AB. The female athlete triad: components, nutrition, issues and health consequences. J Sports Sci. 2007;25(51):561–71.
11. Bonci CM, Bonci LJ, Granger LR, Johnson CL, Malina RM, Milne LW, et al. National Athletic Trainers' Association Position Statement: preventing, detecting and managing disordered eating in athletes. J Athl Train. 2008;43(1):80–108.
12. Melin A, Tornberg AB, Skouby S, Faber J, Ritz C, Sjodin A, et al. The LEAF questionnaire: a screening tool for the identification of female athletes at risk for the female athlete triad. Br J Sports Med. 2014;48:540–5.
13. Mc Nulty KY, Adams CH, Anderson JM, Affenito SG. Development and validation of a screening tool to identify eating disorders in female athletes. J Am Diet Assoc. 2001;101:886–92.
14. Hoch AZ, Pajewski NM, Moraski L, Carrera GF, Wilson CR, Hoffmann RG, et al. Prevalence of the female athlete triad in high school athletes and sedentary students. Clin J Sports Med. 2009;19(5):421–8.
15. Gibbs JC, Williams NI, De Souza MJ. Prevalence of individual and combined components of the female athlete triad. Med Sci Sports Excerc. 2013;45(5):985–95.
16. Micklesfield LK, Hugo J, Johnson C, Noakes TD, Lambert EV. Factors associated with menstrual dysfunction and self-reported bone stress injuries in female runners in the ultra and half-marathons of the Two Oceans. Br J Sports Med. 2007;41:679–83.
17. Barrack MT, Ackerman KE, Gibbs JC. An update on the female athlete triad. Curr Rev Musculoskelet Med. 2013;6:195–204.
18. Barrack MG JC, De Souza MJ, Williams NI, Nichols JF, Rauh MJ, Nattiv A. Higher incidence of bone stress injuries with increasing female athlete triad-related risk factors. Am J Sports Med. 2014;42:949–58.
19. Loucks A. Low energy availability in the marathon and other endurance sports. Sports Med. 2007;37(4-5):348–52.
20. Pollock N, Grogan C, Perry M, Pedlar C, Cooke K, Morrissey D, et al. Bone-mineral density and other features of the female athlete triad in elite endurance runners: a longitudinal and cross-sectional observational study. Int J Sport Nutr Exerc Metab. 2010;20:418–26.
21. Nattiv AL, Manore AB, Sanborm MM, Sundgot-Borden CF, Warren MP. American College of Sports Medicine position stand: the female athlete triad. Am J Sports Med. 2007;39:1867–82.
22. Duckham RPN, Meyer C, Summers GD, Cameron N, Brooke-Wavell K. Risk factors for stress fracture in female endurance athletes: a cross-sectional study. BMJ Open. 2012;2:e001920.

23. Cobb KL, Bachrach LK, Greendale G, Marcus R, Neer RM, Nieves J, et al. Disordered eating, menstrual irregularity and bone mineral density in female runners. Med Sci Sports Exerc. 2002;35(5):711–9.
24. Marcus RCC, Madvig P, Minkoff J, Goddard M, Bayer M, Martin M, et al. Menstrual function and bone mass in elite women distance runners. Annals of Internal Medicine. 1985;102:158–63.
25. Hoch AS, Schimke JE. Prevalence of female athlete triad characteristics in a club triathlon team. Arch Phys Med Rehabil. 2007;88:681–2.
26. Raymond-Barker PPA, Quested E. Assessment of nutritional knowledge in female athletes susceptible to the female athlete triad. J Occup Med Toxicol. 2007;2(10):110–23.
27. Smink FvH D, Hoek HW. Epidemiology, course and outcome of eating disorders. Eating disorders. 2013;26(6):543–8.
28. Barrack MT, Rauh MJ, Barkai H-S, Nichols JF. Dietary restraint and low bone mass in female adolescent endurance runners. Am J Clin Nutri. 2008;87:36–43.
29. Gibbs JC, Williams NI, Scheid JL, Toombs RJ, De Souza MJ. The association of a high drive for thinness with energy deficiency and severe menstrual disturbances: confirmation in a large population of exercising women. Int J Sport Nutr Exerc Metab. 2011;21:280–90.
30. van Gent RN, Siem D, van Middelkoop M, van Os AG, Bierma-Zeinstra SM, Koes BW. Incidence and determinants of lower extremity running injuries in long distance runners: a systematic review. Br J Sports Med. 2007;41:469–80.
31. Fredericson MM,AK. Epidemiology and aetiology of marathon running injuries. Sports Med. 2007;37(4–5):437–9.
32. Hoffman MD, Krishnan E. Health-related and exercise-related medical issues among 1212 ultramarathon runners: baseline findings from the Ultrarunners Longitudinal TRAcking (ULTRA) study. PLOS One. 2014;9(1):e83867. 1–8.
33. Krabak BJW, Waite B, Lipman G. Injury and illness prevention for ultramarathoners. Curr Sports Med Rep. 2013;12(3):183–9.
34. Troy KH, Hoch AZ, Stavrakos JE. Awareness and comfort in treating the female athlete triad: are we failing our athletes? Wisconsin Medical Journal. 2006;105(7):21–4.
35. De Souza MJ, Nattiv A, Joy E, Misra M, Williams NI, Mallinson RJ, et al. 2014 Female Athlete Triad Coalition Consensus Statement on treatment and return to play of the 119: 1st International Conference held in San Francisco, CA, May 2012, and 2nd International Conference held in Indianapolis, IN, May 2013. Clin J Sport Med. 2014;24(2):96–119.

15

Obesity-Related Oxidative Stress: the Impact of Physical Activity and Diet Manipulation

Chun-Jung Huang[1*], Matthew J. McAllister[2], Aaron L. Slusher[1,3], Heather E. Webb[4], J. Thomas Mock[1] and Edmund O. Acevedo[3]

Abstract

Obesity-related oxidative stress, the imbalance between pro-oxidants and antioxidants (e.g., nitric oxide), has been linked to metabolic and cardiovascular disease, including endothelial dysfunction and atherosclerosis. Reactive oxygen species (ROS) are essential for physiological functions including gene expression, cellular growth, infection defense, and modulating endothelial function. However, elevated ROS and/or diminished antioxidant capacity leading to oxidative stress can lead to dysfunction. Physical activity also results in an acute state of oxidative stress. However, it is likely that chronic physical activity provides a stimulus for favorable oxidative adaptations and enhanced physiological performance and physical health, although distinct responses between aerobic and anaerobic activities warrant further investigation. Studies support the benefits of dietary modification as well as exercise interventions in alleviating oxidative stress susceptibility. Since obese individuals tend to demonstrate elevated markers of oxidative stress, the implications for this population are significant. Therefore, in this review our aim is to discuss (i) the role of oxidative stress and inflammation as associated with obesity-related diseases, (ii) the potential concerns and benefits of exercise-mediated oxidative stress, and (iii) the advantageous role of dietary modification, including acute or chronic caloric restriction and vitamin D supplementation.

Key Points

- Acute exercise is a small source of oxidative stress, while chronic exercise elicits protective adaptations against oxidative damage.
- Chronic ingestion of energy-rich foods may contribute to obesity, while acute ingestion may also elicit potentially adverse metabolic responses including oxidative stress.
- Caloric restriction may attenuate oxidative stress and serve as a beneficial weight loss intervention for obese individuals.

Introduction

The prevalence of obesity continues to increase in the USA, with recent reports indicating over 64.1 % of American women and 72.3 % of American men are categorized as overweight and/or obese [body mass index (BMI) ≥ 25 kg/m^2] [1]. Obese individuals have demonstrated markers indicative of oxidative stress, including elevated measures of reactive oxygen species (ROS) [2] and diminished antioxidant defense, which is associated with lower antioxidant enzymes [3]. Oxidative stress is associated with systemic inflammation, endothelial cell proliferation and apoptosis, and increased vasoconstriction, and thus a noteworthy contributing factor to endothelial dysfunction. In concert, this evidence supports the relationship between oxidative stress, endothelial dysfunction, atherosclerosis, and cardiovascular disease (CVD) [4].

Oxidative stress is a general term for cellular damage caused by an imbalance between pro-oxidants such as ROS and/or reactive nitrogen species (RNS) antioxidants. ROS are oxidizing agents generated during cellular metabolism when the chemical reduction of oxygen forms unstable free radicals, characterized by an unpaired electron [4]. ROS are essential for physiological functions such as gene expression, cellular growth, infection defense, and modulating endothelial function

* Correspondence: chuang5@fau.edu
[1]Exercise Biochemistry Laboratory, Department of Exercise Science and Health Promotion, Florida Atlantic University, 777 Glades Road, FH11A-126B, Boca Raton, FL 33431, USA
Full list of author information is available at the end of the article

[4–6]. However, to maintain a physiologically beneficial level of ROS within cells, antioxidants are necessary. Antioxidants are enzymatic and nonenzymatic molecules which significantly delay or prevent the oxidizing damage of ROS through the inhibition of ROS formation and action or by repairing cells which have been damaged by ROS [5].

Furthermore, obesity-induced inflammation is frequently associated with increased oxidative stress (Fig. 1). Specifically, leptin, an adipocyte-derived hormone, is elevated in obese individuals and can induce oxidative stress [7] and plays a key role in mediating a pro-inflammatory state in obesity [8]; and Korda et al. [7] indicated that this physiological link may help to explain the relationship of obesity, oxidative stress, and inflammation. Additionally, the chronic ingestion of lipid-rich meals can also enhance oxidative stress, lead to weight gain, and facilitate the development of insulin resistance [9]. These negative effects can be attenuated with specific nutrient intake strategies including caloric restriction (CR) and the consumption of exogenous antioxidants. Finally, oxidative stress is elevated during physical activity, but likely serves to instigate a positive antioxidant adaptation [10, 11]. In this review, MEDLINE and PUBMED records were searched using the terms obesity, oxidative stress, inflammation, exercise/physical activity, diets, and antioxidants to identify the studies published in the past 10 years pertaining to two factors that impact obesity-related oxidative stress: physical activity intervention and diet manipulation. Therefore, in this review our aim is to discuss (i) the role of oxidative stress and inflammation as associated with obesity-related diseases, (ii) the potential concerns and benefits of exercise-mediated oxidative stress, and (iii) the advantageous role of dietary modification, including acute or chronic CR and vitamin D supplementation.

Obesity: a Link between Oxidative Stress and Inflammation

One of the earliest subclinical stages in the atherosclerotic process is an impairment of endothelium-dependent vasodilation, also known as endothelial dysfunction [12]. A mediator of obesity-induced endothelial dysfunction is the level of oxidative stress. Oxidative stress is an imbalance between antioxidants [e.g., superoxide dismutase (SOD) and glutathione peroxidase (GPX)] and reactive oxygen species [e.g., superoxide (O_2^-), hydrogen peroxide (H_2O_2), and hydroxyl radical (OH^-)] [13]. Under normal physiological conditions, nitric oxide (NO) is a critical homeostatic regulator of the vessel wall and plays a role in the maintenance of vascular tone and reactivity [14]. However, when ROS production is elevated, the process of cell damage occurs and can possibly facilitate the development of CVD [15] which is largely attributed to oxidation of low-density lipoprotein (LDL) [16]. Several

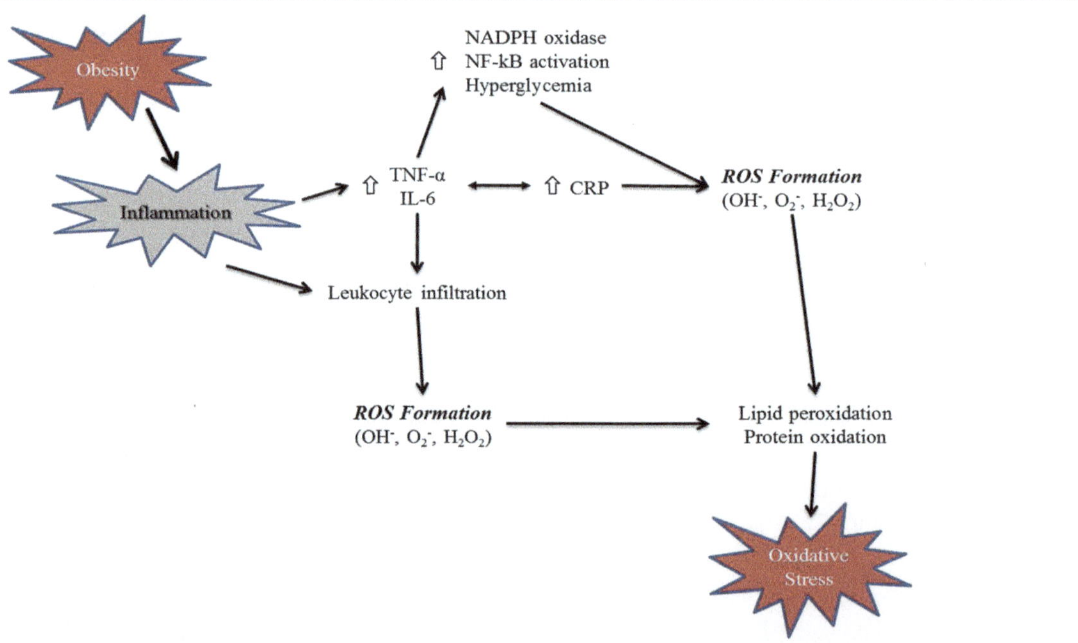

Fig. 1 The link between obesity-induced inflammation and oxidative stress. Increased pro-inflammatory response and leukocyte infiltration in obese populations promote the formation of ROS, resulting in oxidative stress. *NADPH* nicotinamide adenine dinucleotide phosphate, *NF-kB* nuclear factor kappa B, *TNF-α* tumor necrosis factor, *IL-6* interleukin-6, *CRP*, C-reactive protein, *OH⁻*, hydroxyl radical, *O²⁻* superoxide, *H₂O₂* hydrogen peroxide, *ROS* reactive oxygen species

oxidative enzymes such as myeloperoxidase (MPO) and lipoxygenases have been shown to involve in LDL oxidation [17, 18] and are associated with the development of obesity along with inflammation and insulin resistance [19, 20]. Furthermore, increased endogenous activity of antioxidants such as SOD and GPX can decrease the potential for CVD development by regulating ROS and NO production [21, 22]. Importantly, the vascular response to shear stress in obese individuals has been shown to be attenuated [23]. This subsequent attenuation of shear stress has been shown to reduce the activation of endothelial NO synthase (eNOS), resulting in the reduction of NO [24]. The primary sources of ROS in the vasculature are nicotinamide adenine dinucleotide phosphate (NADPH) oxidase, xanthine oxidase, and uncoupled eNOS [25]. Particularly, NADPH oxidase has been found to be the most potent source of O_2^- in the human vasculature [26] and could be activated by LDL and high levels of free fatty acid [27, 28]. Thus, this would help explain the reduced endothelial function in obesity.

More specifically, obese individuals demonstrate elevated markers of ROS, including urinary 8-isoprostanes [2] and decreased antioxidant defenses, represented by lower antioxidant enzymes (e.g., SOD and catalase) [3]. Furthermore, in obese insulin-resistant individuals, the effect of insulin on eNOS is impaired and inducible NO synthase (iNOS) is stimulated, resulting in NO overproduction [29]. Evidence has demonstrated that when expressed iNOS is fully active, it can generate large amount of NO to react with O_2^-, resulting in elevated peroxynitrite ($ONOO^-$), a powerful reactive oxidant [30]. These findings are further supported by Perticone et al. [31] who demonstrated that abdominal fat distribution and insulin resistance are negatively correlated with forearm blood flow in response to acetylcholine infusion in obese individuals.

Although the mechanisms for obesity-induced oxidative stress remain unclear, leptin, an adipocyte-derived hormone, has been considered as an important contributor. Leptin is responsible for regulating energy intake and expenditure and is also known to play a key role in mediating pro-inflammatory state in obese individuals [8]. Korda et al. [7] have shown that elevated leptin induces oxidative stress (e.g., reduced NO and increased O_2^- and $ONOO^-$) in both human endothelial cells and the endothelium of obese mice. Yamagishi et al. [32] have further demonstrated that leptin can increase intracellular ROS generation in microvascular endothelial cells. Thus far, two possible mechanisms have been proposed for the leptin-induced oxidative stress: (i) the stimulation of mitochondrial oxidation of fatty acids [33] and (ii) the elevation of pro-inflammatory cytokines [34].

The pro-inflammatory state of the vessel can negatively impact oxidative stress and play a crucial role in the pathogenesis of obesity-related diseases. Elevated pro-inflammatory cytokines such as tumor necrosis factor (TNF-α) have been shown to downregulate the expression of eNOS (diminishing the dilatory response) in human aortic endothelial cells [34]. Specifically, TNF-α is a potent activator for activation of NADPH oxidase, resulting in the formation of ROS [35]. Picchi et al. [36] also examined the effects of TNF-α administration on oxidative stress response and found that higher O_2^- levels with reduced NO bioavailability in the coronary artery of Zucker obese rats compared to controls.

Interestingly, research has also shown that higher levels of leptin are associated with elevated pro-inflammatory cytokines (e.g., TNF-α and interleukin-6 [IL-6]) [37]. For example, *in vitro* a high dose of leptin has been found to elicit a great amount of TNF-α and IL-6 secretion from activated human peripheral blood mononuclear cells (PBMCs) [38]. In addition, macrophages play a vital role in regulating obese inflammation by the ability to shift T-helper (Th) cell differentiation toward the Th1 subtype, a pro-inflammatory condition [39]. Within the Th1 immune response, the most potent trigger for macrophage-induced ROS production is interferon-gamma (IFN-γ) [40]. Increased ROS such as O_2^-, H_2O_2, and OH^- released by macrophages also provides a positive feedback to upregulate Th1 cell activation [41]. Importantly, leptin has been shown to serve as an immunological adjuvant to efficiently promote Th1 cell response [42]. Thus, inflammation and its subsequent impact on oxidative stress may play a crucial role in the pathogenesis of obesity-related diseases [43, 44].

Oxidative Stress and Physical Activity

Exercise-Induced Oxidative Stress

Exercise-induced oxidative stress has been shown to be dependent upon a number of factors including the mode [the form or type of exercise being utilized (cycling, jogging, and swimming)], intensity [percentage of maximal exercise capacity (VO_{2max})], and duration (total time exercising at a given percentage of VO_{2max}) of exercise being performed [45–49]. For example, concentrations of circulating oxidative stress markers were increasingly elevated at greater exercise intensities (25 vs. 50 vs. 75 % VO_{2peak}) following 30 min stationary cycling [45, 46] as well as at longer durations (120 vs. 60 vs. 30 min) following stationary cycling at 75 % VO_{2peak} [47]. Additionally, the characteristics of the participant (fitness or training levels, gender, and clinical disease status) can impact the resultant amount of oxidization that occurs [50, 51].

Research has shown that both acute aerobic [52–54] and anaerobic [55–57] exercise can result in increased free radical production, propagating a potential increase in oxidative stress. Further, for oxidative stress to occur, the ROS and RNS produced during exercise must exceed the levels of the antioxidant available for cellular defense, thus resulting in oxidative damage to specific biomolecules [58]. As demonstrated in ironman competitors, the level of antioxidant defenses appear to be adequate to mitigate ROS/RNS production which occurs as a result of high-intensity, but shorter-duration exercise bouts (half ironman competitors), whereas in increasing intensity and/or duration of the acute bout (full ironman competitors), antioxidant defenses can no longer be maintained at sufficient levels, thereby resulting in oxidative damage to surrounding tissues [59]. Both single bouts of aerobic and anaerobic exercises (including resistance-type exercise) can induce oxidative stress, as indicated by the presence of oxidized molecules in a variety of tissue types, especially skeletal muscle [56, 57]. While acute bouts of exercise will lead to associated oxidative stress, these increases seem to be necessary in order to allow for an upregulation in endogenous antioxidant defenses, thus providing beneficial effects to the individual engaged in chronic exercise [60].

Interestingly, the mechanism for increased oxidative stress is somewhat different for aerobic and anaerobic activities. During aerobic exercise, mitochondrial respiration has been purported to produce ROS and RNS; whereas during anaerobic exercise and resistance training, it has been suggested that increases in free radical production may be tempered by enzymatic reactions, prostanoid metabolism, and/or altered calcium homeostasis [48, 49]. It has further been suggested that anaerobically induced oxidative stress may also result from the ischemia/reperfusion cycle of muscle contraction and/or immune system responses following muscle damage that occurs with anaerobic exercise [49, 55, 61]. Similar to aerobic exercise, the results of anaerobic investigations are currently unclear whether the observed increases in ROS and RNS represent a necessary stimulus for adaptation or a detrimental event. While the specific underlying factors that dictate the differences in responses between aerobic and anaerobic physical activities vary, the endpoint of both types of exercise is similar, an elevation in ROS and RNS [48, 62]. An elucidation of the distinct mechanisms may support proposals for different remediation strategies or interventions to limit oxidative stress.

Obesity-Related Oxidative Stress

Pro-inflammation has also shown to exert a negative oxidative effect in the skeletal muscle of obese individuals. Obese population exhibit decreased skeletal muscle strength and function compared to healthy weight subjects [63], as well as impaired skeletal muscle mitochondrial respiratory function which contributes to increases in mitochondrial ROS production [64]. Specifically, obese individuals present higher ratios of type II to type I skeletal muscle fibers which have shown to generate two- to threefold more ROS production than type I fibers [64, 65]. Furthermore, Plomgaard et al. [66] demonstrated that TNF-α is solely expressed by type II muscle fibers and serves as a catalyst in skeletal muscle-derived oxidative stress [67]. Additionally, systemic TNF-α administration has been shown to diminish skeletal muscle force production in animal models [68] and directly promotes muscle protein loss [67] via oxidative activation of TNF-α/NF-κB signaling [69]. Interestingly, TNF-α-induced skeletal muscle oxidative stress has been shown to be prevented by antioxidant treatment [67], suggesting that TNF-α may provide a vital target toward correcting obesity-related oxidative stress.

Of special interest is the fact that exercise-induced oxidative stress is exacerbated in obese populations, which has been shown in response to both acute aerobic and resistance exercises. Specifically, the total antioxidant status (TAS) in obese subjects decreased by 8.6 and 17.6 % in response to a single bout of aerobic and resistance exercises, respectively, whereas increases were observed in normal-weight individuals [50]. Furthermore, greater thiobarbituric reactive acid substances (TBARS), a marker of systemic oxidative stress, and lipid hydroperoxide (PEROX) increases were noted in obese subjects [50, 51]. Additionally, despite similar increases in PEROX levels in response to acute aerobic exercise in healthy obese and obese subjects with type 2 diabetes mellitus (T2DM), those with T2DM demonstrated greater decreases in TAS following exercise [70], suggesting a synergistic effect of metabolic dysfunction in further diminishing oxidative stress resistance. The authors suggested these outcomes may be the result of decreased availability of plasma vitamins C and E, elevated systolic blood pressure which may exacerbate vascular production of ROS during exercise, or greater mechanical and metabolic stress imposed by excessive adiposity; however, definitive reasoning remains yet to be elucidated. Finally, a number of assay techniques for the total antioxidant capacity have minimal sensitivity and specificity, thus the results for this measure have limited generalizability.

Physical Activity Intervention

Dietary CR as well as aerobic exercise, anaerobic exercise, and resistance training in association with weight loss has been shown to be advantageous in ameliorating oxidative stress and alleviating inflammation in obesity [71–77]. Specifically, overall oxidative stress, as indicated by TBARS and total PEROX, was reduced in healthy obese adults following 24 weeks of resistance-type circuit training [72], potentially due to increases in maximal oxygen consumption and fat-free mass and/or decreases in total fat mass [73]. Additionally, Oh et al. [75] demonstrated that 12 weeks of moderate- to high-intensity aerobic training decreased TBARS and body weight in obese individuals, while baseline levels of the antioxidant GPX were increased following 6 months of aerobic training in obese women [78]. More importantly, following exercise intervention, acute exercise-induced increases in the oxidative stress marker malondialdehyde (MDA) were attenuated while SOD and GPX levels were increased compared to acute exercise-induced responses pre-training [78].

In the absence of weight loss, 3 months of aerobic training in previously sedentary healthy obese adults resulted in significant reductions in skeletal muscle-specific oxidative stress, as indicated by the urinary excretion marker 4-HNE and systemic 8-isoprostane and increased concentrations of mitochondrial antioxidants [79]. Utilizing a similar protocol, Derives et al. [80] reported similar alterations in systemic oxidative stress; however, no change in skeletal muscle 4-HNE expression was observed, suggesting that oxidative stress improvements also occur in other tissue sources. Furthermore, Youssef et al. [81] demonstrated that 12 weeks of moderate aerobic training in the absence of weight loss was also sufficient to attenuate exercise-induced increases of oxidized LDL (ox-LDL) and MPO following an acute bout of maximal aerobic exercise in overweight and obese adolescent girls compared to pre-training responses. Conversely, exercise without weight loss was not sufficient to improve any markers of oxidative stress in obese adolescents as result of 8-week exercise training, despite utilizing higher intensities of exercise [82]. In addition, none of the aforementioned protocols elicited improvements from a pro- to anti-inflammatory state in obese populations at baseline, suggesting that in obese populations: (i) exercise-induced improvements of systemic or skeletal muscle-specific oxidative stress may be the result of intensity and/or duration of the intervention, and (ii) weight loss may be necessary to alter inflammatory profiles.

Dietary Intervention

Although exercise training independent of weight loss beneficially increases antioxidant defenses and decreases oxidative stress at baseline and in response to exercise, previous studies suggest at least a 10 % reduction in body weight is necessary to reverse pro-inflammatory parameters which contribute to oxidative stress during obesity [71, 82, 83]. Dramatic weight loss (i.e., gastric bypass surgery) in previously obese men and women has been shown to decreases oxidative stress and vital inflammatory markers, such as IL-6, C-reactive protein, and TNF-α, suggesting that weight loss independently can reduce oxidative stress and inflammation [84, 85]. This strategy may not be feasible or advisable to the general population; however, CR serves as an effective alternative. In animal models, 12 weeks of high-fat feeding increased NADPH oxidase, an important marker in the generation of oxidative stress, and accelerated the pathogenesis of endothelial dysfunction [86]. However, following high-fat diet, rodents underwent an additional 12 weeks of CR with and without exercise training, demonstrating a normalization of NADPH oxidase levels and reversal of the pathological progression of endothelial dysfunction. Furthermore, weight reductions of 10 % following 3 months of dietary restriction (500–1000 kcal/day energy deficit) in obese women resulted in increased glutathione reductase [87], while 6 months of hypocaloric diet elicited weight reductions of nearly 20 % which was sufficient to increase GPX and reduce 8-isoprostane, IL-6, and triglyceride levels in a manner associated with BMI reductions [88]. Additionally, alternate-day dietary restriction (20 %) resulted in a significant reduction in body weight and serum 4-HNE and 8-isoproponate while increasing antioxidant concentrations in obese adults [77]. TNF-α concentrations were also reduced after only 4 weeks, results which persisted throughout the 8-week study [77], potentially contributing to reduced production of cellular ROS [67]. Taken together, research suggests that significant weight fluctuations can directly dictate oxidative stress, inflammatory, and antioxidant enzyme profiles, processes which can be ameliorated through dietary weight lose intervention.

In obese individuals, 6 months of dieting coupled with aerobic exercise training designed to elicit a 10 % reduction in body weight also decreased overall oxidative stress [76]. Interestingly, Roberts et al. [89] reported decreases in oxidative stress accompanied with increases in TAS after only 3 weeks of combined strict dietary intervention and daily aerobic training. Despite no significant reductions in body weight, short-term diet and exercise intervention reduced *in vitro* expression of intracellular adhesion molecule (ICAM), a cellular adhesion marker which serves as an independent marker of CVD and vascular health. Furthermore, monocyte-derived monocyte chemoattractant protein-1 (MCP-1) production was attenuated, results which suggest that macrophage recruitment and exacerbation of the inflammatory response may be improved fairly quickly in response to lifestyle modifications in obese individuals.

Whether aerobic exercise may have a synergistic influence on long-term diet-induced improvements in oxidative stress and inflammatory profiles remains unclear. Wycherley et al. [74] demonstrated that while both diet and diet with aerobic exercise improved oxidative stress and NO availability and significantly reduced body weight, no difference between interventions was observed after 12 weeks in obese individuals with T2DM. Conversely, Ozcelik et al. [90] reported that hypocaloric diet coupled with the weight loss supplement orlistat or aerobic exercise resulted in significant decreases in body weight; however, the diet plus exercise group exhibited significant decreases in oxidative stress while no difference was observed in the diet plus orlistat group.

Both aerobic and anaerobic activities possess the potential to result in increased ROS and RNS production and subsequent oxidative stress. While obesity has been shown to exacerbate the oxidative stress response, dietary manipulation and exercise training may serve as an effective intervention to ameliorate oxidative stress profiles. Whether exercise training improves oxidative stress and inflammatory profiles in the absence of weight loss remains unclear; however, strict CR alone or coupled with physical activity intervention demonstrates promise in alleviating oxidative stress in obese individuals when accompanied with weight reduction.

Macronutrient-Specific Postprandial Oxidative Stress

Increasing evidence suggests that *postprandial* metabolic responses along with biomarkers of oxidative stress may provide important information regarding an individual's susceptibility and/or progression of type 2 diabetes as well as other diseases [91, 92]. This is significant since the ingestion of calorie-rich meals may be associated with obesity [93]; however, the ingestion of energy-dense feedings may also elicit potentially deleterious metabolic responses that are independent of chronic weight gain. Several investigations have shown that both the amount [9] and composition [94–96] of macronutrient intake can affect postprandial oxidative stress responses. For example, the ingestion of moderate (75 g) and high (150 g) amounts of dextrose results in minimal oxidative stress as quantified by MDA and H_2O_2 [9]. However, the ingestion of 66 g of fat resulted in a significant increase of these two oxidative stress biomarkers [9], which was likely associated with postprandial superoxide production [97]. Varying results were reported following the ingestion of 33 g of fat [98], indicating that not only the source but also the amount of macronutrient distribution can have an effect on postprandial oxidative stress responses. Investigators have also been reported significant increases in postprandial triglycerides (TAG), MDA, H_2O_2, and nitrate/nitrite following ingestion of a lipid meal compared to iso-caloric meals of varying macronutrient compositions [94]. Lipid-induced postprandial oxidative stress is likely explained by mitochondrial oxygen leakage and ROS generation [97, 99]. These results suggest potential "stress" associated with the ingestion of lipid-rich meals. It is important to note, however, that these responses can be affected by sex [100, 101]. Goldfarb and colleagues have suggested that this may be related to elevated glutathione status in women compared to men [102].

Interestingly, the magnitude of oxidative stress resulting from the ingestion of a lipid-rich meal has been shown to be greater than that resulting from strenuous exercise [103]. McCarthy et al. [103] was the first to investigate and compare oxidative stress responses from high-fat meals and acute bouts of strenuous exercise. Considering that the subjects in this study were exercise trained, it is possible that a training induced upregulated antioxidant defenses that contributed to the nonsignificant increase in oxidative stress in response to the strenuous exercise [103]. The potentially adverse effects associated with chronic ingestion of lipid-rich meals are apparent (weight gain) and may also be associated with additional ill health, including the development of insulin resistance [9]. Appropriate lifestyle modification (e.g., exercise and/or dietary interventions) seem to diminish oxidative stress and may positively influence diabetes [104] and vascular functioning [105].

Dietary Modifications and Oxidative Stress

Caloric restriction has been shown to be a successful weight loss intervention that may also improve markers of oxidative stress [106–109]. CR has been shown to promote longevity [110] as well as attenuate morbidity associated with several chronic diseases such as atherosclerosis, diabetes, cancer, autoimmune diseases, renal, neurodegenerative, and respiratory diseases [111]. This dietary modification has been shown to increase lifespan in rodents [112, 113]; however, these findings may not be universal among all animals. Further, a CR diet may be compared to an *ad libitum* diet which may contribute to excessive caloric intake and weight gain [114]. Hence, the validity for CR to promote longevity in humans currently remains a question due to a lack of longitudinal trials. Common approaches to CR include a relative change of macronutrient intake such as decreased carbohydrate or fat intake [115]. Both of which can be coupled with an increase in dietary protein intake. Of these approaches, a relative increase in dietary protein intake may actually contribute to decreased caloric intake since protein of various types (e.g., egg whites, dairy, lean meats) has been shown to have satiating properties [116]. In addition, although dietary fat is also known to induce satiety, higher fat intakes that are commonly coupled with low-carbohydrate diets [115] are potentially dangerous since this can serve as one source of postprandial oxidative stress [9, 94]. CR is usually practiced with a 20–40 % reduction of *ad libitum* dietary intake [117]. This approach has been shown to reduce biomarkers of oxidative stress such as H_2O_2, protein carbonyls, and nitrotyrosine as well [106–109].

Two hypotheses have been proposed as potential mechanisms behind the benefits of CR [98]. The hormesis hypothesis suggests that CR acts as a low-intensity stressor and thus, improvements in health and longevity can result as a defense against the exposure [118]. In addition, the oxidative damage hypothesis, which is supported in the literature, suggests that CR itself achieves the same goal by decreasing oxidative stress [119, 120]. Dietary fasting has been shown to prevent atherogenesis by improving NO bioavailability [121–123]. The Daniel Fast [98, 110, 124] is one type of dietary fast involving a plant-based feeding plan that restricts intake of animal products, refined foods, white flour, preservatives, additives, sweeteners, caffeine, and alcohol. Bloomer et al. [98] reported several benefits resulting from 21 days of this *ad libitum* dietary intervention. Improvements of oxidative stress biomarkers and antioxidant status were noted which included a significant reduction in MDA, an increase in nitrate/nitrite, and a 9 % increase in Trolox equivalent antioxidant capacity [98]. Also reported were improvements in blood lipids, glucose, insulin, systolic blood pressure, and body weight [98].

Another dietary modification that may increase antioxidant status, and thus protect against oxidative stress, is the increased consumption of selected micronutrients such as polyphenols [125, 126]. A wealth of data has supported the health benefits associated with increased fruit and vegetable consumption [127–130] which is likely related to the polyphenol antioxidant content [125, 126, 131]. Some classes of polyphenols include anthocyanins, lignans, flavonols, flavanones, flavanol monomers, proanthocyanidins, isoflavones, hydroxycinnamic acids, and hydroxybenzoic acids [126, 132]. Low consumption of fruits and vegetables and excessive fat intake serve as a major risk factor for an unfavorable imbalance between oxidants and antioxidants [9] and the development of chronic diseases contributing to morbidity and mortality [126].

Numerous studies have supported the link between the consumption of isolated antioxidants with benefits including improved antioxidant capacity [133], improved glucose metabolism [134], improved vascular function [135, 136], and attenuated LDL oxidation and progression of atherosclerosis [137]. Examples of these nutraceuticals that have been shown to improve various markers of oxidative stress include (but are not limited to) resveratrol [135, 136, 138, 139], α-lipoic acid [133, 140], ubiquinone (CoQ-10) [141], curcumin [134], quercetin [142], naringin [143], and lycopene [144]. Resveratrol and quercetin have been shown to activate sirtuin-1 (SIRT1) [145, 146]. Resveratrol is found in grapes and red wine [145] and is well known for its anticancer properties [147–149]. Several reports have investigated the SIRT1 activation activity of resveratrol and reported antioxidant, anti-inflammatory, antiapoptotic effects, as well as improvements in vascular functioning [135, 136]. Additional reports demonstrate that the deacetylase activity of SIRT1 is involved in proper glucose metabolism [150], indicating a potential implication for the importance of SIRT1 and related antioxidants for the treatment of insulin resistance [151]. CR has also been shown to upregulate SIRT1 activity [151] as well as increase peroxisome proliferator activated receptor (PPAR)-γ coactivator-1α (PGC-1α) activity, which was associated with improved mitochondrial functioning as well as improvements in oxidative stress, insulin resistance, metabolic rate, and body composition [152]. These studies demonstrate the cellular adaptations that occur in response to CR that can impact oxidative stress.

The Potential of Vitamin D

Vitamin D insufficiency has shown to correlate with endothelial dysfunction [153], decreased cardiorespiratory fitness [154], and impaired skeletal muscle health, contributing to muscle weakness and decreased function [155]. Furthermore, these conditions may be reversed with vitamin D supplementation [156, 157]. Low vitamin D levels may also serve as a mechanism contributing to the exacerbation of oxidative stress during obesity, a condition worsened by elevated levels of TNF-α [69]; however, research remains limited. *In vivo*, the active vitamin D metabolite, $1,25(OH)_2D_3$, has been shown to downregulate ICAM-1 expression following peripheral blood mononuclear cell following exposure to TNF-α [158] while serving as an antioxidant at the cellular membrane by decreasing PEROX [159, 160] and increasing TAS as well as oxidative capacity in monocytes [161, 162]. Valcheva et al. [163] recently demonstrated that reactive oxygen species production is enhanced in mice deficient for the vitamin D receptor, while 12 weeks of supplementation decreases circulation markers of oxidative stress as well as improved lipid profiles in type 2 diabetics [164]. In addition, the risk of vitamin D insufficiency is elevated during obesity [165, 166], potentially due to increased sequestering of the steroid in adipose tissue [167]. In fact, for each 1 kg/m^2 increase in BMI, an estimated decrease of 0.74 nmol/L of vitamin D has been observed [168]. Importantly, vitamin D has been shown to inhibit the production of both TNF-α and IL-6 by downregulating the NF-kB pathway [169, 170].

Tzotzas et al. [171] have provided evidence of the relationship of obesity to vitamin D. In their study, a 10 % reduction in weight resulted in increased vitamin D concentrations in previously vitamin D-insufficient obese individuals [171]. Furthermore, obese individuals supplemented with 3332 IU/day of vitamin D during weight loss intervention resulted in larger decreases in plasma TNF-α and IL-6 compared to placebo [172], while 1000 IU/day of vitamin D coupled with diet and exercise resulted in greater increases in VO_{2max} and weight loss compared to either diet or exercise alone [173]. These results suggest a potential attenuation of oxidative stress in obese individuals supplemented with vitamin D, particularly during exercise. Of note, there are no studies that have investigated the potential role of vitamin D supplementation to suppress oxidative stress in obese individuals during weight loss interventions.

Conclusions

Aerobic exercise, utilized to reduce obesity, results in an acute state of oxidative stress. However, it is likely that chronic physical activity provides a stimulus for favorable oxidative adaptations and enhanced physiological performance and physical health [13, 73]. Furthermore, while the specific underlying factors that dictate the differences in responses between aerobic and anaerobic exercises vary, the result for both is an elevation in biomarkers of oxidative stress [46, 62]. The mechanisms that would explain the potential benefits from chronic aerobic and anaerobic exercises have not been elucidated. Some have documented that a training-induced increases in endogenous antioxidant status may protect individuals against oxidative stress [78]. Without greater understanding of the distinct mechanisms, it is difficult to propose a specific activity that would result in a specific benefit or outcome.

Numerous studies support the benefits of dietary modification, including vitamin D supplementation, in alleviating oxidative stress; however, the interaction of obesity and physical activity has not been determined. Various metabolic, inflammatory, and cardiovascular mechanisms likely interact to explain the benefits of these interventions. Most importantly, further mechanistic investigations are necessary to determine the most effective intervention(s) for distinct benefits. It does seem evident that weight loss is significant in the alleviation of oxidative stress.

Oxidative stress is strongly associated with obesity, inflammation, vascular function, and diabetes [104, 105]. Appropriate lifestyle modifications can be taken (e.g., exercise training, dietary interventions) to alleviate oxidative stress. A greater understanding of the mechanisms associated with oxidative stress and disease can be utilized in the development of targeted treatment strategies to improve health.

Competing interest

C-JH, MM, ALS, HEW, JTM, and EOA declare that they have no competing interest, and no financial support was received for the conduct of this study or preparation of this manuscript.

Authors' contributions

All authors participated in the conception and design of the study and also read and approved the final manuscript.

Author details

[1]Exercise Biochemistry Laboratory, Department of Exercise Science and Health Promotion, Florida Atlantic University, 777 Glades Road, FH11A-126B, Boca Raton, FL 33431, USA. [2]Department of Kinesiology, Mississippi State University, Starkville, MS, USA. [3]Department of Kinesiology and Health Sciences, Virginia Commonwealth University, Richmond, VA, USA. [4]Department of Kinesiology, Texas A&M University–Corpus Christi, Corpus Christi, TX, USA.

References

1. Flegal KM, Carroll MD, Ogden CL, Curtin LR. Prevalence and trends in obesity among US adults, 1999-2008. JAMA. 2010;303:235–41.
2. Keaney JF, Larson MG, Vasan RS, Wilson PW, Lipinska I, Corey D, et al. Obesity and systemic oxidative stress clinical correlates of oxidative stress in the Framingham Study. Arterioscler Thromb Vasc Biol. 2003;23:434–9.
3. Olusi S. Obesity is an independent risk factor for plasma lipid peroxidation and depletion of erythrocyte cytoprotectic enzymes in humans. Int J Obes Relat Metab Disord. 2002;26:1159–64.
4. Montezano AC, Touyz RM. Reactive oxygen species and endothelial function–role of nitric oxide synthase uncoupling and Nox family nicotinamide adenine dinucleotide phosphate oxidases. Basic Clin Pharmacol Toxicol. 2012;110:87–94.
5. Kunwar A, Priyadarsini K. Free radicals, oxidative stress and importance of antioxidants in human health. J Med Allied Sci. 2011;1:53–60.
6. Vider J, Laaksonen DE, Kilk A, Atalay M, Lehtmaa J, Zilmer M, et al. Physical exercise induces activation of NF-κB in human peripheral blood lymphocytes. Antioxid Redox Signal. 2001;3:1131–7.
7. Korda M, Kubant R, Patton S, Malinski T. Leptin-induced endothelial dysfunction in obesity. Am J Physiol Heart Circ Physiol. 2008;295:H1514–H21.
8. Wannamethee SG, Tchernova J, Whincup P, Lowe G, Kelly A, Rumley A, et al. Plasma leptin: associations with metabolic, inflammatory and haemostatic risk factors for cardiovascular disease. Atherosclerosis. 2007;191:418–26.
9. Bloomer RJ, Kabir MM, Marshall KE, Canale RE, Farney TM. Postprandial oxidative stress in response to dextrose and lipid meals of differing size. Lipids Health Dis. 2010;9:79.
10. Miyazaki H, Oh-ishi S, Ookawara T, Kizaki T, Toshinai K, Ha S, et al. Strenuous endurance training in humans reduces oxidative stress following exhausting exercise. Eur J Appl Physiol. 2001;84:1–6.
11. Yavari A, Javadi M, Mirmiran P, Bahadoran Z. Exercise-induced oxidative stress and dietary antioxidants. Asian J Sports Med. 2015;6:e24898.
12. Singhal A. Endothelial dysfunction: role in obesity-related disorders and the early origins of CVD. Proc Nutr Soc. 2005;64:15–22.
13. Sies H. Oxidative stress: oxidants and antioxidants. Exp Physiol. 1997;82:291–5.
14. Verma S, Anderson TJ. Fundamentals of endothelial function for the clinical cardiologist. Circulation. 2002;105:546–9.
15. Ji LL, Gomez-Cabrera MC, Vina J. Exercise and hormesis. Ann N Y Acad Sci. 2006;1067:425–35.
16. Zhang P, Xu X, Li X. Cardiovascular diseases: oxidative damage and antioxidant protection. Eur Rev Med Pharmacol Sci. 2014;18:3091–6.
17. Carr AC, McCall MR, Frei B. Oxidation of LDL by myeloperoxidase and reactive nitrogen species reaction pathways and antioxidant protection. Arterioscler Thromb Vasc Biol. 2000;20:1716–23.
18. Takahashi Y, Zhu H, Yoshimoto T. Essential roles of lipoxygenases in LDL oxidation and development of atherosclerosis. Antioxid Redox Signal. 2005;7:425–31.
19. Wang Q, Xie Z, Zhang W, Zhou J, Wu Y, Zhang M, et al. Myeloperoxidase deletion prevents high-fat diet–induced obesity and insulin resistance. Diabetes. 2014;63:4172–85.
20. Neels JG. A role for 5-lipoxygenase products in obesity-associated inflammation and insulin resistance. Adipocyte. 2013;2:262–5.
21. Blankenberg S, Rupprecht HJ, Bickel C, Torzewski M, Hafner G, Tiret L, et al. Glutathione peroxidase 1 activity and cardiovascular events in patients with coronary artery disease. N Engl J Med. 2003;349:1605–13.
22. Fukai T, Folz RJ, Landmesser U, Harrison DG. Extracellular superoxide dismutase and cardiovascular disease. Cardiovasc Res. 2002;55:239–49.
23. Arcaro G, Zamboni M, Rossi L, Turcato E, Covi G, Armellini F, et al. Body fat distribution predicts the degree of endothelial dysfunction in uncomplicated obesity. Int J Obes Relat Metab Disord. 1999;23:936–42.
24. Cheang WS, Wong WT, Tian XY, Yang Q, Lee HK, He G-W, et al. Endothelial nitric oxide synthase enhancer reduces oxidative stress and restores endothelial function in db/db mice. Cardiovasc Res. 2011;92:267–75.
25. Hamilton C, Miller W, Al-Benna S, Brosnan M, Drummond R, McBride M, et al. Strategies to reduce oxidative stress in cardiovascular disease. Clin Sci (Lond). 2004;106:219–34.

26. Griendling KK, Ushio-Fukai M. NADH/NADPH oxidase and vascular function. Trends Cardiovasc Med. 1997;7:301–7.
27. Berry C, Hamilton CA, Brosnan MJ, Magill FG, Berg GA, McMurray JJ, et al. Investigation into the sources of superoxide in human blood vessels angiotensin II increases superoxide production in human internal mammary arteries. Circulation. 2000;101:2206–12.
28. Inoguchi T, Li P, Umeda F, Yu HY, Kakimoto M, Imamura M, et al. High glucose level and free fatty acid stimulate reactive oxygen species production through protein kinase C-dependent activation of NAD(P)H oxidase in cultured vascular cells. Diabetes. 2000;49:1939–45.
29. Dallaire P, Marette A. Obesity-linked insulin resistance: is nitric oxide the missing link. Can J Diabetes. 2004;28:59–66.
30. Pacher P, Beckman JS, Liaudet L. Nitric oxide and peroxynitrite in health and disease. Physiol Rev. 2007;87:315–424.
31. Perticone F, Ceravolo R, Candigliota M, Ventura G, Iacopino S, Sinopoli F, et al. Obesity and body fat distribution induce endothelial dysfunction by oxidative stress protective effect of vitamin C. Diabetes. 2001;50:159–65.
32. S-i Y, Amano S, Inagaki Y, Okamoto T, Takeuchi M, Inoue H. Pigment epithelium-derived factor inhibits leptin-induced angiogenesis by suppressing vascular endothelial growth factor gene expression through anti-oxidative properties. Microvasc Res. 2003;65:186–90.
33. S-i Y, Edelstein D, Du X-l, Kaneda Y, Guzmán M, Brownlee M. Leptin induces mitochondrial superoxide production and monocyte chemoattractant protein-1 expression in aortic endothelial cells by increasing fatty acid oxidation via protein kinase A. J Biol Chem. 2001;276:25096–100.
34. Zhang H, Park Y, Wu J, Chen X, Lee S, Yang J, et al. Role of TNF-alpha in vascular dysfunction. Clin Sci (Lond). 2009;116:219–30.
35. Yan S, Zhang X, Zheng H, Hu D, Zhang Y, Guan Q, et al. Clematichinenoside inhibits VCAM-1 and ICAM-1 expression in TNF-α-treated endothelial cells via NADPH oxidase-dependent IκB kinase/NF-κB pathway. Free Radic Biol Med. 2014;78C:190–201.
36. Picchi A, Gao X, Belmadani S, Potter BJ, Focardi M, Chilian WM, et al. Tumor necrosis factor-α induces endothelial dysfunction in the prediabetic metabolic syndrome. Circ Res. 2006;99:69–77.
37. Zumbach MS, Boehme MWJ, Wahl P, Stremmel W, Ziegler R, Nawroth PP. Tumor necrosis factor increases serum leptin levels in humans. J Clin Endocrinol Metab. 1997;82:4080–2.
38. Zarkesh-Esfahani H, Pockley G, Metcalfe RA, Bidlingmaier M, Wu Z, Ajami A, et al. High-dose leptin activates human leukocytes via receptor expression on monocytes. J Immunol. 2001;167:4593–9.
39. Lumeng CN, Saltiel AR. Inflammatory links between obesity and metabolic disease. J Clin Invest. 2011;121:2111–7.
40. Nathan CF, Murray HW, Wiebe M, Rubin BY. Identification of interferon-gamma as the lymphokine that activates human macrophage oxidative metabolism and antimicrobial activity. J Exp Med. 1983;158:670–89.
41. Murr C, Schroecksnadel K, Winkler C, Ledochowski M, Fuchs D. Antioxidants may increase the probability of developing allergic diseases and asthma. Med Hypotheses. 2005;64:973–7.
42. Cojocaru M, Cojocaru IM, Silosi I, Rogoz S. Role of leptin in autoimmune diseases. Maedica (Buchar). 2013;8:68.
43. Maingrette F, Renier G. Leptin increases lipoprotein lipase secretion by macrophages: involvement of oxidative stress and protein kinase C. Diabetes. 2003;52:2121–8.
44. Youn J-Y, Siu KL, Lob HE, Itani H, Harrison DG, Cai H. Role of vascular oxidative stress in obesity and metabolic syndrome. Diabetes. 2014;63:2344–55.
45. Bloomer RJ, Goldfarb AH, Wideman L, McKenzie MJ, Consitt LA. Effects of acute aerobic and anaerobic exercise on blood markers of oxidative stress. J Strength Cond Res. 2005;19:276–85.
46. Bloomer RJ, Goldfarb AH. Anaerobic exercise and oxidative stress: a review. Can J Appl Physiol. 2004;29:245–63.
47. Goto C, Higashi Y, Kimura M, Noma K, Hara K, Nakagawa K, et al. Effect of different intensities of exercise on endothelium-dependent vasodilation in humans: role of endothelium-dependent nitric oxide and oxidative stress. Circulation. 2003;108:530–5.
48. Goto C, Nishioka K, Umemura T, Jitsuiki D, Sakagutchi A, Kawamura M, et al. Acute moderate-intensity exercise induces vasodilation through an increase in nitric oxide bioavailability in humans. Am J Hypertens. 2007;20:825–30.
49. Bloomer R, Davis P, Consitt L, Wideman L. Plasma protein carbonyl response to increasing exercise duration in aerobically trained men and women. Int J Sports Med. 2007;28:21–5.
50. Vincent HK, Morgan JW, Vincent KR. Obesity exacerbates oxidative stress levels after acute exercise. Med Sci Sports Exerc. 2004;36:772–9.
51. Vincent HK, Vincent KR, Bourguignon C, Braith RW. Obesity and postexercise oxidative stress in older women. Med Sci Sports Exerc. 2005;37:213–9.
52. Davies KJ, Quintanilha AT, Brooks GA, Packer L. Free radicals and tissue damage produced by exercise. Biochem Biophys Res Commun. 1982;107:1198–205.
53. Ashton T, Rowlands CC, Jones E, Young IS, Jackson SK, Davies B, et al. Electron spin resonance spectroscopic detection of oxygen-centred radicals in human serum following exhaustive exercise. Eur J Appl Physiol Occup Physiol. 1998;77:498–502.
54. Ashton T, Young IS, Peters JR, Jones E, Jackson SK, Davies B, et al. Electron spin resonance spectroscopy, exercise, and oxidative stress: an ascorbic acid intervention study. J Appl Physiol. 1999;87:2032–6.
55. Groussard C, Rannou-Bekono F, Machefer G, Chevanne M, Vincent S, Sergent O, et al. Changes in blood lipid peroxidation markers and antioxidants after a single sprint anaerobic exercise. Eur J Appl Physiol. 2003;89:14–20.
56. Bailey DM, Lawrenson L, Mceneny J, Young IS, James PE, Jackson SK, et al. Electron paramagnetic spectroscopic evidence of exercise-induced free radical accumulation in human skeletal muscle. Free Radic Res. 2007;41:182–90.
57. Bailey DM, Young IS, McEneny J, Lawrenson L, Kim J, Barden J, et al. Regulation of free radical outflow from an isolated muscle bed in exercising humans. Am J Physiol Heart Circ Physiol. 2004;287:H1689–H99.
58. Halliwell B. Oxygen radicals: a commonsense look at their nature and medical importance. Med Biol. 1984;62:71–7.
59. Knez WL, Jenkins DG, Coombes JS. Oxidative stress in half and full Ironman triathletes. Med Sci Sports Exerc. 2007;39:283.
60. Fisher-Wellman K, Bloomer RJ. Acute exercise and oxidative stress: a 30 year history. Dyn Med. 2009;8:1.
61. McAnulty SR, McAnulty LS, Nieman DC, Morrow JD, Utter AC, Dumke CL. Effect of resistance exercise and carbohydrate ingestion on oxidative stress. Free Radic Res. 2005;39:1219–24.
62. Hartmann A, Niess AM. Oxidative DNA damage in exercise. In: Sen C, Packer L, Hänninen O. Handbook of oxidants and antioxidants in exercise. New York: Elsevier; 2000. pp. 195–217.
63. Hilton TN, Tuttle LJ, Bohnert KL, Mueller MJ, Sinacore DR. Excessive adipose tissue infiltration in skeletal muscle in individuals with obesity, diabetes mellitus, and peripheral neuropathy: association with performance and function. Phys Ther. 2008;88:1336–44.
64. Hey-Mogensen M, Højlund K, Vind B, Wang L, Dela F, Beck-Nielsen H, et al. Effect of physical training on mitochondrial respiration and reactive oxygen species release in skeletal muscle in patients with obesity and type 2 diabetes. Diabetologia. 2010;53:1976–85.
65. Anderson EJ, Neufer PD. Type II skeletal myofibers possess unique properties that potentiate mitochondrial H_2O_2 generation. Am J Physiol Cell Physiol. 2006;290:C844–C51.
66. Plomgaard P, Penkowa M, Pedersen BK. Fiber type specific expression of TNF-alpha, IL-6 and IL-18 in human skeletal muscles. Exerc Immunol Rev. 2005;11:53–63.
67. Li Y-P, Reid MB. NF-κB mediates the protein loss induced by TNF-α in differentiated skeletal muscle myotubes. Am J Physiol Regul Integr Comp Physiol. 2000;279:R1165–R70.
68. Wilcox P, Wakai Y, Walley K, Cooper D, Road J. Tumor necrosis factor alpha decreases in vivo diaphragm contractility in dogs. Am J Respir Crit Care Med. 1994;150:1368–73.
69. Reid M, Li YP. Cytokines and oxidative signalling in skeletal muscle. Acta Physiol Scand. 2001;171:225–32.
70. Brinkmann C, Chung N, Schmidt U, Kreutz T, Lenzen E, Schiffer T, et al. Training alters the skeletal muscle antioxidative capacity in non-insulin-dependent type 2 diabetic men. Scand J Med Sci Sports. 2012;22:462–70.
71. Bruun JM, Helge JW, Richelsen B, Stallknecht B. Diet and exercise reduce low-grade inflammation and macrophage infiltration in adipose tissue but not in skeletal muscle in severely obese subjects. Am J Physiol Endocrinol Metab. 2005;290:E961–E7.
72. Phillips MD, Patrizi RM, Cheek DJ, Wooten JS, Barbee JJ, Mitchell JB. Resistance training reduces subclinical inflammation in obese, postmenopausal women. Med Sci Sports Exerc. 2012;44:2099–110.
73. Vincent HK, Bourguignon C, Vincent KR. Resistance training lowers exercise-induced oxidative stress and homocysteine levels in overweight and obese older adults. Obesity. 2006;14:1921–30.

74. Wycherley TP, Brinkworth GD, Noakes M, Buckley JD, Clifton PM. Effect of caloric restriction with and without exercise training on oxidative stress and endothelial function in obese subjects with type 2 diabetes. Diabetes Obes Metab. 2008;10:1062–73.
75. Oh S, Tanaka K, Warabi E, Shoda J. Exercise reduces inflammation and oxidative stress in obesity-related liver diseases. Med Sci Sports Exerc. 2013;45:2214–22.
76. Rector RS, Warner SO, Liu Y, Hinton PS, Sun GY, Cox RH, et al. Exercise and diet induced weight loss improves measures of oxidative stress and insulin sensitivity in adults with characteristics of the metabolic syndrome. Am J Physiol Endocrinol Metab. 2007;293:E500–E6.
77. Johnson JB, Summer W, Cutler RG, Martin B, Hyun D-H, Dixit VD, et al. Alternate day calorie restriction improves clinical findings and reduces markers of oxidative stress and inflammation in overweight adults with moderate asthma. Free Radic Biol Med. 2007;42:665–74.
78. Shin Y-A, Lee J-H, Song W, Jun T-W. Exercise training improves the antioxidant enzyme activity with no changes of telomere length. Mech Ageing Dev. 2008;129:254–60.
79. Samjoo I, Safdar A, Hamadeh M, Raha S, Tarnopolsky M. The effect of endurance exercise on both skeletal muscle and systemic oxidative stress in previously sedentary obese men. Nutr Diabetes. 2013;3:e88.
80. Devries MC, Hamadeh MJ, Glover AW, Raha S, Samjoo IA, Tarnopolsky MA. Endurance training without weight loss lowers systemic, but not muscle, oxidative stress with no effect on inflammation in lean and obese women. Free Radic Biol Med. 2008;45:503–11.
81. Youssef H, Groussard C, Lemoine-Morel S, Pincemail J, Jacob C, Moussa E, et al. Aerobic training suppresses exercise-induced lipid peroxidation and inflammation in overweight/obese adolescent girls. Pediatr Exerc Sci. 2015;27:67–76.
82. Kelly AS, Steinberger J, Olson TP, Dengel DR. In the absence of weight loss, exercise training does not improve adipokines or oxidative stress in overweight children. Metabolism. 2007;56:1005–9.
83. Forsythe LK, Wallace JM, Livingstone MBE. Obesity and inflammation: the effects of weight loss. Nutr Res Rev. 2008;21:117–33.
84. Kopp H-P, Kopp C, Festa A, Krzyzanowska K, Kriwanek S, Minar E, et al. Impact of weight loss on inflammatory proteins and their association with the insulin resistance syndrome in morbidly obese patients. Arterioscler Thromb Vasc Biol. 2003;23:1042–7.
85. Gletsu-Miller N, Hansen JM, Jones DP, Go YM, Torres WE, Ziegler TR, et al. Loss of total and visceral adipose tissue mass predicts decreases in oxidative stress after weight-loss surgery. Obesity. 2009;17:439–46.
86. Touati S, Montezano AC, Meziri F, Riva C, Touyz RM, Laurant P. Exercise training protects against atherosclerotic risk factors through vascular NADPH oxidase, ERK1/2 and SAPK/JNK down-regulation in obese rats. Clin Exp Pharmacol Physiol. 2015;42:179–85.
87. Ramezanipour M, Jalali M, Sadrzade-Yeganeh H, Keshavarz SA, Eshraghian MR, Bagheri M, et al. The effect of weight reduction on antioxidant enzymes and their association with dietary intake of vitamins A, C and E. Arq Bras Endocrinol Metabol. 2014;58:744–9.
88. Bougoulia M, Triantos A, Koliakos G. Plasma interleukin-6 levels, glutathione peroxidase and isoprostane in obese women before and after weight loss. Association with cardiovascular risk factors. Hormones (Athens). 2006;5:192–9.
89. Roberts CK, Won D, Pruthi S, Kurtovic S, Sindhu RK, Vaziri ND, et al. Effect of a short-term diet and exercise intervention on oxidative stress, inflammation, MMP-9, and monocyte chemotactic activity in men with metabolic syndrome factors. J Appl Physiol. 2006;100:1657–65.
90. Ozcelik O, Ozkan Y, Karatas F, Kelestimur H. Exercise training as an adjunct to orlistat therapy reduces oxidative stress in obese subjects. Tohoku J Exp Med. 2005;206:313–8.
91. O'Keefe JH, Bell DS. Postprandial hyperglycemia/hyperlipidemia (postprandial dysmetabolism) is a cardiovascular risk factor. Am J Crdiol. 2007;100:899–904.
92. Pastromas S, Terzi A-B, Tousoulis D, Koulouris S. Postprandial lipemia: an under-recognized atherogenic factor in patients with diabetes mellitus. Int J Cardiol. 2008;126:3–12.
93. Rosenheck R. Fast food consumption and increased caloric intake: a systematic review of a trajectory towards weight gain and obesity risk. Obes Rev. 2008;9:535–47.
94. Fisher-Wellman KH, Bloomer RJ. Exacerbated postprandial oxidative stress induced by the acute intake of a lipid meal compared to isoenergetically administered carbohydrate, protein, and mixed meals in young, healthy men. J Am Coll Nutr. 2010;29:373–81.
95. Rebolledo O, Dato SA. Postprandial hyperglycemia and hyperlipidemia-generated glycoxidative stress: its contribution to the pathogenesis of diabetes complications. Eur Rev Med Pharmacol Sci. 2005;9:191–208.
96. Sies H, Stahl W, Sevanian A. Nutritional, dietary and postprandial oxidative stress. J Nutr. 2005;135:969–72.
97. Liu Y, Fiskum G, Schubert D. Generation of reactive oxygen species by the mitochondrial electron transport chain. J Neurochem. 2002;80:780–7.
98. Bloomer RJ, Kabir MM, Trepanowski JF, Canale RE, Farney TM. A 21 day Daniel Fast improves selected biomarkers of antioxidant status and oxidative stress in men and women. Nutr Metab (Lond). 2011;8:17.
99. Ruggiero C, Ehrenshaft M, Cleland E, Stadler K. High-fat diet induces an initial adaptation of mitochondrial bioenergetics in the kidney despite evident oxidative stress and mitochondrial ROS production. Am J Physiol Endocrinol Metab. 2011;300:E1047–E58.
100. Bloomer RJ, Ferebee DE, Fisher-Wellman KH, Quindry JC, Schilling BK. Postprandial oxidative stress: influence of sex and exercise training status. Med Sci Sports Exerc. 2009;41:2111–9.
101. Bloomer RJ, Fisher-Wellman KH. Lower postprandial oxidative stress in women compared with men. Gend Med. 2010;7:340–9.
102. Goldfarb AH, McKenzie MJ, Bloomer RJ. Gender comparisons of exercise-induced oxidative stress: influence of antioxidant supplementation. Appl Physiol Nutr Metab. 2007;32:1124–31.
103. McCarthy CG, Farney TM, Canale RE, Dessoulavy ME, Bloomer RJ. High-fat feeding, but not strenuous exercise, increases blood oxidative stress in trained men. Appl Physiol Nutr Metab. 2013;38:33–41.
104. Giacco F, Brownlee M. Oxidative stress and diabetic complications. Circ Res. 2010;107:1058–70.
105. Ramadan R, Dhawan SS, Syed H, Pohlel FK, Binongo JN, Ghazzal ZB, et al. Effects of clopidogrel therapy on oxidative stress, inflammation, vascular function, and progenitor cells in stable coronary artery disease. J Cardiovasc Pharmacol. 2014;63:369–74.
106. Bevilacqua L, Ramsey JJ, Hagopian K, Weindruch R, Harper M-E. Effects of short-and medium-term calorie restriction on muscle mitochondrial proton leak and reactive oxygen species production. Am J Physiol Endocrinol Metab. 2004;286:E852–E61.
107. Hagopian K, Harper M-E, Ram JJ, Humble SJ, Weindruch R, Ramsey JJ. Long-term calorie restriction reduces proton leak and hydrogen peroxide production in liver mitochondria. Am J Physiol Endocrinol Metab. 2005;288:E674–E84.
108. Hyun D-H, Emerson SS, Jo D-G, Mattson MP, de Cabo R. Calorie restriction up-regulates the plasma membrane redox system in brain cells and suppresses oxidative stress during aging. Proc Natl Acad Sci U S A. 2006;103:19908–12.
109. Zainal TA, Oberley TD, Allison DB, Szweda LI, Weindruch R. Caloric restriction of rhesus monkeys lowers oxidative damage in skeletal muscle. FASEB J. 2000;14:1825–36.
110. Trepanowski JF, Canale RE, Marshall KE, Kabir MM, Bloomer RJ. Impact of caloric and dietary restriction regimens on markers of health and longevity in humans and animals: a summary of available findings. Nutr J. 2011;10:107.
111. S-i I. SIRT1 and caloric restriction: an insight into possible trade-offs between robustness and frailty. Curr Opin Clin Nutr Metab Care. 2009;12:350–6.
112. Goldberg EL, Romero-Aleshire MJ, Renkema KR, Ventevogel MS, Chew WM, Uhrlaub JL, et al. Lifespan-extending caloric restriction or mTOR inhibition impair adaptive immunity of old mice by distinct mechanisms. Aging Cell. 2015;14:130–8.
113. Jové M, Naudí A, Ramírez-Núñez O, Portero-Otín M, Selman C, Withers DJ, et al. Caloric restriction reveals a metabolomic and lipidomic signature in liver of male mice. Aging cell. 2014;13:828–37.
114. Sohal RS, Forster MJ. Caloric restriction and the aging process: a critique. Free Radic Biol Med. 2014;73:366–82.
115. Noakes TD. Low-carbohydrate and high-fat intake can manage obesity and associated conditions: occasional survey. S Afr Med J. 2013;103:826–30.
116. Kremsdorf RA, Hoofnagle AN, Kratz M, Weigle DS, Callahan HS, Purnell JQ, et al. Effects of a high-protein diet on regulation of phosphorus homeostasis. J Clin Endocrinol Metab. 2013;98:1207–13.
117. Cantó C, Auwerx J. Caloric restriction, SIRT1 and longevity. Trends Endocrinol Metab. 2009;20:325–31.

118. Masoro EJ. Caloric restriction and aging: an update. Exp Gerontol. 2000;35:299–305.
119. Gredilla R, Barja G. Minireview: the role of oxidative stress in relation to caloric restriction and longevity. Endocrinology. 2005;146:3713–7.
120. Sohal RS, Weindruch R. Oxidative stress, caloric restriction, and aging. Science. 1996;273:59–63.
121. Nisoli E, Tonello C, Cardile A, Cozzi V, Bracale R, Tedesco L, et al. Calorie restriction promotes mitochondrial biogenesis by inducing the expression of eNOS. Science. 2005;310:314–7.
122. Kondo M, Shibata R, Miura R, Shimano M, Kondo K, Li P, et al. Caloric restriction stimulates revascularization in response to ischemia via adiponectin-mediated activation of endothelial nitric-oxide synthase. J Biol Chem. 2009;284:1718–24.
123. Monda M, Messina G, Scognamiglio I, Lombardi A, Martin GA, Sperlongano P, et al. Short-term diet and moderate exercise in young overweight men modulate cardiocyte and hepatocarcinoma survival by oxidative stress. Oxid Med Cell Longev. 2014;2014:131024.
124. Trepanowski JF, Kabir MM, Alleman Jr RJ, Bloomer RJ. A 21-day Daniel fast with or without krill oil supplementation improves anthropometric parameters and the cardiometabolic profile in men and women. Nutr Metab (Lond). 2012;9:82.
125. Mennen LI, Sapinho D, de Bree A, Arnault N, Bertrais S, Galan P, et al. Consumption of foods rich in flavonoids is related to a decreased cardiovascular risk in apparently healthy French women. J Nutr. 2004;134:923–6.
126. Urquiaga I, Leighton F. Plant polyphenol antioxidants and oxidative stress. Biol Res. 2000;33:55–64.
127. Liu RH. Health benefits of fruit and vegetables are from additive and synergistic combinations of phytochemicals. Am J Clin Nutr. 2003;78:517S–20S.
128. Lotito SB, Frei B. Consumption of flavonoid-rich foods and increased plasma antioxidant capacity in humans: cause, consequence, or epiphenomenon? Free Radic Biol Med. 2006;41:1727–46.
129. Tuso P, Stoll SR, Li WW. A plant-based diet, atherogenesis, and coronary artery disease prevention. Perm J. 2015;19:62–7.
130. Jiang Y, Wu S-H, Shu X-O, Xiang Y-B, Ji B-T, Milne GL, et al. Cruciferous vegetable intake is inversely correlated with circulating levels of proinflammatory markers in women. J Acad Nutr Diet. 2014;114:700–8. e2.
131. Feskanich D, Ziegler RG, Michaud DS, Giovannucci EL, Speizer FE, Willett WC, et al. Prospective study of fruit and vegetable consumption and risk of lung cancer among men and women. J Natl Cancer Inst. 2000;92:1812–23.
132. Manach C, Williamson G, Morand C, Scalbert A, Rémésy C. Bioavailability and bioefficacy of polyphenols in humans. I. Review of 97 bioavailability studies. Am J Clin Nutr. 2005;81:230S–42S.
133. Nickander KK, Mcphee BR, Low PA, Tritschler H. Alpha-lipoic acid: antioxidant potency against lipid peroxidation of neural tissues in vitro and implications for diabetic neuropathy. Free Radic Biol Med. 1996;21:631–9.
134. Zhang D-W, Fu M, Gao S-H, Liu J-L. Curcumin and diabetes: a systematic review. Evid Based Complement Alternat Med. 2013;2013:636053.
135. Csiszar A, Labinskyy N, Podlutsky A, Kaminski PM, Wolin MS, Zhang C, et al. Vasoprotective effects of resveratrol and SIRT1: attenuation of cigarette smoke-induced oxidative stress and proinflammatory phenotypic alterations. Am J Physiol Heart Circ Physiol. 2008;294:H2721–H35.
136. Ungvari Z, Orosz Z, Rivera A, Labinskyy N, Xiangmin Z, Olson S, et al. Resveratrol increases vascular oxidative stress resistance. Am J Physiol Heart Circ Physiol. 2007;292:H2417–H24.
137. Kumar A, Kaur H, Devi P, Mohan V. Role of coenzyme Q10 (CoQ10) in cardiac disease, hypertension and Meniere-like syndrome. Pharmacol Ther. 2009;124:259–68.
138. Kasdallah-Grissa A, Mornagui B, Aouani E, Hammami M, El May M, Gharbi N, et al. Resveratrol, a red wine polyphenol, attenuates ethanol-induced oxidative stress in rat liver. Life Sci. 2007;80:1033–9.
139. Kode A, Rajendrasozhan S, Caito S, Yang S-R, Megson IL, Rahman I. Resveratrol induces glutathione synthesis by activation of Nrf2 and protects against cigarette smoke-mediated oxidative stress in human lung epithelial cells. Am J Physiol Lung Cell Mol Physiol. 2008;294:L478–L88.
140. Stanković MN, Mladenović D, Ninković M, Đuričić I, Šobajić S, Jorgačević B, et al. The effects of α-lipoic acid on liver oxidative stress and free fatty acid composition in methionine–choline deficient diet-induced NAFLD. J Med Food. 2014;17:254–61.
141. Tarry-Adkins JL, Blackmore HL, Martin-Gronert MS, Fernandez-Twinn DS, McConnell JM, Hargreaves IP, et al. Coenzyme Q10 prevents accelerated cardiac aging in a rat model of poor maternal nutrition and accelerated postnatal growth. Mol Metab. 2013;2:480–90.
142. Wang L, Cheng X, Li H, Qiu F, Yang N, Wang B, et al. Quercetin reduces oxidative stress and inhibits activation of c-Jun N-terminal kinase/activator protein-1 signaling in an experimental mouse model of abdominal aortic aneurysm. Mol Med Rep. 2014;9:435–42.
143. Chen J, Guo R, Yan H, Tian L, You Q, Li S, et al. Naringin inhibits ROS-activated MAPK pathway in high glucose-induced injuries in H9c2 cardiac cells. Basic Clin Pharmacol Toxicol. 2014;114:293–304.
144. Fletcher NM, Awonuga AO, Saed MG, Abu-Soud HM, Diamond MP, Saed GM. Lycopene, a powerful antioxidant, significantly reduces the development of the adhesion phenotype. Syst Biol Reprod Med. 2013;60:14–20.
145. Borra MT, Smith BC, Denu JM. Mechanism of human SIRT1 activation by resveratrol. J Biol Chem. 2005;280:17187–95.
146. Lagouge M, Argmann C, Gerhart-Hines Z, Meziane H, Lerin C, Daussin F, et al. Resveratrol improves mitochondrial function and protects against metabolic disease by activating SIRT1 and PGC-1α. Cell. 2006;127:1109–22.
147. Amiri F, Zarnani A-H, Zand H, Koohdani F, Jeddi-Tehrani M, Vafa M. Synergistic anti-proliferative effect of resveratrol and etoposide on human hepatocellular and colon cancer cell lines. Eur J Pharmacol. 2013;718:34–40.
148. Ulasli SS, Celik S, Gunay E, Ozdemir M, Hazman O, Ozyurek A, et al. Anticancer effects of thymoquinone, caffeic acid phenethyl ester and resveratrol on A549 non-small cell lung cancer cells exposed to benzo(a)pyrene. Asian Pac J Cancer Prev. 2013;14:6159–64.
149. Jung K-H, Lee JH, Park JW, Quach CHT, Moon S-H, Cho YS, et al. Resveratrol-loaded polymeric nanoparticles suppress glucose metabolism and tumor growth in vitro and in vivo. Int J Pharm. 2014;478:251–7.
150. Caron AZ, He X, Mottawea W, Seifert EL, Jardine K, Dewar-Darch D, et al. The SIRT1 deacetylase protects mice against the symptoms of metabolic syndrome. FASEB J. 2014;28:1306–16.
151. Kitada M, Koya D. SIRT1 in type 2 diabetes: mechanisms and therapeutic potential. Diabetes Metab J. 2013;37:315–25.
152. Civitarese AE, Carling S, Heilbronn LK, Hulver MH, Ukropcova B, Deutsch WA, et al. Calorie restriction increases muscle mitochondrial biogenesis in healthy humans. PLoS Med. 2007;4:e76.
153. Nemerovski CW, Dorsch MP, Simpson RU, Bone HG, Aaronson KD, Bleske BE. Vitamin D and cardiovascular disease. Pharmacotherapy. 2009;29:691–708.
154. Mowry DA, Costello MM, Heelan KA. Association among cardiorespiratory fitness, body fat, and bone marker measurements in healthy young females. J Am Osteopath Assoc. 2009;109:534–9.
155. Moran DS, McClung JP, Kohen T, Lieberman HR. Vitamin D and physical performance. Sports Med. 2013;43:601–11.
156. Cannell JJ, Hollis BW, Sorenson MB, Taft TN, Anderson J. Athletic performance and vitamin D. Med Sci Sports Exerc. 2009;41:1102–10.
157. Sato Y, Iwamoto J, Kanoko T, Satoh K. Low-dose vitamin D prevents muscular atrophy and reduces falls and hip fractures in women after stroke: a randomized controlled trial. Cerebrovasc Dis. 2005;20:187–92.
158. Martinesi M, Treves C, d'Albasio G, Bagnoli S, Bonanomi AG, Stio M. Vitamin D derivatives induce apoptosis and downregulate ICAM-1 levels in peripheral blood mononuclear cells of inflammatory bowel disease patients. Inflamm Bowel Dis. 2008;14:597–604.
159. Garcion E, Sindji L, Leblondel G, Brachet P, Darcy F. 1, 25-Dihydroxyvitamin D3 regulates the synthesis of γ-glutamyl transpeptidase and glutathione levels in rat primary astrocytes. J Neurochem. 1999;73:859–66.
160. Wiseman H. Vitamin D, is a membrane antioxidant ability to inhibit iron-dependent lipid peroxidation in liposomes compared to cholesterol, ergosterol and tamoxifen and relevance to anticancer action. FEBS Lett. 1993;326:285–8.
161. Cohen MS, Mesler DE, Snipes RG, Gray T. 1, 25-Dihydroxyvitamin D3 activates secretion of hydrogen peroxide by human monocytes. J Immunol. 1986;136:1049–53.
162. Wu C-C, Chang J-H, Chen C-C, Su S-B, Yang L-K, Ma W-Y, et al. Calcitriol treatment attenuates inflammation and oxidative stress in hemodialysis patients with secondary hyperparathyroidism. Tohoku J Exp Med. 2011;223:153–9.
163. Valcheva P, Cardus A, Panizo S, Parisi E, Bozic M, Lopez Novoa JM, et al. Lack of vitamin D receptor causes stress-induced premature senescence in vascular smooth muscle cells through enhanced local angiotensin-II signals. Atherosclerosis. 2014;235:247–55.
164. Eftekhari MH, Akbarzadeh M, Dabbaghmanesh MH, Hassanzadeh J. The effect of calcitriol on lipid profile and oxidative stress in hyperlipidemic patients with type 2 diabetes mellitus. ARYA Atheroscler. 2014;10:82–8.

165. Konradsen S, Ag H, Lindberg F, Hexeberg S, Jorde R. Serum 1, 25-dihydroxy vitamin D is inversely associated with body mass index. Eur J Nutr. 2008;47:87–91.
166. Parikh SJ, Edelman M, Uwaifo GI, Freedman RJ, Semega-Janneh M, Reynolds J, et al. The relationship between obesity and serum 1, 25-dihydroxy vitamin D concentrations in healthy adults. J Clin Endocrinol Metab. 2004;89:1196–9.
167. Wortsman J, Matsuoka LY, Chen TC, Lu Z, Holick MF. Decreased bioavailability of vitamin D in obesity. Am J Clin Nutr. 2007;72:690–3.
168. McGill A-T, Stewart JM, Lithander FE, Strik CM, Poppitt SD. Relationships of low serum vitamin D3 with anthropometry and markers of the metabolic syndrome and diabetes in overweight and obesity. Nutr J. 2008;7:4.
169. Khoo A-L, Chai LY, Koenen HJ, Kullberg B-J, Joosten I, van der Ven AJ, et al. 1, 25-Dihydroxyvitamin D3 modulates cytokine production induced by Candida albicans: impact of seasonal variation of immune responses. J Infect Dis. 2011;203:122–30.
170. Li B, Baylink DJ, Deb C, Zannetti C, Rajaallah F, Xing W, et al. 1, 25-Dihydroxyvitamin D3 suppresses TLR8 expression and TLR8-mediated inflammatory responses in monocytes in vitro and experimental autoimmune encephalomyelitis in vivo. PLoS One. 2013;8:e58808.
171. Tzotzas T, Papadopoulou FG, Tziomalos K, Karras S, Gastaris K, Perros P, et al. Rising serum 25-hydroxy-vitamin D levels after weight loss in obese women correlate with improvement in insulin resistance. J Clin Endocrinol Metab. 2010;95:4251–7.
172. Zittermann A, Frisch S, Berthold HK, Götting C, Kuhn J, Kleesiek K, et al. Vitamin D supplementation enhances the beneficial effects of weight loss on cardiovascular disease risk markers. Am J Clin Nutr. 2009;89:1321–7.
173. Villareal DT, Chode S, Parimi N, Sinacore DR, Hilton T, Armamento-Villareal R, et al. Weight loss, exercise, or both and physical function in obese older adults. N Engl J Med. 2011;364:1218–29.

16

Falls and injuries to Polo players: risk perception, mitigation and risk factors

C M Inness[2] and K L Morgan[1,2*]

Abstract

Polo, one of the world's oldest sports, is played in over 80 countries. It is unique in combining the skills of a person with the agility and performance of an animal in a contact sport. There is only one report of the frequency and type of injuries in this population. Here we report risk perception, mitigation and risk factors for injuries and falls in UK polo players. Data were collected retrospectively from a random sample of 112 UK polo players by telephone questionnaire. Injuries (commonly to a shoulder or wrist) requiring a hospital visit were sustained by 17.3% (95% confidence interval [CI] 9.1–25.5) of players. Falls (odds ratio [OR] 6.6, 95% CI 1.4–31.9) and higher self-assessed fitness levels increased the risk (OR 1.7, CI 1.2–2.4). Use of wrist supports (OR 0.2, CI 0.03–0.9) and gym exercise (OR 0.1, CI 0.02–0.9) reduced it. Falls were reported by 58% (CI 47.3–68.8) of players. Women were less at risk than men (OR 0.3, CI 0.1–0.9). Aiming for a better handicap increased the risk (OR 8.4, CI 1.2–57.0). Pre-season rider and horse training were also risk factors. Helmets are compulsory, but players reported that safety certification was not their most important criterion for helmet selection; 49.4% (CI 38.5–60.3) chose appearance. Attendance of a doctor at polo games was not considered important by 65.4% (CI 55.1–75.8) of players; attendance of paramedics and ambulances was volunteered as being of greater consequence. The findings of this study suggest that the protective effect of wrist supports needs testing, helmet manufacturers should incorporate both style and safety into their designs, and paramedics and ambulances should attend polo games.

Key points

- This is the first study of the perception of risk, mitigation and risk factors for falls and injuries in polo players.
- Injuries requiring hospital attendance were sustained by 17.3% of players; higher self-assessed fitness levels increased the risk; use of wrist supports and gym exercise reduced it.
- Falls were reported by 58% of players; aiming for a better handicap increased the risk; pre-season rider and horse training reduced it.

Background

Polo, one of the world's oldest sports, is unique in merging the skill of a person with the agility and performance of an animal to create a single participant in a contact sport. In this respect, it differs from all other sports. Preventing injuries in these modern-day centaurs offers medics, vets and dentists an unrivalled opportunity to collaborate, but surprisingly there has only been one previous publication on injuries in this population [1]. We have recently reported the prevalence and risk factors for injuries in polo ponies [2]. Here we present the risk and type of injury, risk factors and perception of risk, training and fitness in riders in the same population.

Polo is played in over 80 countries. Two teams of four mounted players hit a 9 cm white plastic ball, at speeds of up to 96 miles per hour, using the wide face of a 48- to 54-inch-long polo mallet with a bamboo shaft and a hardwood head. A goal is scored when the ball passes, at any height, between two posts at each end of the pitch. The game is divided into 7.5 min time periods called 'chukkas'. There can be between four and eight chukkas per game. The winning team is the one that has scored the most goals when adjusted for player handicap. Handicaps range from −2 to 10 and are summed to give a combined team handicap. The lower handicapped team is awarded goals at the start of the game, depending on the handicap difference. Polo is played in arenas

* Correspondence: k.l.morgan@liv.ac.uk
[1]Department of Musculoskeletal Biology, Institute of Ageing and Chronic Disease, University of Liverpool, Leahurst Campus, Neston CH64 7TE, UK
[2]School of Veterinary Sciences, University of Liverpool, Leahurst Campus, Neston CH64 7TE, UK

and outdoors. In the UK, outdoor polo is played on grass pitches from the start of April until the end of September. Membership of the governing body, the Hurlingham Polo Association (HPA), is obligatory. Currently, almost 3,000 full playing members and over 13,000 horses are registered.

Polo is considered a high-risk sport, but in the only previous report, a small prospective study of elite players in Argentina, the incidence of injury was 7.8/1,000 playing hours [1]. This is relatively low when compared with soccer (17–29/1,000 h) [3-5] and rugby (53.8/1,000 h) [6]; however, 64% of these injuries were considered serious. Arm and head injuries were most common and were frequently associated with falls [1]. The only other information on injuries in polo players is clinical reports of unusual cases, such as ulna stress fracture [7] and popliteus muscle rupture [8].

Polo has been advocated as a sport for all ages [9]. The starting point for a 'one health' [10] approach to injury prevention is to determine the frequencies and risk factors for injuries in riders and horses [2] in the same population. Riders' opinions on causes of injury, their perceptions, and mitigation of risk and risk factors are reported here.

Methods

Study design

Telephone interviews were used to collect data on injuries, falls, pre-season training and perceptions of risk to polo owner-players and horses, using a retrospective cohort design. The study unit was the player. Potential participants were contacted by mail and were informed of the study aims and that taking part was voluntary, opinions and data were anonymous and opting out was a prerogative. Telephone interviews were conducted between 26 April and 4 May 2010. The option to opt out was repeated at the beginning of each interview. Any person who was unavailable during this period or was non-contactable after five attempts was considered a non-responder. One person conducted all interviews. The University of Liverpool Veterinary Ethics Committee approved the study.

Study population

The target population was HPA-member, UK-resident, horse-owning polo players, aged over 18 years, with an address and telephone number in the members' database. These criteria were met by 1,181 players. A random sample of 112 was selected without replacement. Players known personally to the interviewer (CMI) were substituted with another randomly selected member. The sample size was calculated to allow estimation of the prevalence of injuries, falls and opinions with 95% confidence and 10% precision, assuming the population prevalence to be 50% and a predicted response rate of 80% [11]. This was estimated to be 89 players. This sample size allowed 95% confidence that one opinion, variable or injury would be detected if its prevalence was 3%.

Questionnaire design

The questionnaire design is detailed elsewhere [2]. Briefly, it had two sections—one related to players, the other to the horses that they owned. It contained closed and open questions. Player–owners were asked about falls and acute injuries sustained in the previous season. Injuries were defined as physical insults sustained during a polo game that required a hospital visit. Respondents were asked about their height, weight and handicap; the range and intensity of their winter exercise; the importance of pre-season training on a 1 to 4 scale (with 1 being the lowest); their self-reported fitness levels on a 1 to 10 scale (with 10 being the highest); their perception of the risk of injury in the first, middle and final thirds of the season; their use of protective apparel; and their opinion on the importance of a doctor attending games, on a 1 to 4 scale. The questionnaire was pre-tested before use and modified accordingly, but there was no external validation.

Data processing and analysis

Data were entered into a Microsoft Access database. Frequency distributions of injuries were described, and exact binomial 95% confidence intervals (CIs) were calculated. Falls and any rider injury were used as binary variables, and the association with different exposure variables was examined. Univariable analyses were carried out using Epi-Info 2007 [12]. Continuous variables were compared using analysis of variance, except where Bartlett's test indicated variance heterogeneity, when Kruskal–Wallis tests were used. Categorical variables were analysed using χ^2 and Fisher's exact tests.

All variables associated with either falls or injuries with p values of <0.1 in univariable analyses were offered to multivariable logistic regression models developed manually using forward stepwise procedures in Stata [13]. Variables were added in the order of their p value, smallest first. Any with p values of <0.05 were retained in the model. Variables with a value approaching 0.05 were retained where the change in the Akaike information criterion (AIC) supported it. Model quality was assessed by the sensitivity, specificity, accuracy and area under the receiver–operating characteristic (ROC) curve and the goodness of fit evaluated by the Hosmer–Lemeshow statistic.

Results

Response rate

The useable response rate was 73% (81/112). Eighty-four polo players responded, but two no longer kept polo ponies and one had kept them in work over winter.

Participants

The participants' mean age was 41.7 years (standard deviation [SD] 10.7), the mean body mass index (BMI) was 24.8 (SD 1.9) and the median handicap was 0 (interquartile range [IQR] 0–1). Each participant owned between 2 and 110 horses, with a median of seven (IQR 5.0–10.0). Eighty percent (CI 71.6–88.9) of respondents were men. Sixty-three percent (CI 52.5–73.5) were responsible for day-to-day horse management, and the remainder employed a groom.

Falls

Fifty-eight percent (CI 47.3–68.8) of players reported falling in the previous season. The median frequency was once (IQR 0–2), but 2.5% (CI 0.0–5.9) of players fell 10 or more times.

Injuries to riders

Fourteen riders (17.3%, CI 9.1–25.5) reported injuries. Wrist and shoulder injuries were most common. The injuries were a broken collar bone (2), shoulder injury, wrist injury (3), damage to tendons in a hand and wrist, dislocated elbow, torn groin ligament, broken rib, 'damaged cartilage', damage to cruciate ligaments, damaged right leg with torn calf muscle and haematoma, pelvic injury x-rayed but not broken, hamstring injury, and arm and fingers hit by a mallet. Three patients reported more than one injury. Players were hit in the mouth by mallets (9.9%, CI 3.4–16.4) and balls (3.7%, CI 0.0–7.8). None required dental treatment. All but 1.2% (CI 0.0–3.6) of players reported bruising after playing, and 56.8% (CI 46–67.6) were bruised regularly.

Pre-season exercise and fitness levels

Just over half of the respondents (54.3%, CI 43.5–65.2) rode during winter, 37% (CI 26.5–47.6) played winter polo and 86.4% (CI 79.0–93.9) reported gym exercise, hockey, running, swimming, yoga, squash, weight training, Pilates, cycling and walking either singly or in combinations. The frequencies of these different types of exercise are shown in Table 1.

Over half of the players (58.0%, CI 47.3–68.8) considered their exercise intensity to be less than the recommended UK adult level of 'moderate exercise for 30 min or more five times per week'. Their median self-assessed fitness to play polo was 5 (IQR 4–7) with a range of 2–10.

When asked for their opinion on the importance of pre-season training, 58% (CI 47.3–68.8) scored it a very important 4; 35.8% (CI 26.5–47.6) scored it 3; 4.9% (CI 0.2–9.7) scored it 2 and 1.2% scored it 1.

Table 1 Frequencies of winter exercise and use of protective apparel reported by players

	Number	Percentage	95% CI
Winter exercise			
Gym exercise	33	40.7	30.0–51.4
Running	18	22.2	13.2–31.3
Swimming	14	17.3	9.1–25.5
Yoga	9	11.1	4.3–18.0
Squash	8	9.9	3.4–16.4
Weight training	7	8.6	2.5–14.8
Pilates	6	7.4	1.7–13.1
Cycling	5	6.2	0.9–11.4
Walking	3	3.7	0.0–7.8
Use of protective apparel			
Knee pads	80	98.8	96.4–100
Goggles	40	49.4	38.5–60.3
Wrist support	28	34.6	24.2–44.9
Face guard	17	21.0	12.1–29.9
Elbow pads	8	9.9	3.4–16.4
Gum shield	5	6.2	0.9–11.4
Back support	3	3.7	0.0–7.8

CI confidence interval.

Use of protective apparel

The use of protective apparel is shown in Table 1. Wearing a helmet is compulsory in the UK, and all respondents reported wearing one. The next most common item was knee pads, followed by goggles, wrist supports, face guards, elbow pads, gum shields and back supports.

Perception of risk

Although it is compulsory for helmets to carry a safety standard mark, only 29.6% (CI 19.7–39.6) of riders considered it the most important aspect of helmet purchase, 49.4% (CI 38.5–60.3) chose appearance and 7.4% (CI 1.7–13.1) chose price.

Perception of risk changed with the stage of the season. Forty-three percent (CI 32.4–54.0) of respondents considered it highest in the first third of the season, compared with 1.2% (CI 0.0–3.6) in the last third. Thirty-seven percent (CI 26.5–47.6) considered the risk constant throughout the season.

The presence of doctors at games was considered of low or very low importance by the majority of participants (65.4%, CI 55.1–75.8), but a significant minority (23.5%, CI 14.2–32.7) considered it highly important. Many participants volunteered the opinion that the attendance of paramedics and an ambulance was of far greater consequence.

Risk factors for injury

Risk factors for serious rider injury are shown in Table 2. Rider age, sex, height, weight, BMI and experience did not influence the risk of injury. In univariable analysis, risk factors were a fall, higher self-scored fitness, participation in gym exercise and yoga, use of wrist supports and the number of days from the start of the year to the first chukka.

After adjustment for confounding, falls were associated with an increased risk of injury (odds ratios [OR] 6.6, CI 1.4–31.9), as was higher self-scored fitness (OR 1.7, CI 1.2–2.4). In contrast, gym exercise reduced the likelihood of injury (OR 0.14, CI 0.03–0.9), as did use of wrist supports (OR 0.17, CI 0.02–0.9). Use of goggles and face protectors had no effect.

The model had sensitivity of 50%, specificity of 92.5%, accuracy of 85.2% and an area under the ROC curve of 0.87. The Hosmer–Lemeshow goodness-of-fit statistic was 4.2 ($p = 0.84$).

Risk factors for falls

Risk factors for falls during polo games are shown in Table 3. In univariable analysis, risk factors for falls were the sex of the rider, yoga and squash as out-of-season exercise, aiming for a lower handicap, cold water hosing of the horse's legs after exercise and the duration of pre-season horse training.

After adjustment for confounding, the odds of women falling was a third of that of men (OR 0.3, CI 0.1–0.9). Players who aimed to improve their end-of-season handicap had eight times the risk (OR 8.4, CI 1.2–57.0) of those who did not aim to improve their handicap. All eight riders who reported playing squash experienced at least one fall, and those who reported doing yoga had 20 times the risk (OR 20.7, CI 1.6–262.6) of those who did not report doing yoga.

Players exercising their horses for longer prior to the first chukka (51.1 versus 43.5 days) were less likely to fall; the OR was 0.93 for every day increase. Riders who cold-water hosed their horses' legs after exercise had six times the risk of falling (OR 6.1, CI 1.5–25.4).

This model had sensitivity of 80.9%, specificity of 73.5%, accuracy of 77.8% and an area under the ROC curve of 0.87. The Hosmer–Lemeshow goodness-of-fit statistic was 7.92 ($p = 0.44$). When squash was excluded from the model, the AIC was 89.8, compared with 82.7 when squash was included; the latter was selected.

Table 2 Risk factors for serious rider injury

Risk factor	Odds ratio	95% CI	*p* value
Fall	6.57	1.35–31.91	0.02
Rider self score of fitness	1.68	1.18–2.40	0.004
Rider exercise: gym	0.14	0.23–0.88	0.035
Rider use of wrist supports	0.17	0.30–0.93	0.04

CI confidence interval.

Table 3 Risk factors for falls during polo games

Risk factor	Odds ratio	95% CI	*p* value
Rider sex: female	0.27	0.08–0.94	0.04
Rider aim to increase handicap	8.36	1.23–56.97	0.03
Rider exercise: yoga	20.73	1.64–262.59	0.02
Rider exercise: squash	NA	Perfect predictor	
Horse: pre-season exercise (per day)	0.93	0.88–0.98	0.012
Horse: cold water hosing	6.10	1.47–25.41	0.013

CI confidence interval, *NA* not applicable.

Discussion

This is the first description of the frequencies and risk factors for injuries and falls in UK polo players. It also records their perceptions of risk and its mitigation.

Polo is recognised as a rough contact sport [1]. Almost all of the players in this study reported bruising after playing. Injuries requiring a hospital visit were less common. The cumulative risk was 17.3% (CI 9.1–25.5), which equates to 519 hospital visits per year in the total population. Shoulder and wrist injuries were most common. This finding is consistent with the only previous report of polo injures [1].

Use of wrist supports was associated with a decreased risk of injury (OR 0.17, CI 0.03–0.93). This applied to all injuries rather than just those involving the wrist. Interpreting this as a proxy measure of risk-averse or safety-conscious riders is not supported by the lack of association between wrist supports and falls. Wrist supports may reduce the effect of forces on the wrist caused by swinging the mallet. This hypothesis is biologically plausible and warrants an intervention study.

Rider fitness was associated with positive and negative risks; perception of self fitness was associated with an increased risk of injury, whereas actual fitness, as measured by gym exercise, was associated with a decreased risk.

Rider falls were common, and they were associated with injury (OR 6.6, CI 1.4–31.9). Fifty-eight percent of players reported falling at least once during the season. Risk factors were the sex of the rider, intention to improve handicap, pre-season pony exercise and days from the start of the year.

Females were half as likely to fall as males (OR 0.3, CI 0.1–0.9). This may be because women are better riders, have better balance, or are more cautious and risk averse during games. It could not be explained by physical attributes, such as height and weight, or riding experience, as falls were not associated with these variables.

Players aiming to improve their handicap were 8.4 (CI 1.2–56.9) times as likely to fall as those who considered that their handicap would remain the same. This may reflect more competitive players pushing themselves and exceeding their limits in order to improve. It was not associated with rider age.

The association between rider falls and the number of days of pre-season pony exercise was a surprise. Riders exercising horses for a mean of 51.1 days (SD 12.2) were at lower risk (OR 0.9, CI 0.9–0.98) of falling than those exercising for 43.5 days (SD 10.9). This suggests that horse preparation is important in preventing rider falls and may reflect improved fitness, reduced excitability or better control. Alternatively, it may be a proxy measure for another variable, e.g. management. It is also possible that this effect was associated with the improved ground conditions later in the calendar year, rather than the time interval itself. When the number of days from the start of the year to the first chukka was examined, it was associated with a decrease in falls at a level close to statistical significance ($p = 0.052$). It is possible that two effects operate here: pre-season pony training and improved ground conditions. The effect of pre-season pony exercise needs further investigation.

Attitude to risk was assessed from priorities in helmet selection, the frequency of wearing protective apparel, perceived periods of highest risk and the perceived importance of attendant medical staff.

Helmets are compulsory, but only 29.6% (CI 19.7–39.6) of riders chose safety as the most important criterion for selection. Almost half of them considered appearance most important. This highlights the need for style and safety considerations in helmet design [14].

The ranking of additional protective apparel was knee pads, goggles, wrist supports and face guards. A small proportion of players used elbow pads, gum shields and back supports.

Players differed in their perception of the stage of the season and the risk of injury. The first third of the season was considered high risk by 43.2% (CI 32.4–54.0), whereas a similar proportion (37.0%, CI 26.5–47.6) considered the risk constant throughout the season. A prospective study would add quantitative data to these perceptions.

Rider opinions on the value of having a doctor present were polarized, with 65.5% scoring it low priority and 23.5% scoring it high priority. The only other study of polo injuries recommended the presence of a trauma-trained doctor at all matches [1]. Although it was not on the questionnaire, the importance of paramedic and ambulance attendance was voiced by a number of riders.

This is the first population-based study of falls and injuries to polo players in the UK. It is small because of the absence of any recognizable funding stream for research on polo, but it followed STROBE (Strengthening the Reporting of Observational Studies in Epidemiology) guidelines to maximize accuracy and generalizability. The usable response rate was lower than anticipated but at 73% was still acceptable. A retrospective cohort design was used, and to maximize recall, the study focused on memorable events, injuries requiring a hospital visit and falls in the previous season. In the UK, this would involve a visit to an Accident and Emergency Department, and this was used as a proxy measure for the injury being both acute and serious. We did not ask for precise details of the injuries, their severity or the injury mechanism, as our focus in this initial study was simply to estimate injury frequency and type. The study was carried out at the beginning of the season because we were also interested in out-of-season training of riders and horses. The results are player reports. Although there was no external validation, the risk of rider injury was similar to that reported previously [1]. Not all respondents were responsible for the day-to-day management of their horses. Thirty-seven percent (CI 26.5–47.6) employed a groom. This may have resulted in inaccuracies but should not have introduced systematic bias.

These UK players differed from those in the only previous report, a prospective study of 34 Argentinean riders [1]. Handicaps ranged from −1 to 7 compared with 7–10 [1], suggesting that the UK players were recreational rather than high performance. At 41.7, the mean age was surprisingly high. This may reflect the inclusion criterion of owning at least one horse. Younger players may have been excluded because their mounts were hired or registered under a parent's name. Horse-owning players were selected because we were also interested in the injuries to horses [2]. It was considered unlikely that players using hired or loaned horses would be able to supply this information. Selecting this population may have biased the overall estimate of injury by excluding younger players.

Polo is interesting from a number of scientific perspectives. The unique relationship between rider and horse in this ancient, unpredictable contact sport offers medics, vets and dentists the opportunity to collaborate in the field of sports injury prevention.

Ethical approval

This study was approved by the University of Liverpool Veterinary Ethics Committee and was performed in accordance with the ethical standards laid down in the 1964 Declaration of Helsinki and its later amendments. All participants gave their informed consent prior to their inclusion in the study.

Acknowledgments

We thank the Hurlingham Polo Association (HPA) and its members for participating in this study. Financial support was provided by the University of Liverpool. CMI is a polo-playing member of the HPA. KLM has no conflict of interest.

References

1. Costa-Paz M, Aponte-Tinao L, Muscolo D. **Injuries to polo riders: a prospective evaluation.** *Br J Sports Med.* 1999; **33**:329–31.
2. Innes CM. Polo pony injuries: player–owner reported risk, perception, mitigation and risk factors. Equine Vet J. Epub 2014 Jul 17. doi:10.1111/evj.12298.
3. Engstrom B, Johansson C, Tornkvist H. **Soccer injuries among elite female players.** *Am J Sports Med.* 1991; **19**:372–5.
4. Rahnama N, Reilly T, Lees A. **Injury risk associated with playing actions during competitive soccer.** *Br J Sports Med.* 2002; **36**:354–59.
5. Walden M, Hagglund M, Orchard J, Kristenson K, Ekstrand J. **Regional differences in injury incidence in European professional football.** *Scand J Med Sci Sports.* 2013; **23**:424–30.
6. Fuller C, Brooks J, Cancea R, Hall J, Kemp S. **Contact events in rugby union and their propensity to cause injury.** *Br J Sports Med.* 2007; **41**:862–7.
7. Clark R, Sizer P, Slauterbeck J. **Stress fracture of the ulna in a male competitive polo player.** *Am J Sports Med.* 2002; **30**:130–2.
8. Winge S, Phadke P. **Isolated popliteus muscle rupture in polo players.** *Knee Surg Sports Traumatol Arthrosc.* 1996; **4**:89–91.
9. Vail J. **Polo for all ages.** *J Psychosoc Nurs.* 2009; **47**:24–7.
10. Morris A. **One medicine: combining veterinary and medical expertise.** *Vet Rec.* 2009; **165**:159–61.
11. Brogan D, Denniston M, Liff J, Flagg E, Coates R, Brinton L. **Comparison of telephone sampling and area sampling: response rates and within-household coverage.** *Am J Epidemiol.* 2001; **153**:1119–27.
12. Dean A, Arner T, Sunki G, et al. *Epi-Info™, a database and statistics program for public health professionals.* Atlanta: CDC; 2011.
13. StataCorp. *Stata statistical software: release 11.* College Station: StataCorp LP; 2009.
14. Czarnecki N, Yoganandan N, Sances A, Pintar F, Reinartz J, Battocletti J. **An evaluation and collective review of helmet standards.** *J Clin Eng.* 1986; **11**:461–7.

17

A cross-cultural re-evaluation of the Exercise Addiction Inventory (EAI) in five countries

Mark D Griffiths[1], Robert Urbán[6], Zsolt Demetrovics[6], Mia B Lichtenstein[3], Ricardo de la Vega[4], Bernadette Kun[6], Roberto Ruiz-Barquín[4], Jason Youngman[5] and Attila Szabo[2*]

Abstract

Research into the detrimental effects of excessive exercise has been conceptualized in a number of similar ways, including 'exercise addiction', 'exercise dependence', 'obligatory exercising', 'exercise abuse', and 'compulsive exercise'. Among the most currently used (and psychometrically valid and reliable) instruments is the Exercise Addiction Inventory (EAI). The present study aimed to further explore the psychometric properties of the EAI by combining the datasets of a number of surveys carried out in five different countries (Denmark, Hungary, Spain, UK, and US) that have used the EAI with a total sample size of 6,031 participants. A series of multigroup confirmatory factor analyses (CFAs) were carried out examining configural invariance, metric invariance, and scalar invariance. The CFAs using the combined dataset supported the configural invariance and metric invariance but not scalar invariance. Therefore, EAI factor scores from five countries are not comparable because the use or interpretation of the scale was different in the five nations. However, the covariates of exercise addiction can be studied from a cross-cultural perspective because of the metric invariance of the scale. Gender differences among exercisers in the interpretation of the scale also emerged. The implications of the results are discussed, and it is concluded that the study's findings will facilitate a more robust and reliable use of the EAI in future research.

Key points

- Cultural factors prevent the actual (score-based) comparison of Exercise Addiction Inventory (EAI) factor scores.
- The EAI is useful for studying the covariates of exercise addiction in all cultures.
- The interpretation of the EAI (and its items) may be different for men and women.

Background

Although the beneficial effects of exercise are well known, there is now a growing literature that a small minority of people can experience various negative consequences of excessive exercising [1]. Research into the detrimental effects of excessive exercise has been conceptualized in a number of similar ways, including 'exercise addiction' [1], 'exercise dependence' [2,3], 'obligatory exercising' [4], 'exercise abuse' [5], and 'compulsive exercise' [6]. To assess the negative effects of excessive exercise, several instruments have been developed and have been extensively reviewed elsewhere [7,8]. Among the most currently used (and psychometrically valid and reliable) instruments are the 'Obligatory Exercise Questionnaire' (OEQ) [4,9], the 'Exercise Dependence Scale' (EDS) [10,11], the 'Exercise Dependence Questionnaire' [12], and the 'Exercise Addiction Inventory' (EAI) [13].

The EAI is a short, 6-item instrument aimed at identifying the risk of exercise addiction that has become widely used over the last few years. The EAI assesses six common symptoms of addictive behaviors [14,15] (i.e. salience, mood modification, tolerance, withdrawal symptoms, conflict, and relapse) and has relatively high internal consistency and convergent validity with the Exercise Dependence Questionnaire [13,16,17]. Not only does the EAI have good reliability and validity, but it is theoretically driven, has clear cut-off scores for operationally defining exercise addiction, and is a much shorter scale than other instruments (helping to reduce the time that participants spend completing research surveys).

* Correspondence: szabo.attila@ppk.elte.hu
[2]Institute of Health Promotion and Sport Sciences, Faculty of Education and Psychology, Eötvös Loránd University, Budapest, Hungary
Full list of author information is available at the end of the article

To date, only one national representative study examining exercise addiction has been carried out [17]. This study surveyed a Hungarian adult population aged 18–64 years ($n = 2{,}710$), and assessed exercise addiction using both the EAI and the EDS. Results showed that 10.1% (EAI) and 6.2% (EDS) of the population were characterized as non-dependent-symptomatic exercisers, while the proportion of the persons at-risk for exercise dependence was 0.5% (EAI) and 0.3% (EDS). Although there has only been one national study, the EAI has been used to assess exercise addiction in a number of different non-nationally representative subsamples, all of which have confirmed the good psychometric properties of the EAI (see Table 1).

In a survey of 451 exercisers, Szabo and Griffiths [18] found that 6.9% of British sport-science students ($n = 261$, aged 19–23 years) were at risk of exercise addiction, as measured by the EAI, compared with 3.6% of British gym users ($n = 194$, aged 17–74 years). Warner and Griffiths [19] reported similar results using the EAI. They found that 8% of British gym users ($n = 100$, aged 18–74 years) were exercise addicts. Lichtenstein et al. [20] validated the EAI in Danish by screening 588 exercisers in fitness and football (aged 14–70 years) who exercised for an average of 8 h per week. They reported that the prevalence of exercise addiction in their sample was 5.8%. Another team led by the same author found that exercise addiction prevalence rates in young male footballers (age 18–39 years) were 7.1%, while the figure was higher in general-fitness participants (9.7%) [21].

Using the EAI, Szabo et al. surveyed two Spanish groups of university athletes, including sport students ($n = 57$) and non-sport students ($n = 90$), and a group of ultra-marathon runners ($n = 95$; mean age of the total sample = 27.5 years) [22]. EAI scores were higher in men than women, and ultra-marathoners scored higher on the EAI than both groups of university athletes. The prevalence of being at risk for exercise addictions was 7–10% in university athletes and 17% in ultra-marathoners. They also reported that the amount of exercise was not directly related to exercise addiction. Allegre et al. surveyed 95 French 'ultra-marathoners' (who typically run 100-km races) using the EAI and reported only three people (3.2%) as at-risk for exercise addiction [23]. Youngman also investigated the risk for exercise addiction in endurance athletes [24]. The sample comprised 1,285 American male and female triathletes (aged 18–70 years). Approximately 20% of triathletes were classed as being at risk for exercise addiction (with 79% exhibiting some symptoms of exercise addiction). Female triathletes were at greater risk for exercise addiction than male triathletes. As the number of weekly training hours or the number of weekly training sessions increased, so did a triathlete's risk for exercise addiction.

There is a need to demonstrate the cross-cultural validity of the construct of exercise addiction and its measurement for both theoretical and practical reasons. Testing the cross-cultural properties can highlight the source of differences in cross-national prevalence rates estimated by the EAI. For a meaningful comparison across groups, measurement equivalence or invariance in the constructs underlying one questionnaire across these groups must be demonstrated [25,26]. Different levels of measurement invariance are defined hierarchically, including dimensional, configural, metric, scalar, and strict factorial [25]. Dimensional invariance refers to there being the same numbers of factors present across the comparison groups (e.g. the same number of factors in the EAI across the countries should be present). Configural invariance refers to the same items being related to each factor. In this case, the same items of EAI should define the same factors across the countries. Metric invariance depicts the equivalence of factor loadings that describe the strength of the associations between the specific items and their specific factors. Statistical analysis can

Table 1 Use of the exercise addiction inventory in previously published studies

Study	Year	Sample	Measures	Prevalence (%) of exercise addiction
Griffiths et al. [16]	2005	University students	EAI (English)	3.0
Szabo and Griffiths [18]	2007	Habitual exercisers and sport-science students	EAI (English)	3.6 (habitual exercisers); 6.9 (sport-science undergraduates)
Youngman [24]	2007	Triathletes	EAI (English)	19.9
Villella et al. [30]	2010	High-school students	EAI (Italian)	8.5
Lejoyeux et al. [31]	2012	Fitness-centre attendees	EAI (French)	29.6
Mónok et al. [17]	2012	Nationally representative sample (population aged 18–64 years)	EAI (Hungarian)	0.5 (general population); 3.2 (regular exercisers)
Lichtenstein et al. [20]	2013	Fitness exercisers and football players	EAI (Danish)	5.8
Menczel et al. [32]	2013	Fitness-centre attendees	EAI (Hungarian)	1.8 + 1.8 who exhibited both exercise addiction and eating disorders
Szabo et al. [22]	2013	University students and athletes	EAI (Spanish)	7–17

EAI Exercise Addiction Inventory.

reveal if the factor loadings of EAI items are statistically equal, demonstrate that the participants respond to the items in the same way, and that the factors have the same meaning across the countries. Metric invariance is a prerequisite to study factor variance and covariances. Scalar invariance refers to the equivalent intercepts of the items. Scalar invariance is required to compare latent means across groups. The scalar invariance of EAI would be a prerequisite to compare means across groups such as gender, countries, or any other groups. The present study therefore aimed to further explore the psychometric properties of the EAI by combining the datasets of a number of surveys carried out in five different countries (Hungary, UK, Spain, US, and Denmark). This was done to test the assumption that the EAI is invariant across countries and that it can be a useful instrument for future cross-cultural research.

Methods

Participants

Data collected in five countries from six previously published studies using the EAI (between 2003 and 2013) were merged to create a new combined dataset (i.e. data from six studies [13,17,18,20,22,24]). These datasets were chosen because all authors, using a non-English version of the EAI worldwide, were contacted for possible collaboration. However, only authors from five nations agreed to share their data and participate in the study. The EAI has also been translated into Italian and French and the authors of these were also invited to collaborate; however, no response was obtained from these researchers therefore no data from those studies were included in the present study. The newly combined dataset provided a sample size of 6,031 participants (2,911 males, 3,095 females, and 25 undisclosed genders). The participant characteristics of each of the six studies are shown in Table 2.

Measures

Age, gender, and EAI scores were the only measures collated for analysis. The EAI is the shortest psychometrically validated questionnaire to date. It comprises only six statements that correspond to the 'components' model of addiction [16]. Each statement is rated on a five-point Likert scale. The statements are coded so that the high scores reflect attributes of addictive exercise behavior: 1 = 'strongly disagree', 2 = 'disagree', 3 = 'neither agree nor disagree', 4 = 'agree', 5 = 'strongly agree'. The six statements that make up the inventory are: (1) "Exercise is the most important thing in my life" (salience); (2) "Conflicts have arisen between me and my family and/or my partner about the amount of exercise I do" (conflict); (3) "I use exercise as a way of changing my mood" (mood modification); (4) "Over time I have increased the amount of exercise I do in a day" (tolerance); (5) "If I have to miss an exercise session I feel moody and irritable" (withdrawal symptoms); and (6) "If I cut down the amount of exercise I do, and then start again, I always end up exercising as often as I did before" (relapse). The EAI cut-off score for individuals considered at-risk of exercise addiction is 24 (out of 30). This cut-off represents those individuals with scores in the top 15% of the total scale score. High scores were considered to be the most problematic for the individual. A score of 13–23 was chosen to be indicative of a potentially symptomatic person, and a score of 0–12 was deemed to indicate an asymptomatic individual.

Table 2 Descriptive statistics of exercise addiction inventory data from six samples in five countries, including age, gender, mean exercise addiction inventory score, and individual item analysis

	Spain	UK	US	Denmark	Hungary	Hungary_2
N	266	294	1272	587	583	2,752
Women [*N* (%)]	90 (33.8)	137 (46.6)	684 (53.7)	293 (39.6)	297 (50.7)	1,556 (56.5)
Age [years; mean (SD)]	27.2 (10.61)	25.5 (10.00)	37.9 (9.44)	28.4 (10.74)	29.7 (11.62)	31.5 (8.48)
Exercise addiction score [mean (SD)]	18.6 (4.07)	16.3 (4.45)	20.7 (3.58)	17.6 (3.93)	15.1 (4.72)	17.7 (4.09)
Cronbach's α	0.70	0.80	0.58	0.66	0.73	0.61
Items						
Exercise is the most important thing in my life	3.23 (0.93)	2.30 (1.00)	2.72 (1.03)	2.85 (0.99)	3.00 (1.06)	3.10 (1.02)
Conflicts have arisen between me and my family and/or my partner about the amount of exercise I do	2.23 (1.22)	1.97 (1.10)	2.99 (1.24)	2.09 (1.15)	1.55 (0.97)	1.63 (1.17)
I use exercise as a way of changing my mood	3.75 (1.02)	3.17 (1.11)	3.88 (0.88)	3.42 (1.11)	3.07 (1.31)	3.31 (1.17)
Over time I have increased the amount of exercise I do in a day	3.56 (1.08)	3.18 (1.05)	4.11 (0.81)	3.59 (1.01)	2.52 (1.31)	3.18 (1.31)
If I have to miss an exercise session I feel moody and irritable	2.75 (1.11)	2.52 (1.06)	3.51 (0.99)	2.73 (1.16)	2.19 (1.18)	2.98 (1.24)
If I cut down the amount of exercise I do, and then start again, I always end up exercising as often as I did before	3.03 (1.03)	3.18 (0.99)	3.60 (0.88)	2.90 (1.04)	2.73 (1.34)	3.53 (1.23)

Table 3 Degree of model fit of the exercise addiction inventory in six samples from five different countries and tests of measurement invariance

	χ^2	*df*	*p*-Value	RMSEA	Cfit of RMSEA	CFI	TLI	SRMR	$\Delta\chi^2$	Δdf	*p*-Value	ΔRMSEA	ΔCFI
Confirmatory factor analysis in each country separately													
Spain	6.1	9	0.727	<0.001	0.946	1.000	1.000	0.022					
UK	32.6	9	<0.001	0.094	0.017	0.942	0.903	0.042					
US	58.4	9	<0.001	0.065	0.051	0.920	0.867	0.033					
Denmark	14.3	9	0.113	0.032	0.828	0.985	0.975	0.024					
Hungary	21.4	9	0.011	0.049	0.491	0.976	0.961	0.027					
Hungary_2	80.5	9	<0.001	0.054	0.266	0.949	0.915	0.027					
Multigroup analyses to test the measurement invariance													
Configural invariance	211.5	54	<0.001	0.055		0.955	0.925	0.029					
Configural vs. metric invariance									114.2	25	<0.001	0.002	0.025
Metric invariance	325.4	79	<0.001	0.057		0.930	0.920	0.051					
Metric vs. scalar invariance									2,140.0	25	<0.001	0.093	0.571
Scalar invariance	2,346.2	104	<0.001	0.150		0.361	0.447	0.136					

The latent variables were identified by fixing one factor loading being equal to 1.
χ^2 Chi-square value of model fit of each model, *df* degree of freedom, *RMSEA* root mean squared error of approximation, *Cfit of RMSEA* is a statistical test that evaluates the statistical deviation of RMSEA from the value 0.05, and non-significant probability values ($p > 0.05$) indicate acceptable model fit; *CFI* comparative fit index, *TLI* Tucker–Lewis index, *SRMR* the standardized root mean square residual, $\Delta\chi^2$ Satorra–Bentler scaled (S–B scaled) χ^2 difference test, Δdf the difference of df in two models compared, *ΔRMSEA* the difference of RMSEA values in two models compared, *ΔCFI* the difference of CFI values in two models compared.

Results

Descriptive statistics

The sample statistics from each of the six studies are presented in Table 3. The samples are varied in sample size, gender distribution, age, and exercise addiction scores.

Testing measurement invariance across countries

In order to test for measurement invariance across countries, a series of multigroup confirmatory factor analyses (CFAs) with increasing constraints were carried out. To compare the degree of fit of the nested models, the traditional $\Delta\chi^2$ test (i.e. the Satorra-Bentler scaled χ^2 difference test) and the recommendations of Cheung and Rensvold [27] and Chen [28] for comparing two nested models were used. Cut-off values of $\Delta\text{CFI} \leq 0.01$ (comparative fit index) and $\Delta\text{RMSEA} \leq 0.015$ (root mean squared error of approximation) were used. The fit indices are reported in Table 3. In order to support dimensional invariance, CFAs of the measurement model in participating countries were separately performed, which resulted in an adequate or acceptable degree of fit. The next step was to test the measurement model freely across all five countries together. This unconstrained solution fitted the data satisfactorily and supported the dimensional and configural invariance. In a further test, the factor loadings were set as equal across countries, and the degree of fit (χ^2) decreased significantly. However, the change in RMSEA was less than the cut-off (≤0.015) but the decrement in CFI was larger than 0.01.

Table 4 Comparisons of factor loadings and intercepts of the individual Exercise Addiction Inventory items in six samples from five different countries

Items	Test of equality of factor loadings				Test of equality of intercepts			
	$\Delta\chi^2$	*p*-Value	ΔRMSEA	ΔCFI	$\Delta\chi^2$	*p*-Value	ΔRMSEA	ΔCFI
Exercise is the most important thing in my life (item 1)	13.0	<0.03	0.001	0.002	225.9	<0.001	0.027	0.063
Conflicts have arisen between me and my family and/or my partner about the amount of exercise (item 2)	13.7	<0.02	0.001	0.003	1,238.5	<0.001	0.069	0.292
I use exercise as a way of changing my mood (item 3)	34.9	<0.001	0.004	0.007	214.7	<0.001	0.005	0.061
Over time I have increased the amount of exercise I do in a day (item 4)	3.7	0.600	0.001	0.004	179.9	<0.001	0.017	0.247
If I have to miss an exercise session I feel moody and irritable (item 5)	15.7	<0.01	0.001	0.003	153.0	<0.001	0.001	0.042
If I cut down the amount of exercise I do, and then start again, I always end up exercising as often as I did before (item 6)	15.6	<0.01	0.001	0.003	140.8	<0.001	0.004	0.068

For the newly proposed decision criteria, to compare two-nested models the cut-off value of ΔCFI is ≤0.01 and the cut-off value for ΔRMSEA is ≤0.015 [27, 28].
$\Delta\chi^2$ Satorra–Bentler scaled (S–B scaled) χ^2 difference test, *ΔRMSEA* the difference of root mean squared error of approximation values in two models compared, *ΔCFI* the difference of comparative fit index values in two models compared.

The factor loading for each item separately was also tested and, based on ΔRMSEA and ΔCFI values having equal loadings, empirical support for the metric invariance of the scale was found (see Table 4). In the third model, the intercepts were set as equal. The degree of fit (χ^2) decreased significantly again. Furthermore, ΔRMSEA and ΔCFI values were much higher than the cut-off, and therefore scalar invariance of the EAI cannot be claimed. We also tried to identify items that were invariant; hence, we tested each item separately. However, all analyses

Table 5 Testing gender invariance of the Exercise Addiction Inventory in five different countries: multigroup analyses in six samples

Model		χ^2	*df*	RMSEA	CFI	$\Delta\chi^2$	Δ*df*	*p*-Value	ΔRMSEA	ΔCFI
Spain										
1.	Configural invariance	25.0	18	0.054	0.968					
	Configural vs. metric invariance					7.9	5	0.164	0.003	0.014
2.	Metric invariance	32.9	23	0.057	0.954					
	Metric vs. scalar invariance					20.5	6	<0.003		
3.	Scalar invariance	53.3	29	0.079	0.887				0.022	0.067
UK										
1.	Configural invariance	52.8	18	0.115	0.920					
	Configural vs. metric invariance					7.9	5	0.161	−0.009	0.007
2.	Metric invariance	60.8	23	0.106	0.913					
	Metric vs. scalar invariance					6.7	6	0.353		
3.	Scalar invariance	67.9	29	0.096	0.910				−0.010	0.003
US										
1.	Configural invariance	68.7	16	0.067	0.915					
	Configural vs. metric invariance					8.6	5	0.127	0.006	0.006
2.	Metric invariance	77.0	23	0.061	0.909					
	Metric vs. scalar invariance					51.8	6	<0.001		
3.	Scalar invariance	127.1	29	0.073	0.835				0.012	0.074
Denmark										
1.	Configural invariance	38.7	18	0.063	0.945					
	Configural vs. metric invariance					1.9	5	0.866	0.013	0.011
2.	Metric invariance	39.6	23	0.050	0.956					
	Metric vs. scalar invariance					44.9	6	<0.001	0.030	0.100
3.	Scalar invariance	83.0	29	0.080	0.856					
Hungary										
1.	Configural invariance	29.8	18	0.047	0.977					
	Configural vs. metric invariance					8.6	5	0.128	0.001	0.006
2.	Metric invariance	38.3	23	0.048	0.971					
	Metric vs. scalar invariance					32.8	6	<0.001	0.021	0.049
3.	Scalar invariance	69.8	29	0.069	0.922					
Hungary_2										
1.	Configural invariance	98.8	18	0.057	0.944					
	Configural vs. metric invariance					13.5	5	<0.002	−0.004	0.006
2.	Metric invariance	111.8	23	0.053	0.938					
	Metric vs. scalar invariance					92.1	6	<0.001	0.013	0.057
3.	Scalar invariance	199.6	29	0.065	0.881					

The latent variables were identified by fixing one factor loading being equal to 1.
df degree of freedom, *RMSEA* root mean squared error of approximation, *CFI* comparative fit index, $\Delta\chi^2$ Satorra–Bentler scaled (S–B scaled) χ^2difference test, Δ*df* the difference of df in two models compared, Δ*RMSEA* the difference of RMSEA values in two models compared, Δ*CFI* the difference of CFI values in two models compared.

resulted in higher change scores than the cut-offs (see Table 4), and therefore none of the items demonstrated equal intercepts across the countries.

Testing measurement invariance between men and women

The gender invariance of the EAI in each country was also separately tested. Among the six samples, the change in degree of fit (χ^2) was not significant after constraining factor loadings to be equal in males and females. Furthermore, ΔRMSEA and ΔCFI values were lower than the cut-off values; therefore, metric invariance was supported. However, the scalar invariance was not supported in all countries because degree of fit (χ^2) decreased significantly in all countries, and ΔRMSEA and ΔCFI values were larger than the cut-off scores (see Table 5).

Discussion

The aim of the present study was to explore the psychometric properties of the EAI by combining six datasets from five different countries (Hungary, UK, Spain, US, and Denmark). The results demonstrated that a one-factor solution was confirmed in data from five countries. The fit indices indicated an excellent degree of fit from data collected in Spain, Denmark, and Hungary, and an adequate level of fit from data collected in the UK and the US. The differences between countries are most likely explained by the undetermined confounding variables due to different sampling methods used by the different research teams. However, testing the factorial structure in the multigroup analysis, the configural invariance was supported; hence, in each country, the one-factor solution is acceptable.

Further analysis of invariance revealed that the liberal criteria for metric invariance supported the equality of factor loadings. Therefore, the covariance analyses are comparable across countries. The scalar invariance is required to compare latent means across groups. This invariance also implies that scales have the same measurement unit and origins; therefore, scores obtained are bias-free and thus can be compared directly [29]. However, analysis of the combined dataset demonstrated that the scalar invariance was not supported across the five countries. This means the intercepts of items were not equal across countries, and that the comparison of EAI scores was biased due to the different use of scales by participants from the five different countries. Put more simply, the EAI factor scores of five countries were not comparable because either the scale was not used in the five countries in the same way, or was not interpreted in the same way by the respondents. However, the covariates of exercise addiction can be studied across countries because the metric invariance was acceptable.

Gender invariance of EAI was also tested in each country separately. Results showed strong support for metric invariance across the gender of exercisers in all samples, but the scalar invariance could not be established. It appears that men and women use starting points of the items (namely intercepts) differently. The consequence of the results obtained is that gender comparison of exercise addiction should be carried out as covariates but that comparison of means directly should be performed cautiously. It can also be considered that different cut-offs should be calculated for men and women.

This is the first study to compare and combine data about exercise addiction (using EAI data) cross-culturally. The study has much strength and is a significant contribution to the exercise addiction literature—particularly in relation to psychometric measurement of the exercise addiction construct. Compared with all previously published studies in the area, the sample size was large and the analysis was both methodical and rigorous. However, there are clearly a number of limitations. The main weakness of the data was that all the data were based on self-report. Such data may be open to recall biases, social desirability biases, and issues surrounding the overall veracity and reliability of the data. The combined dataset and subsequent analyses suggest that the EAI is psychometrically sound but that research teams should be cautious when carrying out cross-cultural research.

Conclusions

Despite some inter-country differences, the EAI is still an appropriate instrument to assess exercise addiction. However, there is a need to carry out further research on invariance, and the need to consider the development of a cross-culturally invariant measure.

Competing interest

Mark Griffiths, Robert Urbán, Zsolt Demetrovics, Mia Lichtenstein, Ricardo de la Vega, Bernadette Kun, Roberto Ruiz-Barquín, Jason Youngman, and Attila Szabo declare that they have no conflicts of interest.

Funding

No financial support was received for the conduct of this study or preparation of this manuscript.

Author details

[1]Nottingham Trent University, Nottingham, UK. [2]Institute of Health Promotion and Sport Sciences, Faculty of Education and Psychology, Eötvös Loránd University, Budapest, Hungary. [3]University of Southern Denmark, Odense, Denmark. [4]Autonomous University of Madrid, Madrid, Spain. [5]University of Miami, Coral Gables, FL, USA. [6]Institute of Psychology, Faculty of Education and Psychology, Eötvös Loránd University, Budapest, Hungary.

References

1. Berczik K, Szabo A, Griffiths MD, Kurimay T, Kun B, Urbán R, et al. **Exercise addiction: symptoms, diagnosis, epidemiology, and etiology.** *Subst Use Misuse.* 2012; **47**:403–17.

2. Cockerill IM, Riddington ME. **Exercise dependence and associated disorders: a review.** *Couns Psychol Q.* 1996; **9:**119–29.
3. Hausenblas HA, Symons DD. **Exercise dependence: a systematic review.** *Psychol Sport Exerc.* 2002; **3:**89–123.
4. Pasman L, Thompson JK. **Body image and eating disturbance in obligatory runners, obligatory weightlifters, and sedentary individuals.** *Int J Eat Disord.* 1988; **7:**759–69.
5. Davis C. **Exercise abuse.** *Int J Sport Psychol.* 2000; **31:**278–89.
6. Dalle Grave R, Calugi S, Marchesini G. **Compulsive exercise to control shape or weight in eating disorders: prevalence, associated features, and treatment outcome.** *Comp Psychiatry.* 2008; **49:**346–52.
7. Allegre B, Souville M, Therme P, Griffiths M. **Definitions and measures of exercise dependence.** *Addict Res Theory.* 2006; **14:**631–46.
8. Kurimay T, Griffiths MD, Berczik K, Demetrovics Z. **Exercise addiction: the dark side of sports and exercise.** In: Baron D, Reardon C, Baron SH, editors. *Contemporary issues in sports psychiatry: a global perspective.* Chichester: Wiley; 2013: p. 33–43.
9. Ackard DM, Brehm BJ, Steffen JJ. **Exercise and eating disorders in college-aged women: profiling excessive exercisers.** *Eat Disord.* 2002; **10:**31–47.
10. Downs DS, Hausenblas HA, Nigg CR. **Factorial validity and psychometric examination of the exercise dependence scale-revised.** *Meas Phys Educ Exerc Sci.* 2004; **8:**183–201.
11. Hausenblas HA, Downs DS. **How much is too much? The development and validation of the exercise dependence scale.** *Psychol Health.* 2002; **17:**387–404.
12. Ogden J, Veale D, Summers Z. **The development and validation of the exercise dependence questionnaire.** *Addict Res Theory.* 1997; **5:**343–55.
13. Terry A, Szabo A, Griffiths M. **The exercise addiction inventory: a new brief screening tool.** *Addict Res Theory.* 2004; **12:**489–99.
14. Brown I. **A theoretical model of the behavioral addictions: applied to offending.** In: Hodge JE, McMurran M, Hollin RC, editors. *Addicted to Crime.* Chichester: Wiley; 1997: p. 13–65.
15. Browns RIF. **Some contributions of the study of gambling to the study of other addictions.** In: Eadington WR, Cornelius JA, editors. *Gambling Behavior and Problem Gambling.* Reno, NV: University of Nevada; 1993: p. 241–72.
16. Griffiths MD, Szabo A, Terry A. **The exercise addiction inventory: a quick and easy screening tool for health practitioners.** *Br J Sports Med.* 2005; **39:**e30.
17. Mónok K, Berczik K, Urbán R, Szabo A, Griffiths MD, Farkas J, Magi A, Eisinger A, Kurimay T, Kökönyei G, Kun B, Paksi B, Demetrovics Z. **Psychometric properties and concurrent validity of two exercise addiction measures: a population wide study.** *Psychol Sport Exerc.* 2012; **13:**739–46.
18. Szabo A, Griffiths MD. **Exercise addiction in British sport science students.** *Int J Ment Health Addict.* 2007; **5:**25–8.
19. Warner R, Griffiths MD. **A qualitative thematic analysis of exercise addiction: an exploratory study.** *Int J Ment Health Addict.* 2006; **4:**13–26.
20. Lichtenstein MB, Christiansen E, Bilenberg N, Støving RK. **Validation of the exercise addiction inventory in a Danish sport context.** *Scand J Med Sci Sports.* 2014; **24:**447–53.
21. Lichtenstein MB, Larsen KS, Christiansen E, Støving RK, Bredahl TVG. **Exercise addiction in team sport and individual sport: prevalences and validation of the exercise addiction inventory.** *Addict Res Theory.* 2014; **5:**431–7.
22. Szabo A, Vega R, Ruiz-Barquín R, Rivera O. **Exercise addiction in Spanish athletes: investigation of the roles of gender, social context and level of involvement.** *J Behav Addict.* 2013; **2:**249–52.
23. Allegre B, Therme P, Griffiths M. **Individual factors and the context of physical activity in exercise dependence: a prospective study of 'ultra-marathoners'.** *Int J Ment Health Addict.* 2007; **5:**233–43.
24. Youngman J. Risk for exercise addiction: a comparison of triathletes training for sprint-, olympic-, half-ironman-, and ironman-distance triathlons. Open Access Diss.. 2007. Available from: http://scholarlyrepository.miami.edu/oa_dissertations/12 Accessed 7 Jul 2014.
25. Gregorich SE. **Do self-report instruments allow meaningful comparisons across diverse population groups? Testing measurement invariance using the confirmatory factor analysis framework.** *Med Care.* 2006; **44:**S78–94.
26. Milfont TL, Fischer R. **Testing measurement invariance across groups: applications in cross-cultural research.** *Int J Psychol Res.* 2010; **3:**111–30.
27. Cheung GW, Rensvold RB. **Evaluating goodness-of-fit indexes for testing measurement invariance.** *Struct Equ Model Multidiscipl J.* 2002; **9:**233–55.
28. Chen FF. **Sensitivity of goodness of fit indexes to lack of measurement invariance.** *Struct Equ Model Multidiscipl J.* 2007; **14:**464–504.
29. He J, van de Vijver F. Bias and equivalence in cross-cultural research. Online Readings in Psychology and Culture; 2012. Available from: http://scholarworks.gvsu.edu/orpc/vol2/iss2/8 Accessed 7 Jul 2014.
30. Villella C, Martinotti G, Di Nicola M, Cassano M, La Torre G, Gliubizzi MD, Messeri I, Petruccelli F, Bria P, Janiri L, Conte G. **Behavioral addictions in adolescents and young adults: results from a prevalence study.** *J Gambl Stud.* 2011; **27:**203–14.
31. Lejoyeux M, Guillot C, Chalvin F, Petit A, Lequen V. **Exercise dependence among customers from a Parisian sport shop.** *J Behav Addict.* 2012; **1:**28–34.
32. Menczel Z, Kovacs E, Farkas J, Magi A, Eisinger A, Kun B, et al. **Prevalence of exercise dependence and eating disorders among clients of fitness centres in Budapest.** *J Behav Addict.* 2013; **2(Suppl. 1):**23–4.

18

ACTN3 R577X polymorphism is not associated with team sport athletic status in Italians

Myosotis Massidda[1*], Valeria Bachis[1], Laura Corrias[1], Francesco Piras[2], Marco Scorcu[2], Claudia Culigioni[1], Daniele Masala[3] and Carla M Calò[1]

Abstract

Background: The *ACTN3* gene may influence performance in team sports, in which sprint action and high-speed movements, regulated by the anaerobic energy system, are crucial to the ultimate success of a match. The aim of this study was to determine the association between the *ACTN3* R577X (rs1815739) polymorphism and elite team sport athletic status in Italian male athletes.

Methods: We compared the genotype and allele frequency of the *ACTN3* R577X polymorphism between team sport athletes ($n = 75$), endurance athletes ($n = 40$), sprint/power athletes ($n = 64$), and non-athletic healthy controls ($n = 192$) from Italy. Genomic DNA was collected using a buccal swab. Extraction was performed according to the manufacturer's directions provided with a commercially available kit (Qiagen S.r.l., Milan, Italy).

Results: Team sport athletes showed a lower frequency of the 577RR genotype compared to the 577XX genotype than sprint/power athletes ($p = 0.044$). However, the *ACTN3* R577X polymorphism was not associated with team sport athletic status compared to endurance athletes and non-athletic controls.

Conclusions: Our results agree with a recent large-scale study involving athletes from Spain, Poland, and Russia. The *ACTN3* R577X polymorphism was not associated with team sport athletic status compared to endurance athletes and non-athletic controls.

Key points

- The study showed that the *ACTN3* R577X polymorphism is not considered a candidate gene to influence the performance of team sport athletes, yet we confirmed that the *ACTN3* 577RR genotype is overrepresented in sprint/power athletes compared to those in team sports.
- As result, this study emphasizes the importance of considering well-defined groups of athletes with a clear reference phenotype in genetic association studies applied to elite sport performance, also suggesting possible inter-individual genetic differences between athletes in the same team sport.

* Correspondence: myosotis.massidda@unica.it
[1]Department of Life and Environmental Sciences, University of Cagliari, SS 554, km 4.500, Monserrato 09042, Italy
Full list of author information is available at the end of the article

Background

Research in the field of genetics among elite athletic performers has focused primarily on the sport at the end point of the sports performance continuum (sprint/power vs. endurance performance), yet the type of sport in which both the aerobic and anaerobic energy systems are important for achieving a high level of performance, such as team sports or endurance sports, has received little attention.

One of the most common targets of investigation has been a single nucleotide polymorphism (SNP) in the *ACTN3* gene, which encodes the alpha-actinin-3 protein [1]. This polymorphism leads to a premature stop codon (X), rather than an arginine (R) at position 577. Alpha-actinin-3 deficiency (*ACTN3* 577XX genotype) occurs in approximately 16% of the global population [1] and is associated with variations in human muscle performance. The alpha-actinin-3 protein is almost exclusively expressed in fast, glycolytic, and type IIX fibers that are responsible for the generation of rapid forceful contractions during activities such as sprinting.

Meta-analyses [2,3] and a recent review [4] of the literature regarding the influence of *ACTN3* on athletic performance suggest that the *ACTN3* 577RR genotype is associated with sprint/power athletes among Caucasians. Recently, Mikami et al. [5] examined a large cohort of elite Japanese athletes ($n = 299$) and found that the *ACTN3* R577X genotype was associated with sprint/power performance among track and field competitors, especially running 100- to 200-m sprints, and that R allele was associated with relative peak power in male collegiate athletes [6]. On the contrary, a recent study of Caucasian and East Asian swimmers did not show an association between *ACTN3* polymorphism and elite swimmer status [7]. The *ACTN3* 577X allele and the 577XX genotype were significantly associated with only certain groups of elite endurance athletes [8-17].

Seto et al. [18] provided a mechanistic explanation for the effects of the *ACTN3* genotype on skeletal muscle performance in elite athletes and on adaptation to changing physical demands in the general population. The authors highlighted the emerging evidence of the roles of alpha-actinin-3 in the regulation of metabolic and signaling pathways, contractile properties, and muscle fiber type. They showed that alpha-actinin-3 deficiency resulted in increased calcineurin activity in mouse and human skeletal muscle and an enhanced adaptive response to endurance training. Only a few studies investigated the association between the *ACTN3* R577X polymorphism and team sport performance. Santiago et al. [19] examined the frequency of this *ACTN3* genotype in 60 top-level professional Spanish soccer players, showing that the percentage distributions of 577RR and 577RX genotypes (48.3% and 36.7%) were significantly higher and lower, respectively, than those in controls ($n = 123$; 28.5% and 53.7%) or endurance athletes ($n = 52$; 26.5% and 52%) ($p = 0.041$). In a previous study [20], we did not find a significant difference in top-level soccer players' ($n = 42$) jump performance among the various genotypes.

Pimenta et al. [21] examined 200 Brazilian professional soccer players and found that 577RR carriers ran 10, 20, and 30 m faster than 577XX carriers. Furthermore, the former scored higher in jump tests compared to both 577RX and 577XX carriers.

Not all the studies, however, found an association between *ACTN3* R577X polymorphism and team sport performance [22-24]. Recently, Garatachea et al. [25] did not find an association between *ACTN3* genotypes and explosive leg power in elite basketball players or with the status of being this type of athlete. Finally, Eynon et al. [26] compared the genotype and allele frequencies of the *ACTN3* R577X polymorphisms in a relatively large cohort of team sport athletes ($n = 205$), endurance athletes ($n = 305$), sprint/power athletes ($n = 378$), and non-athletic controls ($n = 568$) from Europe and found that *ACTN3* R577X polymorphism was not associated with team sport athletic status. However, they did find that the 577RR genotype was overrepresented in sprint/power athletes compared to team sport athletes.

The aim of this study was to analyze the associations between *ACTN3* R577X polymorphisms and elite team sport athletic status in a group of Italian athletes and to compare their genotype distributions with elite sprint/power athletes, endurance athletes, and non-athletic controls.

Methods

A total of 178 Italian male athletes ($n = 74$ team sport athletes, $n = 64$ sprint/power athletes, $n = 40$ endurance athletes) and 190 controls were recruited between 2004 and 2014. All participants were unrelated European men, and all had Caucasian lineage for at least three generations. According to individual best performances, the athletes were divided into two subgroups: 'elite level' (competitors in European/World Championships or in the Olympic Games) and 'national level' (competitors in national-level but not international-level events) (Table 1). Of the athletes, 101 (57%) were classified as elite level and the remaining 77 (43%) were classified as national level.

(i) The team sport athletes ($n = 74$) included 64 soccer players and 10 hockey players. Of these, 8 hockey players competed at international level

Table 1 Genotype and allelic distribution and Hardy Weinberg equilibrium (HWE) among athletes and controls.

	Team sport	Power	Endurance	Control
All (*n*)	74	64	40	190
XX	14%	6%	15%	12%
RX	54%	45%	55%	58%
RR	32%	49%	30%	30%
MAF	0.413	0.289	0.425	0.406
HWE *p* value	0.478	0.549	1.00	0.057
Elite (*n*)	28	43	15	
XX	14%	7%	13%	
RX	61%	35%	60%	
RR	25%	58%	27%	
MAF	0.446	0.250	0.433	
National (*n*)	46	21	25	
XX	15%	5%	20%	
RX	50%	67%	40%	
RR	35%	28%	40%	
MAF	0.394	0.364	0.400	

(World/European Championships), 20 soccer players competed at international level (including five World Championships), while 2 hockey players and 44 soccer players competed at the national level (Italian Professional Championships, 'Serie A').

(ii) The sprint/power athletes ($n = 64$) included 16 track and field sprinters, 1 sprint swimmer, 17 wrestlers, 11 power lifters, and 19 gymnasts. Of these, 11 sprinters, 1 swimmer, 4 wrestlers, 10 power lifters, and 17 gymnasts were in the elite-level group, while 5 sprinters, 13 wrestlers, 1 power lifter, and 2 gymnasts were in the national-level group.

(iii) The endurance athletes ($n = 40$) included 24 track and field long-distance runners and 16 triathletes. Of these, 15 triathletes were in the elite-level group while all runners and 1 triathlete was in the national-level group.

The genotype frequencies among these athletes were compared with those of the randomly selected healthy non-athletic Italian males (controls). The controls were selected if they did not participate regularly in any competitive or structured sport or physical activity.

All participants and their parent/guardian (for minors) provided written informed consent, and the study protocol and informed written consent procedure were approved by the Medical Ethics Committees of the Italian Sports Federations, in accordance with Declaration of Helsinki for Human Research of 1974 (last modified in 2000).

Genomic DNA was extracted from each athlete with a buccal swab during the years 2004 to 2014, according to the manufacturer's directions provided with a commercially available kit (Qiagen S.r.l., Milan, Italy) [27]. Exon 16 of *ACTN3* was amplified through polymerase chain reaction using the following primers:

forward 5′-CTGTTGCCTGTGGTAAGTGGG-3′
reverse 5′-TGGTCACAGTATGCAGGAGGG-3′.

Polymerase chain reaction products were digested with DdeI enzyme. The 577R and 577X alleles (CGA and TGA codons, respectively) were distinguished by the presence (577X) or absence (577R) of a DdeI restriction site in exon 16. Allele 577X shows two fragments with 205 and 85 bp, while allele 557R presents three fragments with 108, 97, and 86 bp. The obtained fragments were separated by 10% polyacrylamide gel electrophoresis and stained with ethidium bromide [27]. To ensure proper internal control, for each genotype analysis, we used positive and negative controls from different DNA aliquots that were previously genotyped with the same method.

Chi-squared tests were used to test for the presence of Hardy-Weinberg equilibrium (HWE). Multinomial logistic regression analyses were conducted to assess the association between genotype and athletic status/competition level. In each case, analyses were made comparing 577XX (reference group) vs. 577RX, 577XX vs. 577RR (co-dominant effect), 577XX vs. 577RR and 577RX combined (dominant effect), and 577XX and 577RX combined (reference group) vs. 577RR (recessive effect). Significance was accepted when $p \leq 0.05$. Chi-squared tests for HWE were conducted using Genepop (v. 9), while statistical analyses were conducted using STATISTICA (Statsoft v. 7)

Results

Table 1 shows the genotype and allele frequency distributions in the non-athletes and athletes divided by group and subgroup. The genotype distributions met HWE (all $p > 0.05$) for all groups of participants.

Our data showed significant differences in genotype frequency between team sport athletes and sprinters (Table 2). Team sport athletes had a lower frequency of the 577RR genotype compared to the 577XX genotype than the sprint/power athletes ($p = 0.044$) (Table 2). In fact, the sprint/power athletes were approximately 1.5 times more likely to have the 577RR genotype (as opposed to the 577XX genotype) than team sport

Table 2 Odds ratios of genotypes for athletes and control groups according to sport type

	Team sports vs. control	Team sports vs. endurance	Team sports vs. sprint/power
XX (ref)			
OR	1	1	1
RX			
OR	0.72	0.99	0.50
CI	0.32 to 1.63	0.23 to 4.18	0.14 to 1.73
p	0.520	1	0.384
RR			
OR	0.79	1.04	0.26
CI	0.33 to 1.89	0.21 to 4.98	0.07 to 0.95
p	0.654	1	*0.044*
RR and RX (XX ref)			
OR	0.75	1.01	0.38
CI	0.34 to 1.63	0.25 to 4.03	0.11 to 1.26
p	0.534	1	0.168
RR (RX and XX ref)			
OR	1.02	1.05	0.48
CI	0.57 to 1.83	0.35 to 3.08	0.23 to 0.96
p	1	1	0.053

OR, odds ratio; CI, confidence interval; *p*, two-tailed *p* value. Significance is assumed when $p < 0.05$. The value in italics is statistically significant.

athletes. No association was observed for any of the genotypes with respect to the level of competition (elite vs. national level) (Table 3).

Discussion

We tested, for the first time, the association between *ACTN3* R577X polymorphism and team sport athletic status in Italian athletes. Our results indicate that team sport athletes have a lower 577RR than 577XX genotype frequency, compared to sprint/power athletes ($p = 0.044$). No significant difference in the *ACTN3* R577X polymorphism genotype distribution was found between the team sport athletes, endurance athletes, and control group. Furthermore, the *ACTN3* R577X genotype distribution was similar between elite-level and national-level team sport athletes, suggesting that this polymorphism is not influential among team sport athletes.

Our findings agree with those of Eynon et al. [26], who recently analyzed elite team sport athletes from three European countries (i.e., Spain, Poland, and Russia) and showed that their performance was not significantly influenced by *ACTN3* R577X polymorphism. Similarly, our results agree with theirs in that team sport athletes were less likely to possess the 577RR genotype than the 577XX genotype compared to power athletes ($p = 0.045$).

The *ACTN3* R577X polymorphism was consistently associated with elite sprint/power status [2,3] and muscle power [6]. The functional consequence of the *ACTN3* R577X polymorphisms on sport performance is supported by the Actn3 knock-out (KO) mouse model [28]. The authors demonstrated that the loss of alpha-actinin expression results in a shift in muscle metabolism toward the more efficient aerobic pathway, with a subsequent increase in running distance achieved before exhaustion during a treadmill test [28]. Moreover, the Actn3 KO mice (*ACTN3* 577XX), compared to wild-type (WT) counterparts, had lower muscle mass (smaller diameter fast-twitch muscle fibers), significantly lesser grip strength, significantly lower anaerobic enzyme activity, and higher oxidative/mitochondrial enzyme activity without a shift in fiber-type distribution [29].

Table 3 Odds ratios of genotypes for elite athletes compared to national-level athletes in team sports

Genotype	Team sport		
	OR	CI	*p*
XX (ref)			
RX	1.293	0.32 to 5.13	1
RR	0.765	0.16 to 3.48	1
RX-RR (XX ref)	1.076	0.28 to 4.07	1
RR (XX-RX ref)	0.625	0.21 to 1.78	0.444

CI, confidence interval; ref, reference; OR, odds ratio.

In team sports, most of the decisive actions during competition are characterized by jumping and/or sprinting, and it is for that reason that we hypothesized that the 577RR genotype would be associated with team sport performance. However, team sports generally involve mixed aerobic-anaerobic demands and players may not need to have extraordinary aerobic/anaerobic capacity. During a soccer game, for example, aerobic metabolism dominates energy delivery [30], yet the most decisive actions, characterized by jumping and sprinting, are supported by anaerobic metabolism. In similar team sports, many factors contribute to success, including muscle power, aerobic endurance, ball skills, and psychological traits. Therefore, muscle power represents just one of several factors that determine a player's ability but a substantial development of this factor is decisive during the crucial phases of a match.

When studying the possible role of genetics in team sports, it should be noted that not all players have similar characteristics in terms of physiological demand because it varies based on the position played. For example, during a rugby match, players perform various activities based on their position [31]. Forwards, rather than backs, are involved in significantly more physical collisions and tackles, experience a greater proportion of high-intensity activity than low-intensity activity, and travel greater distances during a match (9,929 vs. 8458 m) [31], demonstrating that a wide range of skills and physiological demands exist for the different playing positions.

Indeed, while *ACTN3* R577X polymorphism has been previously associated with sprint/power or endurance performance, the results of this study suggest that it is not associated with team sport athletic status.

The most obvious limitation of this study is the sample size. However, the very large population samples required to reach a sufficient statistical power in the field of genetic studies do not harmonize with the limited number of elite athletes for each sport discipline. We believe that the small sample size could be justifiable by the number of top-level athletes and by the homogeneity of the sample in terms of geographical and ethnical origin, recruited for the present study.

Conclusions

In conclusion, our results confirm, for the Italian population, the recent data published by Eynon et al. [26] that *ACTN3* R577X polymorphism is not significantly associated with team sport athletic status, when team sport athletes are compared to endurance athletes and non-athletic controls, and the 577RR genotype is overrepresented in power/sprint athletes compared to team sport athletes.

Competing interests
The authors declare that they have no competing interests.

Authors' contributions
MM conceived of the study, participated in its design, performed statistical analysis, interpretated the results and wrote the manuscript. VB carried out the laboratory analyses. LC carried out the laboratory analyses. FP partecipated in data collection. MS partecipated in the sample selection and data collection. CC carried out the laboratory analyses. DM partecipated in the sample selection and data collection. CMC participated in the study design and its coordination, critically revised the manuscript. All authors read and approved the final manuscript.

Acknowledgements
The authors would like to thank all the staff and athletes within the Italian Sports Federations and Cagliari Calcio Spa who participated in the study and who assisted with data collection. The authors are also grateful to Selvin Squire for English editing.

Author details
[1]Department of Life and Environmental Sciences, University of Cagliari, SS 554, km 4.500, Monserrato 09042, Italy. [2]FMSI CR Sardegna and Cagliari Calcio SpA, Viale Tiziano, Cagliari 70-00196, Italy. [3]University of Cassino, Viale dell'Università, Cassino 03043, Italy.

References
1. North KN, Yang N, Wattanasirichaigoon D, Mills M, Easteal S, Beggs AH, et al. A common nonsense mutation results in alpha-actinin-3 deficiency in the general population. Nat Genet. 1999;21(4):353–4.
2. Alfred T, Ben-Shlomo Y, Cooper R, et al. ACTN3 genotype, athletic status, and life course physical capability: meta-analysis of the published literature and findings from nine studies. Hum Mutat. 2011;32(9):1008–18.
3. Ma F, Yang Y, Li X, Hardy R, Cooper C, Deary IJ, et al. The association of sport performance with ACE and ACTN3 genetic polymorphisms: a systematic review and meta-analysis. PLoS One. 2013;8(1):e54685.
4. Eynon N, Hanson ED, Lucia A, Houweling PJ, Garton F, North KN, et al. Genes for elite power and sprint performance: ACTN3 leads the way. Sports Med. 2013;43(9):803–17.
5. Mikami E, Fuku N, Murakami H, et al. ACTN3 R577X genotype is associated with sprinting in elite Japanese athletes. Int J Sports Med. 2014;35(2):172–7.
6. Kikuchi N, Nakazato K, Min SK, Tsuchie H, Takahashi H, Ohiwa N, et al. The ACTN3 R577X polymorphisms is associated with muscle power in male Japanese athletes. J Strength Cond Res. 2014;28(7):1783-9.
7. Wang G, Mikami E, Chiu LL, DE Perini A, Deason M, Fuku N, et al. Association analysis of ACE and ACTN3 in elite Caucasian and East Asian swimmers. Med Sci Sports Exerc. 2013;45(5):892–900.
8. Yang N, MacArthur DG, Gulbin JP, Hahn AG, Beggs AH, Easteal S, et al. ACTN3 genotype is associated with human elite athletic performance. Am J Hum Genet. 2003;73(3):627–31.
9. Eynon N, Duarte JA, Oliveira J, Sagiv M, Yamin C, Meckel Y, et al. ACTN3 R577X polymorphism and Israeli top-level athletes. Int J Sports Med. 2009;30(9):695–8.
10. Niemi AK, Majamaa K. Mitochondrial DNA and ACTN3 genotypes in Finnish elite endurance and sprint athletes. Eur J Hum Genet. 2005;13(8):965–9.
11. Doring FE, Onur S, Geisen U, Boulay MR, Pérusse L, Rankinen T, et al. ACTN3 R577X and other polymorphisms are not associated with elite endurance athlete status in the Genathlete study. J Sports Sci. 2010;28(12):1355–9.
12. Muniesa CA, González-Freire M, Santiago C, Lao JI, Buxens A, Rubio JC, et al. World-class performance in lightweight rowing: is it genetically influenced? A comparison with cyclists, runners and non-athletes. Br J Sports Med. 2010;44(12):898–901.
13. Saunders CJ, September AV, Xenophontos SL, Cariolou MA, Anastassiades LC, Noakes TD, et al. No association of the ACTN3 gene R577X polymorphism with endurance performance in Ironman Triathlons. Ann Hum Genet. 2007;71(Pt 6):777–81.
14. Scott RA, Irving R, Irwin L, Morrison E, Charlton V, Austin K, et al. ACTN3 and ACE genotypes in elite Jamaican and US sprinters. Med Sci Sports Exerc. 2010;42(1):107–12.
15. Ruiz JR, Fernández del Valle M, Verde Z, Díez-Vega I, Santiago C, Yvert T, et al. ACTN3 R577X polymorphism does not influence explosive leg muscle power in elite volleyball players. Scand J Med Sci Sports. 2011;21(6):e34–41.
16. Shang X, Huang C, Chang Q, Zhang L, Huang T. Association between the ACTN3 R577X polymorphism and female endurance athletes in China. Int J Sports Med. 2010;31:913–6.
17. Yang N, MacArthur DG, Wolde B, Onywera VO, Boit MK, Lau SY, et al. The ACTN3 R577X polymorphism in East and West African athletes. Med Sci Sports Exerc. 2007;39(11):1985–8.
18. Seto JT, Quinlan KGR, Lek M, Zheng XF, Garton F, MacArthur DG, et al. ACTN3 genotype influences muscle performance through the regulation of calcineurin signaling. J Clin Invest. 2013;123(10):4255–63.
19. Santiago C, Gonzalez-Freire M, Serratosa L, Morate FJ, Meyer T, Gómez-Gallego F, et al. ACTN3 genotype in professional soccer players. Br J Sports Med. 2008;42 (1):71–3.
20. Massidda M, Corrias L, Ibba G, Scorcu M, Vona G, Calò CM, et al. Genetic markers and explosive leg-muscle strength in elite Italian soccer players. J Sports Med Phys Fitness. 2012;52(3):328–34.
21. Pimenta EM, Coelho DB, Veneroso CE, Barros Coelho EJ, Cruz IR, Morandi RF, et al. Effect of ACTN3 gene on strength and endurance in soccer players. J Strength Cond Res. 2013;27(12):3286–92.
22. Ginevičienė V, Pranculis A, Jakaitienė A, Milašius K, Kučinskas V. Genetic variation of the human ACE and ACTN3 genes and their association with functional muscle properties in Lithuanian elite athletes. Medicina (Mex). 2011;47(5):284–90.
23. Bell W, Colley JP, Evans WD, Darlington SE, Cooper SM. ACTN3 genotypes of Rugby Union players: distribution, power output and body composition. Ann Hum Biol. 2012;39(1):19–27.
24. Sessa F, Chetta M, Petito A, Franzetti M, Bafunno V, Pisanelli D, et al. Gene polymorphisms and sport attitude in Italian athletes. Genet Test Mol Biomarkers. 2011;15(4):285–90.
25. Garatachea N, Verde Z, Santos-Lozano A, Yvert T, Rodriguez-Romo G, Sarasa FJ, et al. ACTN3 R577X polymorphism and explosive leg-muscle power in elite basketball players. Int J Sports Physiol Perform. 2014;9(2):226–32.
26. Eynon N, Banting LK, Ruiz JR, Cieszczyk P, Dyatlov DA, Maciejewska-Karlowska A, et al. ACTN3 R577X polymorphism and team-sport performance: a study involving three European cohorts. J Sci Med Sport. 2014;17(1):102–6.
27. Mills M, Yang N, Weinberger R, Vander Woude DL, Beggs AH, Easteal S, et al. Differential expression of the actin-binding proteins, a-actinin-2 and -3, in different species: implications for the evolution of functional redundancy. Hum Mol Genet. 2001;10(13):1335–46.
28. MacArthur DG, Seto JT, Raftery JM, Quinlan KG, Huttley GA, Hook JW, et al. Loss of ACTN3 gene function alters mouse muscle metabolism and shows evidence of positive selection in humans. Nat Genet. 2007;39(10):1261–5.
29. MacArthur DG, Seto JT, Chan S, Quinlan KG, Raftery JM, Turner N, et al. An Actn3 knockout mouse provides mechanistic insights into the association between alpha-actinin-3 deficiency and human athletic performance. Hum Mol Genet. 2008;17(8):1076–86.
30. Bangsbo J, Mohr M, Krustrup P. Physical and metabolic demands of training and match-play in the elite football player. J Sports Sci. 2006;24(7):665–74.
31. Meir R, Colla P, Milligan C. Impact of the 10-meter rule change on professional rugby league: implications for training. Strength Condit J. 2001;23:42–6.

19

Influence of playing standard and physical fitness on activity profiles and post-match fatigue during intensified junior rugby league competition

Rich D Johnston[1*], Tim J Gabbett[1,2] and David G Jenkins[2]

Abstract

Background: The aim of this study was to determine whether the fatigue responses to the same intensified rugby league competition differed depending on playing standard and physical fitness.

Methods: Players from a high-standard ($n = 15$) and a low-standard ($n = 16$) junior rugby league team had lower body neuromuscular fatigue, perceptual wellbeing, and blood creatine kinase (CK) assessed over an intensified competition. Global positioning system units measured match activity profiles and rating of perceived exertion-assessed internal loads. Players were divided into high- and low-fitness groups across the two standards based on Yo-Yo intermittent recovery test performance.

Results: Playing intensity increased with playing standard and fitness levels (high-standard = 92 ± 6 m·min^{-1} vs. 88 ± 6 m·min^{-1}; low-standard = 88 ± 2 m·min^{-1} vs. 83 ± 6 m·min^{-1}). Despite greater internal and external loads, high-fitness players showed smaller reductions in lower body power (high-standard effect size [ES] = −0.74; low-standard ES = −0.41). High-standard players had smaller increases in blood CK (77% ± 94% vs. 113% ± 81%; ES = −0.41), primarily due to very small increases in the high-fitness group (50% ± 45%).

Conclusions: Increased fitness leads to greater internal and external workloads during intensified competition, smaller increases in blood CK, and less neuromuscular fatigue. Maximising player fitness should be a primary goal of coaches in order to increase match workloads and reduce post-match fatigue during intensified competition.

Key Points:

- Increased physical fitness results in greater relative and absolute match workloads.
- Increased physical fitness results in less fatigue and muscle damage during an intensified competition.
- Coaching staff should aim to maximise physical fitness in order to optimise match performance and reduce player fatigue.

Keywords: Neuromuscular fatigue; Muscle damage; Contact sports; GPS; Physical demands

Background

Rugby league is a physically demanding sport that involves periods of high-intensity activity (e.g. high-speed running, sprinting, physical contact) interspersed with periods of low-intensity activity (e.g. standing, walking, jogging) [1]. During competition, players typically cover relative distances of 90 to 100 m·min^{-1} [1-3], which increases with playing standard [4]. In addition to these running demands, players frequently engage in physical contact (i.e. tackles, hit-ups, and wrestles) during attack and defence [2]. Gabbett et al. [5] reported that players performed 24 to 47 contact efforts during a game at an average frequency of 0.38 to 1.09 contacts·min^{-1}, although players can perform up to 1.9 ± 0.7 contacts·min^{-1} depending on playing position, phase of play, and field position [6].

Given the intense physical demands of rugby league, match play rugby results in increased markers of muscle

* Correspondence: richard.johnston@acu.edu.au
[1]School of Exercise Science, Australian Catholic University, Brisbane, Queensland 4014, Australia
Full list of author information is available at the end of the article

damage, as well as neuromuscular and perceptual fatigue [7-9]. Whilst this fatigue is generally transient in nature, typically persisting for 24 to 48 h after competition, muscle damage can last for 5 days [8]. As such, during tournaments or periods of congested fixtures when players may be required to play multiple games within a week, insufficient recovery may occur [10]. Indeed, during rugby league [10,11], basketball [12], and soccer tournaments [13], fatigue accumulates, which compromises high-intensity match activities during the latter stages of the competition. Johnston et al. [11] showed that the relative distance covered at high speeds was reduced by 50% and 60% in the final two games of an intensified rugby league tournament. Whilst studies from basketball and soccer suggest that recovery strategies, and in particular cold water immersion, may be useful to minimise fatigue-mediated reductions in performance during intensified competitions [12-14], physical qualities such as high-intensity running ability and lower body strength also appear to play an important role in minimising post-match fatigue in rugby league players [9]. Although physical qualities may attenuate post-match fatigue following regular games [9], it is unclear whether they could help minimise fatigue that may occur during intensified rugby league competition [10,11].

It is well documented that the intensity of match play increases with competitive standard [4,15,16]. Indeed, Gabbett reported that, during a junior rugby league tournament, first division players covered greater metres per minute at both low and high speeds and engaged in a higher frequency of collisions and repeated high-intensity effort (RHIE) bouts than third division players [15]. As such, it would seem logical that increased playing intensity would lead to greater fatigue; however, this may be offset by enhanced physical qualities [9]. As playing standard increases in junior players, so too do physical qualities [17,18], which appear central to minimising post-match fatigue [9]. With this in mind, the aims of this study were to investigate whether there was a difference between (1) fatigue responses based on playing level, (2) fatigue responses based on physical fitness, and (3) match activity profiles based on playing standard and physical fitness during the same intensified rugby league competition. It was hypothesised that players competing in the first division (high-standard) would have smaller increases in fatigue despite increased match intensity than players competing in the third division (low-standard) of the competition. In addition, we hypothesised that players from both high- and low-standard teams with well-developed physical qualities would experience less fatigue and greater workloads over the course of the competition.

Methods

Experimental design

In order to test our hypotheses, a between groups, repeated measures experimental design was used. Players from two junior teams (one high- and one low-standard) were tracked for markers of fatigue (neuromuscular and perceptual wellbeing) and muscle damage (blood creatine kinase [CK]) during an intensified rugby league competition. In addition, global positioning system (GPS) microtechnology provided information on the activity profiles of players during matches. To assess the impact of physical fitness on match activities and post-match fatigue, players were also divided into high- and low-fitness groups based on their Yo-Yo intermittent recovery rest (IRT) level 1 performance.

Participants

Thirty-one junior rugby league players (age 16.5 ± 0.5 years; body mass 79.6 ± 11.6 kg) competing for two separate schools in the 2014 Confraternity Shield tournament volunteered to participate in the study. One team was competing in the first division of the competition and represented the high-standard team (*entire team*, $n = 15$; age 16.6 ± 0.5 years; body mass 78.5 ± 9.9 kg; *high-fitness group*, $n = 8$; age 16.6 ± 0.6 years; body mass 78.2 ± 8.8 kg; *low-fitness group*, $n = 7$; age 16.5 ± 0.6 years; body mass 78.9 ± 11.2 kg), the second team was competing in the third division, representing the low-standard team (*entire team*, $n = 16$; age 16.5 ± 0.6 years; body mass 79.6 ± 13.4 kg; *high-fitness group*, $n = 8$; age 16.3 ± 0.4 years; body mass 77.2 ± 10.8 kg; *low-fitness group*, $n = 8$; age 16.7 ± 0.6 years; body mass 84.8 ± 16.6 kg). The tournament took place in July, 3 months into the competitive season. All players were free from injury at the time of testing and were asked to maintain their normal diet throughout the competition; water was available *ad libitum* throughout. Before the study, players attended a familiarisation session and received an information sheet outlining experimental procedures, and the associated risks and benefits of participation. In accordance with the Code of Ethics of the World Medical Association (Declaration of Helsinki), players received an information sheet outlining experimental procedures; written informed consent was obtained from each player and their legal guardian. The study was approved by the Australian Catholic University ethical review board for human research.

Protocol

Ten days prior to the tournament, the Yo-Yo IRT level 1 was used to assess high-intensity intermittent running ability [19]. The test was performed at 15:00 hrs on a grassed playing surface at the start of a training session; players wore studded boots and training kit to complete the test. The test requires players to complete a 20-m shuttle at progressively faster speeds whilst keeping in time with an audio signal. Between each shuttle, there is a 10-s period of active recovery involving a jog/walk around a cone placed 5 m from the start/finish line. When players failed to keep in time with the audio signals on two consecutive occasions, they were deemed to have failed the test; the last level successfully completed and the corresponding metres covered were used as the final score for the test. The players were asked to maintain their normal diet and refrain from physical activity during the 24 h prior to the test. Some of the players were unfamiliar with the test so the first two levels of the test were incorporated into the warm-up to familiarise players with the test protocol. The typical error of measurement (TE) for this test is 4.9% [19]. A schematic overview of the protocol can be seen in Figure 1.

The first 4 games of the tournament were 40 min (2 × 20 min halves), with the final game being 50 min (2 × 25 min halves) in duration. Two games were played on both days 1 and 2, no games on day 3, and one game on day 4, totalling five games (210 min) over a 4-day period. Baseline measurements of neuromuscular fatigue, muscle damage, and perceived wellbeing were assessed approximately 12 h prior to game 1. Subsequent fatigue and muscle damage measures were taken within 1 h of the final match of each day. On day 3, when no games were played, fatigue measures were assessed at the same time as they were on other days (approximately 14:00 to 16:00 hrs). The average temperature, rainfall, and humidity over the competition period were 20.6°C ± 2.2°C, 0.00 ± 0.00 mm, and 51.0% ± 15.3%, respectively.

Neuromuscular fatigue

Lower body neuromuscular fatigue was assessed using peak power from a single countermovement jump (CMJ) performed on a force platform (Kistler 9290AD Force Platform, Kistler, Amherst, NY, USA) interfaced with a laptop (Acer Aspire 2930, Acer, Telford, UK) running manufacturer-designed software (Quattro-Jump, Kistler, Amherst, NY, USA) [10]. Players kept their hands on their hips throughout the jump; no instruction was given on the depth of the countermovement, but players were asked to jump as high as possible on the experimenter's signal in line with previous methodology [10]. The TE from our laboratory for CMJ peak power is 3.5%. Peak power was used to assess neuromuscular fatigue as it offers good reliability and ensures consistency with previous rugby league literature [8-10,20-22].

Creatine kinase

Whole-blood CK activity was used as a marker of muscle damage. A 30-μl sample of blood was taken from a fingertip and immediately analysed using a colorimetric assay procedure (Reflotron, Boehringer Mannheim, Germany). Before each testing session, the instrument was calibrated in accordance with the manufacturer recommendations. The 'normal' reference range for CK activity, as provided by the manufacturer using this method, is 24 to 195 $IU \cdot l^{-1}$ [7,10,23]. The TE for assessing CK was 3.3%.

Perceptual wellbeing

Each day, perceived wellbeing was assessed by the experimenter asking players to rate feelings of fatigue, lower and upper body muscle soreness, sleep quality, and mood and stress on 0 to 5 Likert scales, with the individual scores summated to give an overall wellbeing score using methods outlined previously [10]. The test re-test reliability for the perceptual wellbeing questionnaire was determined by having 12 rugby league players complete the questionnaire on two separate occasions, 7 days apart following 36 h of no physical activity; the TE for perceptual wellbeing was 3.0%. Additionally, 30 min after each game, rating of perceived exertion (RPE) was recorded using a modified RPE scale (CR-10) to rate how hard players perceived each game. The RPE score was then multiplied by the number of minutes played to determine session RPE as a measure of internal load [24]. This method of assessing internal loads has shown to have appropriate levels of validity and reliability (TE = 4.0%) in rugby league players [25].

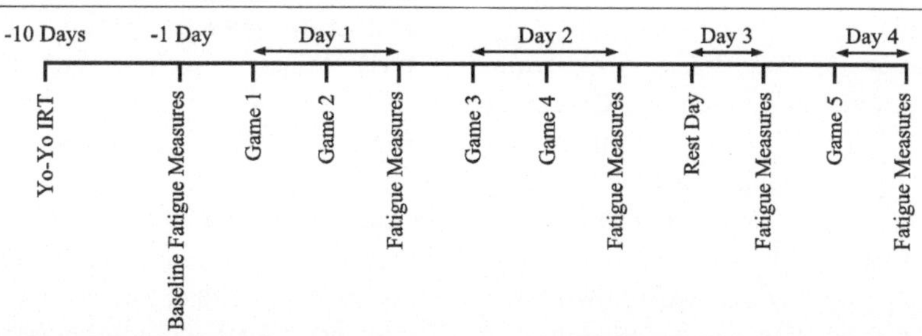

Figure 1 A schematic overview of the data collection protocol. Yo-Yo IRT = Yo-Yo intermittent recovery test (level 1); fatigue measures were conducted within 1 h after the final game of each day and included a countermovement jump, blood creatine kinase, and perceptual wellbeing.

Match activity profiles

Activity profiles during competition were assessed by GPS analysis. Prior to the warm-up before each game, players were fitted with the GPS vest and unit; the unit was switched on and inserted into a padded compartment at the rear of the vest, positioned between the shoulder blades. The GPS units sampled at 10 Hz (Team S4, Catapult Sports, Victoria, Australia) and included a triaxial accelerometer and gyroscope sampling at 100 Hz to provide information on collisions. Data were downloaded to a laptop (Acer Aspire 2930, Acer, Telford, UK) and analysed using software provided by the manufacturer (Sprint, Version 5.1.1, Catapult Sports, Victoria, Australia). Non-playing minutes were omitted from the analysis. Data were categorised into low- (0 to 3.5 $m{\cdot}s^{-1}$), moderate- (3.6 to 5.0 $m{\cdot}s^{-1}$) and high-speed (≥5.1 $m{\cdot}s^{-1}$) movement bands [26]; the total number of collisions was recorded as described previously [1]. In addition, the average speed of each game ($m{\cdot}min^{-1}$) was calculated in relation to the final speed reached by players on the Yo-Yo IRT ($m{\cdot}min^{-1}$) in order to express the speed of the match in relation to the physical capacity of each player. RHIE bouts were classified as three or more maximal acceleration (≥2.78 $m \cdot s^{-2}$), high-speed, or impact efforts with less than 21 s between each effort [1]. These units are reliable for quantifying movements commonplace in rugby league [27-29].

Statistical analysis

In order to determine the influence of physical fitness on match activities and post-match fatigue, players from both the high- and low-standard team were matched for position (forwards and backs) before being divided into low- and high-fitness groups, using a median split, based on Yo-Yo IRT performance. This ensured that there was an even number of forwards and backs in both fitness groups so that the fatigue responses were not influenced by the different match activities performed by each positional group. This provided us with four experimental groups based on Yo-Yo IRT performance: high-standard/high-fitness, high-standard/low-fitness, low-standard/high-fitness, and low-standard/low-fitness.

Differences in fatigue, muscle damage, and activity profiles between the high- and low-standard and high- and low-fitness playing groups and changes over time were determined using traditional null hypothesis testing and magnitude-based inferences. To compare differences in Yo-Yo IRT performance and match activity profiles between high- and low-standard playing groups and fitness levels, a two-way group (high- vs. low-standard) × fitness (high-standard/high-fitness vs. high-standard/low-fitness vs. low-standard/high-fitness vs. low-standard/low-fitness) ANOVA was used. A three-way group (high- vs. low-standard) × time (baseline vs. day 1 vs. 2 vs. 3 vs. 4) × fitness (high-standard/high-fitness vs. high-standard/low-fitness vs. low-standard/high-fitness vs. low-standard/low-fitness) repeated measures ANOVA (SPSS 22.0, SPSS Inc, Chicago, IL, USA) was used to determine changes in neuromuscular fatigue, blood CK, and activity profiles between playing standards and fitness levels. If significant main effects were found, Bonferroni *post hoc* analyses were performed to locate the differences. Changes and differences in perceptual wellbeing and RPE were analysed using a Kruskal-Wallis test. Based on the real-world relevance of the results, magnitude-based inferences were used to assess the meaningfulness of any differences. Firstly, the likelihood that changes in the dependent variables were greater than the smallest worthwhile change was calculated as a small effect size of 0.20 × between subject standard deviation. Based on 90% confidence intervals, the thresholds used for assigning qualitative terms to chances were as follows: <1% almost certainly not; <5% very unlikely; <25% unlikely; <50% possibly not; >50% possibly; >75% likely; >95% very likely; >99% almost certain [30]. The magnitude of difference was considered practically meaningful when the likelihood was ≥75%. Secondly, magnitudes of change in the dependent variables were assessed using Cohen's effect size (ES) statistic [31]. ES of 0.20 to 0.60, 0.61 to 1.19, and ≥1.20 were considered small, moderate, and large, respectively [32]. Data are reported as means ± standard deviation (SD); the significance level was set at $p < 0.05$.

Results

Match activity profiles

Playing standard and activity profiles

There were a number of differences in match activity profiles between the high- and low-standard playing groups (Table 1). The greatest differences were seen in absolute workloads across the five games, primarily due to the high-standard players completing more playing minutes. Despite this, there was still greater relative distance ($p = 0.05$) covered at both high ($p = 0.224$) and moderate speeds ($p = 0.02$) in the high-standard group, more frequent collisions ($p = 0.019$) and RHIE bouts ($p = 0.004$), and greater internal loads highlighted by session RPE ($p = 0.001$). High-standard players covered significantly greater distances on the Yo-Yo IRT ($p = 0.001$). When match speed ($m{\cdot}min^{-1}$) was expressed relative to maximal Yo-Yo IRT speed, there was no difference in match intensity ($p = 0.75$).

Physical fitness and activity profiles

When players from both the high- and low-standard teams were divided into low- and high-fitness groups, there were further differences in physical match performance variables (Table 2). High-fitness players covered more metres per minute of match play across both

Table 1 Physical qualities and average match activity profiles across the tournament between the high- and low-standard team

	High-standard	Low-standard	ES	Likelihood
Playing time (min)	36 ± 6	30 ± 8	0.85	96%, very likely
Distance covered (m)	3,327 ± 588*	2,516 ± 720	1.24	100%, almost certain
Relative distance (m·min^{-1})	90 ± 7*	85 ± 7	0.71	92%, likely
Low-speed activity (m)	2,525 ± 444	2,074 ± 576	0.88	96%, very likely
Low-speed activity (m·min^{-1})	71 ± 5	69 ± 6	0.19	56%, possibly
Moderate-speed running (m)	434 ± 115*	274 ± 94	1.52	100%, almost certain
Moderate-speed running (m·min^{-1})	13 ± 3*	9 ± 2	1.58	100%, almost certain
High-speed running (m)	174 ± 51*	116 ± 58	1.07	99%, very likely
High- speed running (m·min^{-1})	4.3 ± 1.1	3.8 ± 1.0	0.52	81%, likely
Match speed vs. Yo-Yo speed (%)	34 ± 3	34 ± 3	0.05	25%, unlikely
Collisions				
Total (no.)	15 ± 7*	9 ± 3	1.30	100%, almost certain
Total (no./min)	0.4 ± 0.2*	0.3 ± 0.1	0.72	76%, likely
Repeated high-intensity efforts				
Bouts (no.)	3.2 ± 1.8*	1.3 ± 0.6	1.43	100%, almost certain
Bout frequency (no./min)	1 every 17 min*	1 every 23 min	0.62	85%, likely
Internal Loads				
RPE (AU)	5 ± 2	3 ± 1	1.06	98%, very likely
Session RPE (AU)	180 ± 39*	109 ± 37	1.90	100%, almost certain
Physical Qualities				
Yo-Yo IRT (m)	1,420 ± 337*	922 ± 227	1.73	100%, almost certain

Low-speed activity = 0 to 3.5 m·s^{-1}; moderate-speed running = 3.6 to 5.0 m·s^{-1}; high-speed running = ≥5.1 m·s^{-1}. RPE = rating of perceived exertion; session RPE = playing time × RPE; Yo-Yo IRT = Yo-Yo intermittent recovery test level 1. ES = effect size, 0.20 to 0.60, 0.61 to 1.19, and >1.20 were considered small, moderate, and large, respectively. Likelihoods ≥75% are classified as practically meaningful. *Denotes a statistically significant difference ($p < 0.05$) between playing standards.

playing standards and had greater internal loads. High-standard/high-fitness players covered greater distances than all other groups primarily through increased distance covered at moderate speeds ($p < 0.05$). In addition, they engaged in more collisions per minute and RHIE bouts ($p < 0.05$). Whilst there were a number of differences between the high-standard fitness groups, the differences between high- and low-fitness groups were not as great in the low-standard playing group with only moderate differences in relative distance, primarily achieved by greater relative distances covered at low and moderate speeds, and higher internal loads in the high-fitness group. When match speed (m·min^{-1}) was expressed relative to maximal Yo-Yo IRT speed, the high-fitness groups maintained a greater relative intensity across the tournament (high-standard: ES = 0.61; likelihood = 77%, likely; low-standard: ES = 0.22; likelihood = 52%, possibly). The high-standard/high-fitness playing group covered more metres on the Yo-Yo IRT than the low-standard/high-fitness group (ES = 3.88; likelihood = 100%, almost certain). Both high-standard/high-fitness and high-standard/low-fitness players had greater session RPE loads across the competition compared with both low-standard groups ($p = 0.001$).

Fatigue

Playing standard and fatigue

There was little difference in the fatigue responses between the high- and low-standard players across the course of the competition (Figure 2). There were significant reductions in CMJ power over the competition ($p = 0.004$) which peaked on day 2 but only small differences (ES = 0.21 to 0.50; $p = 0.581$) between high- and low-standard players (Figure 2A). Blood CK increased over the competition ($p = 0.01$), peaking on day 2 in both playing groups (Figure 2C). There was a greater overall increase across the competition in the low-standard players (76% ± 94% vs. 113% ± 81%; ES = 0.83, likelihood = 76%, likely; $p = 0.078$), as well as moderately greater increases on day 2 (ES = 0.74, likelihood = 89%, likely; $p = 0.012$) and day 4 (ES = 0.84, likelihood = 99%, very likely; $p = 0.015$). There were significant reductions in perceived wellbeing over the competition (Figure 2B [$p = 0.001$]), which was similar between the high- and low-standard

Table 2 Physical qualities and average match activity profiles across the tournament between high- and low-fitness groups

	High-standard			Low-standard		
	High-fitness	Low-fitness	ES	High-fitness	Low-fitness	ES
Playing time (min)	38 ± 3	33 ± 4	1.41	31 ± 10	30 ± 7	0.16
Distance covered (m)	3,541 ± 278	2,943 ± 735	1.08	2,716 ± 928	2,455 ± 478*	0.35
Relative distance (m·min^{-1})	92 ± 6	88 ± 6	0.73	88 ± 2	83 ± 6*	1.04
Low-speed activity (m)	2,642 ± 318	2,275 ± 537	0.83	2,218 ± 752	2,007 ± 407	0.35
Low-speed activity (m·min^{-1})	70 ± 6	70 ± 3	0.04	72 ± 3	68 ± 6	0.69
Moderate-speed running (m)	503 ± 106	349 ± 104*	1.46	302 ± 88*	258 ± 49*	0.62
Moderate-speed running (m·min^{-1})	13 ± 3	11 ± 2	0.99	10 ± 2*	9 ± 2*	0.36
High-speed running (m)	183 ± 41	149 ± 53	0.74	119 ± 56	117 ± 67	0.03
High-speed running (m·min^{-1})	4.5 ± 1.1	4.0 ± 1.0	0.45	3.8 ± 0.8	3.8 ± 1.3	0.05
Match speed vs. Yo-Yo speed (%)	35 ± 3	33 ± 2	0.61	35 ± 2	34 ± 3	0.22
Collisions						
Total (no.)	19 ± 6	13 ± 7	1.24	10 ± 3*	9 ± 3*	0.35
Total (no./min)	0.5 ± 0.2	0.4 ± 0.1	0.85	0.3 ± 0.1*	0.3 ± 0.1*	0.19
Repeated high-intensity efforts						
Bouts (no.)	4 ± 2	3 ± 1*	0.79	1 ± 1*	1 ± 1*	−0.23
Bout frequency (no./min)	1 every 14 min	1 every 16 min	0.26	1 every 24 min	1 every 22 min	−0.27
Internal Loads						
RPE (AU)	5 ± 2	5 ± 1	−0.02	3 ± 1	3 ± 1	0.24
Session RPE (AU)	196 ± 31	174 ± 37	0.65	116 ± 22*†	100 ± 27*†	0.64
Physical Qualities						
Yo-Yo IRT (m)	1,700 ± 119	1,233 ± 304*	2.02	1,089 ± 188*†	785 ± 155*†	1.76

Low-speed activity = 0 to 3.5 m·s^{-1}; moderate-speed running = 3.6 to 5.0 m·s^{-1}; high-speed running = ≥5.1 m·s^{-1}. RPE = rating of perceived exertion; session RPE = playing time × RPE; Yo-Yo IRT = Yo-Yo intermittent recovery test level 1. ES = effect size, 0.20 to 0.60, 0.61 to 1.19, and >1.20 were considered small, moderate, and large respectively. *Denotes a statistically significant difference ($p < 0.05$) from the high-standard/high-fitness group; †Denotes a statistically significant difference from the high-standard/low-fitness group.

players (−14% ± 17% vs. −17% ± 9%; ES = 0.40, likelihood = 71%, possibly), with no significant difference between playing standards on any day of the competition.

Physical fitness and fatigue

Neuromuscular fatigue: There were reductions in CMJ power (ES = −0.75 to −2.37; $p = 0.052$) for each group over the competition (Figure 3A); these reductions were smallest in the two high-fitness groups from both playing standards ($p = 0.340$), with moderately greater reductions in CMJ power in the high-standard/low-fitness group compared with the high-standard/high-fitness group (ES = 0.74; likelihood = 85%, likely). In the high-standard group, there were greater reductions in CMJ power in the low-fitness players on day 1 (ES = 1.21; likelihood = 100%, almost certain) and day 3 (ES = 0.71; likelihood = 82%, likely). In the low-standard playing group, there was a similar, albeit less pronounced trend, with smaller reductions in CMJ power in the high-fitness group (ES = −0.41; likelihood = 66%, possibly).

Blood creatine kinase: There were increases in CK across the entire tournament for all groups ($p = 0.001$), although the smallest increases were seen in the high-standard/high-fitness group (Figure 3C). Compared with the high-standard/high-fitness group, there were moderately greater increases in blood CK in all other groups across the competition (high-standard/low-fitness group: ES = 0.63; likelihood = 76%, likely; $p = 0.260$; low-standard/high-fitness group: ES = 1.10; likelihood = 90%, likely; $p = 0.623$; low-standard/low-fitness group: ES = 0.95; likelihood = 87%, likely; $p = 0.619$). On days 2 and 3 of the competition, there was a greater increase in CK in the high-standard/low-fitness group (day 2, ES = 0.62; likelihood = 77%, likely; day 3, ES = 0.83; likelihood = 86%, likely), the low-standard/high-fitness group (day 2, ES = 0.93; likelihood = 90%, likely; day 3, ES = 1.00; likelihood = 92%, likely), and the low-standard/low-fitness group (day 3, ES = 1.14; likelihood = 94%, likely). On day 4 of the competition, there were greater increases in CK in both low-standard groups (high-fitness: ES = 0.95; likelihood =

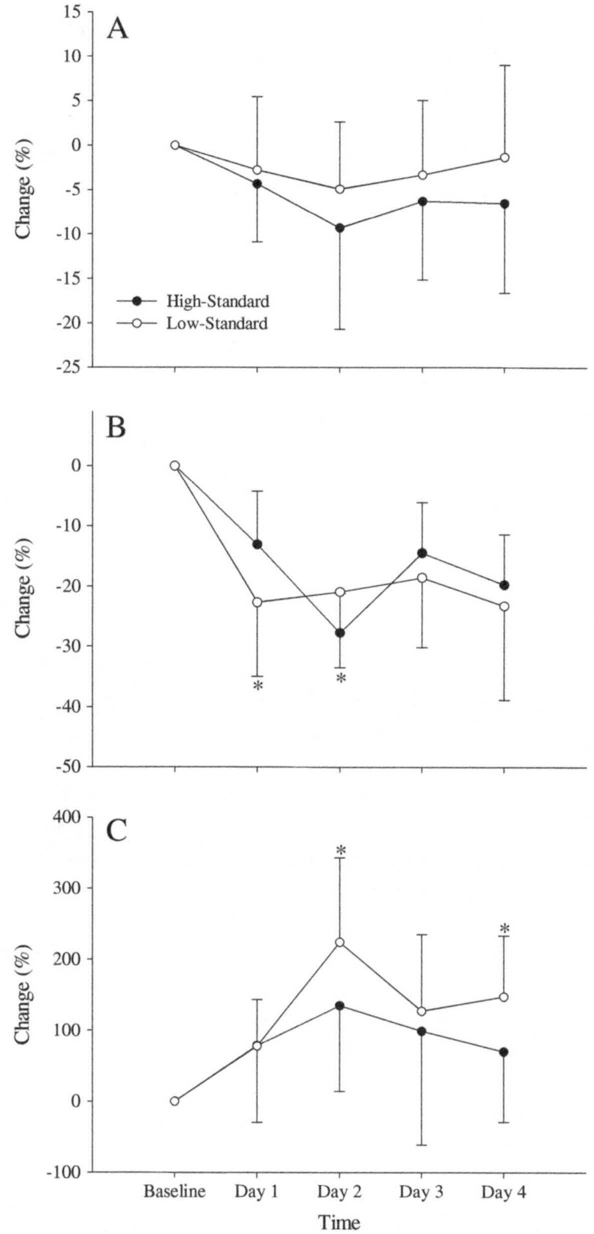

Figure 2 Changes in CMJ peak power, perceptual wellbeing, and blood creatine kinase between high/low-standard playing groups. Changes in **(A)** countermovement jump peak power, **(B)** perceptual wellbeing, and **(C)** blood creatine kinase between the high- and low-standard playing groups over the course of the intensified competition. *Denotes a moderate effect size difference (0.60 to 1.20) between the high- and low-standard playing groups.

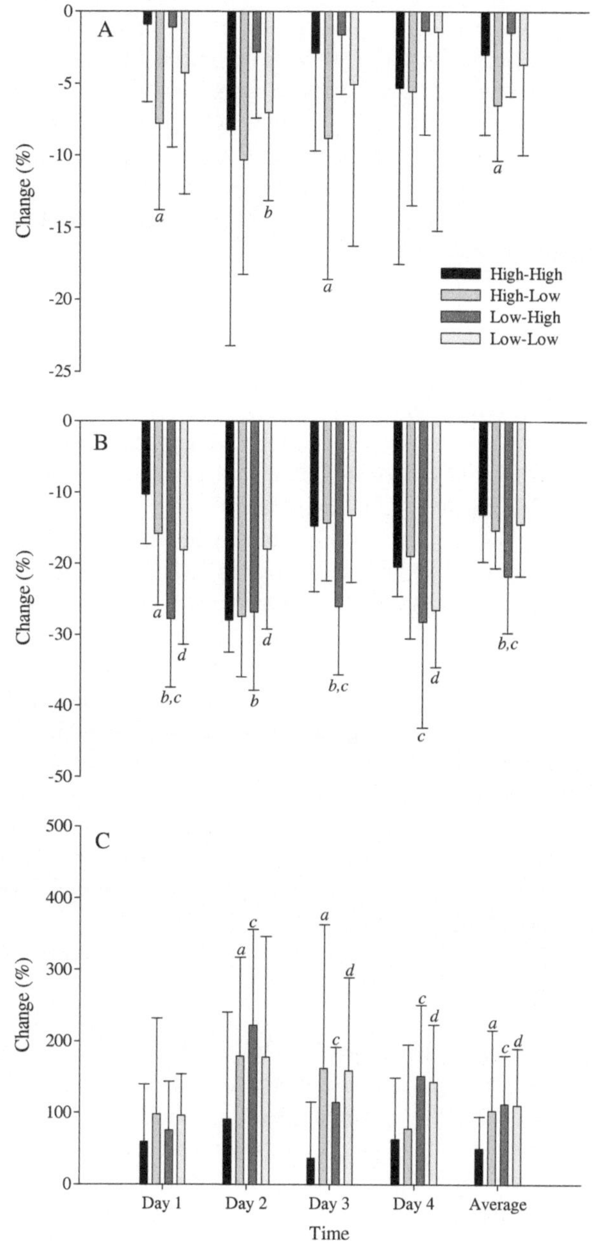

Figure 3 Fatigue changes with players from high- and low-standard playing groups, divided into low- and high-fitness groups. Changes in **(A)** countermovement jump peak power, **(B)** perceptual wellbeing, and **(C)** blood creatine kinase with players from the high- and low-standard playing groups, divided into low- and high-fitness groups over the course of the intensified competition. High-High = high-playing standard/high fitness; High-Low = high-playing standard/low fitness; Low-High = low-playing standard/high fitness; Low-Low = low-playing standard/low fitness. *a* denotes a moderate- to large-effect size difference between High-High and High-Low; *b* denotes a moderate- to large-effect size difference between High-Low and Low-Low; *c* denotes a moderate- to large-effect size difference between High-High and Low-High; and *d* denotes a moderate- to large-effect size difference between High-High and Low-Low.

94%, likely; low-fitness: ES = 0.97; likelihood = 92%, likely).

Perceptual wellbeing: There were reductions in perceptual wellbeing ($p = 0.03$) in each group over the course of the competition (Figure 3B). The greatest reductions were seen in the low-standard/high-fitness group, with similar reductions seen amongst the other groups. On day 1, there were smaller reductions in the high-standard/high-fitness group in comparison to all other groups. On day 2, there were smaller reductions in the low-standard/low-fitness group, with similar reductions amongst the other groups. On day 3, there was some recovery in perceptual wellbeing in all groups except the low-standard/high-fitness group. On day 4, there was little change in the two high-standard playing groups, but there were larger reductions in the low-standard playing groups.

Discussion

This study compared the fatigue responses to intensified junior rugby league competition between playing standards. In addition, the influence that physical fitness had on the fatigue response and match activity profiles was also investigated. Our hypotheses were partially confirmed, with greater playing intensity in the high-standard playing group but little difference in fatigue responses between playing standards, although there was greater increases in blood CK in the low-standard playing group. Our second hypothesis was also partially confirmed with smaller increases in fatigue and blood CK as physical fitness increased despite greater playing intensities. As playing standard increases, so too do the physical demands of competition [15], although this does not appear to translate to increased player fatigue. Higher physical fitness is associated with greater playing intensity during an intensified competition and reduced post-match fatigue and markers of muscle damage.

The high-standard playing group had greater physical fitness than the low-standard group, highlighted by these players covering more metres on the Yo-Yo IRT. This is in accordance with previous research that has shown that as playing standard increases, so too do physical qualities [17,18]. Elevated physical fitness appeared to translate to increases in absolute and relative match workloads. High-standard players covered more metres per minute of match play, which was primarily achieved through greater moderate-speed running. Despite these greater match intensities in the high-standard playing group, when match speed was expressed relative to maximal speed on the Yo-Yo IRT, there was no difference in playing intensity between groups. This suggests that the match speeds in both the high- and low-standard competitions would have placed a similar relative physiological stress on players. On the other hand, the greater internal loads experienced by the high-standard players (highlighted by RPE and session RPE) are suggestive of greater physiological strain during the competition. This could be explained by the increased number of physical collisions and RHIE bouts performed by the high-standard group, which are overlooked by simply assessing match running intensities. Both collisions and RHIE bouts are extremely demanding tasks, both physically and mentally [33,34], and therefore could explain the increased internal loads in the high-standard playing group. These results clearly indicate that as playing standard increases, so too does physical fitness which appears to translate to increases in playing intensity [15,35]. In addition, only assessing the running demands of the game clearly underestimates the physiological loads placed on players.

When players were divided into high-fitness and low-fitness groups across both playing standards based on Yo-Yo IRT performance, there were some differences in absolute and relative playing intensities. In the high-standard group, there was a larger disparity between the high- and low-fitness groups in terms of match workloads. High-fitness players had greater playing minutes, covering more absolute and relative distance, primarily achieved through increased moderate-speed running. The match speeds performed in the high-fitness group were at a greater intensity relative to the maximal Yo-Yo speed. In addition, these players were involved in more collisions and RHIE bouts over the tournament. The differences in the low-standard playing group were less pronounced, with high-fitness players covering more metres per minute, primarily achieved through increased low-speed activity. The large differences in physical performance observed in the high-standard group and smaller differences observed in the low-standard group may be explained by the Yo-Yo IRT scores for each group. In the high-standard players, there was a larger absolute difference in Yo-Yo IRT scores between the high- and low-fitness groups than in the low-standard players. As such, maximising absolute high-intensity running ability, and introducing minimum standards, would be useful in order to maintain performances across the entire playing group.

Despite the increased absolute external and internal loads in the high-standard playing group, there were similar increases in fatigue and markers of muscle damage across the competition between playing standards. These increases in fatigue and markers of muscle damage were greatest over the first 2 days of the competition in both groups when players were involved in two games on each day. This suggests that physical fitness may offer some protective effect against fatigue and markers of muscle damage, which is in accordance with previous research [9]. Although there were greater reductions in CMJ power in the high-standard group, these differences were small in magnitude and did not reach the threshold of practical importance [30]. The similar changes in lower body fatigue between the high- and low-standard teams may be indicative of the similar match speeds relative to maximal Yo-Yo IRT. However, there were smaller increases in blood CK in the high-standard playing group, particularly at the end of days 2 and 4 of the competition. This result is even more significant given that the high-standard playing group was involved in 40% more collisions over the tournament, which are directly linked to elevations in CK [22]. There were also similar reductions in perceptual wellbeing over the competition between the playing standards. Despite greater absolute workloads in the high-standard playing group, there was little difference in the fatigue responses and smaller increases in blood CK across the tournament. This may be due to increased physical fitness in the high-standard playing group. In addition, expressing match speeds in relation to maximal Yo-Yo IRT speed may be a useful metric for determining the relative stress placed on each individual player by the running component of match play.

The protective effects of physical fitness on muscle function and to some extent muscle damage are clear when players were divided into low- and high-fitness groups. Despite greater match speeds in relation to maximal Yo-Yo IRT speed as well as absolute workloads, the high-fitness players in both playing standards exhibited the smallest reductions in CMJ power across the tournament. Previous research has suggested that players with well-developed high-intensity running ability possess greater eccentric strength and the ability to utilise the stretch-shortening cycle [36] which may result in less muscle fatigue [9]. High fitness only appeared to reduce muscle damage in the high-standard group. This group had significantly greater Yo-Yo IRT performance than the low-standard/high-fitness players (1,700 ± 119 m vs. 1,089 ± 188 m) which may suggest that, irrespective of playing intensity, there is a base level of fitness required before muscle damage is reduced through increased fitness. Once again, these high-fitness players performed more collisions than their less fit counterparts, clearly highlighting the protective effect of well-developed physical fitness to elevations in blood CK [9]. There was little difference in perceptual wellbeing between groups, although the low-standard/high-fitness group had greater reductions across the competition. Taken together, well-developed physical fitness appears to reduce post-match fatigue and increase match-playing intensities. As such, coaching staff should aim to maximise fitness prior to intensified competition in order to minimise post-match fatigue.

Whilst this study adds to the body of literature on fatigue in team sport players, our findings are not without their limitations. Only Yo-Yo IRT performance was assessed as a measure of physical fitness. Previous research indicates that lower body strength also impacts on post-match fatigue [9]. Therefore, it is likely that other physical qualities, such as muscular strength, may influence the fatigue response seen following intensified competition. In addition, data collection ceased immediately following the competition. As such, it is unknown whether the recovery time-course differed between groups. Future research addressing these points is warranted.

Conclusions

This study highlighted that as playing standard increases in junior rugby league players, so too does the intensity of match play. Well-developed high-intensity running ability appears to be associated with greater absolute and relative internal and external workloads during competition. Despite increased workloads in players with well-developed physical qualities, these players experienced smaller increases in blood CK and less pronounced reductions in muscle function. As such, increasing fitness in junior players may be one of the most effective strategies for minimising accumulations in post-match fatigue and markers of muscle damage during intensified rugby league competition. Intensified competitions are always likely to occur in junior rugby league and numerous other team sports. Therefore, players should be exposed to demanding training prior to participating in tournaments in an attempt to increase physical fitness and gain a degree of protection against post-match fatigue.

Competing interests

The authors declare that they have no competing interests.

Authors' contributions

TG and DJ helped design the study and write the manuscript. RJ collected and analysed the data and wrote the manuscript. All authors have read and approved the final manuscript.

Acknowledgements

The authors would like to thank the players and coaching staff from St. Thomas More and Padua College for volunteering to take part in the study as well as the organising committee of the Confraternity Shield. No external funding was used in this study.

Author details

[1]School of Exercise Science, Australian Catholic University, Brisbane, Queensland 4014, Australia. [2]School of Human Movement Studies, University of Queensland, Brisbane, Queensland 4072, Australia.

References

1. Gabbett TJ, Jenkins DG, Abernethy B. Physical demands of professional rugby league training and competition using microtechnology. Journal of science and medicine in sport/Sports Medicine Australia. 2012;15(1):80–6. 10.1016/j.jsams.2011.07.004.
2. Sykes D, Twist C, Nicholas C, Lamb K. Changes in locomotive rates during senior elite rugby league matches. J Sports Sci. 2011;29(12):1263–71. 10.1080/02640414.2011.582507.
3. Waldron M, Twist C, Highton J, Worsfold P, Daniels M. Movement and physiological match demands of elite rugby league using portable global positioning systems. J Sports Sci. 2011;29(11):1223–30. 10.1080/02640414.2011.587445.
4. Gabbett TJ. Influence of playing standard on the physical demands of professional rugby league. J Sports Sci. 2013;31(10):1125–38. 10.1080/02640414.2013.773401.

5. Gabbett TJ, Jenkins DG, Abernethy B. Physical collisions and injury in professional rugby league match-play. Journal of science and medicine in sport / Sports Medicine Australia. 2011;14(3):210–5. 10.1016/j.jsams.2011.01.002.
6. Gabbett TJ, Polley C, Dwyer DB, Kearney S, Corvo A. Influence of field position and phase of play on the physical demands of match-play in professional rugby league forwards. Journal of science and medicine in sport / Sports Medicine Australia 2013 doi:10.1016/j.jsams.2013.08.002.
7. Twist C, Waldron M, Highton J, Burt D, Daniels M. Neuromuscular, biochemical and perceptual post-match fatigue in professional rugby league forwards and backs. J Sports Sci. 2012;30(4):359–67. 10.1080/02640414.2011.640707.
8. McLellan CP, Lovell DI, Gass GC. Markers of postmatch fatigue in professional rugby league players. Journal of strength and conditioning research / National Strength & Conditioning Association. 2011;25(4):1030–9. 10.1519/JSC.0b013e3181cc22cc.
9. Johnston RD, Gabbett TJ, Jenkins DG, Hulin BT. Influence of physical qualities on post-match fatigue in rugby league players. Journal of science and medicine in sport / Sports Medicine Australia 2014 doi:10.1016/j.jsams.2014.01.009.
10. Johnston RD, Gibson NV, Twist C, Gabbett TJ, Macnay SA, Macfarlane NG. Physiological responses to an intensified period of rugby league competition. Journal of strength and conditioning research / National Strength & Conditioning Association. 2013;27(3):643–54. 10.1519/JSC.0b013e31825bb469.
11. Johnston RD, Gabbett TJ, Jenkins DG. Influence of an intensified competition on fatigue and match performance in junior rugby league players. Journal of science and medicine in sport / Sports Medicine Australia. 2013;16(5):460–5. 10.1016/j.jsams.2012.10.009.
12. Montgomery PG, Pyne DB, Hopkins WG, Dorman JC, Cook K, Minahan CL. The effect of recovery strategies on physical performance and cumulative fatigue in competitive basketball. J Sports Sci. 2008;26(11):1135–45. 10.1080/02640410802104912.
13. Rowsell GJ, Coutts AJ, Reaburn P, Hill-Haas S. Effect of post-match cold-water immersion on subsequent match running performance in junior soccer players during tournament play. J Sports Sci. 2011;29(1):1–6. 10.1080/02640414.2010.512640.
14. Rowsell GJ, Coutts AJ, Reaburn P, Hill-Haas S. Effects of cold-water immersion on physical performance between successive matches in high-performance junior male soccer players. J Sports Sci. 2009;27(6):565–73. 10.1080/02640410802603855.
15. Gabbett TJ. Influence of playing standard on the physical demands of junior rugby league tournament match-play. Journal of science and medicine in sport / Sports Medicine Australia 2013 doi:10.1016/j.jsams.2013.03.013.
16. McLellan CP, Lovell DI. Performance analysis of professional, semi-professional and junior elite rugby league match-play using global positioning systems. Journal of strength and conditioning research / National Strength & Conditioning Association. 2013. doi:10.1519/JSC.0b013e31828f1d74.
17. Till K, Cobley S, O'Hara J, Brightmore A, Cooke C, Chapman C. Using anthropometric and performance characteristics to predict selection in junior UK rugby league players. Journal of science and medicine in sport / Sports Medicine Australia. 2011;14(3):264–9.
18. Gabbett T, Kelly J, Ralph S, Driscoll D. Physiological and anthropometric characteristics of junior elite and sub-elite rugby league players, with special reference to starters and non-starters. Journal of science and medicine in sport / Sports Medicine Australia. 2009;12(1):215–22. 10.1016/j.jsams.2007.06.008.
19. Krustrup P, Mohr M, Amstrup T, Rysgaard T, Johansen J, Steensberg A, et al. The yo-yo intermittent recovery test: physiological response, reliability, and validity. Med Sci Sports Exerc. 2003;35(4):697–705. 10.1249/01.mss.0000058441.94520.32.
20. McLellan CP, Lovell DI. Neuromuscular responses to impact and collision during elite rugby league match play. Journal of strength and conditioning research / National Strength & Conditioning Association. 2012;26(5):1431–40. 10.1519/JSC.0b013e318231a627.
21. Johnston RD, Gabbett TJ, Jenkins DG, Hulin BT. Influence of physical qualities on post-match fatigue in rugby league players. J Sci Med Sport. 2014(0). doi:http://dx.doi.org/10.1016/j.jsams.2014.01.009.
22. Johnston RD, Gabbett TJ, Seibold AJ, Jenkins DG. Influence of physical contact on neuromuscular fatigue and markers of muscle damage following small-sided games. Journal of science and medicine in sport / Sports Medicine Australia 2013 doi:10.1016/j.jsams.2013.07.018.
23. Twist C, Sykes D. Evidence of exercise-induced muscle damage following a simulated rugby league match. European Journal of Sport Science. 2011;11(6):401–9. 10.1080/17461391.2010.536575.
24. Foster C, Florhaug JA, Franklin J, Gottschall L, Hrovatin LA, Parker S, et al. A new approach to monitoring exercise training. Journal of strength and conditioning research / National Strength & Conditioning Association. 2001;15(1):109–15.
25. Gabbett TJ, Domrow N. Relationships between training load, injury, and fitness in sub-elite collision sport athletes. J Sports Sci. 2007;25(13):1507–19. 10.1080/02640410701215066.
26. Twist C, Highton J, Waldron M, Edwards E, Austin D, Gabbett TJ. Movement demands of elite rugby league players during Australian National Rugby League and European Super League matches. International journal of sports physiology and performance. 2014;9(6):925–30.
27. Boyd LJ, Ball K, Aughey RJ. The reliability of MinimaxX accelerometers for measuring physical activity in Australian football. Int J Sports Physiol Perform. 2011;6(3):311–21.
28. Gabbett T, Jenkins D, Abernethy B. Physical collisions and injury during professional rugby league skills training. Journal of science and medicine in sport / Sports Medicine Australia. 2010;13(6):578–83. 10.1016/j.jsams.2010.03.007.
29. Varley MC, Fairweather IH, Aughey RJ. Validity and reliability of GPS for measuring instantaneous velocity during acceleration, deceleration, and constant motion. J Sports Sci. 2012;30(2):121–7. 10.1080/02640414.2011.627941.
30. Batterham AM, Hopkins WG. Making meaningful inferences about magnitudes. Int J Sports Physiol Perform. 2006;1(1):50–7.
31. Cohen J. Statistical power analysis for the behavioral sciences (rev. ed.). Lawrence Erlbaum Associates, Inc: Hillsdale, NJ, England; 1977.
32. Hopkins WG, Marshall SW, Batterham AM, Hanin J. Progressive statistics for studies in sports medicine and exercise science. Med Sci Sports Exerc. 2009;41(1):3–13. 10.1249/MSS.0b013e31818cb278.
33. Johnston RD, Gabbett TJ. Repeated-sprint and effort ability in rugby league players. Journal of strength and conditioning research / National Strength & Conditioning Association. 2011;25(10):2789–95. 10.1519/JSC.0b013e31820f5023.
34. Johnston RD, Gabbett TJ, Seibold AJ, Jenkins DG. Influence of physical contact on pacing strategies during game-based activities. Int J Sports Physiol Perform. 2014;9(5):811–6. 10.1123/ijspp. 2013-0424.
35. Gabbett TJ, Seibold A. Relationship between tests of physical qualities, team selection, and physical match performance in semi-professional rugby league players. Journal of strength and conditioning research/National Strength & Conditioning Association 2013 doi:10.1519/JSC.0b013e31828d6219.
36. Miyaguchi K, Demura S. Relationships between stretch-shortening cycle performance and maximum muscle strength. Journal of strength and conditioning research / National Strength & Conditioning Association. 2008;22(1):19–24. 10.1519/JSC.0b013e31815f2f94.

20

Strength training in soccer with a specific focus on highly trained players

João R Silva[1,2*], George P Nassis[1] and Antonio Rebelo[2]

Abstract

Background: Data concerning the physical demands of soccer (e.g., activity pattern) suggest that a high level of performance requires well-developed neuromuscular function (NF). Proficient NF may be relevant to maintain and/or increase players' short- (intense periods of soccer-specific activity; accelerations, decelerations, and sprinting) and long-term performance during a match and throughout the season.

Objective: This review examines the extent to which distinct modes of strength training improve soccer players' performance, as well as the effects of concurrent strength and endurance training on the physical capacity of players.

Data sources: A selection of studies was performed in two screening phases. The first phase consisted of identifying articles through a systematic search using relevant databases, including the US National Library of Medicine (PubMed), MEDLINE, and SportDiscus. Several permutations of keywords were utilized (e.g., soccer; strength; power; muscle function), along with the additional scanning of the reference lists of relevant manuscripts. Given the wide range of this review, additional researchers were included. The second phase involved applying six selection criteria to the articles.

(Continued on next page)

* Correspondence: joao.silva@aspetar.com
[1]National Sports Medicine Programme Excellence in Football Project, Aspetar-Qatar Orthopaedic and Sports Medicine Hospital, P.O BOX 29222, Doha, Qatar
[2]Center of Research, Education, Innovation and Intervention in Sport (CIFI2D), Porto, Portugal

(Continued from previous page)

Results and conclusions: After the two selection phases, 24 manuscripts involving a total sample of 523 soccer players were considered. Our analysis suggests that professional players need to significantly increase their strength to obtain slight improvements in certain running-based actions (sprint and change of direction speed). Strength training induces greater performance improvements in jump actions than in running-based activities, and these achievements varied according to the motor task [e.g., greater improvements in acceleration (10 m) than in maximal speed (40 m) running movements and in non-squat jump (SJ) than in SSC-based actions (countermovement jump)]. With regard to the strength/power training methods used by soccer players, high-intensity resistance training seems to be more efficient than moderate-intensity resistance training (hypertrophic). From a training frequency perspective, two weekly sessions of strength training are sufficient to increase a player's force production and muscle power-based actions during pre-season, with one weekly session being adequate to avoid in-season detraining. Nevertheless, to further improve performance during the competitive period, training should incorporate a higher volume of soccer-specific power-based actions that target the neuromuscular system. Combined strength/power training programs involving different movement patterns and an increased focus on soccer-specific power-based actions are preferred over traditional resistance exercises, not only due to their superior efficiency but also due to their ecological value. Strength/power training programs should incorporate a significant number of exercises targeting the efficiency of stretch-shortening-cycle activities and soccer-specific strength-based actions. Manipulation of training surfaces could constitute an important training strategy (e.g., when players are returning from an injury). In addition, given the conditional concurrent nature of the sport, concurrent high-intensity strength and high-intensity endurance training modes (HIT) may enhance a player's overall performance capacity.
Our analysis suggests that neuromuscular training improves both physiological and physical measures associated with the high-level performance of soccer players.

Key points

- Neuromuscular training improves both physiological and physical measures associated with high-level performance.
- It seems that strength and power training programs should target all the force-velocity potential/spectrum of the neuromuscular system.
- Due to the conditioned concurrent nature of the sport, combined strength and combined high-intensity training approaches may constitute a good training approach within a football periodized process.

Review

Introduction

The central goal of strength/power training in a highly competitive sport is to improve the players' specific and relevant athletic activities inherent in their sport. To achieve this outcome, different strength/power training modes with i) distinct movement patterns (traditional resistance exercises, ballistic exercises, plyometrics, weight lifting, and/or sport-specific strength-based actions), ii) different combinations of the temporal organization of strength/power training loads (e.g., microcycle and training session variations), iii) distinct loads, iv) a wide range of movement velocities, v) specific biomechanical characteristics, and vi) different training surfaces have been adopted with the final end point of achieving an improvement in players' performance in relevant motor tasks (e.g., jumping, sprinting, and changing direction) [1-24].

Certain training methods combine different exercise modes (e.g., weight training, plyometric training, and sport-specific force-based actions) and allow for optimal power development and transfer to athletic activities due to both the neural and morphological adaptations typically associated with advanced training [25]. In fact, the intrinsic characteristics of soccer activity patterns (a varied range of motor actions that involve both breaking and propulsive forces as well as distinct contraction modes and velocities that require the all force-velocity potential of the neuromuscular system) that highlight the importance of the principle of specificity in strength and muscle power training cannot be understated [26,27].

A combination of different methods, including high-intensity strength training involving traditional resistance exercises (TRE; squats) and plyometrics [6], TRE and sprint training [10], and complex strength training (CT) [11,15,19], have all recently received considerable attention. Although some similarities exist between the previous modes of strength and power training, there are important differences. In this review, we found that complex training refers to training protocols that are comprised of the alternation of biomechanically comparable strength exercises and sport-specific drills in the same workout (e.g., six repetitions of calf extension exercise at 90% of one repetition maximum (1RM) + 5 s of rest + eight vertical jumps + 5 s of rest + three high ball headers) [25].

By focusing on more effective periodization techniques, researchers have investigated the effectiveness of different loading schemes throughout the power training phase (from high-force/low-velocity end to low-force/high-velocity end or vice versa) [22]. The training-induced effects of exercises with distinct biomechanical and technical characteristics during the plyometric-based component (e.g., purely vertically or a combination of vertically and horizontally oriented exercises [12,16,21,23], as well as the effects of plyometric training on different ground surfaces (grass vs. sand) [12], have both garnered significant attention. Furthermore, the adaptiveness of the functional and muscle structure of professional players (e.g., myosin heavy chain composition) to high-intensity strength training in the isokinetic contraction mode has also been investigated. However, the implementation of this analysis during the off-season resulted in lower ecological validity of these findings [7]. With regard to the search for complementary procedures and/or less stressful interventions, the effects of other methodologies (e.g., effects of electrostimulation training on semi-professional players) on physical fitness have also been investigated [28].

In general, most studies have examined the training-induced performance effects of two [1,6,8,10,14,16,19] to three [2,3,11,12,21,28] sessions per week. Given the multi-component requisites of soccer players' training (e.g., endurance, speed endurance, strength, power, and agility) that coincide with the increased amount of training time, some researchers examined the short-term effect of a lower weekly volume program (one session) [1,15,19] and the effect of training-induced adaptations of different weekly training frequencies (e.g., one vs. two sessions and one session per week vs. one session every second week) on both physiological and performance parameters during pre-season [19] and throughout the in-season in well-trained soccer players [1].

Nevertheless, despite an increase in the body of evidence regarding the applicability of strength/power training programs to routine soccer training, the short-term duration of interventions (e.g., 4 to 12 weeks) [2,3,6,8,10-12,14-16,19,21-23,28], the wide variety of training methods, the distinct season time lines used throughout the pre-season [2,3,6,12,19] and in-season [8,14-16,21,24,28] periods, the different weekly training loads, and the absence of control groups make the drawing of precise conclusions very difficult. With regard to the latter aspect, it is accepted that due to the importance of winning matches, technical staff of semi-professional and professional teams are unable to implement different training scenarios based on research interests. Nevertheless, in this review, our aim is to contribute to the understanding of the present state of the art of strength/power training and concurrent training in soccer to motivate future studies.

Methods

Search strategy: databases and inclusion criteria

The selection of studies was performed in two consecutive screening phases. The first phase consisted of identifying articles through a systematic search using the US National Library of Medicine (PubMed), MEDLINE, and SportDiscus databases. Literature searches were performed from January 2013 until June 2014, and this review comprises papers from 1985 to 2014 ($N_{1985\text{-}2009} = 76$ papers, $N_{2010} = 7$ papers, $N_{2011} = 17$ papers, $N_{2012} = 4$ papers, $N_{2013} = 21$ papers, $N_{2014} = 11$ papers). The following keywords were used in combination: 'elite soccer', 'professional soccer', 'first division soccer,' 'highly trained players,' 'seasonal alterations', 'performance analysis', 'soccer physiology', 'football', 'strength training', 'concurrent training', 'training transfer', 'neuromuscular performance,' 'muscular power', 'jump ability', 'sprint ability', 'agility', 'repeated sprint', 'intermittent endurance'. Further searching of the relevant literature was performed by using the 'related citations' function of PubMed and by scanning the reference lists. The second phase involved applying the selection criteria to the articles. Studies were chosen if they fulfilled the following six selection criteria: (i) the studied athletic population consisted of highly trained soccer players, ii) the players in the sample were not under 17 years of age, (iii) detailed physiological and performance tests were included, iv) the training programs applied were specified, (v) appropriate statistical analyses were used, and (vi) the article was written in the English language and published as an article in a peer-reviewed journal or a peer-review soccer-specific book edition.

Data extraction and presentation

Data related to the players' physiological parameters (e.g., lean leg volume, body fat percentage, running economy, anaerobic threshold, maximum absolute and relative oxygen consumption and strength values, peak and mean power values, and rate force development measures) and performance parameters (e.g., soccer-specific endurance tests, maximal aerobic speed, repeated and single sprint tests, jump ability exercises, agility, and ball speed) were extracted. All data are presented as the percentage of change in the means (Δ) unless otherwise specified.

Search data and study characteristics

The aim of providing players with updated data and training approaches in modern scenarios was fulfilled by 23 of the 24 papers published in the last 10 years. There were a total of 24 manuscripts fulfilling the five selection criteria, and the total sample population consisted of 523 soccer players. The distribution of players by competition level was as follows: 322 adults, 145 U-20 players, 12 U-19 players, and 44 U-18 players.

General physiological considerations of strength/power training

Strength training has become an integral component of the physical preparation for the enhancement of sports performance [29]. While strength is defined as the integrated result of several force-producing muscles performing maximally, either isometrically or dynamically during a single voluntary effort of a defined task, power is the product of force and the inverse of time, i.e., the ability to produce as much force as possible in the shortest possible time [9]. Nevertheless, strength and power are not distinct entities, as power performance is influenced by training methods that maximize both strength and stretch-shortening cycle activity (SSC) [30]. The ability of a muscle to produce force and power is determined by the interaction of biomechanical and physiological factors, such as muscle mechanics (e.g., type of muscle action) and morphological (e.g., muscle fiber type) and neural (e.g., motor unit recruitment) factors, and by the muscle environment itself (e.g., biochemical composition) [31].

The mechanisms underlying strength/power adaptations are largely associated with increases in the cross-sectional area of the muscle (hypertrophy methods) [32]. However, muscular strength increments can be observed without noticeable hypertrophy and serve as the first line of evidence for the neural involvement in the acquisition of muscular strength [32]. Thus, despite the notion that hypertrophy and neural adaptations are the basis of muscle strength development [33], their respective mechanisms of adaptation in the neuromuscular system are distinct [34]. In fact, 'more strength', i.e., the adaptational effect, does not necessarily imply an increase in muscle mass, as several distinct adaptations can lead to the same effect [33]. In this regard, the trainable effects of explosive/ballistic and/or heavy-resistance strength training causing enhanced force/power production have been primarily attributed to neural adaptations, such as motor unit recruitment, rate coding (frequency or rate of action potentials), synchronization, and inter-muscular coordination [31,35,36].

Physiological adaptations in soccer players

Our analysis suggests that the physiological adaptations underlining strength/power training may result in improvements in different motor tasks and performance qualities in high- and low-level players (Table 1 and Figure 1). In fact, independent of the players' standard, an enhanced dynamic [1-7,10,14,22,23] and static maximum force production [4,5,28] and increased muscle power outputs during different physical movements can be obtained through the implementation of strength/power training routines [2-8,14,22,37]. Specifically, increases in 1RM were observed during isoinertial assessments of half-squat exercises [1-3,6,10,14,22], hamstring leg curls, and one-leg step-up bench exercises [10]. Additionally, in our analysis, we observed a large range of improvements in the 1RM of well-trained players after short-term intervention periods (e.g., pre-season, Figure. 1, from 11% to 52% during the squat exercise) with average increments of approximately 21% [1-3,6,22,37,38]. Only Helgerud et al. [37] reported considerably larger gains in 1RM compared with other studies (11% to 26%; Table 1). Moreover, increments in maximal isometric voluntary contraction (MIVC) in the leg press task after CT training [11] and in knee extension strength after electrostimulation [28] and isokinetic training [4,5] have also been reported. Interestingly, not only were improvements in absolute force production (1RM) achieved, but an increased efficiency was also evident after allometric scaling of the results; 1RM per lean leg volume (LLV; 1RM/LLV) improved after high- and moderate-intensity modes of strength training [2], and relative force (maximum force divided by body mass) improved after complex strength training [11].

According to Harris et al. [27], intervention studies should use a specific isoinertial loading scheme, and test protocols should assess performance over the force-velocity continuum to gain a better understanding of the effect of load on muscular function. Moreover, neuromuscular-related qualities, such as impulse, rate of force development (RFD), and explosive strength, can better predict athletic performance; thus, the development of these approaches should be targeted [27]. The functional performance of soccer players seems to be more significantly associated with variables that are measured within the power-training load range (75% to 125% of body weight [BW] in half-squats) at which peak power (PP) is obtained (60% 1RM = 112% of BW) [39]. The PPs of highly trained soccer players were shown to occur with loads of 45% and 60% 1RM during jump- and half-squat exercises, respectively [22,39]. It is likely that superior improvements in power performance may be achieved by working on these optimal power training load ranges [22,39].

One particular muscle strength/power training adaptation involves an increase in the force-velocity relationships and the mechanical parabolic curves of power vs. velocity after high-intensity training programs, both in isoinertial [14] and isokinetic [4] exercises. Ronnestad et al. [6] and Gorostiaga et al. [8] observed increases in the force-velocity curve after high-intensity TRE and explosive-type strength training among professional and amateurs players, respectively. In the former study, the analysis of the pooled groups revealed increases in all measures of PP [6]. It seems that high-intensity strength training significantly increases performance in professional players at both the high-force end (increases in 1RM and sprint acceleration) and the high-velocity end (improvements in peak sprint velocity and four

Table 1 Physiological and functional adaptations to strength training

Study	Level/country/*n* (age)	Type of training	F/D	P	Physiological adaptations	Performance changes
Bogdanis et al., [2]	Professional/Greek/9 (22.9 ± 1.1)	*RST: Program 1* - 8 to 12 upper and lower body exercises + 4 sets of half-squats at 90% 1RM/5 rep/3-min rest between sets/emphasis on maximal mobilization during concentric action	3×/wk/6 wks	PS	↑17.3% 1RM† ↑16.3% 1RM/LLV† ↑6.2% PPO† ↑5.7% F_0 (kg) ↔ V_{opt} (ver.min^{-1}); V_0 (ver.min^{-1}); LLV	↑ ~1.6% 10m sprint † ↑ ~1.9% 40-m sprint ↑ ~2.5% 10 × 10-m Zig-Zag test (45° COD)† ↑ ~2.1% *t*-test† ↑ ~1% Illinois† ↑ ~10% CMJ†
		RST: Program 2 - 8 to 12 upper and lower body exercise + 4 sets of half-squat at 70% 1RM/12 rep/1.5-min rest/emphasis on both eccentric and concentric action with controlled movement speed			↑ 4.2% LLV ↑ 11% 1RM ↑ 6.6% 1RM/LLV ↑4.1% PPO ↔ V_{opt} (ver.min^{-1}); V_0 (ver.min^{-1}); F_0 (kg)	↑ ~1% 10-m sprint↑ ~1.9% 40-m sprint ↑ ~1.3% 10 × 10-m Zig-Zag test (45° COD) ↑ ~1.2% *t*-test ↑ ~0.6% Illinois ↑ ~5.3% CMJ
Bogdanis et al., [3]	Professional/Greek/9 (22.9 ± 1.1)	The *Program 1* adopted in the previous study	3×/wk/6 wks	PS	↑ 5.4% total work in RSA ↑ 10.9% RE ↑ 4.9% VO_2 max ↑ 7% MAS	↑ 29.4% YYIE2 ↑ 10% DTT
		The *Program 2* adopted in the previous study			↑ 4.5% total work in RSA ↑ 6.2% VO_2 max ↑ 5.8% VO_2 max ↔ RE	↑ 21.5% YYIE2 ↑ 9.6% DTT
Loturco et al. [22]	Professional/Brazil/16 (19.8 ± 0.72)	$RST_{(wk1\ to\ wk3)}$: half-squat exercise during first 3 weeks: wk_1 - 4 sets × 8 rep (50% 1RM); wk_2 - 4 sets × 8 rep (65% 1RM); wk_3 - 4 sets × 8 rep (80% 1RM)*Power* $training_{(wk4\ to\ wk6)}$: jump squat exercise: wk_4 - 4 sets × 4 rep (60% 1RM); wk_5 - 4 sets × 5 rep (45% 1RM); wk_6 - 4 sets × 6 rep (30% 1RM)	2×/wk/6 wks	PS	↑ 19.8% 1RM ↑ 18.5% $MP_{60\%\text{-}1RM\text{-}squat}$ ↑ 29.1% $MPP_{45\%\text{-}1RM\text{-}jump\ squat}$	↑ 4.3% 10m sprint ↑ 7.1% SJ ↑ 6.7% CMJ ↔ 30-m sprint
	Professional/Brazil/9 (19.1 ± 0.7)	$RST_{(wk1\ to\ wk3)}$: half-squat exercise during first 3 weeks: wk_1 - 4 sets × 8 rep (50% 1RM); wk_2 - 4 sets × 8 rep (65% 1RM); wk_3 - 4 sets × 8 rep (80% 1RM)*Power* $training_{(wk4\ to\ wk6)}$: jump squat exercise: wk_4 - 4 sets × 6 rep (30% 1RM); wk_5 - 5 sets × 5 rep (45% 1RM); wk_6 - 4 sets × 4 rep (60% 1RM)	2×/wk/6 wks	PS	↑ 22.1% 1RM ↑ 20.4% $MP_{60\%\text{-}1RM\text{-}squat}$ ↑ 31% $MPP_{45\%\text{-}1RM\text{-}jump\ squat}$	↑ 1.6% 10m sprint ↑ 4.5% SJ ↑ 6.9% CMJ ↔ 30-m sprint
Ronnestad et al., [6]	Professional/Norway/6 (22 ± 2.5)	*RST* (half-squats): $wk_{1\ to\ 2}$ (3 sets × 6RM); $wk_{3\ to\ 5}$ (4 sets × 5RM); $wk_{6\ to\ 7}$ (5 sets × 4RM) emphasizing maximal mobilization in concentric phase and slower eccentric phase (i.e. ~2 s).	2×/wk/7 wks	PS	↑ 26% 1RM ↑ 9.9% PPO_{20kg} ↑ 11.1% PPO_{50kg} ↔ PPO_{35kg}	↑3.6% 4BT ↔ CMJ, SJ; 10m sprint; 30-40m sprint; 40m sprint time

Table 1 Physiological and functional adaptations to strength training *(Continued)*

	8 (23 ± 2)	*RST* plus *PT* performed in the same session: *ALB* = [$wk_{1\ to\ 2}$ (3 sets × 8 rep); wk_3 (3 sets × 8 rep); $wk_{4\ to\ 5}$ (3 sets × 10 rep); $wk_{6\ to\ 7}$ (4 sets × 10 rep)]/*DLHJ* = [$wk_{1\ to\ 7}$ (2 sets × 5 rep)]/*SLFH* = [$wk_{1\ to\ 7}$ (2 sets × 5 rep)] maximal intensity, emphasizing fast switch from eccentric to concentric contraction; 1-min rest between sets	2×/wk/7 wks		↑ 23% 1RM ↑ 10% PPO_{20kg} ↑ 8% PPO_{35kg} ↑ 9.5% PPO_{50kg}	↑ 4% 4BT ↑ 9.1% SJ ↑ 0.009% 30- to 40-m sprint time ↑ 1.1% 40-m sprint ↔ CMJ; 10-m sprint
Koundourakis et al., [48]	Professional/Greece/1st league 23 (25.5 ± 1.1)	*Team A* (*high-strength training stress*): *PS*: 11 sessions *RST* + 15 sessions. *SST* + 4 sessions *SAQ* during 7 weeks pre-season; *IN*: 1 sessions RST; 2 sessions SST; 2 sessions SAQ; 1 sessions speed and 1 session reaction speed training during each week of in-season training *RST*: circuit strength training, 10 stations, 4 sets, 10 reps in free weights, 4-min rest between sets; 70% to 80% 1RM; 2 core strength exercises + lunge, squats, steps up on bench with external weight, pullover, arm curls, triceps, and bench press	*PS*: 7 wks *IN*: 35 wks	PS + IN	IN_1: ↑ 5.3% VO_2 max ↑ 16.6% BF IN_2: ↑ 26.4% BF ↔ VO_2 max	IN_1: ↑ 7.7% SJ ↑ 7.2% CMJ ↑ 2.2% 10-m sprint ↑ 1% 20-m sprint IN_2: ↑ 3.8% SJ ↑ 4% CMJ ↑ 1.1%10-m sprint ↑ 0.3% 20-m sprint
	Professional/Greece/1st league 22 (24.7 ± 1.0)	*Team B* (*moderate-strength training stress*): *PS*: 6 sessions RST + 9 sessions SST + 4 sessions. SAQ during 7 weeks pre-season *IN*: 1 session RST/wk; 1 session SST; 1 session SAQ; 1 session speed training during each week of in-season training *RST*: 4 sets; 6 reps, 90% 1RM; explosive action high execution speed; leg extension, hamstring curls chest press, calf raise, pullover arm curls and biceps	*PS*: 7 wks *IN*: 35 wks	PS + IN	*IN_1*: ↑ 3.9% VO_2 max ↑ 16.7% BF IN_2: ↔ VO_2 max; % BF	IN_1: ↑ 8.1% SJ ↑ 7.7% CMJ ↑ 2.8% 10-m sprint ↑ 1.6% 20-m sprint IN_2: ↔ SJ; CMJ; 10- and 20-m sprint
	Professional/Greece/2nd league 22 (23.8 ± 0.9)	*Team C* (*low-strength training stress*) *PS*: 4 session RST + 7 session SST + 4 session SAQ performed during 7 weeks pre-season *IN*: 1 session RST or SST; 1 session SAQ; 1 session speed training during each week of in-season training *RST*: 4 sets; 6 reps, 90% 1RM; explosive action high execution speed, (alternating with SST training every second strength training session); leg extension, hamstring curls chest press, calf raise, pullover arm curls and biceps	*PS*: 7 wks *IN*: 35 wks	PS + IN	IN_1: ↑ 4% VO_2 max ↑ 8.7% BF IN_2: ↔ VO_2 max; % BF	IN_1: ↑ 5.9% SJ ↑ 4.8% CMJ ↑ 1.7% 10-m sprint ↑ 0.7% 20-m sprint IN_2: ↔ SJ; CMJ; 10m and 20-m sprint

Table 1 Physiological and functional adaptations to strength training *(Continued)*

Ronnestad et al., [1]	Professional/Norway/ 7 (22 ± 2)	*RST - PS*: $wk_{1\ to\ 3}$ (1st session - 3 × 10RM + 2nd session - 3 × 6RM); $wk_{4\ to\ 6}$ (1st session - 3 × 8RM + 2nd session - 3 × 5RM); $wk_{7\ to\ 10}$ (1st session - 3 × 6RM + 2nd session - 3 × 4RM); *IN*: $wk_{11\ to\ 22}$ (1 session wk - 3 × 4RM) half-squats emphasizing maximal mobilization in concentric phase and slower eccentric phase	2×/wk/10 wks + 1×/wk/12 wks	PS + IN	PS: ↑ 19% 1RM IN: ↔ 1RM	PS: ↑ 1.8% 40-m sprint ↑ 3.3% SJ ↔ CMJ; IN: ↔ 40-m sprint; SJ; CMJ
	Professional/Norway/ 7 (26 ± 2)	*RST - PS*: $wk_{1\ to\ 3}$ (1st session - 3 × 10RM + 2nd session - 3 × 6RM); $wk_{4\ to\ 6}$ (1st session - 3 × 8RM + 2nd session - 3 × 5RM); $wk_{7\ to\ 10}$ (1st session - 3 × 6RM + 2nd session - 3 × 4RM); *IN*: $wk_{11\ to\ 22}$ (1 session each 2 wk - 3 × 4RM) half-squats emphasizing maximal mobilization in concentric phase and slower eccentric phase	2×/wk/10 wks + 0.5×/wk/12 wks	PS + IN	PS: ↑ 19% 1RM IN: ↓ 10% 1RM	PS: ↑ 1.8% 40-m sprint ↑ 3.3% SJ ↔ CMJ; IN: ↓ 1.1% 40-m sprint ↔ SJ; CMJ
Chelly et al.,[14]	Junior/NS/11 (17.3 ± 0.5)	*RST* - back half-squat 1st - 1 set × 7 rep 70% 1RM 2nd - 1 set × 4 rep 80% 1RM 3rd - 1 set × 3 rep at 85% 1RM 4th - 1 set × 2 rep 90% 1RM	2×/wk/8 wks	IS	↑ 25% 1RM ↑ 7.2% Wpeak ↔ LMV; TMV, MTCSA	↑ 23% Vfirst step ↑ 7.1% Vfirst 5-m ↑ 12% Vmax ↑ 4.7% 5J ↑ 10% SJ ↔ CMJ; MPV
Kotzamanidis et al., [10]	NS/Greece/12 (17.0 ± 1.1)	*RST* plus *SP* 10-min after strength session: 3 exercises [(Back half-squat at 90° (BHS); step up on a bench with one leg (SU); leg curls for hamstrings (LCH)] $wk_{1\ to\ 4}$ = 4 sets × 8RM + 4 × 30-m; $wk_{5\ to\ 8}$ = 4 sets × 6RM + 5 × 30 m; wk_9 = 4 sets × 3RM + 6 × 30-m; 3-min rest between sets/3-min rest between sprint rep/10-min interval between strength and sprint program	2×/wk/9 wks	ND	↑ 8.6% 1RM of BHS ↑ 17.5% 1RM of SU ↑ 18% 1RM of LCH	↑ 7.8% SJ† ↑ 6.6% CMJ† ↑ 3.5% 30-m sprint† ↔ DJ40cm
	11 (17.1 ± 1.1)	Only perform the previous defined RST program	2×/wk/9 wks		↑ 10% 1RM of BHS ↑ 16.7% 1RM of SU ↑ 16.1% 1RM of LCH	↔ SJ†; CMJ†; DJ40cm; 30-m sprint†
Los Arcos et al., [23]	Professional/Spain/ 11 (20.3 ± 1.9)	*RST plus vertical-oriented exercises* (*VS*): *RST* (1 to 2 exercises session) - double (70% to 76% PPO) and single leg (30% to 35% PPO) half-squats (2 sets × 5 reps) and calf exercises (50% to 60% PPO; 2 sets × 5 reps); *VS* (1 to 2 exercises session) - double and single leg CMJ to box (1 to 3 sets × 3 to 5 reps); vertical jump with load (5% BM; 3 sets × 4 reps); skipping and vertical jump (3 sets × 3 reps); drop vertical jump single leg (2 to 3 sets × 3 reps)	12 sessions/ 5 wks + 3 wks	PS + IS	↑ 12.6% PPO (kg) ↑ 8.1% IT ($km.h^{-1}$)	↔ 5- and 15-m sprint; CMJ; CMJ D; CMJ ND

Table 1 Physiological and functional adaptations to strength training *(Continued)*

	Professional/Spain/11 (19.6 ± 1.9)	*RST plus vertical and horizontal oriented exercises (VHS)*: *RST*: same protocol; *VHS* (1 to 2 exercises session) - sled walking (5 sets × 1 reps × 10 m; 50% to 55% BM); hip extension wall drill single and double (2 sets × 5 reps); horizontal jump with load (3 sets × 3 to 4 reps; 5% BM); drop horizontal jump single leg (2 to 3 sets × 3 reps); sled-towing (maximal speed, 7.5%; 10 m); double-triple jump (1 × 5 reps)	12 sessions/ 5 wks + 3 wks	PS + IS	↑ 12.2% PPO (kg) ↑ 3.4% IAT ($km.h^{-1}$)	↑ 3.3% CMJ†; ↔ 5- and 15-m sprint; CMJ D; CMJ ND
Aagaard et al., [4]	Elite/Denmark/24 (NS)	*High-resistance isokinetic strength training* 4 sets × 8RM	32 sessions/ 12 wks	OS	↑ 10% to 26% CON $IKE_{(0,\ 4.18\ and\ 5.24\ rad/s)}$ ↑ 9% to 14% CON $IKE_{50°\ (0\ and\ 0.52\ rad/s)}$ ↑ 5% to 29% $PPO_{↑\ 3.14\ rad/s}$ ↑ 5% to 29% $PPO_{50°(↑\ 3.14\ rad/s)}$ ↑ 24% to 42% CON $IKE_{Vpeak(↑\ 5.24\ rad/s)}$ ↑ 18% to 32% $PPO_{Vpeak\ (↑\ 5.24\ rad/s)}$ ↑ $MIVC_{KE\ (50°)}$	↔ $BS_{without\ run\ up}$
		Low-resistance isokinetic strength training in isokinetic mode (low-intensity high speed contraction group) 4 sets × 24RM			↑ 9% CON $IKE_{(2.09\ rad/s)}$ ↔ PPO; $PPO_{50°}$; $MIVC_{50°knee\ extension}$; CON $IKE_{at\ Vpeak}$; $PPO_{Vpeak\ ↑\ 5.24\ rad/s}$	↔ $BS_{without\ run\ up}$
		Functional strength training in the form of loaded kicking movements without ball 4 sets × 16RM			↑ 7% to 13% CON $IKE_{(0.52\text{-}2.09\text{-}3.14\ rad/s)}$ ↑ 9-14% CON $IKE_{50°\ (0\ and\ 0.52\ rad/s)}$ ↑ 7% $PPO_{(4.18\ rad/s)}$ ↑ 9-12% $PPO_{50°\ (0.52\text{-}2.09\ to\ 3.14\ rad/s)}$ ↔ CON IKE_{Vpeak}; $PPO_{Vpeak(↑\ 5.24 rad/s)}$	↔ $BS_{without\ run\ up}$
Maio Alves et al., [19]	Elite/Portugal/9 (17.4 ± 0.6)	*CT*: *1st station*: 6 rep of 90° squats at 85% 1RM then 1 set of 5-m high skipping, in a straight line and then 5-m sprint. 2nd station: 6 rep of calf extension at 90% 1RM then 8 vertical jumps and then 3 high ball headers. 3rd station: 6 rep of leg extension exercise at 80% 1RM then 6 jump from the seated position than 3 drop jumps (60 cm), executing a soccer heading.				↑ 9.2% 5m sprint ↑ 6.2% 15m sprint ↑12.6% SJ ↔ CMJ; 505 agility tests
	8 (17.4 ± 0.6)	The same *CT* training but performed 2× a week				↑ 9.2% 5m sprint ↑ 6.2% 15m sprint ↑12.6% SJ) ↔ CMJ; 505 agility tests

Table 1 Physiological and functional adaptations to strength training *(Continued)*

Mujika et al., [15]	Elite/Spain/10 (18 ± 0.5)	*CT: 1st session* - introduction session of hill sprinting (8% slope); 2nd session - dedicated to sled pulling sprint training, towing ~18% BM; 3rd, 4th, and 5th session (weeks 3 to 5) 3 series of 4 reps of calf rises (~35% BM) and parallel squats (~50% BM) and 2 repetitions per leg of hip flexions (~15% BM); 6th session - stair climbing: 18× (18 steps × 22.5 cm)/120-s rec (alternating single leg, double leg, single, double, frontal, and lateral step). Weight training emphasizing maximal concentric mobilization. Strength and power exercises in sessions 3 to 5 immediately followed soccer-specific activities such as jumps, accelerations, ball kicks, and offensive and defensive actions				↑~2.8% 15m sprint† ↔ CMJ; CMJWAS; CMJ15-S; Agility 15m;
	10 (18 ± 0.7)	*Sprint training*: 1st and 2nd session - 2× (4× 30-m); 3rd and 4th session- 3× (4× 30-m); 5th and 6th session- 4× (4× 30-m); 90-s rec between rep/180-s rec between sets				↔ CMJ; CMJWAS; CMJ15-S; Agility 15m; 15m sprint
Manopoulos et al., [11]	Amateurs/NS/10 (19.9 ± 0.4)	*CT*: $wk_{1\text{-}2}$: general strength (10 exercises/ 3 sets/15 to 20 rep); $wk_{3\text{-}4}$: 3 sets/6 rep (5 different exercises as skipping, jumping on one leg and on both legs, jumping running forwards, backwards and to the side, jumping obstacles and kicking); $wk_{5\text{-}10}$: (a) 3 sets × 6 instep kicks within a time of 5 s (b) 6 kicking's with a 5-m run-up approach against resistance provided by a rubber band (RRB) attached on the ankle of the swinging leg (c) 3 × 10-min/5- or 8-a SSG, with or without loads (d) series of modified exercise sequences: *1st*) 6 kicking's (RRB), 3 jumps, isometry trunk with a player on the back (PB) in a semi-seated position for 6 s, 4 sideward jumps; *2nd*) 6 leg extensions RRB, 3 headers, isometry ankle musculature, carrying PB for 6 s, 1 kicking; *3rd*) 6 knee flexion repetitions RRB, 4 sideward jumps, 3 × 5-m sprints and a soccer kick	3×/wk/10 wks	NS	↑ 13.9% $MIVC_{leg\ press}$ ↑ 14% MIVC/BW ↑ 29.1% F_{60} ↑ 17.2% F_{100} ↑ 30% EMG VL	↑ ~4% 10-m sprint ↑ ~10% $BS_{with\ run\ up}$ ↔ MCS

Table 1 Physiological and functional adaptations to strength training *(Continued)*

Impellizzeri et al., [12]	Amateurs/Italian/37 (25 ± 4)	*PT* on grass; *vertical jumping*: 15 sets in wk_1; 20 sets wk_2; 25 sets in $wk_{3\ to\ 4}$; always 10 rep per wk; *bounding*: 3 sets wk_1; 4 sets wk_2; 5 sets per wk in $wk_{3\text{-}4}$; always 10 rep per wk; *broad jumping*: 5 sets × 8 rep wk_1; 5 sets wk_2; 7 sets wk_3; 7 sets wk_4; always 10 rep per $wk_{2\text{-}4}$; *drop jump*: 3 sets × 5 rep wk_1; 5 sets × 9 rep wk_2; 6 sets × 15 rep per wk in $wk_{3\text{-}4}$; rec 15 to 30 s between repetitions 1 to 2 min between sets	3×/wk/4 wks	PS		↑ 3.7% 10-m sprint ↑ 2.8% 20-m sprint ↑ 4.7% SJ ↑ 14.5% CMJ† ↑ 9% CMJ/SJ†
		Same *PT* protocol but performed on a different ground surface (sand)				↑ 4.3% 10-m sprint ↑ 2.5% 20-m sprint ↑ 10% SJ† ↑ 6.4% CMJ; ↑ 3.7% CMJ/SJ
Sedano et al., [21]	Elite U-19/Spain/11 (18.4 ± 1.1)	*PT*: jump over hurdles: 16 to 26 sets/5 rep; horizontal jumps: 16 to 26 sets/5 rep; lateral jumps over hurdles: 16 to 26 sets/5 rep; wk_1 - 270 jumps; $wk_{2,4,9}$ - 300 jumps; $wk_{3,8}$ - 240 jumps; $wk_{5,7}$ - 330 jumps; wk_6 - 180 jumps; wk_{10} - 390 jumps; 30-s rec between sets of 5 rep and 5 min after 4 sets of 5 reps	3×/wk/10 wks	IS		↑ 8% CMJ ↑ 5% CMJWAS ↑ 5.8% BSdl ↑ 6.4% BSndl ↑ 0.32% 10-m sprint ↔ SJ;
Thomas et al., [16]	Semi-professional/UK/12 (17 ± 0.4)	*PT*: $DJ_{40group}$ session began at 80 foot contacts and progressed to 120 by end of training program	2×/wk/6 wks	IS		↑ ~5% CMJ ↑ ~5% 505 agility test ↔ 5-, 10-, 15-, and 20-m sprint time
		PT: CMJ_{group} session began at 80 foot contacts and progressed to 120 by end of training program				↑ ~7% CMJ ↑ ~10% 505 agility test ↔ 5-, 10-, 15-, and 20-m sprint time
Gorostiaga et al., [8]	Amateurs/Spain/10 (17.3 ± 0.5)	*Explosive-strength training* (low load weight training and plyometric and sprint exercises): full squat-lift (2 to 3 sets/2 to 6 rep/ 20 to 52 kg) and power clean (3 to 4 sets/ 3 to 4 rep/16 to 28 kg) 2×/wk; vertical CMJ to box (3 to 5 sets/5 to 8 rep/only in $wk_{1\ to\ 8}$); hurdle vertical jumps (3 sets/4 rep/only in the $wk_{9\ to\ 11}$); sprints (1 set/3 to 5 rep/15 to 40 m) performed 1×/wk; 2-min rec between sets and exercises	2×/wk/11 wks	IS	↔ $Hr_{13\text{-}14\ km.h-1(bpm)}$; ↔ $La_{13\text{-}14\ km.h-1(mM)}$	↑ 5.1% CMJ ↑ 7.5% CMJ_{20kg} ↑ 13.9% CMJ_{30kg} ↔ 5- and 15-m sprint; $CMJ_{40\text{-}50\text{-}60\text{-}70kg}$

Table 1 Physiological and functional adaptations to strength training *(Continued)*

Billot et al., [28]	Amateurs/French/10 (20 ± 2)	*ES*: 2-min session on both quadriceps femoris muscle (36 contractions per session); knee fixed at 60° (0° corresponding to full extension of the leg); EMS 3 s long followed by a rest period of 17 s (duty cycle 15%); intensity range 60 to 120 mA (higher than 60% of muscle voluntary contraction)	3×/wk/5 wks	IS	↑ 22.1% ECC IKE $_{(-60°.s-1)}$ ↑ 9.9% CON IKE $_{(60°.s-1)}$ ↑ 23.2% CON IKE $_{(240°.s-1)}$ ↑ 27.1% $MIVC_{KE\ (60°)}$	↑ 9.6% BS $_{without\ run\ up}$ ↑ 5.6% BS $_{with\ run\ up}$ ↔ SJ; CMJ; CMJWAS; 10-m sprint; $V_{10\ m}$

↑, significant improvement; ↓, significant decrement; ↔, no significant alterations; †, significant differences between groups; ~, approximately and data extracted from graphs; NS, not specified; F/D, frequency and duration of training protocols; P, period of the soccer season; rec, recovery; RST, resistance strength training; PT, plyometric training; SP, sprint training; wk, week; PS, performed during preseason; IS, performed during in-season; ND, not defined; rep., repetitions; 1RM, one repetition maximum; 1RM/LLV, maximal strength in half-squat strength per lean leg volume; PPO, peak power output; F_0, individual theoretical maximal force generated at zero pedal speed; V_{opt}, speed were the highest value of power is achieve; V_0, maximal cycling speed corresponding to zero load; LLV, lean leg volume; m, meters; COD, change of direction; $CMJ_{(10\text{-}20\text{-}30\text{-}40\text{-}50\text{-}60\text{-}70kg)}$, countermovement jump with or without external (load); RSA, repeated sprint ability test; RE, running economy; VO_2 max, maximal oxygen consumption; MAS, maximal aerobic speed; YYIE2, Yo-Yo intermittent endurance test level 2; DTT, Holff's dribbling track test; $MP_{60\%\text{-}1RM\text{-}squat}$, mean power; $MPP_{45\%\text{-}1RM}$, jump squat; mean propulsive power; SJ, squat jump; ALB, alternate leg bound; DLHJ, double leg hurdle jump; SLFH, single leg forward hop; 4BT, four bounce test; SST, soccer-specific strength; SAQ, speed, agility and quickness; BF, body fat; Wpeak, leg cycling peak power; LMV, leg muscle volume; TMV, thigh muscle volume; MTCSA, mean thigh cross-sectional area; $V_{first\ step}$, velocity during the first step after the start of sprint test; $V_{first5\text{-}m}$, average running velocity during the first 5 m of the sprint test; Vmax, maximal running velocity; 5J, five jump test; MPV, maximal pedaling velocity; BHS, back half-squat at 90°; SU, step up on a bench with one leg; LCH, leg curls for hamstrings; DJ40cm, drop jump from 40-cm height; VH, vertical oriented exercises; VHS, vertical and horizontal oriented exercises; BM, body mass; IAT, individual anaerobic threshold; CMJ D, countermovement jump dominant leg; CMJ ND, countermovement jump non-dominant leg; OS, off-season; CON $IKE_{(0,\ 4.18\ and\ 5.24\ rad/s)}$, concentric isokinetic knee extensor peak torque (angular velocity); CON $IKE_{50°\ (0\ and\ 0.52\ rad/s)}$, concentric isokinetic knee extensor peak torque at 50° knee extension (angular velocity); $PPO_{\uparrow 3.14\ rad/s}$, peak power at angular velocity higher than 3.14 rad/s; $PPO_{50°(\uparrow 3.14\ rad/s)}$, peak power at 50° knee extension (angular velocity); CON $IKE_{Vpeak(\uparrow 5.24\ rad/s)}$, concentric isokinetic knee extensor peak torque exerted at the instance of peak velocity (angular velocities higher than 5.24 rad/s); $PPO_{Vpeak\ (\uparrow 5.24\ rad/s)}$, peak power output exerted at the instance of peak velocity (angular velocities higher than 5.24 rad/s); $MIVC_{50°\ knee\ extension}$, maximal isometric voluntary contraction of knee extensors (angle); BS $_{with\ or\ without\ run\ up}$, ball speed after kicking with or without previous run up; CT, complex strength training; CMJWAS, counter movement jump with arm swing; $CMJ_{15\text{-}s}$, counter movement jump during 15-s period; RRB, resistance provided by a rubber band; SSG, small sided game; PB, player on the back; $MIVC_{leg\ press}$, maximal isometric voluntary contraction in the leg press machine (knee and hip angles of 110° and 90°, respectively; 180° = full extension); MIVC/BW, maximal force divided by body weight; $F_{60\text{-}100}$, maximal force value during the first 60 or 100 ms of the contraction; EMG VL, electromyography activity of vastus medialis of the swinging leg (phase 3) normalized relatively to the maximal EMG value during kick; MCS, maximal cycling speed; CMJ/SJ, eccentric utilization ratio; BSdl, ball speed after kicking with dominant leg; BSndl, ball speed after kicking with non-dominant leg; UK, United Kingdom; $Hr_{13\text{-}14\ km.h\text{-}1(bpm)}$, - heart rate at 13 and 14 $km.h^{-1}$; $La_{13\text{-}14\ km.h\text{-}1(mM)}$, blood lactate concentration at 13 and 14 $km.h^{-1}$; V_{10m}, velocity at 10-m sprint.

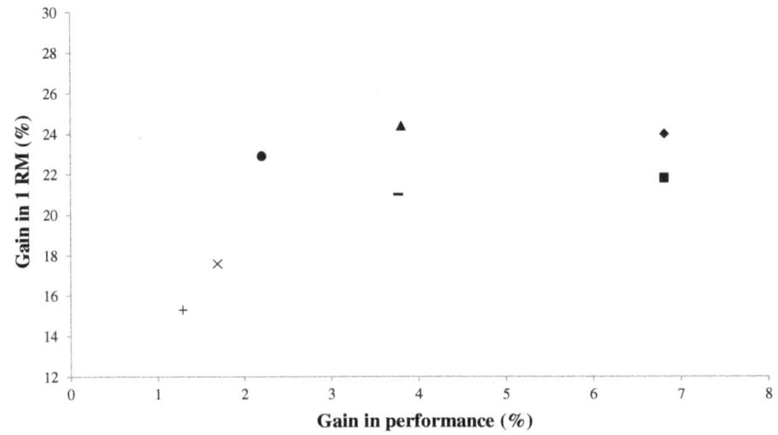

Figure 1 The gains in strength and different motor abilities of high-level players after 5 to 10 weeks. Squares represent the average squat jump performance [1,6,14,22]; rhombi represent the average countermovement jump performance [2,22,37]; triangles represent the average four bounce test performance [6]; circles represent the average 10-m sprint performance [2,22,37,38]; x symbols represent the average 40-m sprint performance [1,2,6]; + symbols represent the average change in direction ability [2,38]; and lines represent the average of all the previous motor tasks.

bounce test; 4BT) but only as long as the subjects perform concurrent plyometric and explosive exercises during their soccer sessions [6]. Furthermore, Los Arcos et al. (2013) recently found that professional players performing 5 weeks of pre-season and 3 weeks of in-season strength/power training increased the load at which PP was achieved during the half-squat exercise [11]. Additionally, 10 weeks of complex strength training, consisting of soccer-specific strength and skill exercises (soccer kick), improved measures of explosive strength and RFD during the isometric leg press in low-level players, with an increase in the electromyography (EMG) activity of certain muscles involved in the task also reported [11].

Adaptations in sport-specific efforts

The effectiveness of a strength/power program is evaluated by the magnitude of sport-specific improvements. Although the predominant activities during training and matches are performed at low and medium intensities, sprints, jumps, duels, and kicking, which are mainly dependent on the maximum strength and anaerobic power of the neuromuscular system, are essential skills [40]. Power and speed usually support the decisive decision-making situations in professional football, e.g., straight sprinting is the most frequent physical action in goal situations [41]. Furthermore, a high degree of stress is imposed on the neuromuscular system of players to enable them to cope with these essential force-based actions required during training and competition (e.g., accelerations and decelerations) [42,43].

Although not universally confirmed, there is evidence of associations between the measures of maximal (1RM) [44] and relative strength (1RM/BM) [45], as well as between certain muscle mechanical properties, such as peak torque [46,47] and PP [39], and the ability of soccer players to perform complex multi-joint dynamic movements, e.g., jumping and sprinting actions. Independently of a player's level, strength-related interventions represent a powerful training stimulus by promoting adaptations in a wide range of athletic skills (e.g., jumping, Table 1, Figures 1, 2 and 3 and Additional file 1: Figure S1-5) [2,3,6,8,10,12,14,15,19,21-23,48] and soccer-specific skills (soccer kick) [21,28] (Tables 1 and 2). Interestingly, the addition of a long-term strength/power training program to normal soccer training routines seems to result in a higher long-term increase in the physical performance of elite youth players [45,49]. Furthermore, to have a clear picture of the effect of strength training on physical performance, different motor tasks should be assessed; jumping, sprinting, and change of direction abilities may represent separate and independent motor abilities, and concentric and slow SSC jumping actions are shown to be relatively independent of fast SSC abilities [50].

Sprint ability

With regard to adaptations in sprint qualities (e.g., acceleration and maximal speed, Table 1 and Additional file 1: Figure S1), improvements in different sprint distances (5- to 40-m distances) [1,2,6,10-12,14,15,19,21,22,48,51] have been reported in different levels of players. On average, highly trained players [1,2,6,22,37,38] need to increase their 1RM half-squat by 23.5% to achieve an approximately 2% improvement in sprint performance at 10- and 40-m distances (Figure 2). Excluding the study of Helgerud et al. [37], which reported significantly larger increments in strength, studies have demonstrated

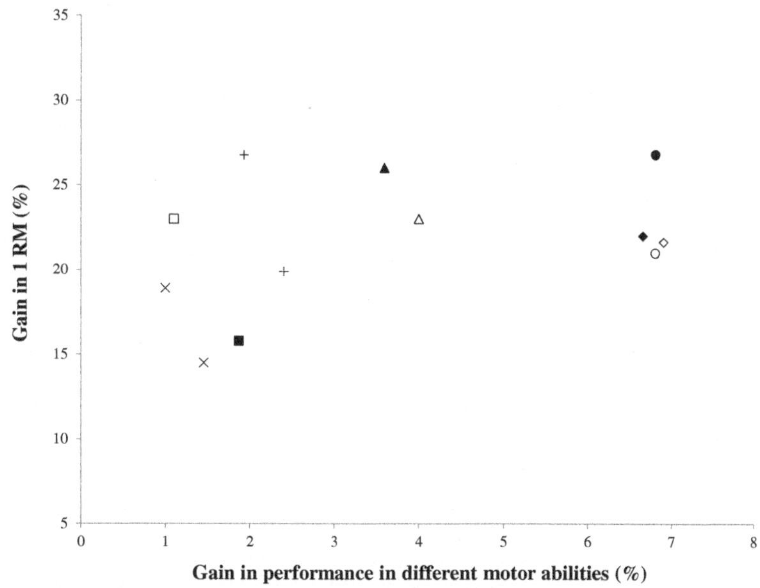

Figure 2 Gains in strength and motor abilities of high level players after different training modes (5 to 10 weeks). x and dashed x symbols represent the change of direction ability performance after traditional resistance exercises programs (TRE) [2] and combined programs (COM) [38], respectively; filled and unfilled squares represent the 40-m sprint performance after TRE [1,2] and COM [6], respectively; + and dashed + symbols represent the 10-m sprint performance after TRE [2,37] and COM [22,38], respectively; filled and unfilled triangles represent the four bounce test performance after TRE [6] and COM [6], respectively; filled and unfilled rhombi represent the squat jump performance after TRE [1,14] and COM [6,22], respectively; and filled and unfilled circles represent the countermovement jump performance after TRE [2,37] and COM [22], respectively.

that lower increments in 1RM (19%) are required to achieve a similar improvement in sprint performance (1.9%) after short-term training interventions (in average, an 18% increments in 1RM resulted in a 2% average improvements in 10-m sprint performance [2,22,38] and 17% average increments in 1RM resulted in 1.6% improvements in 40-m distance time [1,2,6]). Nevertheless, improvements in sprint performance have not been entirely confirmed [1,6,8,10,16,22,28]. Notwithstanding, factors associated with the training status of various players, players' background, and/or the characteristics of the training modes adopted should be considered as the most likely factors. For example, the sole performance of one type of plyometric exercise [16] and of electrostimulation training [28], which has an apparent lower level of specificity, may explain, at least in part, the lack of transfer of training adaptations to dynamic and complex activities, where the coordination and force production of different body muscles, as is the case of sprint performance, are essential.

Jump ability

Our analysis suggests that strength/power training induces adaptations in the jump abilities of high-level players (Table 1 and Figure 1 and Additional file 1: Figure S2). On average, 24.4% 1RM improvements during squats result in a CMJ increase of approximately 6.8% [2,22,37]. Lower performance improvements in four bounce test (4-BT; 3.8%) were found with similar increments in 1RM (24.5%) [6], and similar improvements in SJ (6.8%) occurred with an average 1RM increase of 21.8% [1,6,14,22]. Curiously, the plotted data of all studies assessing the improvement in jump abilities in high-level players revealed that, on average (Figure 2, Additional file 1: Figure S5), a 23.5% 1RM increase may result in a 6.2% improvement in jump ability tasks after 6 to 10 weeks of strength/power training [1,2,6,14,22,37]. The previous results suggest that, on average, higher increments in force are needed to improve CMJ to the same extent as SJ (figure 1). This result may reflect the fact that the current programs were not able to increase (at the same relative rate) performance ability in the positive and negative phases of the SSC component and may explain, at least in part, the smaller improvements in sprint performance.

Improvements in the squat jump (SJ) [1,10,12,14,19,22], four bounce test (4BT) [6], five jump test (5-JT) [14], countermovement jump test (CMJ) [2,8,10,12,16,21,22], CMJ with free arms [21], and eccentric utilization ratio (CMJ/SJ) [12] have been observed in different players. Nevertheless, contradictions regarding improvements in SJ after plyometric [21] and in CMJ after high-intensity strength protocols performed by well-trained players can be found in the literature [1,14]. Additionally, no significant increases in CMJ were observed after CT involving workouts with high [19] or low loads [15] or in drop jumps from a 40-cm height (DJ_{40}) [10] following TRE and TRE plus sprint training.

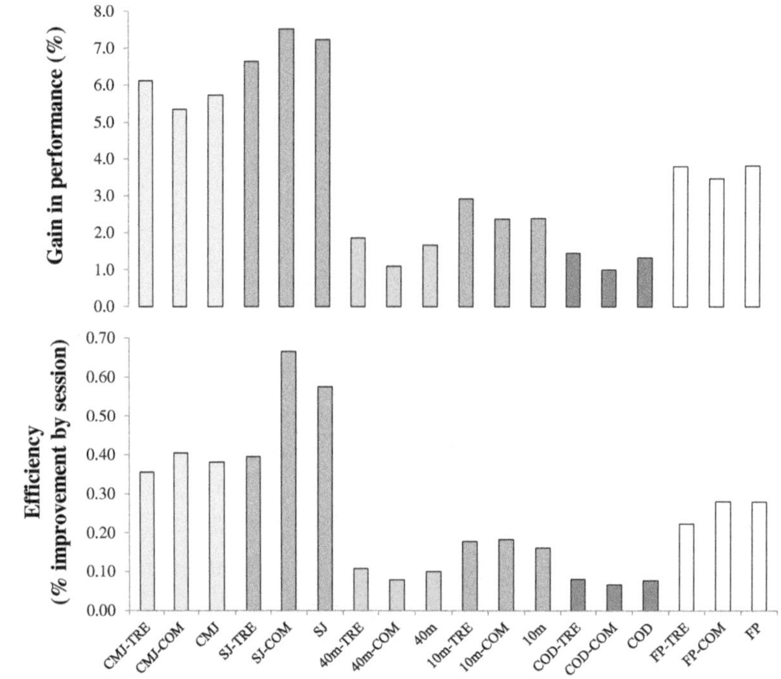

Figure 3 Percentage of improvement by training program and training session. Percentage of improvement by training program and training session after traditional resistance exercises programs (TRE), combined programs (COM), and strength/power training programs in the different motor tasks and overall functional performance (FP) of high-level players. Countermovement jump (CMJ) after TRE (CMJ-TRE) [2,20,37]; CMJ after COM (CMJ-COM) [22,23,38]; CMJ [2,20-23,37,38]; squat jump (SJ) after TRE (SJ-TRE) [1,14]; SJ after COM (SJ-COM) [6,19,22]; SJ [1,6,14,19,22]; 40-m sprint performance after TRE (40m-TRE) [1,2]; 40-m sprint performance after COM (40m-COM) [6]; 40-m sprint performance (40-m) [1,2,6]; 10-m sprint performance after TRE (10m-TRE) [2,20,37]; 10-m sprint performance after COM (10m-COM) [22,38]; 10-m sprint performance (10m) [2,20-22,37,38]; change of direction ability (COD) after TRE (COD-TRE) [2]; COD after COM (COD-COM) [38]; COD [2,38]; FP after TRE (FP-TRE) [1,2,6,14,20,37]; FP after COM (FP-COM) [6,19,22,23,38]; and FP [1,2,6,14,19-23,37,38].

Change of direction speed (COD)

According to the literature, it is difficult to discern which force/power qualities (e.g., horizontal and lateral) and technical factors influence event- or sport-specific COD ability [52]. To date, limited research has been conducted on agility/COD adaptations, with even less known about high-level athletes. Despite the limitations initially described see Introduction our results suggest that, on average, an increase of 15% in 1RM results in a 1.3% improvement in COD abilities after 5 to 6 weeks of training (Table 1; Figure 1 and Additional file 1: Figure S3) [2,38]. Bogdanis et al. [2] observed that applying TRE-targeting hypertrophic or neural adaptations was effective in increasing COD (Table 1, Additional file 1: Figure S3). Nevertheless, improvements in COD performance evaluated by the 505 agility test after different plyometric techniques [16] were not found after CT [19]. Additionally, in a study by Mujika et al. [15] where players performed CT, no improvements in COD, evaluated by the agility 15-m test, were observed. The spectrum of possible factors associated with this discrepancy in results is ample and includes the players' background and initial training status, the different training periods during which the intervention was carried out, the structure of the training intervention, game exposure, and distinct force/power qualities and technical factors that influence event- or sport-specific COD. For example, the study of Maio Alves et al. [19] was implemented during pre-season, and the research of Thomas et al. [16] was carried out during in-season. Consequently, the accumulated effect of COD actions performed during training sessions and games may influence these results [46,53]. Although the players are from the same age groups, the differences in the competitive levels of the players from previous studies should not be ignored. Moreover, the lack of improvements in COD after in-season CT that are reported by Mujika et al. [15] may be related to the fact that only six sessions were performed in a 7-week period. As will be further analyzed ('Training efficiency'), this fact, among others, may suggest that higher training volumes may be necessary to induce adaptations in COD.

Sport-specific skills

One of the most important indicators of a successful soccer kick is the speed of the ball. Studies involving

Table 2 Physiological and functional adaptations to concurrent strength and endurance training

Study	Level/country/*n* (age)	Type of training	D	P	Physiological adaptations	Performance changes
Nunez et al., [13]	Semi-professional/Spain/ 16 (28 ± 3.7)	*ST* and *ET* - a sequence of general, special, and specific exercises incorporated in different training blocks. ET followed the time-line sequence of variable trajectory, medium extensive, intensive, and short intensive intervals. ST followed the sequence of maximal holds, fast holds, horizontal, and vertical jumps. ET block (2 sessions ET + 1 session ST) ST block (1 session ET + 2 session ST)	4 blocks of 12 wks	S		↑ 73% to 80% Probst test ↑ 11.1% to 16.2% SJ ↑ 8% to 8.7% CMJ ↑ 6% to 7% CMJWAS
Wong et al., [20]	Professional/Hong-Kong/ 9 (24.6 ± 1.5)	*ST*: 5 exercises; high-pull, jump squat, bench press, back half-squat, and chin-up; 4 sets at 6RM with 3-min rest between sets)*SE*:16 x 15 s at 120% of MAS with 15-s rest	2×/wk/8 wks	PS		↑ 4% VJ, ↑ 5.9% T_{10m} ↑ 2.8% T_{30m} ↑ 19.7% YYIR1, ↑ 3.1% MAS ↑ 9.2% $MAS_{distance}$
Lopez-Segovia et al., [18]	Elite/Spain/ U-19	*ET*: high-intensity runs, physical-technical circuits and SSG, with maximal intensity during 4-6-min periods.*ST*: jumps with and without external training loads, half-squats and full-squats. The speed of movement ranged from 0.8 to 1.2 $m.s^{-1}$. ST complemented with sprint exercises with loads (5 kg) including change of direction movements, and 15- to 20-m take-offs with resisted sled-towing (10 kg)	2×/wk/16 wks	PS-IS		↑ 6.8% $CMJ_{(20\ kg)}$ ↑ 5.8% $Fsquats_{20kg}$ ↑ 7.1% $Fsquats_{30kg}$ ↑ 5.2% $Fsquats_{40kg}$ ↓ 2.3% T_{20m} ↓ 2.4% T_{30m} ↓ 3.2% $T_{st/10\text{-}20\text{-}m}$ ↓ 1.6% $T_{st/10\text{-}30\text{-}m}$ ↓ 2.6% $T_{st/20\text{-}30\text{-}m}$
Helgerud et al., [37]	Elite/Spain/23 (25; range 20 to 31)	ET: 4 × 4 min at a treadmill (5.5% inclination) 90% to 95% HRmax separated by 3-min jogging at 50% to 60% HRmax ST: 4 sets × 4RM half-squats 90° with 3-min rest between sets	2×/wk/8 wks	PS	↑ 8.6% VO_2 max ↑ 3.7% $RE_{(11km.h)}$ ↑ 52% $1RM_{HS}$ ↑ 49% 1RM/BW	↑ 3.2% T_{10m} ↑ 1.6% T_{20m} ↑ 5.2% CMJ
Jovanovic et al. [24]	Elite junior/Croatia/50 (19)	RST: 2 session a wk targeting the major muscle groups (e.g., legs, back, and chets) with workouts focusing power development (e.g., jump squat, squats, and bench throws) with loads up to 75% to 85% 1RM; SAQ: 3 sessions a wk, work:rest ratio of 3:2; ET: 1 session a wk, 4 × 4 min at 90% to 95% HRmax, 3 min rec 55% to 65% HRmax)	8 wks (1st 8 wks in-season)	IS		↑ 2.1% T_{5m} ↑ 3.7% T_{10m} ↑ 1% CMJ ↑ 0.8% CJS ↔ SJ, maximal CMJ
McGawley and Andersson [38]	Semi-professional and professional players/ Sweden/9 (23 ± 4)	ET + ST Tuesday: RSA + speed endurance (e.g., 2× [7× (30 s on/90 s off)] ~95%, 3-min rest: reps 3 and 6 with ball) + 2nd session: RST (e.g., 3 × 5 cleans, 2 × 10 squats, 3 × 10 nordic hamstrings, 2 × 10 core rotations, 3 × 10 barbell rowing; 75%. 60- to 90-s rest); Thursday: (e.g., 2× [8× 45 s on/12 s off) agility/SAQ circuit] ~95% + 1 session functional strength (e.g., 2 × 8 lunges,	3×/wk/5 wks	PS	↑ 7.6% fat (%) ↑ 6% fat (kg) ↑ 1.5% lean mass (%) ↑ 3% lean mass (kg) ↑ 18.7% 1RM half-squat ↑ 28.5% 1RM lunge ↑ 97.3% iliopsoas (°) ↑ 5.3% hamstrings (°)	↑ 1.4% T_{10m} ↑ 7% CMJ ↑ 1.1% agility ↑ 1.9% RSA ↑ 19.6% perf dec RSA ↑ 15.4% YYIR2 ↑ 65.3% chins ↑ 14.5% hanging sit-ups

Table 2 Physiological and functional adaptations to concurrent strength and endurance training *(Continued)*

		2 × 10 hamstrings kicks, 2 × 8 sideway lunges, 2 × 10 standing chest press, 2 × 10 crunches: 75%, 60 to 90s rest); Friday: (e.g., dribble track 4 × 4 min/3 min active rest; 90% to 95%, alternate ball) + 1 session PT (e.g., 3 × 4 Borzov jumps/3 × 10 core rotations; 3 × 6 bounding jumps/3 × 20 ball bounces; 3 × 15 toe bounding/3 × 20 fast shifting lunges)				
	Semi-professional and professional players/ Sweden/ 9 (23 ± 4)	ST + ET the same daily training but the inverse order (1st, the strength training and after endurance training)	3×/wk/7 wks	PS	↑ 7.1% fat (%) ↑ 5.2% fat (kg) ↑ 1.6% lean (%) ↑ 3.6% lean (kg) ↑ 19.1% 1RM half-squat ↑ 19.1% 1RM lunge ↑ 165.2% iliopsoas (°) ↑ 10.3% hamstrings (°)	↑ 2.2% T_{10m} ↑ 1.9% CMJ ↑ 0.9% agility ↑ 0.8% RSA ↑ 16.8% perf dec RSA ↑ 22.9% YYIR2 ↑ 22.9% chins ↑ 9.7% hanging sit-ups

↑, significant improvement; ↓, significant decrement; ↔, no significant alterations; ~, approximately; NS, not specified; F/D, frequency and duration of training protocols; P, period of the soccer season; ST, strength training; ET, endurance training; SJ, squat jump; CMJ, countermovement jump; CMJWAS, countermovement jump with arm swing; MAS, maximal aerobic speed; VJ, vertical jump; $Fsquats_{(20\text{-}40kg)}$, speed of movement during full squats exercise (range of the external load); $T_{5\text{-}30m}$, sprint performance; $T_{st/10\text{-}30}$, sprint performance in predetermined split distances; VO_2 max, maximal oxygen consumption; RE $_{(11km.h)}$, running economy (velocity); $1RM_{HS}$, one repetition maxim in half-squat strength exercise; 1RM/BW, strength per kilogram of body weight; rec, recovery; CJS, continuous jumps with legs extended; YYIR1, Yo-Yo intermittent recovery level one; $MAS_{distance}$, maximal aerobic distance; SSG, small-sided game; $CMJ_{(20kg)}$, countermovement jump (external load); SAQ, speed, agility and quickness; HRmax, maximal heart rate; IS, performed during in-season; RSA, repeated sprint ability; PT, plyometric training; perf dec RSA, performance decrement in the repeated sprint ability test; YYIR2, Yo-Yo intermittent recovery level 2.

amateur players observed that CT [11] and electrostimulation training [28] increase ball speed with [11,28] and without (Table 1) run up [28]. Nevertheless, these improvements were examined in lower standard players. Moreover, elite U-19 players performing plyometric training increased ball speed with the dominant and non-dominant leg [21]. Other studies involving elite players performing different modes of strength training (isokinetic strength training or functional training) did not report improvements in ball speed [4,5]. Nevertheless, in studies performed during the off-season period, training stimulus consists of the exercise mode of the experimental designs and no other types of soccer routines are undertaken. Thus, the results should be analyzed with caution as the scenarios for training transfer to occur during this period are constricted (off-season); the increases in certain strength parameters were not reflected in positive transference to consecutive gains in ball speed.

Comparing different training variables in strength/power interventions in soccer

The multi-factorial constructs of soccer performance (technical, tactical, and physical performance) and their associated components bring a higher complexity to the designing of the training process. In fact, professionals involved in the preparation of soccer teams have to reflect on several questions associated with the manipulation of the individual variables that affect each of these relevant constructs and how they can affect each other. With regard to physical performance, several potential questions arise: What are the most beneficial movement patterns and type of training? How many sessions do athletes need to improve and maintain the performance outcome? Does ground surface have an effect on adaptations? We will analyze these and other relevant questions in the following sections.

Force production and movement pattern specificity: traditional resistance exercises vs. combined programs

Our analysis suggests that the activity patterns of applied exercises may influence performance outcomes (Figures 2 and 3 and Additional file 1: Figure S4 to S5). Therefore, we compared programs involving mainly traditional resistance exercises (TREs) with programs that combine different activity patterns during the training intervention (COM; programs including TRE and ballistic exercises, plyometrics, weight lifting, body weight exercises, and/or sprint training during training cycles). Despite the fact that some limitations can be ruled out from this type of analysis (e.g., differences in session and weekly training volumes and load, the density of different intrinsic activity patterns, and the 1RM percentage used during the loaded exercises), we believe that it will aid in challenging research designs in this field.

Effects on sprint performance On average, despite TRE resulting in superior strength gains compared with COM, greater performance improvements in the 10-m sprint are observed after COM (TRE = in average, 26.8% increments in 1RM resulted in 1.93% average improvements in 10-m sprint [2,37]; COM = in average, 19.9% increments in 1RM resulted in 2.4% average improvements in 10-m sprint [2,22,38]; Figure 2 and Additional file 1: Figure S5). However, our analysis suggests the opposite with regard to 40-m sprint performance (TRE = in average, 15.8% increments in 1RM resulted in 1.9% average improvements in 40-m time [1,2] COM = in average, 23% increments in 1RM resulted in 1.1% average improvements in 40-m sprint time [6]). Nevertheless, all pooled data suggest that despite the TRE result of greater increases in 1RM (26%) than COM (21%), this may not translate into superior improvements in the sprint performance of high-level players (1.9% TRE vs. 2.1% COM; Additional file 1: Figure S4).

Effects on jump ability By performing the same analysis for jump ability exercises (Figure 2 and Additional file 1: Figure S5), we found that there is a tendency toward greater strength increases after TRE (in average, 26.8% increments in 1RM resulted in 6.8% average improvements in CMJ; in average, 22% increments in 1RM resulted in 6.7% average enhancement in SJ; in average, 25% increments in 1RM resulted in 6% average improvements in 4BT) that are not translated into superior performance gains compared with the results observed following COM (in average, 21% increments of 1RM resulted in 6.8% average improvements in CMJ; in average, 22% increments in 1RM resulted in 6.9% average enhancements in SJ; in average, 22% increments of 1RM resulted in 6.4% average improvements in 4BT). In fact, all pooled data show that greater improvements in jump ability may be obtained with lower strength increases after COM than TRE only (Additional file 1: Figure S5; in average, 21.6% increments in 1RM resulted in 6.4% average improvements in jump ability and a 25% average increments in 1RM resulted in 6% average improvements in jump ability, respectively). This higher efficacy of transfer of strength gains to performance improvements after COM seems to be more evident in SSC jump ability (CMJ). Taking into consideration, among other factors, the described associations between physiological and mechanical characteristics (e.g., post-activation potentiation and peak torque) and CMJ and running-based actions in professional players [44,46,54], this fact may suggest that COM may represent a superior method for improving sport-specific actions compared with TRE alone. Additional studies on this topic are necessary.

Effects on COD ability Given the scarcity of literature assessing the effect of COD training modes and the reported small to moderate associations between strength and power variables with COD performance and different characteristics (e.g., test duration, COD number, and primary application of force throughout the test) of the agility tests commonly used to evaluate COD [52], conclusions should be drawn with caution. In fact, within programs involving only TRE, as will be discussed later in this review ('Manipulation of loading schemes'), it seems that manipulating different mechano-biological descriptors of strength/power stimuli may influence performance adaptations in COD actions [2]. Nevertheless, our analysis shows that, on average, lower strength increases after TRE [2] produce greater performance improvements in the agility *t*-test than after COM [38] (in average, 14.2% increments in 1RM resulted in 1.7% average improvements in *t*-test and a 19.9% average increment in 1RM resulted in 1% average improvement in *t*-test, respectively; Figure 2).

Two studies are particularly relevant with regard to this topic: TRE vs. TRE plus plyometrics [6] and TRE vs. TRE plus sprint training [10]. In the study of Ronnestad et al. [6], although no significant differences between groups were observed, the group of players who utilized combined approaches broadly improved their performance. Additionally, Kotzamanidis et al. [10] observed that the jump and sprint performance of low-level players only improved in the combined program approach. Thus, it seems that combining heavy and light load training schemes may be an effective method for improving muscular function and may be particularly useful when force application is required in a wide range of functional tasks [27].

Training efficiency To estimate the improvement in the different motor tasks and in overall functional performance, as well as the efficiency (efficiency = percentage of improvement/number of training sessions) of strength/power interventions and the effects of the different types of programs (TRE vs. COM) on specific motor tasks and functional performance, we performed an analysis involving all studies in highly trained players where performance outcomes were reported despite no references to changes in force production (Figure 3). Despite the limitations already highlighted, our analysis suggests that even though TRE slightly increases overall functional performance, the efficiency (gains by session) is lower than in COM modes. These uncertainties make this research topic particularly crucial. In summary, considering the high demands of high-level competition, the increase in different motor tasks (1.3% to 7.2%) and overall functional performance (4%) observed in highly trained players following strength/power training programs makes strength/power programs an essential training component. In general, it seems that strength/power training induces greater improvements in jump abilities than in running-based activities. Moreover, combining resistance- and speed-training or plyometric- and soccer-specific strength programs in the same session seems to be more effective than the resistance-training program alone [6,10,48].

Manipulation of loading schemes

Bogdanis et al. [2,3] analyzed the effects of high-repetition/moderate-load (hypertrophy) and low-repetition/high-load (neural adaptations) programs on anthropometric, neuromuscular, and endurance performance. These last studies [2,3] and others [4,5,23] suggest that the manipulation of different mechano-biological descriptors of strength/power stimuli (e.g., load magnitude, number of repetitions) is associated with different physiological and performance adaptations in highly trained soccer players. The hypertrophic mode was associated with increases in lower limb muscle mass, while the neural mode was more effective in improving 1RM/LLV, sprint, and COD performance [2]. In another study, Bogdanis et al. [3] found that even though both groups (hypertrophic group vs. neural group) improved the total work performed during a repeated cycle ergometer sprint test (RST; 10 × 6-s sprint with 24-s passive recovery), the neural mode group had a significantly greater improvement in work capacity during the second half (sprint 6 to 10; 8.9% ± 2.6%) compared with the first half of RST (sprint 1 to 5; 3.2% ± 1.7%). These results suggest that the neural mode confers a higher fatigue resistance during RST [3]. In addition, the mean power output expressed per lean leg volume (MPO/LLV) was better maintained during the last six sprint post-training only in the neural group, and there was no change in MPO/LLV in the hypertrophic group in the RST [3]. These results suggest, at least in part, a better efficacy of neural-based programs in high-level players [2,3] that could be linked to several adaptive mechanisms that are not associated with increases in muscle volume. However, the most likely adaptations are at the neuro-physiological level, i.e., changes in the pattern of motor unit recruitment and increases in rate coding [2,32].

Other researchers observed that physiological and performance outcomes can be independent of the kinetics of the power loading scheme used (from the high-force/low-velocity end to the low-force/high-velocity end and vice versa) because the loading scheme components spanned the optimal power training spectrum [22].

Contraction modes

The analysis of the impact of high- vs. low-intensity isokinetic strength vs. functional strength showed that professional players who performed a high-load, low angular velocity program had a higher improvement in maximal isometric and isokinetic strength and in PP at different knee angles and velocities [4,5]. Although the increases in dynamic muscle strength were generally associated with the specific velocities used in the training programs, the high-load/low-velocity group also exhibited improvements in muscle force and power at high knee extension velocities [4,5]. Although several explanations can be offered to clarify the greater adaptations associated with a wide range of velocities observed after the high-load/low-velocity strength training program, the most likely explanation is the occurrence of changes in neural and morphological factors associated with this type of training (e.g., increases in RFD, muscle mass, and/or fiber pennation angle).

Training frequency

As previously mentioned, high-level soccer players are usually involved in weekly matches of national leagues and are often involved in international commitments, thus limiting the time available for fitness training. Maio Alves et al. [19] found that different weekly volumes (two vs. one session per week) of complex training performed by high-level junior players resulted in similar improvements in sprint, jump, and COD ability. Ronnestad et al. [1] observed that one high-intensity strength training session per week during the first 12 weeks of the in-season period represented a sufficient training stimulus for maintaining the pre-season (two sessions per week for 10 weeks) gains in strength, jump, and sprint performance of professional players. However, a lower weekly in-season volume (one session every two weeks) only prevented detraining in jump performance [1]. Accordingly, a recent study [48] involving a larger sample of players showed that professional teams subject to distinct weekly strength training stress (all performed one resistance strength session a week) exhibit higher neuromuscular performance in the middle of the season than at the start of the season. Nevertheless, only the team that performed a higher number of sessions targeting the neuromuscular system showed improved neuromuscular performance during the second phase of the season. Despite the distinct individual variables that constituted the weekly resistance training session performed by the teams (e.g., percentage of 1RM, number of repetitions and exercises), differences in strength/power training stress were mainly due to the higher employed volume of both soccer-specific strength and sprint sessions [48]. This result again established the important role of the specificity of the training stimulus. Given the important role of circulating levels of androgens in strength and power performance, it is relevant to mention that only the high neuromuscular training scheme positively affected the circulation and activation (increase in 3a Diol G) of the androgen pool (total testosterone) [48].

However, Mujika et al. [15] observed that a low volume of combined forms of strength/power training is more effective in improving sprint performance (15-m sprint time) than the sole performance of lower volumes of sprint training in elite U-19 players.

Manipulation of biomechanical components of plyometric-based exercises

Performance outcomes may also be influenced by the biomechanical nature of the exercises employed in a single or combined program. Los Arcos et al. [23] observed that weight training plus plyometric and functional exercises involving vertically and horizontally oriented movements were more effective in enhancing the CMJ performance of highly trained players than exercises involving purely vertically oriented movements. Nevertheless, both groups improved their PP and showed small, although non-significant, improvements in 5- and 15-m sprint performance [23]. In contrast, Thomas et al. [16] examined that both plyometric training involving drop jumps or CMJs were effective in improving the jump (CMJ) and COD ability (505 agility test) of semi-professional players, regardless of the lack of change in short sprint distances. It is important to highlight that although no between-group differences were reported, the improvements in COD ability were twofold greater in the CMJ group. Nevertheless, given the age group of the players (U-18), it is important to be cautious in extrapolating these findings to professional adult players.

Training surface

There is also evidence that the ground surface used during plyometrics (sand vs. grass) may influence adaptations [12]. Impellizzeri et al. [12] observed that performing plyometrics on grass produced greater effects in CMJ and in the eccentric utilization ratio CMJ/SJ than when performed on sand. However, a trend toward higher adaptations was observed in SJ when the training program was performed on sand (Table 1). Additionally, sand was found to induce lower levels of muscle soreness compared with grass [12]. The fatigue development and recovery kinetics during and after a game have been well characterized in recent years. A reduction in the players' ability to produce force toward the end of the match and in the match recovery period, an increase in some indirect markers of muscle damage, and longer periods of post-match muscle soreness have all been described [55-68]. In light of these findings, it may be expected that sandy surfaces may be a good alternative for the execution of plyometric programs during periods of high-volume, high-intensity, or high-frequency training (e.g., pre-season) and when athletes are recovering from injury and trying to regain physical capacity. In fact, in addition to improving neuromuscular capabilities, sand has been shown to produce lower levels of muscle soreness compared with grass [12]. Accordingly, compared with natural grass or artificial turf, the performance of dynamic powerful actions on sand, despite the known higher energy expenditures and metabolic power values, results in smaller impact shocks and limited stretching of the involved muscles [69].

Interference between concurrent strength and endurance training

Concurrent training involves the incorporation of both resistance and endurance exercises in a designed, periodized training regime [70]. The current dogma is that muscle adaptations to RE are blunted when combined with endurance [71], resulting in lower strength and power gains than those achieved by resistance exercise alone. When the modes of strength and endurance training focus on the same location of adaptation (e.g., peripheral adaptations), the muscle is required to adapt in distinctly different physiological ways [72]. However, when the modes of strength/power and endurance training are at opposite ends of the biomechanical and neuro-coordinative spectrum, the anatomical and performance adaptations may be reduced, and the accuracy of the intended movement, fluidity, and elegance that characterize excellence may be compromised. In fact, it is the entire spectrum of characteristics (e.g., metabolic and neuro-coordinative) of the upstream stimulus (resistance vs. endurance exercise; RE vs. E) that determines the downstream events necessary for training adaptations to occur. The range of factors that may be associated with the interference phenomenon or the incapability of achieving/maintaining higher levels of strength/power during concurrent strength and endurance training is ample and spans from excessive fatigue or increments in catabolic environments to differences in motor unit recruitment patterns, possible shifts in fiber type, and conflicts with the direction of adaptation pathways required by the muscle [34,70,72,73].

Molecular events

RE stimulates a cascade of events leading to the induction or inhibition of muscle atrophy [74]. From a molecular standpoint, these adaptations result from the downstream events promoted by the phosphatidylinositol 3-kinase/protein kinase B/mammalian target of rapamycin (PI3-k/Akt/mTOR) pathway [74,75]. However, three kinases [p38 mitogen-activated protein kinase (MAPK), AMP-activated protein kinase (AMPK), and calmodulin-dependent protein kinase] are particularly relevant in the signaling pathways that mediate skeletal muscle adaptations to endurance-based training [75,76].

A few studies highlight the notion that both translation efficiency and protein synthesis may be compromised due to the incompatibility of the two different intracellular signaling networks, i.e., activation of AMPK during endurance exercise impairs muscle growth by inhibiting mTOR [74,75]. Nevertheless, other studies revealed that endurance performed after RE did not compromise the signaling pathways of RE (mTORC1-S6K1) [71] and may amplify the adaptive response of mitochondrial biogenesis [76]. Moreover, the translational capacity for protein synthesis can be reinforced rather than compromised when aerobic exercise precedes RE and molecular events are not compromised; mTOR and P70S6K shown greater phosphorylation in response to concurrent aerobic exercise compared with RE alone [77]. Furthermore, chronic concurrent aerobic exercise and RE may increase aerobic capacity and promote a greater increase in muscle size than RE alone [78]. Nevertheless, taking into account the complexity and the several molecular interactions that constitute the cascade of events associated with resistance and endurance exercise, conclusions should be drawn with caution. Additionally, studies have been performed primarily in healthy adults (physically active college students, moderately trained and recreationally active subjects) and not high-level athletes; although not universally confirmed, athletes with more extensive training backgrounds may have distinct phenotypes [79-81] and genotypes than normally active subjects [82]. Moreover, to the authors' best knowledge, there is no research concerning how the distinct genotypes that can be found within a high-level group of athletes [82-84] may influence the individual responses to concurrent training.

Methodological considerations

Given the divergent physiological nature of strength and endurance training [34], the methodology applied, the volume and frequency of training, and the target goal all play key roles in increasing the degree of compatibility between these two key physical fitness determinants [34,72]. Slow long-duration sustained aerobic conditioning (SLDC) has been shown to be potentially detrimental to the overall performance of athletes involved in power sports and, for example, may have a negative impact on strength and power development [85]. Excessive training volumes may contribute to high metabolic stress, leading to high levels of substrate depletion and catabolic states (e.g., increased cortisol responses) [85]. Furthermore, SLDC may compromise recovery and regeneration, leading to a progression in the overtraining continuum [85]. Moreover, the high levels of oxidative stress (e.g., damaging proteins, lipids, and DNA) that are associated with high-volume training may increase reactive oxygen species (ROS) production to a level that overcomes the positive adaptations that may be triggered by ROS, i.e., there is a range in which ROS may represent an optimal redox state for greater performance, as with force production capacity [86]. Additionally, these previous factors associated with SLDC that limit force production may compromise skill acquisition by reducing the quality of execution (e.g., the technical ability of force application) and, thus, motor learning [85]. It is reasonable to consider that there may be certain mechanisms associated with the combination of training modalities that produce positive improvements and are additive in nature [87].

A low-volume, high-intensity approach, such as sprint interval training, may favor an anabolic environment (e.g., growth hormone, insulin-like growth factor-I, IGF binding protein-3, and testosterone) [88-92], maintain a muscle fiber phenotype associated with strength and power capabilities [93], and increase endurance and neuromuscular-related outcomes [94-96]. In fact, HIT and/or combined forms of HIT seem to promote adaptations in skeletal muscle and improvements in laboratory and field endurance-related parameters that are comparable to the effects of high-volume endurance training [94,97-101] and may improve muscle power-based actions [94,102]. Interestingly, the type of previously observed hormonal responses to HIT (e.g., sprint interval training) [88-92] constitutes one of the paradigms of resistance exercise biology, namely, an increase in cellular signaling pathways as well as satellite cell activation that contributes to an increase in translation and transcription processes associated with protein synthesis [74]. In this regard, supramaximal interval training is shown to be superior to high-intensity interval training for concurrent improvements in endurance, sprint, and repeated sprint performance in physically active individuals [103].

Does the magnitude of neuromuscular involvement during training sessions reduce possible incompatibilities associated with concurrent training? Are the biomechanical and neuro-coordinative demands (e.g., accelerations/decelerations impacting mechanical load and neuromuscular demands) of different training modes with similar physiological responses the same (e.g., 4 × 4-min interval running with 2-min rest vs. 4 × 4-min SSG with 2-min rest vs. 4 × 4-min intermittent situational drill with 2-min rest)? It is possible that, from a biomechanical and neuromuscular standpoint, more specific training methods to develop strength/power and endurance performance with higher biomechanical and neuromuscular demands may improve both adaptations and performance outcomes, as well as reduce the negative effect of this interference from a molecular point of view; human-based studies to date are far from agreement regarding the molecular interference after acute concurrent exercise [70]. In fact, strength/power and HIT are characterized by brief intermittent bouts of intense muscle contractions. Questions related to training transfer should be observed with greater attention when extrapolating the applicability of concurrent training to sport-specific settings. In fact, several factors can influence the transfer of strength training in endurance performance and the impact of endurance workloads on strength and power performances [104].

Soccer: a concurrent modality

A soccer player's performance is intimately associated with the efficiency of different energy-related systems [105-107]. During the season, players perform intense programs with multiple goals of increasing strength, power, speed, speed endurance, agility, aerobic fitness, and game skills [108]. In fact, despite the predominant activity patterns of the game being aerobic in nature, the most deterministic factors of match outcome depend on anaerobic mechanisms [41]. It is common sense that the most intense match periods and worst-case match scenarios are associated with periods of high mechanical and metabolic stress. In fact, recently developed techniques of match analysis provide a body of evidence that supports the belief that neuromuscular demands of training and competition are higher than initially suspected (e.g., accelerations/decelerations) [42,43,109] and give further support to the viewpoint that strength/power-related qualities are crucial for high-level performance.

There is a belief that by stressing the neuromuscular system, adaptive mechanisms that are neurological, morphological, and biomechanical in nature will be triggered, thus increasing the player's neuromuscular performance and providing him/her with a superior short- and long-term endurance capacity [17,110-113]. In this regard, associations between neuromuscular qualities (e.g., CMJ peak power) and intermittent endurance exercise [114] and repeated sprint ability performance [115] have also been observed. Moreover, there has been evidence supporting the association between team success and jump abilities (e.g., CMJ and SJ) [116]. Additionally, starter players demonstrate higher strength [108] and power performance capabilities than non-starters [117], and greater neuromuscular capabilities have been associated with game-related physical parameters and lower fatigue development during matches [118]. Moreover, Meister et al. [119] observed that after a match congestion period, players with a higher exposure time show better scores in certain neuromuscular parameters (CMJ, drop jump height, and drop jump contact) than players with a lower exposure time, although this result is not significant. Interestingly, recent reports revealed that neuromuscular-based actions, such as sprinting, have improved more in recent years than physiological endurance parameters. Professional players tested during the 2006 to 2012 seasons actually had a 3.2% lower VO_2 max than those tested during 2000 to 2006 [120,121]. Although with the obvious limitations and the universal consensus of the importance of aerobic fitness in soccer, these observations suggest that anaerobic power is *'stealing space'* from aerobic power with regard to the constructs relevant in soccer performance. All of these previous facts highlight the role of neuromuscular exercise during soccer training and suggest that soccer routines should be performed concurrently as they are concurrent by nature. In fact, the physiological systems associated with endurance fitness development and maintenance are generally largely targeted in any match competition, friendly game, tactical exercise, circuit technical drills that often involve frequent displacements, and/or small side game exercises performed during a 90-min soccer competition/training session [106,122,123].

Physiological and performance adaptations

The summary of changes in physiological and functional parameters resulting from concurrent strength and endurance training are presented in Table 2. Wong et al. [20] observed that 8 weeks of pre-season high-intensity strength training and SE resulted in a significant improvement in endurance markers, soccer-specific endurance (SSE), and soccer-specific neuromuscular (SSN) parameters. Helgerud et al. found that 8 weeks of other modes of HIT (aerobic high-intensity training) and high-intensity strength training during the preseason of non-elite [51] and elite [37] football players improved VO_2 max (8.6% and 8.9%), running economy (3.5% and 4.7%), and 1RM during half-squat strength exercise (52%), respectively. Moreover, the 10- and 20-m sprint performance (3.2% and 1.6%, respectively) and CMJ (5.2%) of elite players also improved [37]. These strength improvements occurred with minor increases in body mass (average 1%) and a substantial increase in relative strength [37]. More recently, McGawley et al. [38] found that a high-frequency program (three times a week) of concurrent high-intensity running-based training with strength/power-based training in the same session resulted in a positive training effect on all evaluated measures, ranging from flexibility, anthropometric, endurance, and neuromuscular-related parameters (Table 2). Moreover, these results suggested that the order of completion of the program, E + RE or RE + E, did not influence the performance adaptations. These results [38] and others [2,37] may support, at least in part, the better compatibility between high-intensity modes of strength and endurance training.

It is reasonable to assume that the players in the studies examining the effects of strength training programs (Table 1) had performed training with significantly high weekly endurance-based loads (e.g., preseason). In this regard, Bogdanis et al. [3], when examining the strength training effects of the hypertrophic and neural modes in professional soccer players during pre-season, reported that the weekly cycle also involved a considerable amount of interval training and small-sided games, which have been described as effective methodologies targeting endurance fitness and SSE development (for a review, see [95,122]). The authors [3] observed that both aerobic fitness parameters (e.g., VO_2 max and MAS) and SSE, evaluated by the Yo-Yo intermittent endurance test and Hoff's dribbling track test, respectively, were significantly improved in both groups (Table 1). Furthermore, other researchers [23] found that strength/power training performed in parallel with endurance training resulted in improvements in the individual anaerobic threshold and muscle/power parameters. Additionally, the performance of explosive-type strength training with routine soccer training did not interfere with the aerobic capacity of amateur young players [8], e.g., sub-maximal blood lactate values. These findings suggest that performing concurrent strength/power training and routine soccer training is advisable because, in addition to an increase in neuromuscular performance and the anabolic environment, this training did not interfere with the development of aerobic capacity [8]. Nevertheless, the question of whether this compatibility is related to the type of endurance and strength performed is highlighted in the distinct between-group results presented in the study of Bogdanis et al. [3], e.g., point 'Manipulation of loading schemes', where only the neural group significantly improved with respect to running economy and a trend toward a better performance in the YYIE2 in the neural group than in the hypertrophic group was reported.

In another study [13], semi-professional male soccer players performed both endurance and strength sessions as part of the annual periodization (four cycles of 12 weeks). This type of periodization was effective in improving both the endurance performance (Probst test) and SSN parameters, e.g., CMJ. These results suggested that no adaptation conflicts occur when one or two sessions of strength/power and endurance are simultaneously combined during a soccer training cycle (endurance block composed of two endurance training sessions and one strength training session and vice versa).

Additionally, Lopez-Segovia et al. [18] examined training adaptations in elite U-19 players during a 4-month period. The training program consisted of four sessions per week, targeting the improvement of player's aerobic performance. Training was complemented with one or two specific strength training sessions per week performed at the start of the training session. This type of periodization improved loaded CMJ performance and the speed of movement in full squats, with loads ranging from 20 to 40 kg. Nevertheless, significant decrements in different sprint abilities were found. According to the researchers, the lack of improvement in the former sprint variables was attributed to the high volume of aerobic work performed.

Nevertheless, an increase in MAS (3.2%) was observed after the intervention period [18].

Conclusions

Our analysis suggests that, independent of the methodology applied (Table 1) and the form of concurrent endurance and strength/power training (Table 2), pre-season training resulted in an improvement in physiological and soccer-specific and non-specific performance parameters. The large responsiveness to training may be associated with the fact that most of the studies were conducted during an early stage of pre-season, with off-season detraining negatively affecting several physical attributes, such as anthropometric characteristics (e.g., decreases in LBM and increases in BF) [124-126], endurance-related markers [53,101,126,127], soccer-specific endurance [101,128], and neuromuscular parameters [126,129]. With this in mind, the overall conclusion of the analyzed literature is that the addition of strength/power training programs to routine soccer training favors a more integral physical fitness development of the player. The associated improvements in physiological (e.g., 1RM/LLV, PP) and performance (e.g., jump, sprint, COD) parameters may, at least in part, increase a player's ability to cope with training and competition demands. Our analysis suggests that high-intensity strength training (HIST) may be a more efficient method than moderate-intensity methods (hypertrophic). In addition, the compatibility between strength and endurance training may be greater when high-intensity or explosive strength training is combined with high-intensity endurance training to favor a more soccer-specific phenotype.

One of the most sensitive periods of training implementation is the in-season period. As the match is the most important part of the soccer-training schedule, technical staff often view the in-season periodization with particular prudence. They want to maintain or even increase the pre-season gains obtained throughout the short pre-season period (5 to 7 weeks). However, they face the constant dilemma of determining the proper dose/response that allows for the cycle of training-recovering/competing-recovering to be effective; a high volume of training and/or competition interspersed by insufficient recovery favors fatigue development [130], resulting in a transition from a functional to a non-functional overreaching state or, in more severe cases, an overtraining state [131,132]. Unfortunately, studies implemented during in-season are scarce [1,8,13-16,18,21,24,28,48]; seven were conducted with U-19 players, and only four were conducted with adult soccer players [1,13,28,48]. Our analysis suggests that two weekly sessions allow for highly trained players to obtain significant performance enhancements and that one session a week is sufficient to avoid in-season detraining. It may be possible that, in parallel with a higher volume of neuromuscular training (soccer-specific strength/power-based efforts), further in-season improvements could be observed. Moreover, manipulations of the training surface could constitute an important strategy (e.g., players returning from injury and the management of biochemical and perceptual disturbances).

We found that the results of high-force increments vs. low-performance enhancements and the respective efficiency of the programs (jump vs. running-based actions and non-SSC abilities (SJ) vs. SSC-based actions (e.g., CMJ)) suggest that current approaches may overlook some essential aspects required to achieve an increase in a player's performance capacities. According to Komi [133], an effective SSC is obtained with 'a well-timed pre-activation of the muscle(s) before the eccentric phase, a short and fast eccentric phase, and an immediate transition (short delay) between stretch (eccentric) and shortening (concentric phase).' The observed increments in force production will most likely occur to a greater extent in the positive phase of the SSC. We suggest that to achieve greater improvements, weight training should be combined with more soccer-specific strength exercises (e.g., the player's ability to use strength and power effectively and consistently [134], allowing for the application of force/power in a larger range of planes (horizontal) and specific angles). Therefore, a conditioning method such as Speed, Agility and Quickness (SAQ) may be useful, as it incorporates plyometric and soccer-specific strength exercises and can, therefore, constitute a good conditioning tool for this type of outcome (acting on the entire spectrum of the SSC and on the transition from eccentric to concentric movements; it should be kept in mind that plyometric training is a technique demonstrated to increase musculo-tendinous stiffness, which can optimize power output in explosive movements) [135]. The greater ecological validity of COM approaches make combined methods a preferred training strategy for strength training in soccer; targeting the intra- and inter-muscular aspects of athletic performance should occur in parallel and begin at the start of the preparation period. In fact, hypertrophy and general power exercises can enhance sports performance, but optimal transfer from football-specific activities also requires football-specific exercise programs [29] in which the biomechanical and neuro-coordinative patterns of sport-specific motor tasks are taxed.

In summary, the analyzed literature suggests that the training of neuromuscular function and its combination with soccer-specific endurance results in improvements in non-specific (e.g., anthropometric characteristics, relative strength, and VO_2 max) and soccer-specific endurance and neuromuscular parameters (e.g., YYIER, RSA, and sprint).

Additional file

Additional file 1: Figure S1. The gains in strength and sprint performance of high-level players after 5 to 10 weeks. Squares represent the 10-m distance [2,22,37,38]; circles represent the 20-m distance [37]; rhombi represent the 40-m distance [1,2,6]; + symbols represent the average of all distances; triangles represent the average of the 10-m distance; and lines represent the average of the 40-m distance. **Figure S2.** The gains in strength and jump performance of high-level players after 6 to 10 weeks. Squares represent the squat jump performance (SJ) [1,6,14,22]; triangles represent the countermovement jump (CMJ) performance [2,22,37]; rhombi represent the four bounce test (4BT) performance [6]; lines represent the five jump test [14]; circles represent the average CMJ; x symbols represent the average SJ performance; and + symbols represent the average 4BT performance. **Figure S3.** The gains in strength and change of direction ability of high-level players after 5 to 6 weeks. Squares represent the *t*-test performance [2,38]; circles represent the Zig-Zag test performance [2]; and rhombi represent the Illinois agility test performance [2]. Red-filled triangles represent average of all tests. **Figure S4.** The gains in strength and overall sprint performance of high-level players following traditional resistance exercise programs (TRE; 6 to 10 weeks) and combined programs (COM; 5 to 7 weeks). Filled circles represent the TRE results; empty circles represent the COM results; red-filled circles represent the average TRE [1,2,37]; empty red circles represent the average COM [6,22,38]. **Figure S5.** The gains in strength and overall jump ability of high-level players following traditional resistance exercise programs (TRE; 6 to 10 weeks) and combined programs (COM; 6 to 7 weeks). Blue-filled and unfilled triangles represent the countermovement jump (CMJ) results after TRE and COM, respectively; red-filled and unfilled triangles represent the squat jump (SJ) results after TRE and COM, respectively; green-filled and unfilled triangles represent the four bounce test (4BT) results after TRE and COM, respectively; yellow-filled triangles represent the five jump test (5JT) results after TRE; blue-filled and unfilled circles represent the average CMJ results after TRE [2,37] and COM [22], respectively; red-filled and unfilled circles represent the average SJ results after TRE [1,14] and COM [6,22], respectively; black-filled and unfilled circles represent the average overall jump ability increases after TRE [1,2,6,14,37] and COM [6,22], respectively.

Competing interests
The authors declare that they have no competing interests.

Authors' contributions
All authors read and approved the final manuscript.

Acknowledgments
No funding was used to assist in the preparation of this review.

References
1. Ronnestad BR, Nymark BS, Raastad T. Effects of in-season strength maintenance training frequency in professional soccer players. J Strength Cond Res. 2011;25(10):2653–60.
2. Bogdanis GC, Papaspyrou A, Souglis A, Theos A, Sotiropoulos A, Maridaki M. Effects of hypertrophy and a maximal strength training programme on speed, force and power of soccer players. In: Reilly T, Korkusuz F, editors. Science and Football VI. The proceedings of the sixth world congress on science and football. New York: Routledge; 2009. p. 290–5.
3. Bogdanis GC, Papaspyrou A, Souglis AG, Theos A, Sotiropoulos A, Maridaki M. Effects of Two Different Half-Squat Training Programs on Fatigue During Repeated Cycling Sprints in Soccer Players, Journal of strength and conditioning research / National Strength & Conditioning Association. 2011. May 12.
4. Aagaard P, Trolle M, Simonsen E, Bangsbo J, Klausen K. High speed knee extension capacity of soccer players after different kinds of strength trainning. In: Reilly T, Clarys J, Stibbe A, editors. Science and Footbal II. London: F & FN Spon; 1993. p. 92–4.
5. Trolle M, Aagaard P, Simonsen E, Bangsbo J, Klausen K. Effects of strength trainning on kicking performance in soccer. In: Reilly T, Clarys J, Stibbe A, editors. Science and Footbal II. London: F & FN Spon; 1993. p. 95–7.
6. Ronnestad BR, Kvamme NH, Sunde A, Raastad T. Short-term effects of strength and plyometric training on sprint and jump performance in professional soccer players. J Strength Cond Res. 2008;22(3):773–80.
7. Andersen JL, Klitgaard H, Bangsbo J, Saltin B. Myosin heavy chain isoforms in single fibres from m. vastus lateralis of soccer players: effects of strength-training. Acta Physiol Scand. 1994;150(1):21–6.
8. Gorostiaga EM, Izquierdo M, Ruesta M, Iribarren J, Gonzalez-Badillo JJ, Ibanez J. Strength training effects on physical performance and serum hormones in young soccer players. Eur J Appl Physiol. 2004;91(5–6):698–707.
9. Hoff J, Helgerud J. Endurance and strength training for soccer players: physiological considerations. Sports Med. 2004;34(3):165–80.
10. Kotzamanidis C, Chatzopoulos D, Michailidis C, Papaiakovou G, Patikas D. The effect of a combined high-intensity strength and speed training program on the running and jumping ability of soccer players. J Strength Cond Res. 2005;19(2):369–75.
11. Manolopoulos E, Papadopoulos C, Kellis E. Effects of combined strength and kick coordination training on soccer kick biomechanics in amateur players. Scand J Med Sci Sports. 2006;16(2):102–10.
12. Impellizzeri FM, Rampinini E, Castagna C, Martino F, Fiorini S, Wisloff U. Effect of plyometric training on sand versus grass on muscle soreness and jumping and sprinting ability in soccer players. Br J Sports Med. 2008;42(1):42–6.
13. Nunez VM, Da Silva-Grigoletto ME, Castillo EF, Poblador MS, Lancho JL. Effects of training exercises for the development of strength and endurance in soccer. J Strength Cond Res. 2008;22(2):518–24.
14. Chelly MS, Fathloun M, Cherif N, Ben Amar M, Tabka Z, Van Praagh E. Effects of a back squat training program on leg power, jump, and sprint performances in junior soccer players. J Strength Cond Res. 2009;23(8):2241–9.
15. Mujika I, Santisteban J, Castagna C. In-season effect of short-term sprint and power training programs on elite junior soccer players. J Strength Cond Res. 2009;23(9):2581–7.
16. Thomas K, French D, Hayes PR. The effect of two plyometric training techniques on muscular power and agility in youth soccer players. J Strength Cond Res. 2009;23(1):332–5.
17. Aagaard P, Andersen JL. Effects of strength training on endurance capacity in top-level endurance athletes. Scand J Med Sci Sports. 2010;20:39–47.
18. Lopez-Segovia M, Palao Andres JM, Gonzalez-Badillo JJ. Effect of 4 months of training on aerobic power, strength, and acceleration in two under-19 soccer teams. J Strength Cond Res. 2010;24(10):2705–14.
19. Maio Alves JM, Rebelo AN, Abrantes C, Sampaio J. Short-term effects of complex and contrast training in soccer players' vertical jump, sprint, and agility abilities. J Strength Cond Res. 2010;24(4):936–41.
20. Wong PL, Chaouachi A, Chamari K, Dellal A, Wisloff U. Effect of preseason concurrent muscular strength and high-intensity interval training in professional soccer players. J Strength Cond Res. 2010;24(3):653–60.
21. Sedano S, Matheu A, Redondo JC, Cuadrado G. Effects of plyometric training on explosive strength, acceleration capacity and kicking speed in young elite soccer players. J Sports Med Phys Fitness. 2011;51(1):50–8.
22. Loturco I, Ugrinowitsch C, Tricoli V, Pivetti B, Roschel H. Different loading schemes in power training during the preseason promote similar performance improvements in Brazilian elite soccer players. J Strength Cond Res. 2013;27(7):1791–7.
23. Los Arcos A, Yanci J, Mendiguchia J, Salinero JJ, Brughelli M, Castagna C. Short-term training effects of vertically and horizontally oriented exercises on neuromuscular performance in professional soccer players. Int J Sports Physiol Perform. 2014;9(3):480–8.
24. Jovanovic M, Sporis G, Omrcen D, Fiorentini F. Effects of speed, agility, quickness training method on power performance in elite soccer players. J Strength Cond Res. 2011;25(5):1285–92.
25. Ebben WP, Watts P. A review of combined weight training and plyometric training modes: Complex training. Strength Cond J. 1998;20:18–27.
26. Saez de Villarreal E, Requena B, Izquierdo M, Gonzalez-Badillo JJ. Enhancing sprint and strength performance: combined versus maximal power, traditional heavy-resistance and plyometric training. J Sci Med. 2013;16(2):146–50.
27. Harris N, Cronin J, Keogh J. Contraction force specificity and its relationship to functional performance. J Sports Sci. 2007;25(2):201–12.
28. Billot M, Martin A, Paizis C, Cometti C, Babault N. Effects of an electrostimulation training program on strength, jumping, and kicking capacities in soccer players. J Strength Cond Res. 2010;24(5):1407–13.
29. Young W. Transfer of strength and power training to sports performance. Int J Sports Physiol Perform. 2006;1:74–83.

30. Schmidtbleicher D. Training for power events. In: Chem PV, editor. Strength and Power in Sports. Boston: Blackwell Scientific; 1992. p. 381-95
31. Cormie P, McGuigan MR, Newton RU. Developing maximal neuromuscular power: Part 1–biological basis of maximal power production. Sports Med. 2011;41(1):17–38.
32. Gabriel DA, Kamen G, Frost G. Neural adaptations to resistive exercise: mechanisms and recommendations for training practices. Sports Med. 2006;36(2):133–49.
33. Toigo M, Boutellier U. New fundamental resistance exercise determinants of molecular and cellular muscle adaptations. Eur J Appl Physiol. 2006;97(6):643–63.
34. Hakkinen K, Alen M, Kraemer WJ, Gorostiaga E, Izquierdo M, Rusko H, et al. Neuromuscular adaptations during concurrent strength and endurance training versus strength training. Eur J Appl Physiol. 2003;89(1):42–52.
35. Hakkinen K, Komi PV, Alen M. Effect of explosive type strength training on isometric force- and relaxation-time, electromyographic and muscle fibre characteristics of leg extensor muscles. Acta Physiol Scand. 1985;125(4):587–600.
36. Aagaard P, Simonsen EB, Andersen JL, Magnusson P, Dyhre-Poulsen P. Increased rate of force development and neural drive of human skeletal muscle following resistance training. J Appl Physiol. 2002;93(4):1318–26.
37. Helgerud J, Rodas G, Kemi OJ, Hoff J. Strength and endurance in elite football players. Int J Sports Med. 2011;32(9):677–82.
38. McGawley K, Andersson PI. The order of concurrent training does not affect soccer-related performance adaptations. Int J Sports Med. 2013;34(11):983–90.
39. Requena B, Gonzalez-Badillo JJ, de Villareal ES, Ereline J, Garcia I, Gapeyeva H, et al. Functional performance, maximal strength, and power characteristics in isometric and dynamic actions of lower extremities in soccer players. J Strength Cond Res. 2009;23(5):1391–401.
40. Cometti G, Maffiuletti NA, Pousson M, Chatard JC, Maffulli N. Isokinetic Strength and Anaerobic Power of Elite, Subelite and Amateur Soccer Players. Int J Sports Med. 2001;22:45–51.
41. Faude O, Koch T, Meyer T. Straight sprinting is the most frequent action in goal situations in professional football. J Sports Sci. 2012;30(7):625–31.
42. Osgnach C, Poser S, Bernardini R, Rinaldo R, di Prampero PE. Energy cost and metabolic power in elite soccer: a new match analysis approach. Med Sci Sports Exerc. 2010;42(1):170–8.
43. Gaudino P, Iaia FM, Alberti G, Strudwick AJ, Atkinson G, Gregson W. Monitoring training in elite soccer players: systematic bias between running speed and metabolic power data. Int J Sports Med. 2013;34(11):963–8.
44. Wisloff U, Castagna C, Helgerud J, Jones R, Hoff J. Strong correlation of maximal squat strength with sprint performance and vertical jump height in elite soccer players. Br J Sports Med. 2004;38(3):285–8.
45. Keiner M, Sander A, Wirth K, Schmidtbleicher D. Long-term strength training effects on change-of-direction sprint performance. J Strength Cond Res. 2014;28(1):223–31.
46. Silva JR, Magalhaes JF, Ascensao AA, Oliveira EM, Seabra AF, Rebelo AN. Individual match playing time during the season affects fitness-related parameters of male professional soccer players. J Strength Cond Res. 2011;25(10):2729–39.
47. Dauty M, Potiron Josse M. Correlations and differences of performance between soccer players, professionals, young players and amateurs, from the 10-meter sprint test and knee isokinetic assessment. Sci Sports. 2004;19:75–9.
48. Koundourakis NE, Androulakis N, Spyridaki EC, Castanas E, Malliaraki N, Tsatsanis C, et al. Effect of different seasonal strength training protocols on circulating androgen levels and performance parameters in professional soccer players. Hormones. 2014;13(1):578–83.
49. Sander A, Keiner M, Wirth K, Schmidtbleicher D. Influence of a 2-year strength training programme on power performance in elite youth soccer players. Eur J Sport Sci. 2013;13(5):445–51.
50. Salaj S, Markovic G. Specificity of jumping, sprinting, and quick change-of-direction motor abilities. J Strength Cond Res. 2011;25(5):1249–55.
51. Helgerud J, Kemi OJ, Hoff J. Pre-season concurrent strength and endurance development in elite soccer players. In: Hoff J, Helgerud J, editors. Football (soccer): new developments in physical training research. Trondheim: NTNU; 2002. p. 55–66.
52. Brughelli M, Cronin J, Levin G, Chaouachi A. Understanding change of direction ability in sport: a review of resistance training studies. Sports Med. 2008;38(12):1045–63.
53. Caldwell BP, Peters DM. Seasonal variation in physiological fitness of a semiprofessional soccer team. J Strength Cond Res. 2009;23(5):1370–7.
54. Requena B, Saez-Saezde Villarreal E, Gapeyeva H, Ereline J, Garcia I, Paasuke M. Relationship between postactivation potentiation of knee extensor muscles, sprinting and vertical jumping performance in professional soccer players. J Strength Cond Res. 2011;25(2):367–73.
55. Reilly T, Rigby M. Effect of an warm-down following competitive soccer. In: Spinks W, Reilly T, Murphy J, editors. Science and Football IV. London/New York: E&F. N. Spon; 2002. p. 226–9.
56. Mohr M, Krustrup P, Bangsbo J. Fatigue in soccer: a brief review. J Sports Sci. 2005;23(6):593–9.
57. Bangsbo J, Iaia FM, Krustrup P. Metabolic response and fatigue in soccer. Int J Sports Physiol Perform. 2007;2(2):111–27.
58. Reilly T, Drust B, Clarke N. Muscle fatigue during football match-play. Sports Med. 2008;38(5):357–67.
59. Rampinini E, Bosio A, Ferraresi I, Petruolo A, Morelli A, Sassi A. Match-related fatigue in soccer players. Med Sci Sports Exerc. 2011;43(11):2161–70.
60. Magalhaes J, Rebelo A, Oliveira E, Silva JR, Marques F, Ascensao A. Impact of Loughborough Intermittent Shuttle Test versus soccer match on physiological, biochemical and neuromuscular parameters. Eur J Appl Physiol. 2010;108(1):39–48.
61. Rebelo N, Krustrup P, Soares J, Bangsbo J. Reduction in intermittent exercise performance during a soccer match. J Sport Sci. 1998;16:482–3.
62. Silva JR, Ascensao A, Marques F, Seabra A, Rebelo A, Magalhaes J. Neuromuscular function, hormonal and redox status and muscle damage of professional soccer players after a high-level competitive match. Eur J Appl Physiol. 2013;113(9):2193–201.
63. Krustrup P, Ortenblad N, Nielsen J, Nybo L, Gunnarsson TP, Iaia FM, et al. Maximal voluntary contraction force, SR function and glycogen resynthesis during the first 72 h after a high-level competitive soccer game. Eur J Appl Physiol. 2011;111(12):2987–95.
64. Thompson D, Nicholas CW, Williams C. Muscular soreness following prolonged intermittent high-intensity shuttle running. J Sports Sci. 1999;17(5):387–95.
65. Rahnama N, Reilly T, Lees A, Graham-Smith P. Muscle fatigue induced by exercise simulating the work rate of competitive soccer. J Sports Sci. 2003;21(11):933–42.
66. Andersson H, Raastad T, Nilsson J, Paulsen G, Garthe I, Kadi F. Neuromuscular fatigue and recovery in elite female soccer: effects of active recovery. Med Sci Sports Exerc. 2008;40(2):372–80.
67. Greig M. The influence of soccer-specific fatigue on peak isokinetic torque production of the knee flexors and extensors. Am J Sports Med. 2008;36(7):1403–9.
68. Ispirlidis I, Fatouros IG, Jamurtas AZ, Nikolaidis MG, Michailidis I, Douroudos I, et al. Time-course of changes in inflammatory and performance responses following a soccer game. Clin J Sports Med J Acad Sport Med. 2008;18(5):423–31.
69. Gaudino P, Gaudino C, Alberti G, Minetti AE. Biomechanics and predicted energetics of sprinting on sand: hints for soccer training. J Sci Med Sport. 2013;16(3):271–5.
70. Fyfe JJ, Bishop DJ, Stepto NK. Interference between concurrent resistance and endurance exercise: molecular bases and the role of individual training variables. Sports Med. 2014;44(6):743–62.
71. Apro W, Wang L, Ponten M, Blomstrand E, Sahlin K. Resistance exercise induced mTORC1 signaling is not impaired by subsequent endurance exercise in human skeletal muscle. Am J Physiol Endocrinol Metab. 2013;305(1):E22–32.
72. Docherty D, Sporer B. A proposed model for examining the interference phenomenon between concurrent aerobic and strength training. Sports Med. 2000;30(6):385–94.
73. Kraemer WJ, Patton JF, Gordon SE, Harman EA, Deschenes MR, Reynolds K, et al. Compatibility of high-intensity strength and endurance training on hormonal and skeletal muscle adaptations. J Appl Physiol. 1995;78(3):976–89.
74. Spiering BA, Kraemer WJ, Anderson JM, Armstrong LE, Nindl BC, Volek JS, et al. Resistance exercise biology: manipulation of resistance exercise programme variables determines the responses of cellular and molecular signalling pathways. Sports Med. 2008;38(7):527–40.
75. Hawley JA. Molecular responses to strength and endurance training: are they incompatible? Appl Physiol Nutr Metab. 2009;34(3):355–61.
76. Wang L, Mascher H, Psilander N, Blomstrand E, Sahlin K. Resistance exercise enhances the molecular signaling of mitochondrial biogenesis induced by endurance exercise in human skeletal muscle. J Appl Physiol. 2011;111(5):1335–44.
77. Lundberg TR, Fernandez-Gonzalo R, Gustafsson T, Tesch PA. Aerobic exercise alters skeletal muscle molecular responses to resistance exercise. Med Sci Sports Exerc. 2012;44(9):1680–8.
78. Lundberg TR, Fernandez-Gonzalo R, Gustafsson T, Tesch PA. Aerobic exercise does not compromise muscle hypertrophy response to short-term resistance training. J Appl Physiol. 2013;114(1):81–9.

79. Edwards AM, Clark NA. Thermoregulatory observations in soccer match play: professional and recreational level applications using an intestinal pill system to measure core temperature. Br J Sports Med. 2006;40(2):133–8.
80. Cazzola R, Russo-Volpe S, Cervato G, Cestaro B. Biochemical assessments of oxidative stress, erythrocyte membrane fluidity and antioxidant status in professional soccer players and sedentary controls. Eur J Clin Invest. 2003;33(10):924–30.
81. Brites FD, Evelson PA, Christiansen MG, Nicol MF, Basilico MJ, Wikinski RW, et al. Soccer players under regular training show oxidative stress but an improved plasma antioxidant status. Clin Sci (Lond). 1999;96(4):381–5.
82. Egorova ES, Borisova AV, Mustafina LJ, Arkhipova AA, Gabbasov RT, Druzhevskaya AM, et al. The polygenic profile of Russian football players. J Sports Sci. 2014;32(13):1286–93.
83. Pimenta EM, Coelho DB, Veneroso CE, Barros Coelho EJ, Cruz IR, Morandi RF, et al. Effect of ACTN3 Gene on Strength and Endurance in Soccer Players. J Strength Cond Res. 2013;27(12):3286–92.
84. Mustafina LJ, Naumov VA, Cieszczyk P, Popov DV, Lyubaeva EV, Kostryukova ES, et al. AGTR2 gene polymorphism is associated with muscle fibre composition, athletic status and aerobic performance. Exp Physiol. 2014;99(8):1042–52.
85. Elliott MC, Wagner PP, Chiu L. Power athletes and distance training: physiological and biomechanical rationale for change. Sports Med. 2007;37(1):47–57.
86. Reid MB. Invited Review: redox modulation of skeletal muscle contraction: what we know and what we don't. J Appl Physiol. 2001;90(2):724–31.
87. McNamara JM, Stearne DJ. Effect of concurrent training, flexible nonlinear periodization, and maximal-effort cycling on strength and power. J Strength Cond Res. 2013;27(6):1463–70.
88. Meckel Y, Nemet D, Bar-Sela S, Radom-Aizik S, Cooper DM, Sagiv M, et al. Hormonal and inflammatory responses to different types of sprint interval training. J Strength Cond Res. 2011;25(8):2161–9.
89. Wahl P. Hormonal and Metabolic Responses to High Intensity Interval Training. J Sports Med Doping Stud. 2013;3(1):e132.
90. Wahl P, Mathes S, Achtzehn S, Bloch W, Mester J. Active vs. passive recovery during high-intensity training influences hormonal response. Int J Sports Med. 2014;35(7):583–9.
91. Wahl P, Mathes S, Kohler K, Achtzehn S, Bloch W, Mester J. Acute metabolic, hormonal, and psychological responses to different endurance training protocols. Horm Metab Res. 2013;45(11):827–33.
92. Zinner C, Wahl P, Achtzehn S, Reed JL, Mester J. Acute hormonal responses before and after 2 weeks of HIT in well trained junior triathletes. Int J Sports Med. 2014;35(4):316–22.
93. Gunnarsson TP, Christensen PM, Holse K, Christiansen D, Bangsbo J. Effect of additional speed endurance training on performance and muscle adaptations. Med Sci Sports Exerc. 2012;44(10):1942–8.
94. Ingebrigtsen J, Shalfawi SA, Tonnessen E, Krustrup P, Holtermann A. Performance effects of 6 weeks of aerobic production training in junior elite soccer players. J Strength Cond Res. 2013;27(7):1861–7.
95. Iaia FM, Rampinini E, Bangsbo J. High-intensity training in football. Int J Sports Physiol Perform. 2009;4(3):291–306.
96. Wahl P, Guldner M, Mester J. Effects and sustainability of a 13-day high-intensity shock microcycle in soccer. J Sports Sci Med. 2014;13(2):259–65.
97. Gibala MJ, Little JP, van Essen M, Wilkin GP, Burgomaster KA, Safdar A, et al. Short-term sprint interval versus traditional endurance training: similar initial adaptations in human skeletal muscle and exercise performance. J Physiol. 2006;575(Pt 3):901–11.
98. Burgomaster KA, Hughes SC, Heigenhauser GJ, Bradwell SN, Gibala MJ. Six sessions of sprint interval training increases muscle oxidative potential and cycle endurance capacity in humans. J Appl Physiol. 2005;98(6):1985–90.
99. Gibala M. Molecular responses to high-intensity interval exercise. Appl Physiol Nutr Metab. 2009;34(3):428–32.
100. Jensen L, Bangsbo J, Hellsten Y. Effect of high intensity training on capillarization and presence of angiogenic factors in human skeletal muscle. J Physiol. 2004;557(Pt 2):571–82.
101. Christensen PM, Krustrup P, Gunnarsson TP, Kiilerich K, Nybo L, Bangsbo J. VO2 kinetics and performance in soccer players after intense training and inactivity. Med Sci Sports Exerc. 2011;43(9):1716–24.
102. Dupont G, Akakpo K, Berthoin S. The effect of in-season, high-intensity interval training in soccer players. J Strength Cond Res. 2004;18(3):584–9.
103. Cicioni-Kolsky D, Lorenzen C, Williams MD, Kemp JG. Endurance and sprint benefits of high-intensity and supramaximal interval training. Eur J Sport Sci. 2013;13(3):304–11.
104. Issurin VB. Training transfer: scientific background and insights for practical application. Sports Med. 2013;43(8):675–94.
105. Reilly T. Energetics of high-intensity exercise (soccer) with particular reference to fatigue. J Sports Sci. 1997;15(3):257–63.
106. Bangsbo J, Mohr M, Krustrup P. Physical and metabolic demands of training and match-play in the elite football player. J Sports Sci. 2006;24(7):665–74.
107. Stolen T, Chamari K, Castagna C, Wisloff U. Physiology of soccer: an update. Sports Med. 2005;35(6):501–36.
108. Kraemer WJ, French DN, Paxton NJ, Hakkinen K, Volek JS, Sebastianelli WJ, et al. Changes in exercise performance and hormonal concentrations over a big ten soccer season in starters and nonstarters. J Strength Cond Res. 2004;18(1):121–8.
109. Akenhead R, Hayes PR, Thompson KG, French D. Diminutions of acceleration and deceleration output during professional football match play. J Sci Med Sport. 2013;16(6):556–61.
110. Nummela AT, Paavolainen LM, Sharwood KA, Lambert MI, Noakes TD, Rusko HK. Neuromuscular factors determining 5 km running performance and running economy in well-trained athletes. Eur J Appl Physiol. 2006;97(1):1–8.
111. Saunders PU, Telford RD, Pyne DB, Peltola EM, Cunningham RB, Gore CJ, et al. Short-term plyometric training improves running economy in highly trained middle and long distance runners. J Strength Cond Res. 2006;20(4):947–54.
112. Paavolainen L, Hakkinen K, Hamalainen I, Nummela A, Rusko H. Explosive-strength training improves 5-km running time by improving running economy and muscle power. J Appl Physiol. 1999;86(5):1527–33.
113. Paavolainen LM, Nummela AT, Rusko HK. Neuromuscular characteristics and muscle power as determinants of 5-km running performance. Med Sci Sports Exerc. 1999;31(1):124–30.
114. Castagna C, Impellizzeri F, Chamari K, Carlomagno D, Rampinini E. Aerobic fitness and Yo-Yo continous and intermittent tests performances in soccer players: A correlation study. J Strength Cond Res. 2006;20(2):320–5.
115. Brocherie F, Girard O, Forchino F, Al Haddad H, Dos Santos GA, Millet GP. Relationships between anthropometric measures and athletic performance, with special reference to repeated-sprint ability, in the Qatar national soccer team. J Sports Sci. 2014;17:1–12.
116. Arnason A, Sigurdsson SB, Gudmundsson A, Holme I, Engebretsen L, Bahr R. Physical fitness, injuries, and team performance in soccer. Med Sci Sports Exerc. 2004;36(2):278–85.
117. Sporis G, Jovanovic M, Omrcen D, Matkovic B. Can the official soccer game be considered the most important contribution to player's physical fitness level? J Sports Med Phys Fitness. 2011;51(3):374–80.
118. Silva JR, Magalhaes J, Ascensao A, Seabra AF, Rebelo AN. Training status and match activity of professional soccer players throughout a season. J Strength Cond Res. 2013;27(1):20–30.
119. Meister S, Faude O, Ammann T, Schnittker R, Meyer T. Indicators for high physical strain and overload in elite football players. Scand J Med Sci Sports. 2013;23(2):156–63.
120. Tonnessen E, Hem E, Leirstein S, Haugen T, Seiler S. Maximal aerobic power characteristics of male professional soccer players, 1989-2012. Int J Sports Physiol Perform. 2013;8(3):323–9.
121. Haugen TA, Tonnessen E, Seiler S. Anaerobic performance testing of professional soccer players 1995-2010. Int J Sports Physiol Perform. 2013;8(2):148–56.
122. Hill-Haas SV, Dawson B, Impellizzeri FM, Coutts AJ. Physiology of small-sided games training in football: a systematic review. Sports Med. 2011;41(3):199–220.
123. Owen AL, Wong del P, McKenna M, Dellal A. Heart rate responses and technical comparison between small- vs. large-sided games in elite professional soccer. J Strength Cond Res. 2011;25(8):2104–10.
124. Reinke S, Karhausen T, Doehner W, Taylor W, Hottenrott K, Duda GN, et al. The influence of recovery and training phases on body composition, peripheral vascular function and immune system of professional soccer players. PLoS One. 2009;4(3):e4910.
125. Sotiropoulos A, Travlos AK, Gissis I, Souglis AG, Grezios A. The effect of a 4-week training regimen on body fat and aerobic capacity of professional soccer players during the transition period. J Strength Cond Res. 2009;23(6):1697–703.
126. Koundourakis NE, Androulakis NE, Malliaraki N, Tsatsanis C, Venihaki M, Margioris AN. Discrepancy between Exercise Performance, Body Composition, and Sex Steroid Response after a Six-Week Detraining Period in Professional Soccer Players. PLoS One. 2014;9(2):e87803.
127. Mohr M, Krustrup P, Bangsbo J. Physiological characteristics and exaustive exercise performance of elite soccer players. Med Sci Sports Exerc. 2002;34(5):S24. Supplement 1, May.

128. Krustrup P, Mohr M, Nybo L, Jensen JM, Nielsen JJ, Bangsbo J. The Yo-Yo IR2 test: physiological response, reliability, and application to elite soccer. Med Sci Sports Exerc. 2006;38(9):1666–73.
129. Ostojic S. Seasonal alterations in body composition and sprint performance of elite soccer players. J Exerc Physiol Online. 2003;6(3):24–7.
130. Filaire E, Lac G, Pequignot JM. Biological, hormonal, and psychological parameters in professional soccer players throughout a competitive season. Percept Mot Skills. 2003;97(3 Pt 2):1061–72.
131. Kraemer WJ, Ratamess NA. Hormonal responses and adaptations to resistance exercise and training. Sports Med. 2005;35(4):339–61.
132. Schmikli SL, de Vries WR, Brink MS, Backx FJ. Monitoring performance, pituitary-adrenal hormones and mood profiles: how to diagnose non-functional over-reaching in male elite junior soccer players. Br J Sports Med. 2012;46(14):1019–23.
133. Komi PV, Gollhofer A. Stretch reflexes can have an important role in force enhancement during SSC exercise. J Appl Biomech. 1997;13:451–60.
134. Bangsbo J. The physiology of soccer - with special reference to intense intermittent exrcise. Acta Physiol Scand. 1994;150:615. suppl.
135. Wilson JM, Flanagan EP. The role of elastic energy in activities with high force and power requirements: a brief review. J Strength Cond Res. 2008;22(5):1705–15.

21

Spontaneous Entrainment of Running Cadence to Music Tempo

Edith Van Dyck[1*], Bart Moens[1], Jeska Buhmann[1], Michiel Demey[1], Esther Coorevits[1], Simone Dalla Bella[2] and Marc Leman[1]

Abstract

Background: Since accumulating evidence suggests that step rate is strongly associated with running-related injuries, it is important for runners to exercise at an appropriate running cadence. As music tempo has been shown to be capable of impacting exercise performance of repetitive endurance activities, it might also serve as a means to (re)shape running cadence. The aim of this study was to validate the impact of music tempo on running cadence.

Methods: Sixteen recreational runners ran four laps of 200 m (i.e. 800 m in total); this task was repeated 11 times with a short break in between each four-lap sequence. During the first lap of a sequence, participants ran at a self-paced tempo without musical accompaniment. Running cadence of the first lap was registered, and during the second lap, music with a tempo matching the assessed cadence was played. In the final two laps, the music tempo was either increased/decreased by 3.00, 2.50, 2.00, 1.50, or 1.00 % or was kept stable. This range was chosen since the aim of this study was to test spontaneous entrainment (an average person can distinguish tempo variations of about 4 %). Each participant performed all conditions.

Results: Imperceptible shifts in musical tempi in proportion to the runner's self-paced running tempo significantly influenced running cadence ($p < .001$). Contrasts revealed a linear relation between the tempo conditions and adaptation in running cadence ($p < .001$). In addition, a significant effect of condition on the level of entrainment was revealed ($p < .05$), which suggests that maximal effects of music tempo on running cadence can only be obtained up to a certain level of tempo modification. Finally, significantly higher levels of tempo entrainment were found for female participants compared to their male counterparts ($p < .05$).

Conclusions: The applicable contribution of these novel findings is that music tempo could serve as an unprompted means to impact running cadence. As increases in step rate may prove beneficial in the prevention and treatment of common running-related injuries, this finding could be especially relevant for treatment purposes, such as exercise prescription and gait retraining.

Key Points:

- Music tempo can spontaneously impact running cadence.
- A basin for unsolicited entrainment of running cadence to music tempo was discovered.
- The effect of music tempo on running cadence proves to be stronger for women than for men.

* Correspondence: edith.vandyck@ugent.be
[1]IPEM, Department of Arts, Music and Theatre Sciences, Ghent University, Technicum Blok 2, Sint-Pietersnieuwstraat 41, Ghent, Belgium
Full list of author information is available at the end of the article

Background

Approximately 56 % of recreational runners sustain a running-related injury each year [1]. About 50 % of all running-related injuries occurs at the knee and is most often due to the inability of the lower extremity joints to adequately control the loads applied during initial stance [2–4]. A number of strategies designed to reduce loads to these joints have been suggested, with one of the most common ones applying an increased step rate. Subtle increases in step rate have for instance been shown to substantially reduce the loading to the hip and knee joints during running and may therefore prove beneficial in the prevention and treatment of common running-related injuries [5]. However, less is known about the specific strategies that can be employed to change step rate. In this study, a novel strategy using music as a tool to impact step rate is examined. The means by which music might serve as an adequate tool for manipulating running cadence is discussed below.

A great deal of runners exercise while listening to music. This should not come as a surprise, since music listening during sport activities is believed to capture attention [6], distract from fatigue and discomfort [7], prompt and alter mood states [8, 9], enhance work output [10, 11], increase arousal [12], relieve stress [13], stimulate rhythmic movement [14], and evoke a sense of power and produce power-related cognition and behaviour [15]. Simpson and Karageorghis [16], for instance, examined the effect of music on a 400-m sprint performance while controlling for pre-performance mood. It was shown that music resulted in better sprint performance compared to the no music control. In another study, Styns et al. [17] observed that participants walked faster with music than with metronome ticks, while Bood et al. [18] showed that time to exhaustion was significantly longer with acoustic stimuli than without when participants were asked to run to exhaustion on a treadmill. Results of studies such as these suggest that music could be applied to physical activities, such as walking or running, with a considerable positive effect.

The idea that music can serve as a strategy for coping with physical exertion has been linked to the *parallel processing model*, which focuses on the limited human attention capacity [19, 20]. This implies that the focus of an exerciser is shifted to external events in an effort to reduce the perception of neural exertion signals coming from the muscles, joints, and cardiopulmonary systems [21]. However, it appears that external musical cues can only be the focus of attention in the case of low-to-moderate physiological awareness and perceived exertion. When the workload becomes too high, the exerciser's attention is typically shifted towards the painful or fatiguing effects of the exercise [19, 20, 22–24]. In general, music has shown to be most effective to exert ergogenic and distractive effects when it is used to accompany self-paced exercise [8, 25–27]. In addition, it is believed that particularly motivational music can successfully uplift mood state and increase work capacity [9, 28, 29].

Besides the motivational factor, exercise that is repetitive in nature is believed to benefit mostly from music that is synchronized with the tempo of the exerciser's movements; endurance can be extended, and performers exercise at higher intensities when moving in synchrony with musical stimuli [29]. It has been suggested that this effect of synchronized music is due to its ability to reduce the metabolic cost of exercise by enhancing neuromuscular or metabolic efficiency [28, 30]. Regular corporeal patterns demand less energy to imitate, due to the lack of timely adjustments within the kinetic pattern but also because of an increased level of relaxation resulting from the precise expectancy of the forthcoming movement [31]. As such, a point of reference is created that is able to attract and swiftly entrain recurring motor pattern efficiency [30, 32]. Synchronization is typically understood as an intentional mechanism, which is highly task constrained [33]. Most previous research on the impact of synchronized music on exercise performance generally focused on instructed or imposed synchronization, e.g. [12, 16–18, 29]. However, it is also the case that synchronization can occur spontaneously [33]. Previous studies have highlighted the natural or spontaneous predisposition of humans to respond to rhythmical qualities of music [34, 35], but much less is known about the capabilities of exercisers, and especially runners, to spontaneously synchronize with the tempo of musical stimuli. Yet, spontaneous entrainment of one tempo with another is only believed to occur when the strength of the coupling is able to overcome possible contrasts in natural movement period or tempo [36]. For a given coupling strength, unintentional entrainment only occurs within a specific range of period differences, reflecting the system's entrainment basin [33, 37–40].

The effect of music on repetitive endurance activities also depends on the specific tempo of the musical stimulus. Waterhouse et al. [41] revealed that cyclists' covered distance, power, and pedal cadence increased when faster music was presented, while slowing down the music tempo resulted in decreases of these measures. Edworthy and Waring [8] explored the effect of music tempo (and loudness) on treadmill running and demonstrated that an increase in the tempo, and to a lesser extent the loudness of the stimulus, resulted in an increase in running speed. In the light of findings such as those described above, it is quite plausible that music tempo could also serve as a means to influence running cadence. And as a link between step rate and hip and knee joint loading has been established before [5], results of this study could be particularly relevant with regard to the prevention and treatment of running-related injuries.

The aim of this study was to validate the impact of music tempo on running cadence. We hypothesized that recreational runners would adapt their self-paced running cadence to imperceptible changes in musical tempi and, thus, entrain spontaneously with the music tempo. Furthermore, we believed that the degree of entrainment would decrease with increasing changes in music tempo and, thus, that a basin for unintentional entrainment of running cadence to music tempo exists. As it has been shown that unintentional coordination typically manifests as relative or intermittent coordination (i.e. movements are attracted to a 0 or 180° but are not phase locked) [36, 37, 42], rather than phase-locked steps, *entrainment* refers to the amount of steps taken in a tempo sufficiently close to the music tempo (max. 1 % difference between running cadence and music tempo). Besides, since previous research often reported better results for women compared to men regarding music-to-movement coordination [11, 43], we expected female participants to display larger levels of entrainment. Finally, as it has been demonstrated that only when physiological awareness and perceived exertion are relatively low that music can distract from fatigue and discomfort [19, 22], the relationship between the level of entrainment and the degree of perceived exertion was examined.

Methods

Ethics Statement

The study was approved by the Ethics Committee of the Faculty of Arts and Philosophy of Ghent University, and all procedures followed were in accordance with the statements of the Declaration of Helsinki. In addition, all participants signed a form to declare that they participated voluntarily; that they had received sufficient information concerning the tasks, the procedures, and the technologies used; that they had the opportunity to ask questions; and that they were aware of the fact that running movements were measured, for scientific and educational purposes only.

Participants

To establish sample size, a power analysis for a repeated-measures design was conducted using G*Power 3.1.9.2 [44]. Based on the effect sizes reported in comparable studies [16, 18, 28], the analysis indicated that minimally 14 participants for an α of 0.05 and a power of 0.80 would be required. Sixteen healthy adult participants (nine females) took part in the study. The test group consisted of recreational runners with an average age of 22.25 years (SD = 2.14), a mean body mass of 66.56 kg (SD = 9.32), and an average height of 1.74 m (SD = 0.10), who reported to be fit to run about 10 km. The majority (62.50 %) had received musical training (Fisher's exact test showed no significant association between gender and musical background, $\chi^2(1) = 2.05$, $p = .30$). All participants reported that running is an activity that forms a part of their lives, with varying degrees of frequency (12.50 % runs multiple times a week; 56.25 % runs about once a week; 31.25 % runs about once a month; 0 % runs about once a year or not at all). Of all participants, 50 % reported to typically train with music, 32.25 % generally runs without music, and 18.75 % runs both with and without musical accompaniment.

Stimuli

Previous research indicated that the natural running cadence for recreational runners lies somewhere between 130 and 200 steps per minute (SPM) [45]. On that account, a music database consisting of songs in the tempo range of 130–200 beats per minute (BPM) was created. A group of 19 students from Ghent University, all recreational runners, were asked to provide a list of at least ten songs they believed to be motivational to run to. From that specific list of music, the database for the experiment was created. In total, 117 songs with a clear beat and correct tempo range were pre-selected (see Table 1). In the course of the selection process, it was verified that the tempo of each song remained stable throughout the entire track. Using Audacity software (http://audacity.sourceforge.net), intros without clear beats were cut from the stimuli. BeatRoot [46] was applied to track the beats of each song in order to ensure that only songs between 130 and 200 BPM were included, while ReplayGain was used to normalize perceived loudness and minimize possible imbalances in sound pressure level.

Apparatus

Participants were equipped with two iPods (fourth generation), one attached at each ankle. Using the Sensor Monitor Pro application on the iPods, data from accelerometers and gyroscopes was streamed wirelessly at 100 Hz to the main processing computer. A Wi-Fi hotspot (TP-Link N750) with special 3-dB gain antennas for longer range was used for maintaining a stable connection between the computer and sensors. Some minimal jitter and lag in the data stream were neutralized using a 500-ms buffer before processing.

Incoming sensor data was processed by a customized version of D-Jogger [47], a music alignment framework that selects and tempo-adapts music to runners' gait frequencies using kinematic sensor input (Additional file 1). Music tempi were manipulated using a phase vocoder, which time stretches music without pitch

Table 1 List of musical stimuli

ID	Artist	Song	Label(s)	Year published	Tempo (BPM)
1	Epica	Illusive Consensus	Transmission	2003	132
2	Gregory Porter	On My Way to Harlem (Radio Edit)	Motema	2012	138
3	Interpol	Slow Hands	Matador	2004	139
4	The Supremes	I Hear a Symphony	Motown	1965	139
5	Van Halen	Ain't Talkin' 'Bout Love	Warner Bros	1978	139
6	Combichrist	Electrohead	Out of Line/Metropolis	2007	140
7	dEUS	The Soft Fall	PIAS	2012	140
8	P!nk	Who Knew	LaFace	2006	140
9	Noisettes	Never Forget You	Mercury/Vertigo	2009	141
10	Rammstein	Benzin	Motor	2005	142
11	Royksopp	Tricky Tricky	Astralwerk/EMI	2009	142
12	Deftones	My Own Summer (Shove It)	Maverick/Warner Bros	1997	143
13	16 Horsepower	Outlaw Song	Jetset	2006	144
14	Coldplay	In My Place	Parlophone	2002	144
15	The Hickey Underworld	Future Words	PIAS	2009	145
16	ABBA	Waterloo (English Version)	Polar/Epic	1973	146
17	Steppenwolf	Born to Be Wild	Dunhill/RCA	1967	146
18	The Sisters of Mercy	Alice	Merciful Release	1982	146
19	School Is Cool	The World Is Gonna End Tonight	Not on label	2011	147
20	Tom Odell	I Know	Columbia/In the Name Of	2012	147
21	Trixie Whitley	Irene	Unday Records	2013	147
22	Aphex Twin	Flim	Warp/Sire/WEA	1997	148
23	Bruce Springsteen	Dancing In the Dark	Columbia	1984	148
24	Nneka	Heartbeat	Yo Mama's Recording	2008	148
25	Alt-J	Breezeblocks	Infectious	2012	149
26	Marco Borsato	Ik leef niet meer voor jou	Polydor	1995	149
27	A Perfect Circle	Thinking of You	Virgin	2000	150
28	Editors	An End Has a Start	Kitchenware/FADER	2007	150
29	Florence and The Machine	Dog Days Are Over	Island	2009	150
30	Guns N' Roses	It's So Easy	Geffen Records/Interscope	1987	150
31	Katy Perry	E.T.	Capitol	2010	150
32	Pearl Jam	Lightning Bolt	Monkeywrench/Republic	2013	151
33	The Killers	Spaceman	Island/Vertigo	2008	151
34	Bloc Party	Flux	Wichita/Vice	2007	152
35	Elton John	Saturday Night's Alright (For Fighting)	MCA/DJM	1973	152
36	P!nk	Are We All We Are	RCA	2012	152
37	De Staat	Sweatshop	Cool Green Recordings	2011	153
38	Ike & Tina Turner	Nutbush City Limits	United Artists	1973	153
39	Kings of Leon	Sex On Fire	RCA	2008	153
40	OutKast	B.O.B.	LaFace/Arista	2000	153
41	The Black Eyed Peas	Pump It	Interscope	2005	153
42	Massive Attack	Teardrop	Circa/Virgin	1998	154
43	Kaiser Chiefs	Never Miss a Beat	B-Unique/Universal	2008	155
44	Morphine	Honey White	Rykodisc	1995	155

Table 1 List of musical stimuli *(Continued)*

45	The Pipettes	Your Kisses Are Wasted On Me	Memphis Industries/Cherrytree	2006	155
46	The Strokes	Juicebox	RCA	2006	155
47	Hooverphonic	Mad About You (Orchestra Version)	Columbia	2012	156
48	Nirvana	In Bloom	DGC	1991	156
49	The Van Jets	Ricochet	Belvédère	2005	156
50	Air	Surfing On a Rocket	Virgin	2004	157
51	Millencolin	No Cigar	Epitaph	2000	157
52	The Beach Boys	Surfin' USA	Capitol	1963	157
53	Shaggy	Boombastic	Virgin	1995	158
54	Jones & Stephenson	The First Rebirth (Original Mix)	Prolekult	1994	159
55	Kings of Leon	California Waiting	RCA/HandMeDown	2003	159
56	Michael Sembello	Maniac	Warner Bros	1983	159
57	OutKast	Hey Ya! (Radio Mix Club Mix)	LaFace	2003	159
58	Beyonce	Halo	Columbia	2008	160
59	Birdman & Lil Wayne	Stuntin' Like My Daddy (Street)	Cash Money/Universal	2006	160
60	Customs	Justine	Noisesome/EMI	2009	160
61	Mastodon	Spectrelight	Reprise/Roadrunner	2011	160
62	TNGHT	Higher Ground	Warp/LuckyMe	2012	160
63	P.O.D.	Alive	Atlantic	2001	161
64	Queens of the Stone Age	Little Sister	Interscope	2005	161
65	'T Hof Van Commerce	Baes (Radio Edit)	Plasticine	2012	162
66	Black Sabbath	Paranoid	Vertigo	1970	162
67	Blondie	One Way or Another	Chrysalis	1978	162
68	Karate	Ice or Ground	Southern	2002	162
69	Moby	Feeling So Real	Mute/Elektra	1995	162
70	Orchestral Manoeuvres In the Dark	Electricity	Factory	1979	162
71	U96	Love Religion (Video Edit)	Guppy/Motor	1995	162
72	Wham!	Wake Me Up Before You GoGo	Columbia	1984	162
73	Bomfunk MC's	Freestyler	Sony Music Finland/Epidrome	1999	163
74	Jamaica	Cross the Fader	Downtown	2011	164
75	Midlake	Antiphon	Bella Union	2013	164
76	Muse	Survival	Helium 3/Warner Music Group	2012	164
77	Sugababes	About You Now	Island	2007	164
78	Ella Fitzgerald	A-Tisket, A-Tasket	Golden Options	2008	165
79	Ike & Tina Turner	River Deep Mountain High	Philes	1966	165
80	Green Day	Boulevard of Broken Dreams	Reprise	2004	166
81	Pixies	Where Is My Mind	4 AD	1988	166
82	Rammstein	Mann gegen Mann	Universal	2005	166
83	Arctic Monkeys	Do I Wanna Know	Domino	2013	170
84	Chet Faker	I'm Into You	Opulent/Remote Control	2012	170
85	Joy Division	Disorder	Factory	1979	170
86	Panic! At the Disco	I Write Sins Not Tragedies	Fueled by Ramen/Decaydance	2005	170
87	Queens of the Stone Age	No One Knows	Interscope	2002	170
88	The All-American Rejects	My Paper Heart	Doghouse/DreamWorks	2002	170
89	Foo Fighters	The Pretender	Roswell/RCA	2007	172

Table 1 List of musical stimuli *(Continued)*

90	Netsky	Love Has Gone	Hospital	2012	172
91	Paramore	Misery Business	Fueled by Ramen	2007	172
92	The Streets	Fit But You Know It	Locked On/679	2004	172
93	DJ Fresh	Hot Right Now (Radio Edit)	Ministry of Sound	2012	174
94	Interpol	A Time To Be So Small	Matador	2004	174
95	Kanye West	Homecoming (feat. Chris Martin)	Roc-A-Fella/Def Jam	2008	174
96	Rudimental	Waiting All Night (feat. Ella Eyre)	Asylum	2013	174
97	Kelis & Andre 3000	Millionaire	Virgin	2004	176
98	Technohead	I Wanna Be a Hippy	Mokum	1995	177
99	Komatsu	Comin'	Lighttown Fidelity	2011	178
100	Mo' Horizons	Pe Na Estrada (Radio Edit)	Agogo	2008	178
101	Tony Bennett & Lady Gaga	The Lady Is a Tramp	Sony Music Entertainment	2011	179
102	One Direction	Kiss You	Syco/Columbia	2012	180
103	Red Hot Chili Peppers	Can't Stop	Warner Music	2002	182
104	The Pointer Sisters	I'm So Excited	Planet	1982	184
105	Ok Go	Don't Ask Me	Capitol	2002	186
106	Joan Jett & The Blackhearts	I Love Rock 'N Roll	RAK	1975	188
107	Wheatus	Teenage Dirtbag	Columbia	2000	188
108	Absynthe Minded	Pretty Horny Flow	Abeille Musique	2008	190
109	Eminem	Berzerk	Aftermath Entertainment/Shady/ Interscope	2013	190
110	Macklemore & Ryan Lewis	Thrift Shop (feat. Wanz)	Macklemore LLC/ADA	2012	190
111	Roxette	The Look	EMI	1988	190
112	Isbells	As Long As It Takes	Zeal	2009	197
113	Beyonce	Crazy In Love (feat. Jay-Z)	Columbia/Music World	2003	198
114	Rihanna	Pon de Replay	Def Jam	2005	198
115	Gorillaz	Stylo (Radio Edit) [feat. Mos Def & Bobby Womack]	Parlophone/Virgin	2010	200
116	Wallace Vanborn	Atom Juggler	PIAS	2010	200
117	Linkin Park	In the End	Warner Bros	2000	210

modification. D-Jogger was adapted to match the experimental protocol (detect running cadence, playback tempo-matched music to this reference, increase or decrease music tempo). The system logged all data and calculations in real time. Finally, the resulting auditory stimuli were sent back to the participant using a Sennheiser HDR130 audio transmitter (with a range of up to 100 m). The participant perceived the music through Sennheiser HD60 headphones connected to the transmitter (attached to the upper arm). The delay due to the wireless audio transmission was negligible.

Experimental Procedure and Set-up

The experiment took place in the Flanders Sports Arena of Ghent, Belgium. In order to select motivational music adapted to each runner's personal taste, participants performed the Brunel Music Rating Inventory 2 (BMRI-2) test [48] at the start of the experiment. In this test, they were asked to rate all items of the music database by answering six questions about the motivational aspects of each song. Each item referred to an action, a time, a context, and a target (e.g. "The rhythm of this song would motivate me during a running exercise") [49]. Participants responded on a seven-point Likert scale anchored by 1 ("strongly disagree") and 7 ("strongly agree"). Afterwards, participants filled out a questionnaire on personal background, music education, and sports training. At the same time, for each participant individually, the 20 songs that had obtained the highest scores during the BMRI-2 test were loaded into the D-Jogger system.

Subsequently, participants were equipped with the iPods, the wireless headphone, and the audio transmitter. Each participant was asked to run on a 200-m running track for four laps continuously, for 12 times.

Participants were instructed to run at their own comfortable tempo. No information was distributed concerning the real purpose of the experiment, and all participants ran in solo conditions. After each set of four laps, a break of approximately 5 min was introduced to enable the participant to recover sufficiently. Meanwhile, they were asked to indicate how heavy the effort had been during the exercise. This was rated on a Rating of Perceived Exertion (RPE) Scale [50], ranging from 6 ("no exertion at all") to 20 ("maximal exertion").

To get acquainted with the experimental set-up, the first set of four laps consisted of a practice set during which no music was played. Each of the 11 following four-lap sequences consisted of (1) a lap without music, (2) a lap with tempo-matched music, and (3) two laps with tempo-changed music. In the first lap, the participant ran at his/her self-paced cadence without musical accompaniment. In the second lap, music with a tempo matching the cadence assessed during the final 20 s of the previous lap was played. The musical stimulus consisted of the song that obtained the highest score during the BMRI-2 test with a tempo that differed maximally 5 % from the running cadence of the participant. After the song was selected, its tempo was adjusted to exactly match the mean running cadence. Finally, during the third and fourth laps, the tempo of the music was adjusted according to one of the 11 tempo-changed conditions.

In each of the 11 four-lap sequences, a different condition was tested. During the two final laps with tempo-changed music, the music tempo was adjusted to either −3.00, −2.50, −2.00, −1.50, −1.00, 0.00, +1.00, +1.50, +2.00, +2.50, or +3.00 % of its original one, played during the second lap. This range was chosen since an average person can distinguish tempo variations from about 4 % [51] and since the aim of this study was to test spontaneous or unintentional entrainment. The different conditions were randomized over the experiment in such a way that each participant performed all conditions but no participants performed the conditions in the same order. To ensure that they were not aware of the actual objective, participants filled out a questionnaire regarding their perception of the purpose of the experiment at the end. Responses did not indicate that they were aware of the experiment's real purpose.

Data Analysis

Cadence Adaptation

Running cadence was calculated using the iPods' acceleration data. In order to check the degree of cadence increase/decrease, running cadence (SPM) recorded during the laps with tempo-changed music (*tempo-changed laps* or TCL) was compared to the cadence captured during the lap with tempo-matched music (*tempo-matched lap* or TML) and will be further referred to as *cadence adaptation.* As the tempo was gradually shifting during that period, the first 5 s of the laps with tempo-changed music was discarded. The final 20 s of those laps was also ignored as participants possibly altered their running behaviour due to the anticipated ending of the final lap (e.g. slowing down or speeding up).

$$\text{Cadence adaptation } (\%) = \frac{\text{avg(SPM\_TCL)}}{\text{avg(SPM\_TML)}}$$

Entrainment

A second measure of interest concerned the percentage of tempo-entrained steps during the laps with tempo-changed music. A step taken in a tempo sufficiently close to the music tempo (max. 1 % difference between SPM and BPM) at that specific moment is regarded as a tempo-entrained step. The tempo entrainment score is the percentage of tempo-entrained steps of the total amount of steps.

Results

Running Cadence

This study tested whether the changes in music tempo would affect running cadence. A Kolmogorov-Smirnov test (KS test) showed that the assumption of normality was met, $D(161) = 0.04$, $p > .05$. A $11 \times 2 \times 2$ repeated measures ANOVA with tempo condition as within-subject factor and gender and musical training as between-subject factors revealed a significant main effect of condition on cadence adaptation, $F(10, 40) = 6.50$, $p < .001$. Contrasts revealed a linear relation between condition and cadence adaptation, $F(1, 4) = 94.56$, $p < .001$, $r^2 = .96$. The evolution of cadence adaptation over the different conditions is shown in Fig. 1.

There was no significant effect of gender, indicating rather similar levels of cadence adaptation for males and females, $F(1, 4) = 6.51$, $p = .06$, $r^2 = .62$. However, there was a significant interaction effect between tempo condition and gender, $F(10, 40) = 3.40$, $p < .01$. As can be seen in Fig. 2, although for both males and females running cadence increased (or decreased) with increases (or decreases) in music tempo, these adjustments were more pronounced for women than for men. In addition, there was no significant effect of musical training, $F(1, 4) = 6.48$, $p = .06$, $r^2 = .62$, which indicated that participants without musical training displayed similar levels of cadence adaptation as participants with a musical background. Finally, no significant interaction effect was found between musical training and tempo condition, $F(10, 40) = 1.79$, $p = .10$ (see Fig. 3).

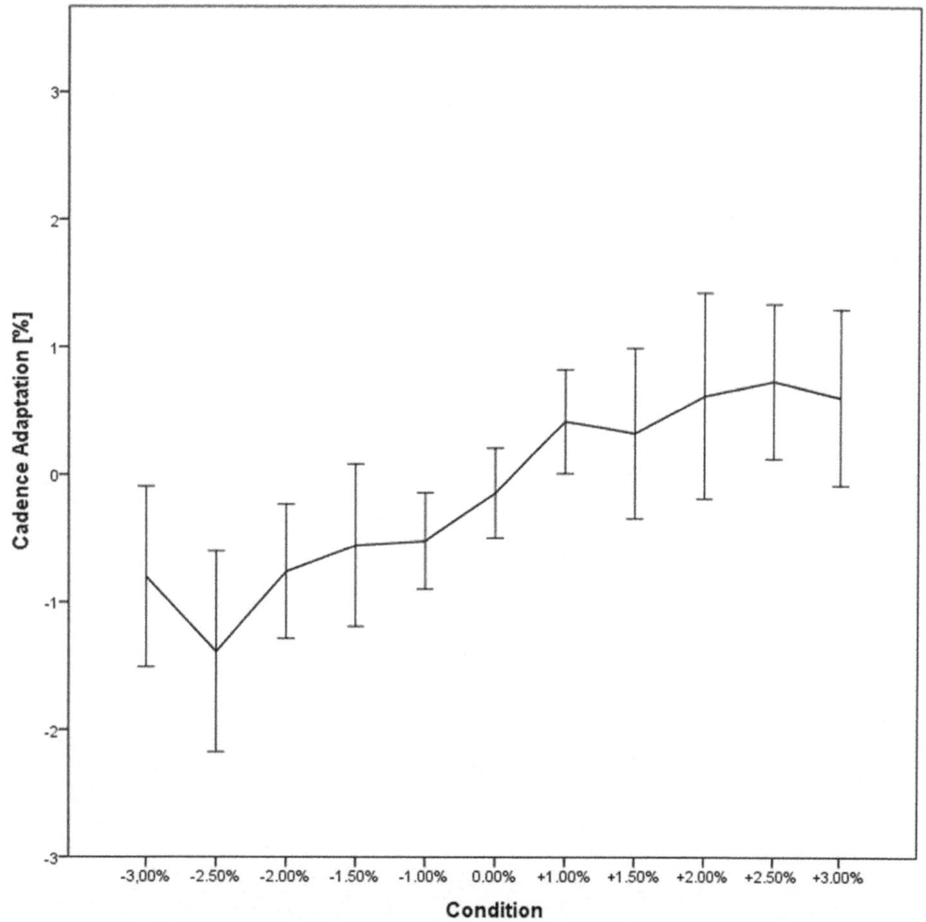

Fig. 1 Mean tempo and cadence adaptation for the different conditions. Data presented is mean ± SE

Entrainment Basin

In order to trace a possible basin for entrainment, the effect of the conditions on the level of tempo entrainment was tested. KS tests showed that the entrainment values were significantly non-normal, $D(161) = 0.15$, $p < .001$. Friedman's ANOVA showed a significant effect of condition on tempo entrainment, $\chi^2(10) = 19.27$, $p < .05$. Wilcoxon tests were used to follow up this finding, and all conditions were compared against the control condition (0 % of tempo change). A Bonferroni correction was applied, and all effects are thus reported at a .005 level of significance. It appeared that, compared to the control condition (Median (Mdn) = 74.25), tempo entrainment was significantly lower in the +2.50 % condition ((Mdn = 12.48), $Z = -2.92$, $r^2 = .53$) and tended to be lower in the +3.00 % ((Mdn = 14.01), $Z = -2.41$, $p = .016$, $r^2 = .36$) and −3.00 % conditions ((Mdn = 6.97), $Z = -2.48$, $p = .013$, $r^2 = .38$). Figure 4 represents the mean tempo entrainment for every single condition.

It is noteworthy that the entrainment basin did not differ significantly between females and males (see Fig. 5). However, the mean level of entrainment appeared to be higher for females as compared to their male counterparts. When testing this assumption, a Mann-Whitney test indeed revealed significantly higher levels of tempo entrainment for female participants (Mdn = 60.05) compared to their male counterparts (Mdn = 39.10), $U = 10.00$, $Z = -2.28$, $p < .05$, $r^2 = .32$. It was also tested whether a link between musical training and entrainment could be found. However, no significant difference was found between participants with (Mdn = 50.73) or without musical background (Mdn = 38.24) regarding their level of entrainment, $U = 18.00$, $Z = -1.30$, $p = .19$, $r^2 = .11$.

Perceived Exertion

It was also checked whether the level of entrainment could be related to the degree of perceived exertion. For this purpose, a two-tailed Spearman's correlation test was performed on entrainment values and ratings on the RPE scale. However, no significant relationship between perceived exertion and entrainment was found, $r_s = -.04$, $p = .58$.

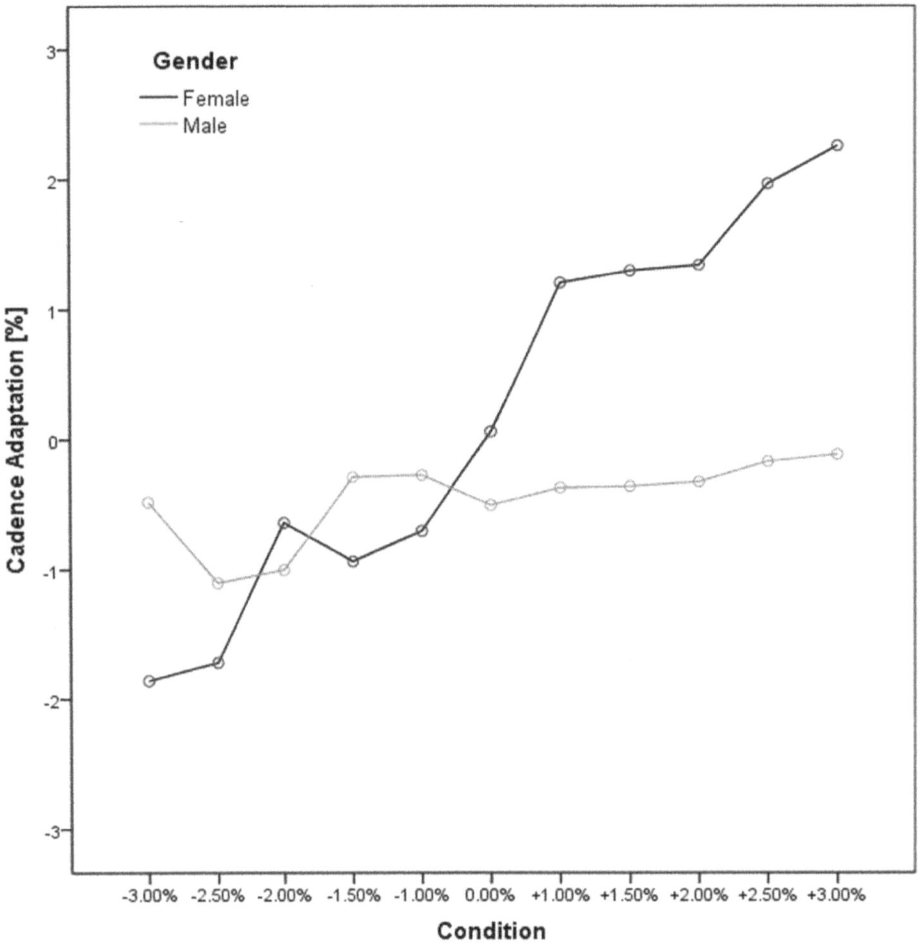

Fig. 2 Interaction plot of estimated marginal means calculated for cadence adaptation at both gender levels

Discussion

The aim of this study was to examine whether music tempo could serve as a means to influence running cadence. Results indeed unveiled a significant relationship between imperceptible alterations in music tempo, in proportion to recreational runners' self-paced running cadence, and cadence adaptation. In other words, faster music resulted in an increase, while slower music led to a decrease in running cadence. This effect can be explained through the idea of a sensorimotor mechanism that aligns footfall to musical beats. Adjustment of the footfalls to the beats relies on a phase-error correction mechanism of expected sensory outcomes [52]. Consequently, our study confirms results of previous research stressing the effect of music tempo on exercise performance [8, 11, 41, 53, 54]. This particular study also extends preceding research, as in this case, the effect on running cadence was tested using imperceptible changes in musical tempi with no explicit instructions regarding entrainment with the music. In contrast, in past research, participants were generally instructed to couple movement to music. Even if this was not the case, employed tempo variations usually proved to be too large to be unnoticeable. For example, Waterhouse, Hudson, and Edwards [41] compared cycling performance to normal, fast (increase of 10 %), and slow music (decrease of 10 %). Edworthy and Waring [8] examined treadmill-running behaviour when listening to music with a tempo of either 200 or 70 BPM, while Karageorghis et al. [53] employed tempi of 80, 120, and 140 BPM in their study on walking. In contrast, a maximum deviation of 3 % from the original music tempo was implemented in this particular study, as the amount of variation in tempo that an average person can distinguish is situated around 4 % [51]. Consequently, novel insights were presented in this study, as it was shown that recreational runners are able to adapt their running cadence (up to 2 % of the original cadence) to tempo changes in music (up to 3 % of the original tempo) without being aware of this attunement and without being instructed to do so. This finding supports the notion that an individual tends to synchronize spontaneously to an auditory rhythm

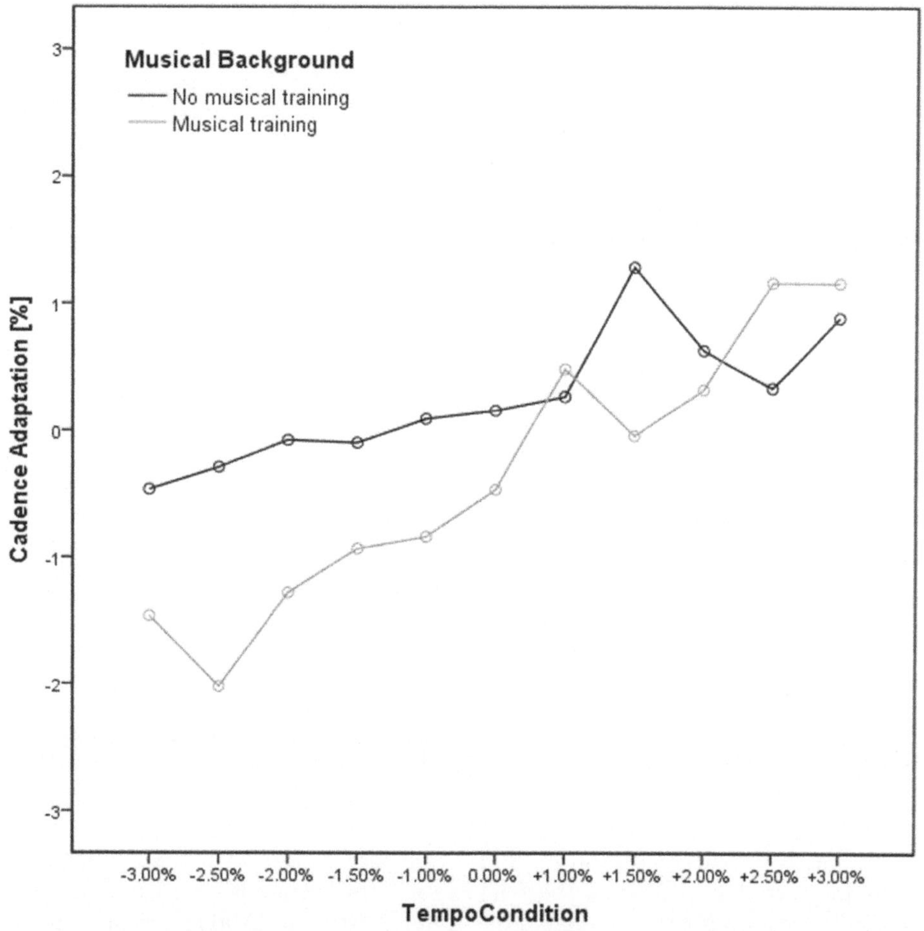

Fig. 3 Interaction plot of estimated marginal means calculated for cadence adaptation at both musical background levels

occurring in the environment [37, 39, 52] and is in agreement with the natural predisposition of humans to respond to rhythmical qualities of music [34, 35].

It was also tested whether a basin for spontaneous entrainment of running cadence to music tempo could be found. Previous research has suggested that a range of period differences exists over which entrainment of movements of an individual with an environmental rhythm generally occurs and that beyond this range the occurrence of unintentional coordination is highly unlikely [33, 36–40]. Results indeed revealed a significant decrease in the level of entrainment in combination with increasing deviations from the original music tempo. The degree of entrainment with the tempo of the music dropped significantly as soon as tempo increases of 2.50 % were introduced but also tended to drop at decreases of 3.00 %. This could be explained by the fact that when deviations (especially increases) from the original, self-selected, and thus comfortable running tempo got larger, the effort required from the runner increased and at a certain point probably required too much effort, resulting in significantly lower levels of entrainment. As such, our results are in line with the idea of an entrainment basin for spontaneous coordination [33, 36–40]. However, our findings also contrast with those of Mendonça et al. [54], showing that for uninstructed synchronization of walking to music, participants did not adapt their step frequency to music that differed 5 to 10 % above and under their nominal step frequency, while they did adjust when synchronization was instructed. This could imply that a wider basin might be found for instructed entrainment to music tempo, while spontaneous entrainment occurs only when smaller deviations from the original tempo are introduced. But this is subject to some speculation and might benefit from further research.

Music is believed to only successfully distract from fatigue and discomfort when physiological awareness and perceived exertion are relatively low [19, 20, 22–24]. Therefore, in order to control for possible effects of

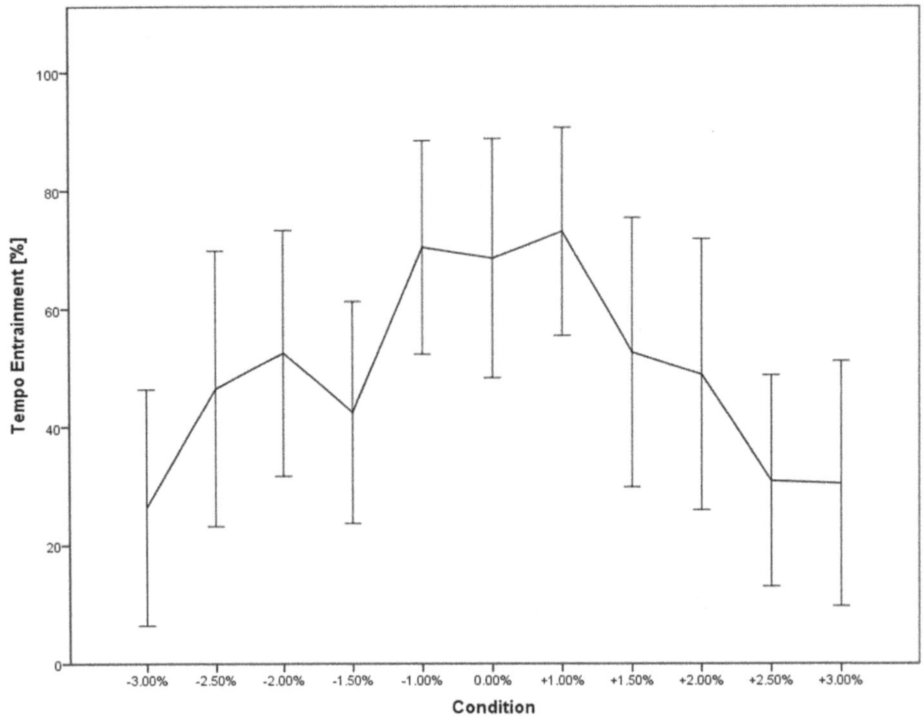

Fig. 4 Entrainment basin displaying mean tempo entrainment for the different conditions. Data presented is mean ± SE

perceived exertion, after each set of four laps, a break of approximately 5 min was introduced. Besides, the relationship between the degree of perceived exertion and the level of entrainment was also examined in the analysis. Nevertheless, no significant relationship between perceived exertion and entrainment was found. This could be due to the fact that, in general, participants did not perceive the task as extremely light or exceptionally hard but mostly rated their perceived exertion as intermediate. A reason for this might be that runners ran at their comfort tempo and no large shifts in the tempo of the music were incorporated in the study, but it might also be partly due to the introduction of the breaks after each condition. Besides, most previous research demonstrating decreasing levels of influence of music on attentional processes at higher exercise intensities tested this effect using asynchronous music, e.g. [19, 20, 22–24]. Whether this also applies to synchronous music still remains rather unclear, although, in their study on the effect of synchronous music on treadmill running, Terry et al. [29] did indicate lower levels of perceived exertion, assessed at moderate-to-high work intensities, for synchronous music compared to the no-music control. Yet, the magnitude of the differences in rating of perceived exertion proved to be rather small.

Another hypothesis referred to gender. We expected female participants to exhibit larger levels of entrainment in comparison with their male counterparts. Indeed, significantly higher levels of tempo entrainment were observed for females. In addition, although the effect of the music tempo on running cadence was unveiled for both males and females, changes in running cadence as a result of deviations in music tempi were more pronounced for female runners than for male ones, which suggests that women were more influenced by tempo changes than men. These findings resonate with the general belief that women are more responsive to musical stimuli [11, 41, 34, 55].

One should bear in mind that the current study focused on self-paced running, and thus, the type of exercise under study concerned one that is of low-to-moderate intensity. When studying activities with higher levels of intensity, music might not have a comparable effect on the exercisers' performance, as when high workloads are undertaken, the exerciser's attention could be shifted towards the painful or fatiguing effects of the exercise [19, 20, 22–24]. However, although most previous research on high-intensity exercise did not show any remarkable effects of music tempo, exemplary studies that have unveiled such effects do exist as well. In a study by Rendi, Szabo, and Szabo [10], for example, where exercisers were asked to perform a 500-m rowing sprint, in which physiological awareness is high, it was shown that fast-tempo music increased arousal and, in turn, performance, even during high-intensity sprints, while music with

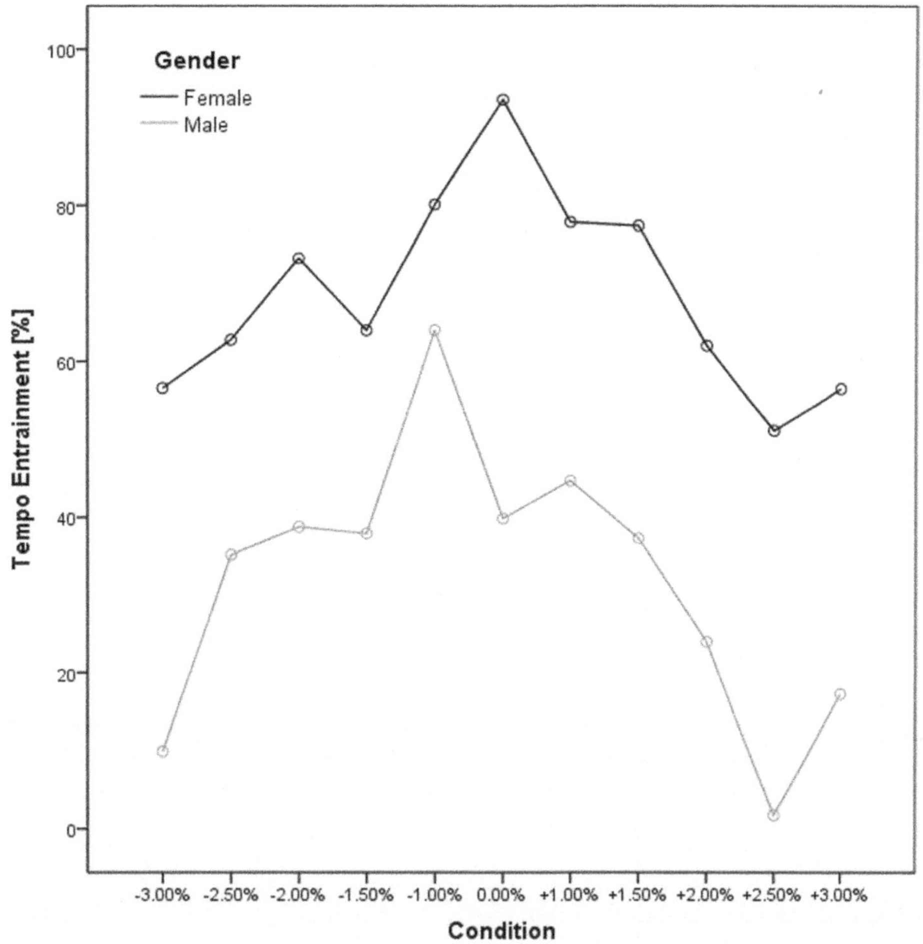

Fig. 5 Interaction plot of estimated marginal means calculated for tempo entrainment at both gender levels

a slow tempo did not generate such stimulating effects. Further exploration of the impact of music tempo on sport activities with high workloads would be beneficial.

It could also be questioned whether spontaneous, thus uninstructed, entrainment is generally more beneficial with regard to exercise performance than instructed entrainment. It could be suggested that when synchronization is spontaneous, it may require less attentional resources, thus leading to even more important benefits (e.g. leaving free attentional resources to realize other tasks). Besides, exercise training could be simplified when instruction would prove to be redundant. On the other hand, it has been indicated that instructed synchronization is a form of active attentional manipulation, which has been shown to have more positive effects, at least in the form of perceived exertion and exercise efficiency [12, 28]. However, as this question has not been solved yet, the discussion whether spontaneous synchronization is more beneficial compared to instructed (or even imposed) synchronization should be unravelled in future studies.

In this particular study, recreational runners were tested. However, since music is believed to be more beneficial for recreational compared to trained exercisers [56], different results might have been obtained if competitive runners were tested. Previous research on treadmill running indicated that less trained exercisers might depend to a greater extent on the positive feeling states generated by music, while trained exercisers generally tend to focus on the tasks and specifics of their training [57, 58]. Furthermore, as (either recreational or professional) runners do not typically tend to run distances of 800 m consecutively, interrupted by short brakes, it might be interesting to investigate whether the effect of music tempo is sustained over the course of longer, interrupted distances. Whether the entrainment basin for recreational runners would differ from that of professional runners and whether its effects are sustained over longer distances could be tested in future research.

Conclusions

To conclude, it was unveiled that music tempo could serve as an unprompted means to re(shape) running cadence of recreational runners. This influence was shown to have a certain range, which suggests that maximal effects of music tempo can only be obtained up to a certain level of tempo change and proved to be stronger for female compared to male runners. As modifying step rate may prove beneficial in the prevention and treatment of common running-related injuries, this novel finding could be especially relevant for treatment purposes, such as exercise prescription and gait retraining.

Competing Interests

The authors declare that they have no competing interests.

Authors' Contributions

Conceived the study: EVD, BM, JB, MD, and ML. Performed the experiments: EVD, BM, JB, and EC. Analysed the data: EVD, BM, and SDB. Wrote and/or revised the paper: EVD and BM. All authors read and approved the final manuscript.

Acknowledgements

The authors wish to thank the Flanders Sports Arena of Ghent, for making it possible to use their running track. The authors also acknowledge BeatHealth (contract #610633), a collaborative project funded by the European Commission under the Seventh Framework Programme, and the Methusalem project, awarded by the Flemish Government, for funding this study.

Author details

[1]IPEM, Department of Arts, Music and Theatre Sciences, Ghent University, Technicum Blok 2, Sint-Pietersnieuwstraat 41, Ghent, Belgium. [2]EuroMov, Movement 2 Health Laboratory (M2H), University of Montpellier, 700 Avenue du Pic Saint Loup, Montpellier, France.

References

1. van Gent RN, Siem D, van Middelkoop M, van Os AG, Bierma-Zeinstra SM, Koes BW. Incidence and determinants of lower extremity running injuries in long distance runners: a systematic review. Br J Sports Med. 2007;41:469–80.
2. Taunton JE, Ryan MB, Clement DB, McKenzie DC, Lloyd-Smith DR, Zumbo BD. A retrospective case-control analysis of 2002 running injuries. Br J Sports Med. 2002;36:95–101.
3. Ferber R, Noehren B, Hamill J, Davis I. Competitive female runners with a history of iliotibial band syndrome demonstrate atypical hip and knee kinematics. J Orthop Sports Phys Ther. 2010;40:52–8.
4. Noehren B, Davis I, Hamill J. ASB clinical biomechanics award winner 2006 prospective study of the biomechanical factors associated with iliotibial band syndrome. Clin Biomech. 2007;22:951–6.
5. Heiderscheit BC, Chumanov ES, Michalski MP, Wille CM, Ryan MB. Effects of step rate manipulation on joint mechanics during running. Med Sci Sports Exerc. 2011;43:296–302.
6. Priest DL, Karageorghis CI. A qualitative investigation into the characteristics and effects of music accompanying exercise. Eur Phys Educ Rev. 2008;14:347–66.
7. Yamashita S, Twai K, Aktmoto T, Sugawara J, Kono I. Effects of music during exercise on RPE, heart rate and the autonomic nervous system. J Sports Med Phys Fitness. 2006;46:425–30.
8. Edworthy J, Waring H. The effects of music tempo and loudness level on treadmill exercise. Ergonomics. 2006;49:1597–610.
9. Shaulov N, Lufi D. Music and light during indoor cycling. Percept Motor Skills. 2009;108:597–607.
10. Rendi M, Szabo A, Szabó T. Performance enhancement with music in rowing sprint. Sport Psychol. 2008;22:175–82.
11. Priest DL, Karageorghis CI, Sharp NCC. The characteristics and effects of motivational music in exercise settings: the possible influence of gender, age, frequency of attendance, and time of attendance. J Sports Med Phys Fitness. 2004;44:77–86.
12. Lim HBT, Karageorghis CI, Romer LM, Bishop DT. Psychophysiological effects of synchronous versus asynchronous music during cycling. Med Sci Sports. 2014;46:407–13.
13. Särkämö T, Tervaniemi M, Laitinen S, Forsblom A, Soinila S, Mikkonen M, et al. Music listening enhances cognitive recovery and mood after middle cerebral artery stroke. Brain. 2008;131:866–76.
14. Atkinson G, Wilson D, Eubank M. Effects of music on work-rate distribution during a cycling time trial. Int J Sports Med. 2004;25:611–5.
15. Hsu DY, Huang L, Nordgren LF, Rucker DD, Galinsky AD. The music of power: perceptual and behavioral consequences of powerful music. Soc Psychol Personal Sci. 2014; doi:10.1177/1948550614542345
16. Simpson SD, Karageorghis CI. The effects of synchronous music on 400-m sprint performance. J Sports Sci. 2006;24:1095–102.
17. Styns F, van Noorden L, Moelants D, Leman M. Walking on music. Hum Mov Sci. 2007;26:769–85.
18. Bood RJ, Nijssen M, van der Kamp J, Roerdink M. The power of auditory-motor synchronization in sports: enhancing running performance by coupling cadence with the right beats. Plos One. 2013; doi:10.1371/journal.pone.0070758
19. Rejeski WJ. Perceived exertion: an active or passive process? J Sport Exerc Psychol. 1985;7:371–8.
20. Nethery VM. Competition between internal and external sources of information during exercise: influence on RPE and the impact of the exercise load. J Sports Med Phys Fitness. 2002;42:172–8.
21. Tenenbaum G. A social-cognitive perspective of perceived exertion. In: Tenenbaum G, Eklund R, editors. Handbook of sport psychology. 3rd ed. Hoboken: Wiley; 2007. p. 560–77.
22. Tenenbaum G. The study of perceived and sustained effort: concepts, research findings, and future directions. In: Hackfort D, Duda J, Lidor R, editors. Handbook of research on applied sport psychology. Morgantown: Fitness Information Technology; 2005. p. 335–49.
23. Razon S, Basevitch I, Land W, Thompson B, Tenenbaum G. Perception of exertion and attention allocation as a function of visual and auditory conditions. Psychol Sport Exerc. 2009;10:636–43.
24. Hutchinson JC, Tenenbaum G. Attention focus during physical effort: the mediating role of task intensity. Psychol Sport Exerc. 2007;8:233–45.
25. Karageorghis CI. The scientific application of music in sport and exercise. In: Lane AM, editor. Sport and exercise psychology. London: Hodder Education; 2008. p. 109–37.
26. Cohen SL, Paradis C, LeMura LM. The effects of contingent-monetary reinforcement and music on exercise in college students. J Sport Behav. 2007;30:146–60.
27. Elliott D, Carr S, Orme D. The effect of motivational music on sub-maximal exercise. Eur J Sport Sci. 2005;5:97–106.
28. Karageorghis CI, Mouzourides D, Priest DL, Sasso T, Morrish D, Whalley C. Psychophysical and ergogenic effects of synchronous music during treadmill walking. J Sport Exerc Psychol. 2009;31:18–36.
29. Terry PC, Karageorghis CI, Mecozzi Saha A, D'Auria S. Effects of synchronous music on treadmill running among elite triathletes. J Sci Med Sport. 2012;15:52–7.
30. Kenyon GP, Thaut MH. Rhythm-driven optimization of motor control. Recent Res Dev Biomech. 2003;1:29–47.
31. Smoll FL, Schultz RW. Accuracy of motor behaviour in response to preferred and nonpreferred tempos. J Hum Mov Stud. 1982;8:123–38.
32. Rossignol S, Melvill-Jones G. Audiospinal influences in man studied by the H-reflex and its possible role in rhythmic movement synchronized to sound. Electroencephalogr Clin Neurophysiol. 1976;41:83–92.
33. Richardson MJ, Marsh KL, Schmidt RC. Effects of visual and verbal interaction on unintentional interpersonal coordination. J Exp Psychol: Human Percept Perform. 2005;31:62–79.

34. Karageorghis CI, Terry PC, Lane AM. Development and validation of an instrument to assess the motivational qualities of music in exercise and sport: the Brunel Music Rating Inventory. J Sports Sci. 1999;17:713–24.
35. Large EW. On synchronizing movements to music. Hum Mov Sci. 2000;19:527–66.
36. von Holst E. Relative coordination as a phenomenon and as a method of analysis of central nervous system function. In: Martin R, editor. The collected papers of Erich von Holst, The behavioral physiology of animal and man, vol. 1. Coral Gables: University of Miami Press; 1973. p. 33–135.
37. Lopresti-Goodman SM, Richardson MJ, Silva PL, Schmidt RC. Period basin of entrainment for unintentional visual coordination. J Mot Behav. 2008;40:3–10.
38. Schmidt RC, Richardson MJ. Dynamics of interpersonal coordination. Berlin: Springer; 2008.
39. Schmidt RC, Richardson MJ, Arsenault CA, Galantucci B. Visual tracking and entrainment to an environmental rhythm. J Exp Psychol: Human Percept Perform. 2007;33:860–70.
40. Strogatz SH. Nonlinear dynamic and chaos: with applications to physics, biology, chemistry, and engineering. Cambridge: Perseus Books; 1994.
41. Waterhouse J, Hudson P, Edwards B. Effects of music tempo upon submaximal cycling performance. Scand J Med Sci Sports. 2010;20:662–9.
42. Kelso JAS. Dynamic patterns: the self-organization of brain and behavior. Cambridge: MIT Press; 1995.
43. Van Dyck E, Moelants D, Demey M, Deweppe A, Coussement P, Leman M. The impact of the bass drum on human dance movement. Music Percept. 2013;30:349–59.
44. Faul F, Erdfelder E, Lang AG, Buchner A. G*Power 3: a flexible statistical power analysis program for the social, behavioral, and biomedical sciences. Behav Res Methods. 2007;39:175–91.
45. Karageorghis CI, Terry PC, Lane AM, Bishop DT, Priest DL. The BASES expert statement on use of music in exercise. J Sports Sci. 2012;30:953–6.
46. Dixon S. Evaluation of the audio beat tracking system BeatRoot. J New Music Res. 2007;36:39–50.
47. Moens B, Muller C, van Noorden L, Franek M, Celie B, Boone J, et al. Encouraging spontaneous synchronisation with DJogger, an adaptive music player that aligns movement with music. Plos One. In press.
48. Karageorghis CI, Priest DL, Terry PC, Chatzisarantis NLD, Lane AM. Development and validation of an instrument to assess the motivational qualities of music in exercise: the Brunel Music Rating Inventory-2. J Sports Sci. 2006;24:899–909.
49. Ajzen I, Fishbein M. Attitude-behavior relations: a theoretical analysis and review of empirical research. Psychol Bull. 1977;84:888–918.
50. Borg G. Borg's perceived exertion and pain scales. Human Kinetics: Champaign; 1998.
51. Levitin D. This is your brain on music: the science of a human obsession. New York: Dutton; 2006.
52. Repp BH, Su YH. Sensorimotor synchronization: a review of recent research (2006-2012). Psychon Bull Rev. 2013;20:403–52.
53. Karageorghis C, Jones L, Low D. Relationship between exercise heart rate and music tempo preference. Res Quart Exerc Sport. 2006;77:240–50.
54. Mendonça C, Oliveira M, Fontes L, Santos J. The effect of instruction to synchronize over step frequency while walking with auditory cues on a treadmill. Hum Mov Sci. 2014;33:33–42.
55. Pellett TL. Children's stereotypical perceptions of physical activities: a K–12 analysis. Percept Motor Skills. 1994;79:1128–30.
56. Karageorghis CI, Priest DL. Music in the exercise domain: a review and synthesis (Part II). Int Rev Sport Exerc Psychol. 2012;5:67–84.
57. Brownley KA, McMurray RG, Hackney AC. Effects of music on physiological and affective responses to graded treadmill exercise in trained and untrained runners. Int J Psychophysiol. 1995;19:193–201.
58. Mohammadzadeh H, Tartibiyan B, Ahmadi A. The effects of music on the perceived exertion rate and performance of trained and untrained individuals during progressive exercise. Facta Univ Phys Educ Sport. 2008;6:67–74.

22

ACTN3 Polymorphism: Comparison Between Elite Swimmers and Runners

Sigal Ben-Zaken[1*], Alon Eliakim[2], Dan Nemet[2], Moran Rabinovich[1], Eias Kassem[3] and Yoav Meckel[1]

Abstract

Background: The human *ACTN3* gene encodes α-actinin-3, an actin-binding protein with a pivotal role in muscle structure and metabolism. A common genetic single nucleotide polymorphism (SNP) at codon 577 of the *ACTN3* results in the replacement of an arginine (R) with a stop codon (X). The R allele is a normal functional version of the gene, whereas the X allele contains a sequence change that completely stops production of functional α-actinin-3 protein. The *ACTN3* R577X polymorphism was found to be associated with power athletic performance especially among track and field athletes. The aim of the current study was to compare allelic and genotype frequencies of the ACTN3 R577X polymorphism among runners and swimmers specializing in different distances, and >non-athletic controls.

Methods: One hundred and thirty-seven runners, 91 swimmers and 217 controls, participated in the study. Runners were assigned to two subgroups according to their event specialty—long-distance runners (LDR) and short-distance runners (SDR). Swimmers were also assigned to two subgroups according to their main swimming event—long-distance swimmers (LDS) and short-distance swimmers (SDS). Genomic DNA was extracted from peripheral EDTA-treated anti-coagulated blood using a standard protocol. Genotypes were determined using the Taqman allelic discrimination assay.

Results: Runners' genotype and allele differed significantly between LDR, SDR, and controls, with the lowest prevalence of RR genotype and R allele among LDR. XX genotype and X allele prevalence was significantly higher among LDR compared to the other groups ($p < 0.01$ for all). On the other hand, swimmers' genotype and allele frequencies did not differ significantly between subgroups (LDS and SDS). Yet, LDS had significantly higher RR genotype and R allele frequencies compared to LDR.

Conclusions: The findings suggest that while ACTN3 R577X polymorphism is a genetic polymorphism that may distinguish between SDR and LDR, it cannot differentiate significantly between SDS and LDS.

Trial Registration: ClinicalTrials.gov: NCT01319032

Key Points:

- *ACTN3* R577X polymorphism is largely associated with running events specialization, with high prevalence of RR genotype and R allele frequency among short-distance runners compare to long-distance runners.
- Unlike in running, *ACTN3* R577X polymorphism is not associated with swimming specialization.
- The inability of the *ACTN3* R577X polymorphism to distinguish between swimmers specializing in different events, presumably since other factors such as body physique, technique, tactics, etc., are more likely to determine such a distinction.

Keywords: ACTN3; Genetic polymorphism; Runners; Swimmers

* Correspondence: sigalbz@wincol.ac.il
[1]Genetics and Molecular Biology Laboratory, The Zinman College of Physical Education and Sports Sciences at the Wingate Institute, Netanya 42902, Israel
Full list of author information is available at the end of the article

Background

Athletic performance is a multifactorial trait, determined by a range of genetic and environmental factors. Most of the genetic polymorphisms considered to be related to athletic performance were investigated in case-control retrospective studies [1], which did not reveal the biological mechanism responsible for the influence of this polymorphism on athletic performance. Moreover, most of these polymorphisms are intronic and non-functional.

The *ACTN3* R577X (rs1815739) polymorphism is an exception in this sense, since it is a well-studied functional polymorphism. The human *ACTN3* gene encodes α-actinin-3, an actin-binding protein with a structural role at the sarcomeric Z-line in glycolytic (type II, fast-twitch) muscle fibers, and plays an increasingly evident role in the regulation of muscle metabolism [2]. A common genetic single nucleotide polymorphism (SNP) at codon 577 of the *ACTN3* results in the replacement of an arginine (R) with a stop codon (X) [3]. The R allele is a normal functional version of the gene, whereas the X allele contains a sequence change that completely stops production of functional α-actinin-3 protein [3]. Therefore, XX homozygotes do not express ACTN3 at all in their muscles [2]. In the knockout mouse, it is clear that ACTN3 deficiency alters skeletal muscle function [2].

Yang et al. [4] demonstrated, for the first time, a significant association between the ACTN3 genotype and athletic performance. They found that both male and female elite sprint athletes have significantly higher frequencies of the 577R allele compared to controls. Since then ACTN3 R577X has been studied in various cohorts. Some articles have reported a strong association between the RR genotype and elite power performance [5–8]. While ACTN3 R carriage may enhance power performance, ACTN3 XX might contribute to endurance performance [9, 10]. However, reports on Asians and Africans suggested that ACTN3 deficiency might not be associated with endurance performance [11, 12]. A recent meta-analysis of 88 articles did not find a significant association for ACTN3 RR genotype with physical performance (odds ratio (OR), 1.03; 95 % confidence interval (CI), 0.92–1.15). However, when the analysis was restricted to power events, a significant association was observed (OR, 1.21; 95 % CI, 1.03–1.42) [13]. Overall, association studies on ACTN3 R577X polymorphism and power performance show consistent results across multiple athlete cohorts [14]. Moreover, unlike many polymorphisms, the ACTN3 R577X polymorphism is a functional polymorphism, with the XX genotype resulting in complete loss of function. A mechanistic explanation for the role of ACTN3 in power performance can be found in the α-actinin-3 knockout (KO) mouse. Compared with wild-type mice, the muscles of the KO mouse exhibit reduced muscle mass, due to decreased diameter of fast muscle fibers, significant decrease in grip strength, higher endurance, and a shift towards increased activity of mitochondrial oxidative metabolism [9, 10]. All of these placed the ACTN3 R577X polymorphism as a pivotal polymorphism explaining power athletic performance [14].

Interestingly, while the ACTN3 R577X polymorphism has been studied extensively among track and field athletes (especially runners), its contributions to performance in swimming, a sport that muscle strength plays also a key role [15], had received little attention. In swimming, muscular strength dictates how much force muscles are able to apply to the water, which in turn propels the body forward. Therefore, muscular strength is of great importance in order to produce speed in sprint swimming, while in endurance swimming muscular strength is required to perform repeated submaximal contractions over time. The few studies that investigate ACTN3 R577X prevalence among swimmers did not find significant association between the ACTN3 R577X polymorphism and swimming performance among Caucasian, East Asians [16], or Spanish swimmers [17]. Among Taiwanese, the R allele was significantly higher in female international sprint swimmers than in national sprint swimmers or the general population [5].

Therefore, the aim of the current study was to compare allelic and genotype frequencies of the ACTN3 R577X polymorphism among runners and swimmers specializing in different distances, and non-athletic controls. We hypothesized that similarly to runners, the R allele will be more frequent among sprint swimmers and the X allele more frequent among endurance swimmers.

Methods

Participants

One hundred and thirty-seven track and field athletes (98 males and 39 females, age 17–50) and 91 swimmers (60 males and 31 females, age 16–49) participated in the study. The track and field athletes were assigned to two subgroups according to their event specialty, as follows: 1) long-distance runners (5000 m marathon runners—LDR) ($n = 65$) and 2) power event athletes (100–200 m sprinters and long jumpers—SDR) ($n = 72$). The swimmers were also assigned to two groups according to their main swimming event, as follows: 1) long-distance swimmers (800–1500 m swimmers—LDS) ($n = 43$) and 2) short-distance swimmers (50–100 m swimmers—SDS) ($n = 48$). All athletes were ranked among the top Israeli results in their event and had competed in national and/or international level meets on a regular basis. Sixty-seven track and field athletes were classified as international athletes (participants in European and World Championships, and Olympic Games). The Israeli runners' criteria for participation in the Olympic Games and World championships are ranking in places 1–12 in the former European championship or 1–16 in the former world championship (both should be no more than 2 years prior to the upcoming event), or setting the international result criteria A at least once. For participation in a European championship, the runners should fulfill the above criteria or set the international result criteria B at least twice. The international results criteria A and B are standard results published yearly by the IAAF (The International Association of Athletic Federation, http://www.iaaf.org/). These standard results are intended to qualify athletes to be eligible to compete in Olympics and World Championships. The A standard is the most difficult to achieve. The B standard is easier to achieve, and usually, national athletic association uses it also as a criterion to international competition participation.

Thirty-one swimmers were classified as international athletes (participants in European and World Championships, and Olympic Games). The Israeli swimmers result criteria for participation in the European and World championships and in the Olympic Games are the average result of the 16th place in the former three respective championships. These criteria indicate a remarkable difference between the international and national level athletes in the present study. The control group consisted of 217 (137 males and 80 females, age 19–29) non-athletic healthy individuals who were not engaged in competitive sport. Characteristics of the athletes and controls are presented in Table 1.

The study was approved by the Institutional Review Board of the Hillel Yaffe Medical Center, Hadera, Israel, according to the Declaration of Helsinki. A written informed consent was obtained from all participants.

Genotyping

Genomic DNA was extracted from peripheral EDTA-treated anti-coagulated blood using a standard protocol. Genotypes were determined using the Taqman allelic discrimination assay. The Assay-by-Design service (www.appliedbiosystem.com) was used to set up a Taqman allelic discrimination assay for the ACTN3 (rs1815739 C1747T). Primer sequences were as follows: forward, GCACGATCAGTTCAAGGCAAC; reverse, GCTGAGGGTGATGTAGGGATTG. Probe sequences were for C1747T: forward, VIC-CGAGGCTGACCGAGAG; reverse, FAM-CCGAGGCTGACTGAGAG. The PCR reaction mixture included 5 ng genomic DNA, 0.125 μl TaqMan assay (40*, ABI), 2.5 μl Master mix (ABI), and 2.375 μl water. PCR was performed in 96 well PCR plates in an ABI 7300 PCR system (Applied Biosystems Inc., Foster City, CA, USA) and consisted of initial denaturation for 5 min at 95 °C, and 40 cycles with denaturation of 15 s at 95 °C and annealing and extension for 60 s at 63 °C. The results were analyzed by the ABI Taqman 7900HT using the sequence detection system 2.22 software (Applied Biosystems Inc).

Statistical Analysis

The SPSS statistical package, version 20.0, was used to perform all statistical evaluations (SPSS, Chicago, IL, USA). A chi-squared test was used to confirm that the observed genotype frequencies were in Hardy-Weinberg equilibrium and to compare alleles and genotype frequencies between athletes and controls, as well as between athletes from different sports (e.g., runners vs. swimmers) and different competitive groups (e.g., sprinters vs. endurance). If observed or expected values included a cell value of 5, we used Fisher's exact test to compare alleles and genotype frequencies.

Results

The complete data on allele and genotype frequencies are presented in Table 2. The genotype subtype did not differ by age or sex. The ACTN3 genotype distribution was in agreement with the Hardy-Weinberg equilibrium in all groups ($p = 0.87$ for LDR, $p = 0.84$ for SDR, $p = 0.99$ for LDS, $p = 0.78$ for SDS, and $p = 0.13$ for controls).

Runners' genotype and allele frequencies are presented in Fig. 1. The runners' genotype differed significantly between long-distance runners, short-distance runners, and controls ($p < 0.01$ for LDR vs. SDR, LDR vs. controls, and SDR vs. controls). The long-distance runners had the lowest frequency of RR genotype (20.0 % compared to 40 % among SDR). This frequency was similar to the RR genotype frequency among controls (22.1 %). On the other hand, the XX genotype frequency was significantly higher among LDR (35.4 %) compared to the other groups, SDR (16.7 %), and controls (18.4 %). LDR had a significantly higher frequency of X allele (57.7 %) compared to SDR (38.2 %, $p < 0.01$). SDR had significant higher R allele frequency (61.8 %) compared to LDR (42.3 %, $p < 0.001$) and controls (51.8 %, $p < 0.05$).

The swimmers' genotype and allele frequencies are presented in Fig. 2. The swimmers' genotype and allele frequencies did not differ significantly between the specialization subgroups (LDS and SDS). Yet, the swimmers' genotype frequency differed significantly from the controls ($p < 0.05$). LDS' and SDS' RR genotype frequencies (37.5 and 37.2 %, respectively) were significantly higher compared to controls' RR genotype frequency (22.1 %, $p < 0.01$ for LDS vs. controls and $p < 0.03$ for SDS vs. controls). LDS had higher XX genotype frequency (18.7 %) compared to SDS (11.6 %), but this difference did not reach statistical significance.

We compared allele and genotype frequencies between athletes specializing in endurance-type events from different sports (e.g., LDS vs. LDR) and between athletes specializing in power-type events from different sports (e.g., SDS vs. SDR). LDS had significantly higher RR genotype and R allele frequency (37.4 and 59.3 %,

Table 1 Athletes and controls' data

Group	Number	Main event	M/F	Top/national level	Age (mean + SD, range)
Runners					
Long distance	65	5000 m marathon	50/15	21/44	31.4 + 9.2 (17–50)
Power event (sprinters and jumpers)	72	100–200 m, jumps	48/24	23/49	30.1 + 12.7 (17–50)
Swimmers					
Long distance	43	800–1500 m	27/16	15/28	23.6 + 7.9 (16–49)
Short distance	48	50–100 m	33/15	16/32	23.3 + 8.3 (16–48)
Controls	217	nr	137/80	nr	26.4 + 5.8 (19–29)

nr not relevant

respectively) compared to LDR (20.0 and 42.3 %, respectively) ($p < 0.04$ and $p < 0.04$ for RR genotype and R allele frequency, respectively) (Fig. 3). The power-type athletes' genotype and allele frequencies did not differ significantly between SDR and SDS.

Discussion

The main finding of the current study is that while the ACTN3 R577X polymorphism was largely associated with a distinction between runners specializing in sprint events compared to runners specializing in long-distance events, this difference was not found among swimmers specializing in sprint events compared to swimmers specializing in long-distance events.

Athletic events can be divided by the distance or time of the activity. Other parameters, like power, speed, and endurance, are also used to characterize specific sports. Track and field is a good example of the use of these descriptors and their activity time frames in differentiating between events based on energetic resources. Endurance-type athletic events are characterized by relatively low-intensity, long-lasting exercise that relies primarily on the aerobic energy-generating process [18]. The term aerobic refers to the use of oxidative phosphorylation to adequately meet energy demands during exercise [19]. In contrast, strength, power, and speed-type athletic events are characterized by intense efforts lasting a short time and by the use of anaerobic metabolism as the energy source.

The ACTN3 R577X polymorphism is a well-documented genetic marker that enables sport scientists to distinguish between a genetic predisposition towards excellence in power-type events or in endurance-type events [14]. Indeed, in the present study we found a significant difference in ACTN3 R577X polymorphism prevalence among LDR compared to SDR, with a high prevalence of 40.3 and 61.8 % for RR genotype and R allele frequency in SDR compared to 20.0 and 42.3 % for RR genotype and R allele frequency in LDR. This finding may suggest that the ACTN3 R577X polymorphism

Table 2 The ACTN3 R577X genotype and allele frequencies in all groups

Group	Number	Genotype			Allele frequency	
		R/R	R/X	X/X	R allele	X allele
Runners						
Long distance	65	13(20.0)*,**	29(44.6)*,**	23(35.4)*,**	55(42.3)¥, ¥¥	75(57.7)¥, ¥¥
Short distance	72	29(40.3)***	31(43.1)***	12(16.7)***	89(61.8)¥¥¥	55(38.2)¥¥¥
Total	187	57(30.5)	86(46.0)	44(23.5)	200(53.5)	174(46.5)
Swimmers						
Long distance	48	18(37.5)#, ^	18(37.5)#	12(25.0)#	57(57.0)&	43(43.0)&
Short distance	43	16(37.2)^^	22(51.2)	5(11.6)	55(62.5)	33(37.5)
Total	91	34(37.4)	40(43.9)	17(18.7)	108(59.3)	74(40.7)
Controls	217	48(22.1)	129(59.4)	40(18.4)	225(51.8)	209(48.2)

Values are absolute (relative frequencies in parentheses)
*$\chi^2(2) = 8.50$, $p < 0.01$, genotype frequency, LDR vs. controls
**$\chi^2(2) = 9.29$, $p < 0.01$, genotype frequency, LDR vs. SDR
***$\chi^2(2) = 9.41$, $p < 0.01$, genotype frequency, SDR vs. controls
#$\chi^2(2) = 8.01$, $p < 0.02$, genotype frequency, LDS vs. controls ($\chi^2(1) = 6.14$, $p < 0.01$, RR genotype, SDS vs. controls
^$\chi^2(1) = 4.25$, $p < 0.04$, RR genotype, LDR vs. LDS
^^$\chi^2(1) = 4.97$, $p < 0.03$, RR genotype, SDS vs. controls
¥¥$\chi^2(1) = 10.42$, $p < 0.001$, allele frequency, LDR vs. SDR
¥¥¥$\chi^2(1) = 4.32$, $p < 0.05$, allele frequency, SDR vs. controls
&$\chi^2(1) = 4.30$, $p < 0.04$, allele frequency, LDR vs. LDS

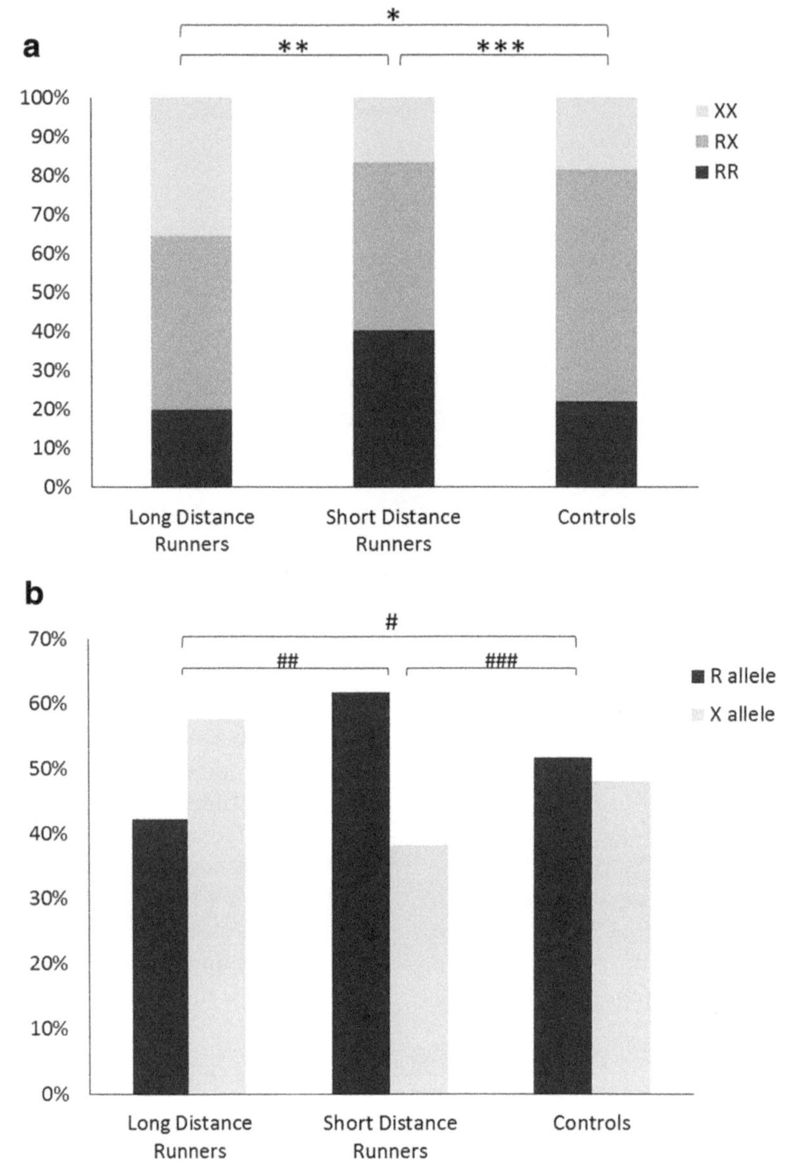

Fig. 1 The ACTN3 R577X polymorphism **a** genotype frequencies, **b** allele frequencies in track and field athletes and controls. *$\chi^2(2) = 8.50$, $p < 0.01$, genotype frequency, LDR vs. controls. **$\chi^2(2) = 9.29$, $p < 0.01$, genotype frequency, LDR vs. SDR. ***$\chi^2(2) = 9.41$, $p < 0.01$, genotype frequency, SDR vs. controls. #$\chi^2(1) = 3.64$, $p = 0.06$, allele frequency, LDR vs. controls. ##$\chi^2(1) = 10.42$, $p < 0.001$, allele frequency, LDR vs. SDR. ###$\chi^2(1) = 4.32$, $p < 0.05$, allele frequency, SDR vs. controls

enables to distinguish between two types of track and field events—a "pure power event" and a "pure endurance event." Yet, for a higher resolution distinction like the one needed to distinguish between middle-distance runners (MDR) and LDR performance, or between MDR and SDR performance, other genetic markers or profiles may be needed. This assumption should be examined in future studies. Since swimming events are also divided by the distance or time of the activity, one would assume that swimming events can also be classified into "endurance-type events" and "power-type events." Subsequently, the genetic background that influences a track and field athlete's capability to excel in one sport discipline (e.g., sprint running) rather than another (e.g., long-distance running) would, presumably, be similar to the genetic background that influences a swimmer's capability to excel in a specific sport discipline. However, in contrast to our hypothesis, no significant association was found in the present study between the ACTN3 R577X polymorphism and swimming performance. This finding is consistent with previous reports that failed to find an association between the ACTN3 R577X polymorphism and swimming performance in Caucasians, East Asians [16], and Spanish swimmers [17]. In contrast, R allele was significantly

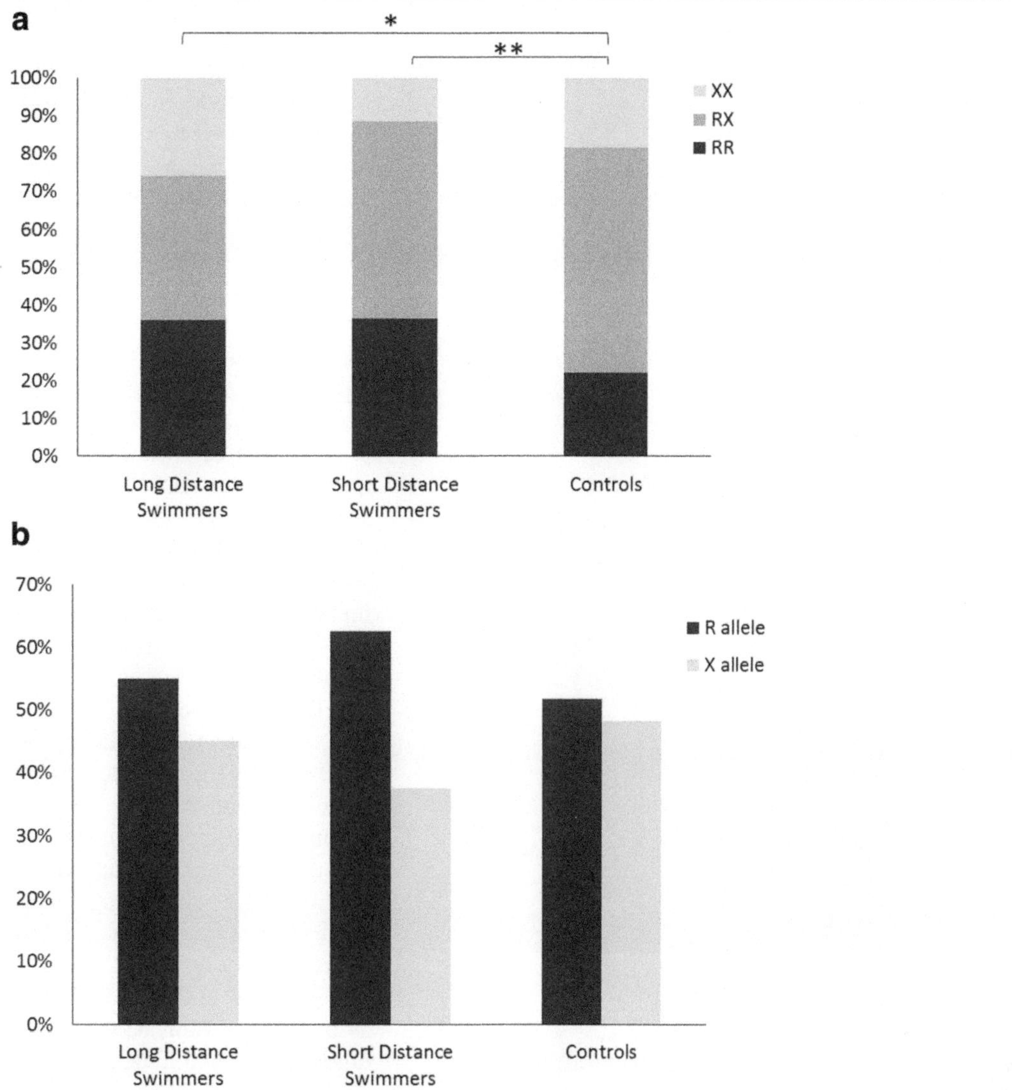

Fig. 2 The ACTN3 R577X polymorphism (**a** genotype frequencies, **b** allele frequencies) in swimmers and controls. *$\chi^2(2) = 8.01$, $p < 0.02$, genotype frequency, LDS vs. controls. **$\chi^2(1) = 4.97$, $p < 0.03$, RR genotype, SDS vs. controls

higher in Taiwanese female international sprint swimmers compared to national-level sprint swimmers and the general population [5].

ACTN3 plays a pivotal role in muscle metabolism, structure, and fiber-type distribution [2, 20], and therefore it has a direct effect on the ability to perform in elite power events. However, based on the present findings, it may be that none of these are detrimental to swimming. It may be that the aspect of power performance affected by the polymorphism is less important in swimming relative to other sports, possibly because of the relatively lower stress put on muscles supported in water and the lack of eccentric contractions [21]. Moreover, in swimming the produced power is lower compared to land activities of similar duration [22]. Efficiency is a critical factor in this sport, which includes several aspects of technique. Swimming is a highly skilled sport, where the neural and biomechanical skills are the greatest contributor for force production [22–24]. Overall, in swimming, the athlete's technique and body physique have a greater impact on performance than in other sports such as running.

In line with this, we have previously found a strong significant correlation ($r = 0.74$) between 100 m and the 2000 m swim times suggesting that swimming times are largely affected by swimming technique and by the swimmers' size (particularly limb length) [25]. These may, at least partially, mask metabolic differences between swimmers, enabling technically skilled and/or tall swimmers to excel at all swimming distances. These relationships are unique for swimming, and this assumption can be supported by the past records of top world-class swimmers, such as Ian Thorpe (world record holder in

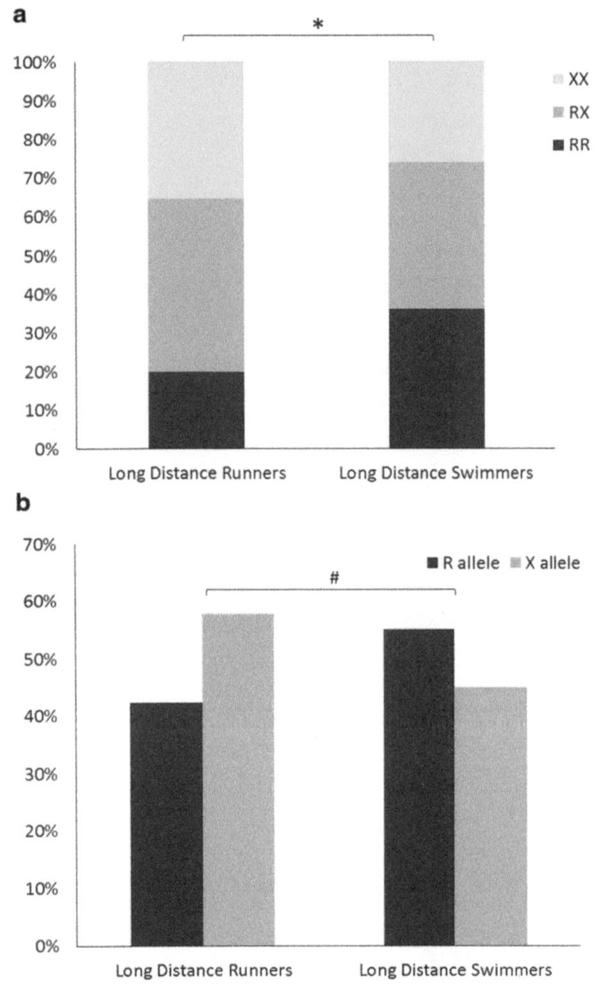

Fig. 3 The ACTN3 R577X polymorphism (**a** genotype frequencies, **b** allele frequencies) in endurance athletes (LDR and LDS). $*\chi^2(1) = 4.25$, $p < 0.04$, RR genotype, LDR vs. LDS. $\#\chi^2(1) = 4.30$, $p < 0.04$, allele frequency, LDR vs. LDS

the 100-m relay and individual 200, 400, and 800 m) and Grant Hackett (world record holder in 200-m relays and individual 400, 800, and 1500 m), as well as others who excel in both short and long swimming distances. A similar phenomenon is very uncommon among runners. To the best of our knowledge, this relationship between short- and long-distance performances in swimming has not been reported previously in other sport types.

Lastly, there is the possibility that a type II error accounts for the fact that we do not see an association between the ACTN3 R577X polymorphism and swimming performance. Large studies with the power to detect significant associations at genome-wide level have not yet been conducted. Although a meta-analysis of the association between ACTN3 and sprint/power athlete status demonstrated evidence for a real association [13, 26], many studies—mainly with small sample sizes—have failed to observe any association between ACTN3 variants and sporting performance.

It should be noted that both LDS and SDS had a higher RR genotype frequency (38.0 and 36.4 %, respectively) compared to controls (22.1 %). This result implies that both LDS and SDS may benefit from ACTN3 R allele existence, strengthening the notion of no clear ACTN3 polymorphism differences between power and endurance swimmers. Moreover, RR genotype and R allele frequency were higher among LDS (38.0 and 57.0 % for RR genotype and R allele frequency, respectively) compared to LDR (20.0 and 42.3 % for RR genotype and R allele frequency, respectively). This may be explained by differences in the specific activity duration of competitive swimming and running. The longest Olympic swim (1500 m ~ 15 min duration) is much shorter than the longest Olympic running race (marathon ~2 h 10-min duration), and therefore ACTN3 power characteristics are needed for long-distance swimmers. It is possible that if open-water swimmers (Olympic race—10K) had been included among the long-distance swimmers in the present study, the differences in the R allele frequency between LDS and LDR would disappear. When comparing the short-duration events, there is also a difference in the specific activity duration of competitive swimming and running. The 100-m distance covered in swimming at approximately 50 s, while the same distance covered in running at approximately 10 s. As a result, a sprint runner relies mostly on anaerobic energy sources, while a sprint swimmer uses also aerobic energy components. Therefore, the SDS and the LDS share some common features, and the ACTN3 RR genotype is not suitable as a distinguishing genetic marker between them, as it does for SDR and LDR.

Conclusions

To conclude, the findings of the present study propose that while the ACTN3 R577X polymorphism is a genetic polymorphism that may distinguish between SDR and LDR, it cannot differentiate significantly between SDS and LDS. This suggests that the power of a specific genetic factor to serve as the sole divider between athletes of different specialties—aerobic or anaerobic—is limited. It seems that body physique, technique, tactics, and psychological factors are more likely to influence and determine such a distinction, especially in certain sport types, like swimming.

Competing Interests

The authors declare that they have no competing interests.

Authors' contributions

SBZ carried out the genetic analysis, performed the statistical analysis, participated in study design and coordination and drafted the manuscript. AE conceived of the study, and drafted the manuscript. DM conceived of the study, and drafted the manuscript MR participated in study design and coordination. EK participated in study design and coordination. YM conceived of conceived of the study, participated in its design and coordination, and drafted the manuscript. All authors read and approved the final manuscript.. All authors read and approved the final manuscript.

Acknowledgements
The authors thank Mr. Roi Mor for the technical assistance. This research was supported by the Zinman College for Physical Education and Sport Sciences at Wingate Institute.

Author details
[1]Genetics and Molecular Biology Laboratory, The Zinman College of Physical Education and Sports Sciences at the Wingate Institute, Netanya 42902, Israel. [2]Child Health and Sports Center, Pediatric Department, Meir Medical Center, Sackler School of Medicine, Tel-Aviv University, Tel-Aviv, Israel. [3]Pediatric Department, Hillel-Yafe Medical Center, Hadera, Israel.

References

1. Bray MS, Hagberg JM, Pérusse L, Rankinen T, Roth SM, Wolfarth B, et al. The human gene map for performance and health-related fitness phenotypes: the 2006-2007 update. Med Sci Sports Exerc. 2009;41:35–73. http://www.ncbi.nlm.nih.gov/pubmed/19123262.
2. Berman Y, North KN. A gene for speed: the emerging role of alpha-actinin-3 in muscle metabolism. Physiology (Bethesda). 2010;25:250–9. http://www.ncbi.nlm.nih.gov/pubmed/20699471.
3. North KN, Yang N, Wattanasirichaigoon D, Mills M, Easteal S, Beggs AH. A common nonsense mutation results in alpha-actinin-3 deficiency in the general population. Nat Genet. 1999;21:353–4. http://www.ncbi.nlm.nih.gov/pubmed/10192379.
4. Yang N, MacArthur DG, Gulbin JP, Hahn AG, Beggs AH, Easteal S, et al. ACTN3 genotype is associated with human elite athletic performance. Am J Hum Genet. 2003;73:627–31. http://www.pubmedcentral.nih.gov/articlerender.fcgi?artid=1180686&tool=pmcentrez&rendertype=abstract.
5. Chiu L-L, Wu Y-F, Tang M-T, Yu H-C, Hsieh L-L, Hsieh SS-Y. ACTN3 genotype and swimming performance in Taiwan. Int J Sports Med. 2011;32:476–80. http://www.ncbi.nlm.nih.gov/pubmed/21472630.
6. Eynon N, Duarte JA, Oliveira J, Sagiv M, Yamin C, Meckel Y, et al. ACTN3 R577X polymorphism and Israeli top-level athletes. Int J Sports Med. 2009;30:695–8. http://www.ncbi.nlm.nih.gov/pubmed/19544227.
7. Papadimitriou ID, Papadopoulos C, Kouvatsi A, Triantaphyllidis C. The ACTN3 gene in elite Greek track and field athletes. Int J Sports Med. 2008;29:352–5. http://www.ncbi.nlm.nih.gov/pubmed/17879893.
8. Paparini A, Ripani M, Giordano GD, Santoni D, Pigozzi F, Romano-Spica V. ACTN3 genotyping by real-time PCR in the Italian population and athletes. Med Sci Sports Exerc. 2007;39:810–5. http://www.ncbi.nlm.nih.gov/pubmed/17468578.
9. MacArthur DG, Seto JT, Chan S, Quinlan KGR, Raftery JM, Turner N, et al. An Actn3 knockout mouse provides mechanistic insights into the association between alpha-actinin-3 deficiency and human athletic performance. Hum Mol Genet. 2008;17:1076–86. http://www.ncbi.nlm.nih.gov/pubmed/18178581.
10. MacArthur DG, Seto JT, Raftery JM, Quinlan KG, Huttley GA, Hook JW, et al. Loss of ACTN3 gene function alters mouse muscle metabolism and shows evidence of positive selection in humans. Nat Genet. 2007;39:1261–5. http://www.ncbi.nlm.nih.gov/pubmed/17828264.
11. Shang X, Huang C, Chang Q, Zhang L, Huang T. Association between the ACTN3 R577X polymorphism and female endurance athletes in China. Int J Sports Med. 2010;31:913–6. http://www.ncbi.nlm.nih.gov/pubmed/20936592.
12. Yang N, MacArthur DG, Wolde B, Onywera VO, Boit MK, Lau SYM-A, et al. The ACTN3 R577X polymorphism in East and West African athletes. Med Sci Sports Exerc. 2007;39:1985–8. http://www.ncbi.nlm.nih.gov/pubmed/17986906.
13. Ma F, Yang Y, Li X, Zhou F, Gao C, Li M, et al. The association of sport performance with ACE and ACTN3 genetic polymorphisms: a systematic review and meta-analysis. PLoS One. 2013;8:e54685. http://www.pubmedcentral.nih.gov/articlerender.fcgi?artid=3554644&tool=pmcentrez&rendertype=abstract.
14. Eynon N, Hanson ED, Lucia A, Houweling PJ, Garton F, North KN, et al. Genes for elite power and sprint performance: ACTN3 leads the way. Sports Med. 2013;43:803–17. http://www.ncbi.nlm.nih.gov/pubmed/23681449.
15. Bloomfield J, Blanksby BA, Ackland TR, Elliott BC. The anatomical and physiological characteristics of pre-adolescent swimmers, tennis players and non-competitors. Aust J Sci Med Sport. 1985;17:19–23.
16. Wang G, Mikami E, Chiu L-L, DE Perini A, Deason M, Fuku N, et al. Association analysis of ACE and ACTN3 in elite Caucasian and East Asian swimmers. Med Sci Sports Exerc. 2013;45:892–900. http://www.ncbi.nlm.nih.gov/pubmed/23190598.
17. Ruiz JR, Santiago C, Yvert T, Muniesa C, Díaz-Ureña G, Bekendam N, et al. ACTN3 genotype in Spanish elite swimmers: no "heterozygous advantage". Scand J Med Sci Sports. 2013;23:e162–7. http://www.ncbi.nlm.nih.gov/pubmed/23317015.
18. Plowman SA, Smith DL. Exercise physiology for health, fitness, and performance. In: 3rd edition, Emily Lupash editor. Exercise Physiology for Health, Fitness, and Performance. Lippincott Williams & Wilkins, 2007: 61.
19. McArdle WD, Katch FI, Katch VL. Essentials of exercise physiology. In: 4th edition, Emily Lupash editor. Essentials of exercise physiology. Lippincott Williams & Wilkins, 2006: 204.
20. Moran CN, Yang N, Bailey MES, Tsiokanos A, Jamurtas A, MacArthur DG, et al. Association analysis of the ACTN3 R577X polymorphism and complex quantitative body composition and performance phenotypes in adolescent Greeks. Eur J Hum Genet. 2007;15:88–93. http://www.ncbi.nlm.nih.gov/pubmed/17033684.
21. Demura S, Aoki H, Yamamato Y, Yamaji S. Comparison of strength values and laterality in various muscle contractions between competitive swimmers and untrained persons. Health (Irvine Calif). 2010;2:1249–54.
22. Toussaint HM, Truijens M. Power requirements for swimming a world-record 50-m front crawl. Int J Sports Physiol Perform. 2006;1:61–4. http://www.ncbi.nlm.nih.gov/pubmed/19114739.
23. Ferreira MI, Barbosa TM, Neiva HP, Marta CC, Costa MJ, Marinho DA. The effect of gender, energetics and biomechanics on swimming masters performance. J Strength Cond Res. 2015; 1 http://www.ncbi.nlm.nih.gov/pubmed/25635608.
24. Trappe S, Costill D, Thomas R. Effect of swim taper on whole muscle and single muscle fiber contractile properties. Med Sci Sports Exerc. 2001;33:48–56. http://www.ncbi.nlm.nih.gov/pubmed/11194111.
25. Meckel Y, Bishop DJ, Rabinovich M, Kaufman L, Nemet D, Eliakim A. The relationship between short- and long-distance swimming performance and repeated sprint ability. J Strength Cond Res. 2012;26:3426–31. http://www.ncbi.nlm.nih.gov/pubmed/22207257.
26. Alfred T, Ben-Shlomo Y, Cooper R, Hardy R, Cooper C, Deary IJ, et al. ACTN3 genotype, athletic status, and life course physical capability: meta-analysis of the published literature and findings from nine studies. Hum Mutat. 2011;32:1008–18. http://www.pubmedcentral.nih.gov/articlerender.fcgi?artid=3174315&tool=pmcentrez&rendertype=abstract.

Synchronized personalized music audio-playlists to improve adherence to physical activity among patients participating in a structured exercise program: a proof-of-principle feasibility study

David A Alter[1,2,4,8,10*], Mary O'Sullivan[2,10], Paul I Oh[2,4,10], Donald A Redelmeier[1,3,4,8,10], Susan Marzolini[2,10], Richard Liu[2,10], Mary Forhan[2,9,10], Michael Silver[2,10], Jack M Goodman[2,5,10] and Lee R Bartel[6,7,10]

Abstract

Background: Preference-based tempo-pace synchronized music has been shown to reduce perceived physical activity exertion and improve exercise performance. The extent to which such strategies can improve adherence to physical activity remains unknown. The objective of the study is to explore the feasibility and efficacy of tempo-pace synchronized preference-based music audio-playlists on adherence to physical activity among cardiovascular disease patients participating in a cardiac rehabilitation.

Methods: Thirty-four cardiac rehabilitation patients were randomly allocated to one of two strategies: (1) no music usual-care control and (2) tempo-pace synchronized audio-devices with personalized music playlists + usual-care. All songs uploaded onto audio-playlist devices took into account patient personal music genre and artist preferences. However, actual song selection was restricted to music whose tempos approximated patients' prescribed exercise walking/running pace (steps per minute) to achieve tempo-pace synchrony. Patients allocated to audio-music playlists underwent further randomization in which half of the patients received songs that were sonically enhanced with rhythmic auditory stimulation (RAS) to accentuate tempo-pace synchrony, whereas the other half did not. RAS was achieved through blinded rhythmic sonic-enhancements undertaken manually to songs within individuals' music playlists. The primary outcome consisted of the weekly volume of physical activity undertaken over 3 months as determined by tri-axial accelerometers. Statistical methods employed an intention to treat and repeated-measures design.

Results: Patients randomized to personalized audio-playlists with tempo-pace synchrony achieved higher weekly volumes of physical activity than did their non-music usual-care comparators (475.6 min vs. 370.2 min, $P < 0.001$). Improvements in weekly physical activity volumes among audio-playlist recipients were driven by those randomized to the RAS group which attained weekly exercise volumes that were nearly twofold greater than either of the two other groups (average weekly minutes of physical activity of 631.3 min vs. 320 min vs. 370.2 min, personalized audio-playlists with RAS vs. personalized audio-playlists without RAS vs. non-music usual-care controls, respectively, $P < 0.001$). Patients randomized to music with RAS utilized their audio-playlist devices more frequently than did non-RAS music counterparts ($P < 0.001$).

(Continued on next page)

* Correspondence: david.alter@ices.on.ca
[1]Institute for Clinical Evaluative Sciences, 2075 Bayview Avenue, Toronto, ON M4N 3M5, Canada
[2]University Health Network Cardiovascular Prevention and Rehabilitation Program, Toronto Rehabilitation Institute-University Health Network, 550 University Avenue, Toronto, Canada
Full list of author information is available at the end of the article

(Continued from previous page)

Conclusions: The use of tempo-pace synchronized preference-based audio-playlists was feasibly implemented into a structured exercise program and efficacious in improving adherence to physical activity beyond the evidence-based non-music usual standard of care. Larger clinical trials are required to validate these findings.

Trial registration: ClinicalTrials.gov ID (NCT01752595)

Key points

- The integration of tempo-pace synchronized preference-based music audio-playlists into structured exercise program resulted in significantly greater weekly physical activity volumes than did non-music usual-care.
- Differences in weekly physical activity volumes were greatest among those receiving rhythmic auditory stimuli embedded into their audio-music playlists.
- A group's average weekly physical activity positively correlated with their use of audio-playlist devices.

Background

Physical activity has irrefutable benefits to quality of life and survival [1,2]. However, suboptimal uptake and adherence undermines the survival and health benefits associated physical activity in real-world settings [3]. Among patients with established cardiovascular disease, structured exercise programs have been used to promote the self-management and adherence of physical activity, [4] but their effectiveness has also been undermined by high rates of behavioural attrition to physical activity [5,6]. Strategies to improve adherence to physical activity among such populations have proven challenging often yielding inconsistent results [6,7].

Music rhythmicity has been shown to modulate the perceptions and ergonomics of physical activity [8-16]. Postulated mechanisms of action have included neural-entrainment effects and movement cueing step-cadence regulation [8,17-30]. When coupled with individual preferences, such music may further enhance motivation, improve affect, induce distraction and attenuate patients' perceptions of effort during exercise [19,21,26,27,31-33]. While integrated mobile music audio-devices are widely available, no study has explored the feasibility and efficacy of using synchronized preference-based music audio-playlists to improve adherence to physical activity.

The objective of the Music Activity INTervention for Adherence Improvement through Neurological entrainment (MAINTAIN) study was to explore the feasibility and efficacy of implementing tempo-pace synchronized personalized audio-playlist devices to improve adherence to physical activity among patients participating in a structured exercise program. All patients received usual care (cardiac rehabilitation). Patients were randomized to either usual-care alone (i.e. no-music) or an integrated music strategy consisting of personalized customizable audio playlists uploaded onto iPods® whose song selections were comprised of tempos (beats per minute) which matched the individuals' pre-specified walking/running pace as prescribed by the structured exercise program itself. As part of our proof-of-concept feasibility study, among patients randomized to the integrated music strategy, we evaluated the incremental feasibility and efficacy of embedding additional rhythmic sonic enhancements to the customized audio-playlists (herein termed rhythmic auditory stimulation (RAS)) to explore whether beat-accentuation could further improve exercise adherent behaviours over and above non RAS synchronous music [29].

Methods

Research setting

Cardiac rehabilitation served as our test-case setting for structured exercise for several reasons: First, it is an established evidence-based guideline-driven structured exercise and lifestyle modification program which has been shown to improve survival in cardiovascular disease [34] and therefore represents an ideal minimum 'gold-standard' level of care for all patients irrespective of treatment allocation. Second, exercise prescriptions, based in part on initial cardiopulmonary assessments, guide an individual's exercise pace. Third, as with other structured exercise programs, cardiac rehabilitation is associated with significant behavioural attrition, which are characterized by high-rates of programmatic drop-out and poor adherence to the self-management of physical activity [35]. Accordingly, a music tempo-pace synchronization strategy theoretically lends itself to the cardiac rehabilitation environment because it can help regulate, maintain and reinforce the exercise pace as prescribed by the program itself.

All study patients had established cardiac disease and were actively participating in the Cardiovascular Prevention and Rehabilitation Program at the Toronto Rehabilitation Institute-University Health Network (TRI-UHN) [35]. Patients were originally referred into the program by physicians or through automated referrals following cardiac hospitalization. All patients received cardiopulmonary and anthropometric baseline assessments and attended on-site exercise classes once per week. An assigned case-manager prescribed aerobic and resistance exercise activities to be conducted at home on at least four additional days per week. Each patient who attended the program was followed for 6 months, and re-evaluated at month 3 and month 6.

Sample eligibility criteria

We included English-speaking patients with known cardiovascular disease participating in cardiac rehabilitation. Exclusion criteria consisted of patients with a history of head trauma/seizures (a relative contraindication to RAS) [36] and those unable to wear headphones due to hearing impairment or hearing aids to ensure that patients had sufficient exposure to the music intervention. Patients were recruited during the third-class of the program (corresponding to a pre-screening period of 3 weeks from program onset).

Study enrollment was restricted by funding. However, we projected that such resource restrictions would still allow for sufficient enrollment to yield a minimum effective sample size that would be sufficient for primary outcome analyses, even after factoring in an anticipated drop-out rate of 10% per group (see sample size justification below) [4,5,37].

The recruitment process began in a group setting, consisting of a cardiac rehabilitation class comprised of between 20 and 25 patients. Patients were informed about the trial within a 5 min presentation following patients' third pre-scheduled cardiac rehabilitation class. In total, 139 patients were screened for the study. Enrollment was confined to the first 34 patients who volunteered and met inclusion/exclusion criteria (all 34 patients who volunteered met eligibility criteria). There were no significant differences in the age and gender of study sample as compared with the non-consenting cardiac rehabilitation classes from which they had been recruited (Additional file 1).

Study design

The study was primarily designed as a proof-of-concept feasibility study to explore the implementation and efficacy of integrating personalized music preferences and tempo-pace synchronization into a structured exercise program.

We incorporated a randomized experimental design. The randomization process incorporated a two-step process in which patients were first randomized to music audio-playlists vs. no music audio-playlists (i.e. 2:1 ratio of music vs. no-music audio-playlist, respectively). Among those randomly allocated to music playlists, patients were further randomized (in 1:1 fashion) to RAS vs. no RAS groups. All patients irrespective of music received usual-care (cardiac rehabilitation). The incorporation of a two-step rather than one-step randomization process allowed us to first explore our primary hypothesis: namely, personalized audio-playlists with tempo-pace synchronization would result in improved adherence to physical activity as compared with a gold-standard non-music usual-care control. The second step in the randomization process allowed us to more specifically explore the implementation of RAS (vs. no RAS) among those initially randomized to music audio-playlists, and do so in blinded fashion.

All randomization incorporated the use of a random-number generator; patient names and study numbers were kept within sealed envelopes during the randomization process to preserve blinding of the randomized-group allocation process.

MAINTAIN was designed to examine the incremental effects of music playlists on the usual-care programmatic delivery of cardiac rehabilitation administered by case managers irrespective of MAINTAIN's treatment allocation. Case managers involved in the administration of cardiac rehabilitation were blinded to all metrics related to the study. In addition to the minimum standard of cardiac rehabilitation care, all three randomized groups received tri-axial accelerometer activity monitors (PAM® Personal Activity Monitor, Model AM300, Pam, Doorwerth, The Netherlands) and self-reported physical activity diaries for use throughout the entire study duration. Each individual irrespective of randomization interacted with the study coordinator every 2 weeks for a 3- to 5-min duration to collect and upload activity diaries and information obtained through the audio-playlist device. During these encounters, patients randomized to music (with or without RAS) had the opportunity to request additional playlists or modifications to playlists that reflected changes in an individual's prescribed exercise pace (if appropriate); such changes were then uploaded on the subsequent scheduled encounter.

Music playlists, tempo-pace synchronization and RAS implementation

Patients randomized to personalized music playlists also received a personalized audio playlist device (iPod® mp3 players), which were preloaded with a playlist of music that satisfied their pre-specified music genre and artist preferences. Music preferences were ascertained at the outset of the study. Patients were asked for examples of music genres (e.g. styles such as rock, jazz, pop, classical, country/western, folk), artists, albums and songs they preferred to listen to, and preferred not to listen to, while exercising.

All music assembled within playlists was synchronized to approximate an individual's prescribed exercise pace. Specifically, commercially available songs selected for music playlists were chosen such that tempos were within ±10 beats per minute of a subject's exercise step-pace as specified by the initial exercise prescription. The incorporation of a maximum 10 beat per minute pace-tempo threshold was based on pre-trial pilot data and qualitative feedback on motivation and perceived exertion with music during exercise. Moreover, evidence suggests that a 10 beat per minute or less tempo-pace calibration difference falls within thresholds by which patients can feasibly adjust their walking/running pace to accommodate to sonic and music rhythms by subconsciously increasing or decreasing their strides accordingly [18]. Exercise pace was ascertained by determining the number of steps taken within a quarter mile in a time duration as ascertained by the cardiac rehabilitation program. The number of steps taken per minute at a target pace was used to generate the optimal tempo of music required for tempo-pace synchronization. Each quarter note was intended to correspond with one paced step. We created a database comprising over 14,500 songs of various genre, artist, title, song duration and music tempo. The music tempo of each song was determined using commercially available software (cadence® software) [38].

The process of RAS enhancement adapted the methodology used by Chen et al. in which each quarter note beat was enhanced through the addition of an audible rhythmic sound [39]. RAS enhancements were conducted in a random subset of songs within an individual's playlist (comprising up to 50% of an individual's personalized playlist). Patients were not told which songs were RAS-enhanced, or which of the two music groups (RAS vs. no RAS) they were allocated to. Our rationale for leaving some of the songs unmodified was to help us ascertain, through focus-group interviews (see below), whether patients could distinguish between RAS and non-RAS songs uploaded into their individual playlist. Pre-study pilot testing further informed the frequencies and volumes used for RAS enhancement. Our intent was to implement RAS enhancement at frequencies and volumes just beyond minimal detection levels without detracting from the authenticity of the music playlists. The RAS-enhancement process first imported the original mp3 playlist audio files into Logic ® 9.0 recording software. RAS-enhancements were conducted using sounds of drums (kick-drum, snares, hihats and rides) through the addition of secondary tracks and digital keyboard MIDI-drum instruments, played concurrently with the original playlist file. Each song was then 'sonically modified' manually to accentuate and enhance the quarter-notes through the use of lower and/or higher frequency drum instruments. Lower frequency drum sounds (e.g. kick-drum at 50 to 100 Hz) were generally maintained at volumes of between 1 and 5 dB louder than the original recording, whereas higher frequency drum sounds (e.g. snare or hihat at 1,000 to 5,000 Hz) were generally maintained at volumes of between 1 and 5 dB lower than the reference original music track. RAS-enhanced mp3 songs were then re-mixed and mastered as a WAV file (44 kbit/24 bit) and subsequently compressed into an mp3 file and uploaded into the RAS iPods® playlist so that maximum 'headphone' volumes were similar to the original audio-recordings. In short, RAS enhancements accentuated the frequencies of externally embedded rhythmic components relative to the other frequencies and sounds of the original audio-file, without altering the total volume of the sound recording itself (Additional file 2).

The sonic attributes of those randomized to RAS enhancement resulted in significantly higher peak frequencies, more abrupt slopes of peak frequencies, selected higher peak volume frequencies relative to baseline and lower frequency levels at peak frequencies (Additional file 3).

Data on baseline variables included age, gender, body mass index (measured weight and height), functional capacity, self-reported depression-score, self-efficacy, referral indication, cardiovascular risk factors and prior disease. Depressive symptoms were ascertained using the Centre for Epidemiological Studies - Depression Scale (CES-D), while exercise self-efficacy was ascertained using the Stanford Self-Efficacy scale; both measures have been validated [40,41]. In addition to data collected through empirical methods, information about the perceived impact (if any) that music had on patient participation in their prescribed exercise program was collected through the use of small group interviews in which participants were asked to describe their exercise experience. Specifically, participants were asked for their opinion about the impact of listening to music on their exercise behaviour. Participants were interviewed in small group settings within their respective treatment allocation arms.

The study was reviewed and approved by the Toronto Rehabilitation Institute-University Health Network Research Ethics Board. All procedures followed were in accordance with the Helsinki Declaration of 1975, as revised in 2008 (5).

Outcomes

The primary outcome was defined as the weekly average volume of physical activity (i.e. mean weekly minutes of physical activity as measured using tri-axial accelerometers) throughout the 3-month study. Sample size estimates incorporated the methods by Hedeker for repeated measures (weekly activity levels) and assumed a correlation of 0.4 in activity levels over 12 weekly interventions [42]. The minimum effective sample size targeted for this study was 10 patients in each of the three groups, which would allow for 80% power to detect a clinically large size mean differences (i.e. 50% or 250 min per week of physical activity) between the music and no music treatment groups, assuming a two-tailed alpha of 0.05. The sample size was only powered sufficiently to account for group-level differences using a repeated-measures design but underpowered to account for variations within and between individuals. Secondary outcome measures consisted of the weekly volume of intensity-specific physical activity as defined as high-intensity,

(≥7 metabolic equivalents), moderate intensity (3 to 6.9 metabolic equivalents) or low intensity (<3 metabolic equivalents), based on the PAM® personal activity monitor. Validation of the PAM® accelerometer has been published elsewhere [43].

Statistical analyses

Given the staged sequential randomization process, statistical analyses first compared usual-care with the combined music intervention groups (with RAS and no RAS combined). Only if significant differences in weekly physical activity volumes between music and non-music groups existed, did we examine differences in outcomes across the three intervention groups (usual-care vs. playlists without RAS vs. playlists with RAS).

The study utilized an intention to treat analysis. Categorical differences in baseline characteristics and outcomes were first evaluated between music and non-music groups incorporating Fishers' exact test, or Mann-Whitney tests where appropriate. If significant differences between music and non-music groups existed, we then evaluated for differences in baseline characteristics and outcomes across all three groups, employing Fishers' exact test and Kruskal-Wallis Test where appropriate.

Generalized Linear Modelling was used to fit the data using maximum likelihood equations (PROC GENMOD), and the first-order autoregressive function was used to examine weekly mean volume of physical activity across intervention groups, while accounting for repeated measures in weekly assessments.

Several sensitivity analyses were conducted which are described within the 'Results' section. Two-tailed $P < 0.05$ was defined as statistically significant. All statistical tests utilized SAS™ Version 9.3 (Cary, NC, USA).

Results

Baseline sample characteristics

The average age of the study sample was 63 years; 70% were male. Most patients were married, overweight and self-confident (i.e. high self-efficacy) in their abilities to self-manage cardiovascular disease and exercise. There were no significant differences in baseline physical activity volume between the music and non-music groups (Table 1) or across the three treatment arms (i.e. no-music, music without RAS, music with RAS) (Additional file 4).

Non-significant intergroup difference in functional capacity and other baseline factors did exist. These were predominantly attributable to the recruitment of two outliers who were randomly allocated to the non-music usual-care control and to the RAS study arms where baseline VO_{2peak} among outliers resided at the extremes of fitness. One such patient was recruited to non-music usual-care, who was 82 years old and had a baseline VO_{2peak} of 8.9 mL·kg·min^{-1}, while another patient, who was recruited to the music-playlist (with RAS) group, was 47 years old and had a baseline VO_{2peak} of 33.5 mL·kg·min^{-1}.

Among the 34 participants, 3 patients dropped out of the study. Two were recruited to the music without RAS group and dropped out within 2 weeks of randomization (one patient never receiving any audio playlist device or activity monitor, while the other patient received both devices but was confirmed to have never used either the audio playlist device or activity monitor). One patient randomized to music playlists with RAS dropped out at week 5 of the study due to musculoskeletal limitations.

Audio-playlist preferences and use

Table 2 represents the difference between music-playlists with RAS and without RAS enhancements. Patients randomized to playlists without RAS enhancement had slower walking pace and tempos of music, greater preferences towards contemporary (top 40 pop, hip-hop, dance), and fewer preferences for rock (classic and hard rock), jazz and classical music. The number of audio-plays was significantly higher among patients randomized to music playlists with RAS-enhancements than without (780.7 vs. 174.0 audio-plays, RAS vs. non-RAS groups, respectively, $P < 0.001$).

Thematic content analysis of participant responses ($n = 13$) during the small group interviews found that 100% of the patients who used their audio-playlist devices identified music as being a key factor that helped them achieve their appropriate levels of intensity and duration of exercise. There were no differences in the perceived impact of music on exercise between RAS and non-RAS groups.

Outcomes

The weekly volume of total physical activity, as measured objectively using tri-axial accelerometer activity monitors, was higher among patients randomized to the group receiving personalized audio-playlists with tempo-pace synchrony as compared with non-music usual-care (Table 3, Figure 1). The improved physical activity volumes among patients randomized to personalized audio-playlists with tempo-pace synchrony was driven by the group receiving RAS-enhanced music playlists (average weekly minutes of physical activity of 631.3 min vs. 320 min vs. 370.2 min, music playlists with RAS vs. music playlists without RAS vs. usual-care, $P < 0.001$). Moreover, higher average weekly pertained to all intensity levels of physical activity (Table 4, Additional file 5) and was sustainable over time (Figure 2). The average number of weekly audio-plays per group strongly correlated with a group's weekly average volume of physical activity ($r = 0.61$, $P < 0.001$), (Figure 3). There were no significant differences in weekly volumes of physical activity between the RAS unenhanced music group and the non-music usual-care controls, although this may have been explained by the limited use of audio-playlists among the non-RAS music arm.

Table 1 Baseline characteristics of the study population

	No music Control ($n = 11$)	Music RAS/non-RAS combined ($n = 23$)	*P* value*
Socio-demographic characteristics			
Age, mean years (STD)	66.4 (12.8)	61.5 (10.3)	0.25
Male (%)	6 (54.6)	17 (77.3)	0.24
Married (%)	7 (63.6)	20 (90.9)	0.15
Clinical factors			
Diabetes (%)	1 (9.1)	6 (30)	0.18
Past or current smoker (%)	5 (45.5)	12 (54.6)	0.62
Body mass index, mean (kg/m^2) (STD)	27.7 (4.5)	28.6 (3.6)	0.56
Prior myocardial infarction (%)	2 (27.3)	5 (25)	0.89
Hypertension (%)	5 (45.5)	10 (50)	1.0
Lung disease (%)	2 (18.2)	4 (20)	0.90
Behavioural factors			
CES-Depression score, mean (STD)	6.25 (8.6)	9.6 (8.9)	0.62
Stanford self-efficacy, mean (STD)	80.6 (18.6)	86.5 (12.6)	0.37
Cardiac self-efficacy, mean (STD)	76.4 (19.4)	80.1 (14.9)	0.62
High behavioural risk[a] (%)	5 (45.5)	12 (54.6)	1.0
Physical factors			
Baseline VO_2, mean mL/kg/min (STD)	18.2 (5.7)	20.3 (5.0)	0.28
Week-1 volume of total activity, mean minutes (STD)	352.8 (408.5)	487.6 (379.6)	0.42
Week 1 volume of vigorous activity, mean minutes (STD)	1.45 (2.1)	5.4 (15.0)	0.98
Week 1 volume of moderate activity, mean minutes (STD)	105 (122.3)	162.3 (151.9)	0.31
Week 1 volume of light activity, mean minutes (STD)	246.4 (295.7)	320.7 (248.1)	0.68
Week 1 calorie burn, mean kcal (STD)	314.0 (359.4)	453.4 (366.9)	0.42

Baseline characteristics according to randomization group: No music controls vs. Music playlists (RAS and non-RAS combined). RAS, rhythmic auditory stimulation; STD, standard deviation. *P value tests for statistical difference between two groups (i.e. Control vs. Music-Playlist RAS/non-RAS combined); statistical tests for continuous variables used the Kruskal-Wallis Test, while statistical tests for categorical outcomes utilized Fisher's Exact Test. [a]Defined based on a BMI >30 kg/m^2 or a CES-depression score of >15.

Sensitivity analyses

Several sensitivity analyses were undertaken as follows:

First, all analyses using Generalized Longitudinal Models were repeated, accounting for variations within and between patients. Our results were similar. Namely, weekly total physical activity volume remained significantly higher among patients randomized to the music intervention, especially among those with RAS-enhancement (dose-response differences across the three groups of 121.6 min of weekly total activity, $P = 0.04$). Moreover, the relationship persisted among intensity-specific physical activity, including vigorous physical activity (dose response differences across the three groups of 4.5 min of weekly vigorous activity, $P = 0.08$).

Second, the positive relationship between music intervention and physical activity adherence remained significant among high-risk subgroups (defined *a priori* based on a BMI exceeding 30 kg/m^2 and a CES-Depression score exceeding 15 [37]) and did so irrespective of the employment of different thresholds for risk and/or the inclusion of individual's predicted likelihood of program drop-out based on on-site attendance (Additional file 6).

Third, to determine when differences in weekly physical activity volume emerged over time, we subdivided the weekly intervals into three equivalent time intervals (weeks 0 to 4; weeks 5 to 8; weeks 9 to 12) and repeated the analyses accordingly. Significant group-specific differences in physical activity diverged and become statistically significant only after week 5, (i.e. group-specific differences during weeks 0 to 4, weeks 5 to 8, and weeks 9 to 12, $P = 0.22$, $P = 0.0004$, $P < 0.0001$, respectively), suggesting that improvements in physical activity behaviours associated with RAS were sustainable.

Finally, to explore whether differences in baseline characteristics explained group-differences in outcomes, two additional sensitivity analyses were performed. The first analysis adjusted for baseline characteristics by

Table 2 Music tempo-pace synchronization, preferences and utilization

	No music control (*n* = 11)	Music audio-playlist without RAS (*n* = 11)	Music audio-playlist with RAS (*n* = 11)	*P* value*
Playlist tempo-pace synchronization				
Exercise walking/running pace, mean steps/min (range)	N/A	110.7 (91 to 128.7)	122.0 (112 to 133)	0.03
Tempo range of music within playlist, mean BPM (range)	N/A	111 (81 to 139)	123 (105 to 168)	0.01
Patient playlist preferences				
Contemporary (e.g. top 40 pop, hip-hop, dance)	N/A	24%	11%	<0.001
Rock	N/A	18%	33%	
Country-Western	N/A	24%	17%	
Jazz, blues	N/A	6%	11%	
Classical	N/A	12%	22%	
Other (includes no stated preferences)	N/A	18%	6%	
Music-playlist utilization				
Average number of audio-plays	0	174 (186)	780.7 (943.7)	<0.001

According to randomized group: No music control vs. music audio-playlist without RAS vs. music audio-playlist with RAS enhancement. RAS, rhythmic auditory stimulation; BPM, beats per minute; N/A, not available. *P value tests for statistical differences across groups based on the Kruskal-Wallis Test or Chi-squared test.

forcing baseline covariates into the model. Group effects in total weekly activity remained significant, even after adjusting for age, marital status and baseline cardiopulmonary fitness ($P = 0.05$) - group-specific differences in baseline characteristics which were most imbalanced despite randomization. The second excluded the two patient outliers described above whose baseline VO_{2peak} fell at the extremes (8.9 and 33.5 mL/kg/min). The removal of these two patients resulted in similar VO_{2peak} across the three groups (19.1 $mL{\cdot}kg{\cdot}min^{-1}$ vs. 19.1 $mL{\cdot}kg{\cdot}min^{-1}$ vs. 19.8 $mL{\cdot}kg{\cdot}min^{-1}$ in the control group vs. music without RAS vs. music playlist with RAS, respectively) and did not meaningfully alter our results. Group differences in physical activity still favored the group receiving music audio-playlists with RAS ($P = 0.02$).

Discussion

Our study demonstrated the feasibility and efficacy of implementing a tempo-pace synchronized preference-based audio-playlist strategy to improve adherence to physical activity among patients receiving cardiac rehabilitation. Patients randomized to personalized audio-playlists with tempo-pace synchronized music embarked on significantly greater amounts of weekly physical activity and experienced lower declines in weekly physical activity than did their non-music usual-care counterparts. Differences in physical activity among those randomized to music playlists were driven predominantly by the group randomized to RAS, where attainment in weekly physical activity volumes were twofold higher than those randomized to music but without RAS enhancements. Improvements in the weekly volume of physical activity associated with RAS increased over time, were sustainable, applied to all intensity-levels of physical activity and were as pronounced among high-risk as it was among low-risk subgroups.

Our study builds on existing music-exercise literature in several additional ways. First, to the best of our knowledge, ours is the first study to have examined the longitudinal adherence-effects of an exercise-music strategy within a structured exercise program. Until now, the

Table 3 Average weekly physical activity among those randomized to music playlists vs. No music control

	No music Control (*n* = 11)	Music RAS and no RAS combined (*n* = 22)	*P* value*
Weekly estimated caloric expenditures, mean kcal (STD)	339.6 (307.2)	435.0 (407.4)	<0.001
Weekly volume of total activity, mean minutes (STD)	370.2 (332.5)	475.6 (446.0)	<0.001
Weekly volume of vigorous activity, mean minutes (STD)	2.22 (4.3)	8.5 (19.6)	<0.001
Weekly volume of moderate activity, mean minutes (STD)	123.3 (130.9)	142.3 (142.7)	0.06
Weekly volume of light activity, mean minutes (STD)	244.7 (230.7)	324.8 (326.3)	<0.001

*P value tests for statistic difference between two groups (i.e. Music with or without RAS vs. Control). Weekly physical activity incorporated Generalized Linear Equations. Process and clinical outcomes incorporated the Kruskal-Wallis Test. Statistical tests for differences in categorical variables used Fishers' Exact test. STD, standard deviation.

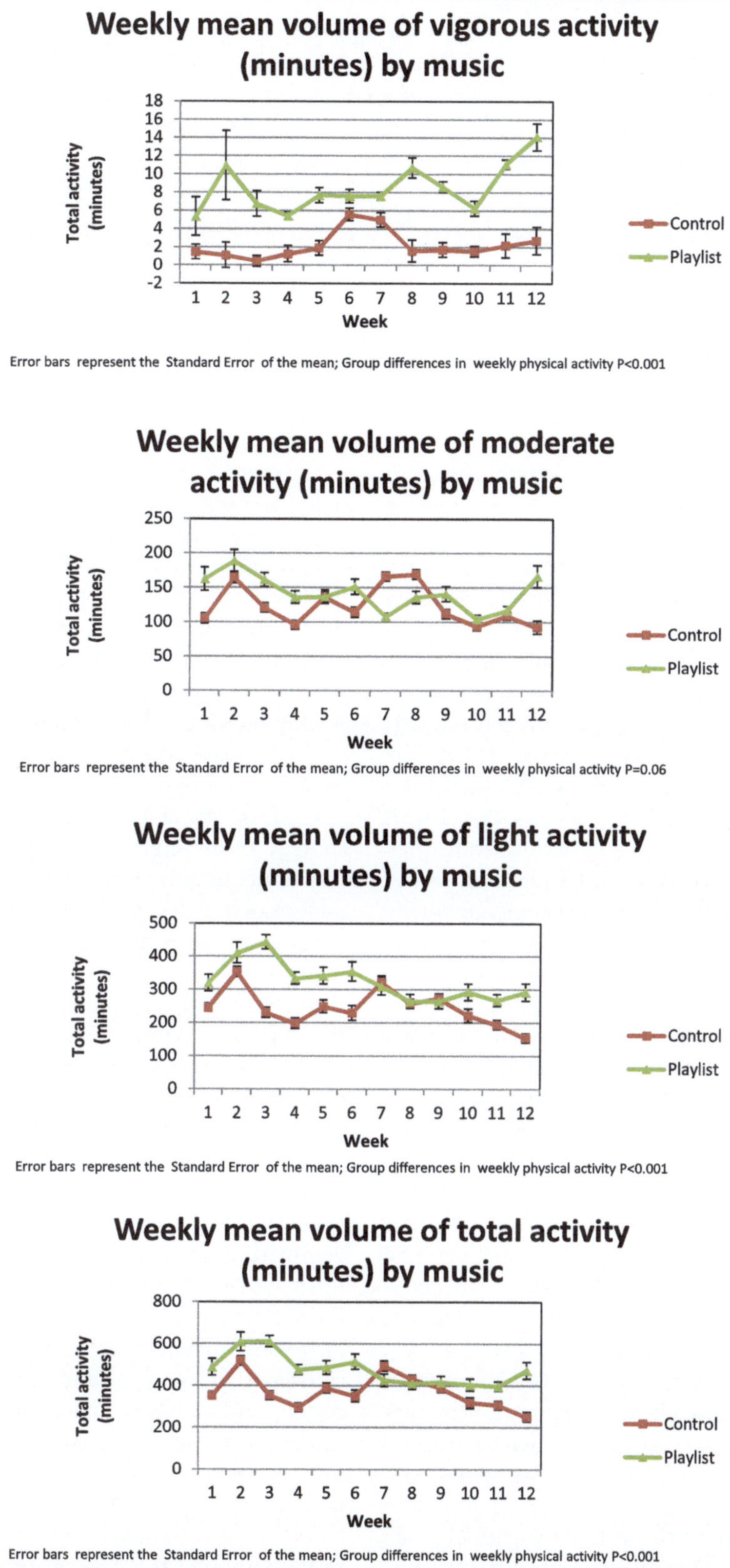

Figure 1 Weekly volume of physical activity, stratified by physical activity intensity. Vigorous activity (top graph); moderate activity (second from the top); light activity (third from the top); total activity (bottom graph). Non-music control (labelled 'Control': red line), music audio-playlist groups (irrespective of rhythmic auditory stimulation) (labelled 'Playlist': green line).

Table 4 Average weekly physical activity volume

	No music control (*n* = 11)	Music audio-playlist without RAS (*n* = 11)	Music audio-playlist with RAS (*n* = 11)	*P* value*
Average weekly caloric expenditures, mean kcal (STD)	339.6 (307.2)	295.3 (327.8)	574.8 (431.9)	<0.001
Average weekly volume of total activity, mean minutes (STD)	370.2 (332.5)	320 (355.2)	631.3 (473.8)	<0.001
Average weekly volume of vigorous activity, mean minutes (STD)	2.22 (4.3)	5.7 (15.1)	11.3 (23.0)	<0.001
Average weekly volume of moderate activity, mean minutes (STD)	123.3 (130.9)	99.6 (120.4)	185.1 (150.7)	< 0.001
Average weekly volume of light activity, mean minutes (STD)	244.7 (230.7)	214.6 (254.7)	435 (352.6)	<0.001

According to randomized group: No music control vs. music audio-playlist without RAS vs. music audio-playlist with RAS enhancement. RAS, rhythmic auditory stimulation; STD, standard deviation. **P* value tests for statistical differences across the three groups (i.e. Control vs. Playlist vs. Playlist-RAS enhanced). Self-managed activity incorporated Generalized Linear Equations. Process and clinical outcomes incorporated the Kruskal-Wallis Test. Statistical tests for differences in categorical variables used Fishers' Exact test.

vast majority of studies exploring the effects of music in exercise have been cross-sectional in design and/or narrow in outcome ascertainment, with most studies limited to ergonomic and/or perceptual outcomes [8-16,44-46]. Second, we employed a novel integrated audio-playlist strategy where patient preferences informed the choices of musical genres and artists but where exercise pace restricted the playlist selection to those songs whose music tempos approximated individuals' program-prescribed steps per minute. Third, our study demonstrated that RAS-enhancements, which were designed to accentuate the auditory cues associated with tempo-pace synchrony [24,27], were accomplished feasibly using commercially available customized playlists. Moreover, such RAS-enhanced playlists were incrementally efficacious in improving long-term physical activity behaviours. Finally, ours, to the best of our knowledge, is the first to compare the behavioural outcomes associated with a personalized music strategy against an evidence-based gold-standard usual-care control, which itself, has been associated with a 20% improvement in long-term survival [4].

Available evidence suggests that tempo-pace synchronous music can reduce exercise-perceived exertion, increase exercise endurance, augment exercise intensity and extend the duration of exercise [19,21,26,27,31-33]. The effects of synchronized music on exercise function have been shown to be greater when music is aligned with individual music preferences. Such alignment can augment affect and enhance intrinsic motivation [31,32,47-49]. Affect augmentation along with the incorporation of other self-regulatory behavioural self-management techniques (i.e. goal-setting, self-monitoring) [50] may have narrowed the intention-motivation-behavioural gap associated with exercise through improved automaticity and organization [51]. While there is supportive evidence suggesting that the combination of affect augmentation with rhythmic synchronization could impact physical activity behaviour [11,21,23,52,53], no study had ever directly tested this hypothesis until now.

Alternate explanations for higher weekly physical activity volumes among those randomized to RAS may have existed. Most importantly, patients randomized to tempo-pace synchronized music with RAS enhancements listened to their audio-devices nearly fourfold more than those who received tempo-pace audio-music devices without RAS enhancements. The correlation between average weekly audio-playcounts and average weekly physical activity volumes precluded us from disentangling the efficacy of audio music playlist devices in general, from tempo-pace synchrony or RAS.

The feasibility of integrating a tempo-pace synchronization strategy into commercially available music in a manner which takes into account personal patient preferences underscores the *potential* for 'real-world' application. All songs comprising an individual's personalized playlist contained tempos that were calibrated to within 10 beats per minute of a patient's prescribed exercise pace - a calibration that falls within 'tempo-pace' asynchronous thresholds where stride length can be modified to accommodate changes in music tempo without perceptual differences in effort [18]. The tempos of commercially available music were ascertained using widely available automated software application tools that are widely available on the web. The implementation of RAS sonic-enhancements to commercially available music was also implemented in a feasible manner by embedding digital auditory stimuli into the existing original sound recordings using MIDI keyboard instruments and commercially available recording software. The original audio-files and the superimposed digital stimuli were then re-mixed into one composite sound recording. One challenge encountered was the fact that the tempos of the original sound recording (i.e. music files within an individual's audio-playlist) were rarely recorded in quantized fashion. As a result, small fluctuations in the tempo of the original recordings existed. To overcome this limitation, sonic enhancements were added manually and played along in real time with the original audio-recording. Additional manual modifications allowed

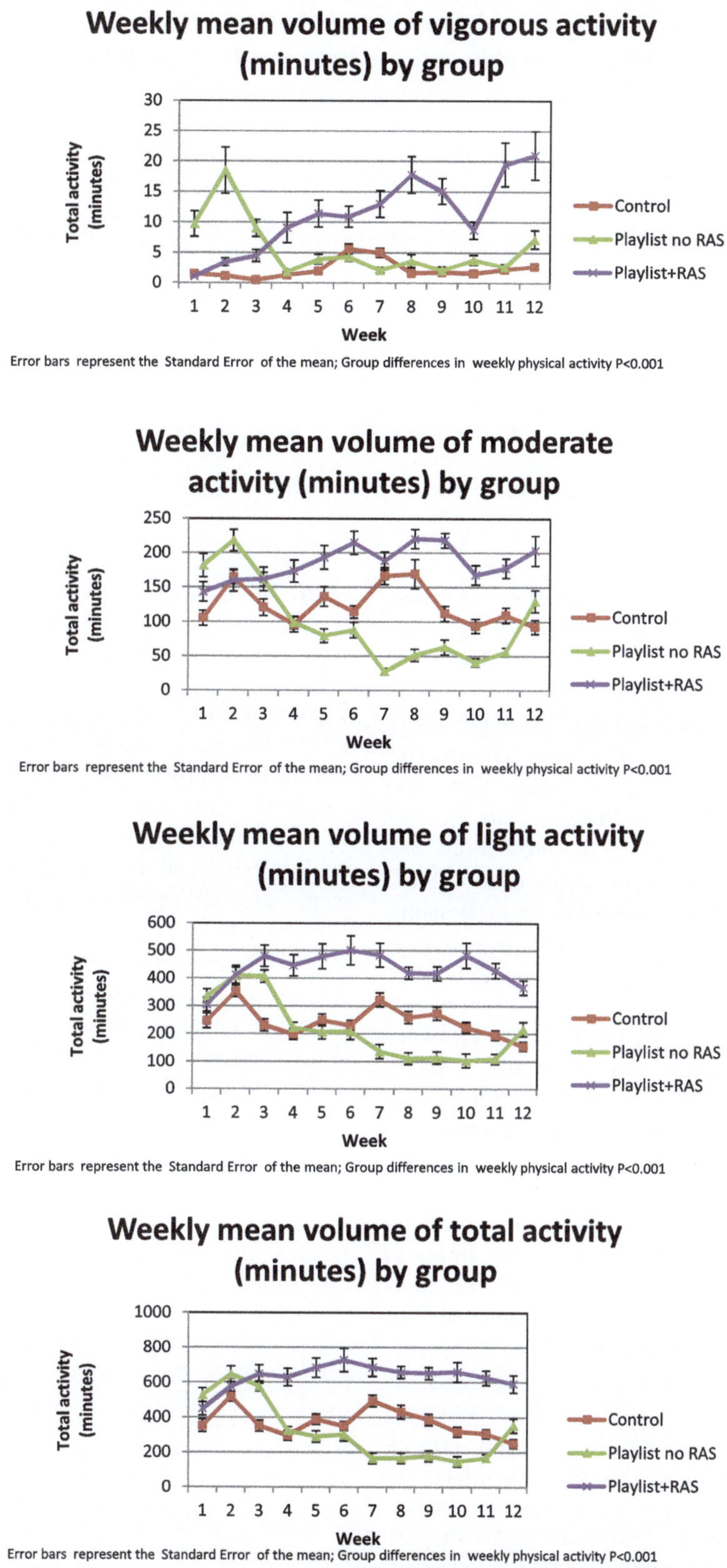

Figure 2 Weekly volume of physical activity, stratified by physical activity intensity. Vigorous activity (top graph); moderate activity (second from the top); light activity (third from the top); total activity (bottom graph). Non-music control (labelled 'Control': red line), music audio-playlist without RAS (labelled 'Playlist': green line), music audio-playlist with RAS (labelled 'Playlist + RAS': purple). RAS, rhythmic auditory stimulation.

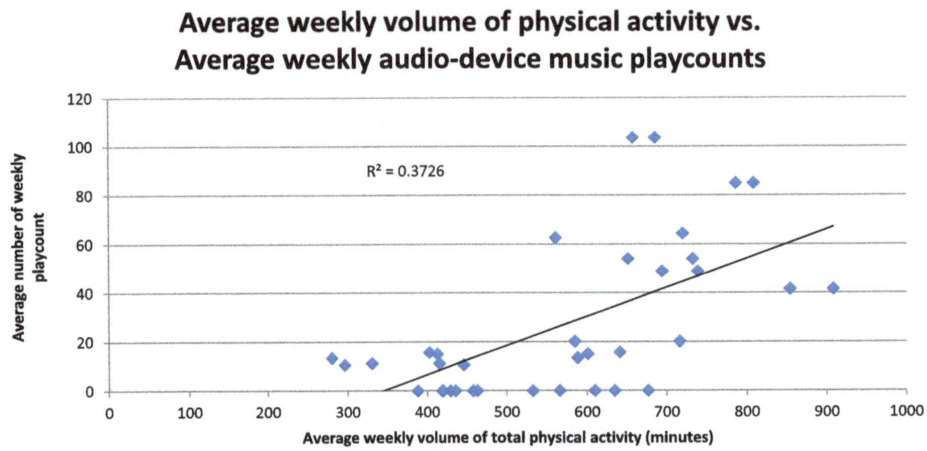

Figure 3 Average weekly volume of physical activity vs. average number of weekly audio-device music playcounts. The graph demonstrates the correlation between a group's average weekly volume of physical activity (in minutes) and a group's average number of weekly playcounts from the audio-playlist devices ($r = 0.61$, $P < 0.001$).

us to optimize the tempo-synchrony between RAS and the original sound music recording where necessary. Future research will need to explore how such methodology can be better automated and standardized.

Our study was designed as a proof-of-principle feasibility study. However, there were several noteworthy study limitations that deserve consideration. First, the sample size of our study was small. Second, with the exception of RAS enhancements which did incorporate patient blinding, the study was largely un-blinded. Third, despite our randomized design, imbalances in baseline characteristics existed across groups. While such imbalances were not statistically significant per se, it is possible that residual confounding may have existed and accounted for some or all of our results. Finally, differences in music preferences, genres and music tempos may have partially explained the variations in exercise adherence between RAS and non-RAS groups [18,54,55].

Notwithstanding such caveats, we believe our findings justify the need for further research through rigorously designed clinical trials. If reproducible, such findings could have potentially transformative health implications. For example, the average difference of 105.4 min in weekly physical activity between those receiving and not receiving music playlists, if sustained, would correlate with a projected life-expectancy gain of 2.5 years for an average male 65-year-old patient [56,57]. Given that benefits of music playlists were equally applicable among those patients who were at higher risk of cardiac rehabilitation programmatic drop-out than those at lower behavioural attrition risk, the absolute survival benefits may be even greater among those most behaviourally disengaged. With their modest associated costs, the use of preference-based music audio playlist devices (i.e. approximately $75 per patient in our study) could also have important cost-effectiveness implications as a health-policy strategy to improve physical activity adherence in the population [58,59].

Conclusions

In conclusion, our results demonstrated the integration of personalized music playlists with tempo-pace synchronization into a structured exercise program was feasible and efficacious at improving adherence to physical activity. Those randomized to audio-music playlists with RAS enhancements attained significantly greater weekly volumes of physical activity than the evidence-based non-music usual standard of care. Such findings may have important clinical application when attempting to engage otherwise behaviourally disengaged populations into structured physical activity programs. Further research is required to reproduce such findings in larger real-world settings.

Competing interests

The authors declare that they have no competing interests.

Authors' contributions

DA, MO, LB, SM, and JG contributed to the development and writing of the study protocol. All authors contributed to the drafting of this manuscript. All authors read and approved the final manuscript.

Authors' information

Dr. Alter is a Career Investigator with the Heart and Stroke Foundation of Ontario. Dr. Alter also holds a Research Chair in Cardiac and Metabolic Rehabilitation, Toronto Rehabilitation Institute-University Health Network, University of Toronto.

Acknowledgements

We would like to acknowledge PAM® for generously providing the tri-axial accelerometer activity monitors for this study. We are also indebted to the tremendous effort, enthusiasm and support by all of the case managers and staff at the Cardiac Rehabilitation and Secondary Prevention program, Toronto Rehabilitation Institute. We would also like to express our gratitude for the support of the Toronto Rehabilitation Foundation and the Ontario Centres of Excellence. Mary O'Sullivan was funded by a grant received by the Ontario Centres of Excellence.

Funding

This study was funded by the Ontario Centres of Excellence. The research was supported by the Cardiac Rehabilitation and Secondary Prevention Program, Toronto Rehabilitation Institute-University Health Network as well as by the Institute for Clinical Evaluative Sciences (ICES). ICES is funded by an annual grant from the Ontario Ministry of Health and Long-Term Care (MOHLTC). The opinions, results and conclusions reported in this paper are those of the authors and are independent from the funding sources. No endorsement by ICES or the Ontario MOHLTC is intended or should be inferred.

Author details

[1]Institute for Clinical Evaluative Sciences, 2075 Bayview Avenue, Toronto, ON M4N 3M5, Canada. [2]University Health Network Cardiovascular Prevention and Rehabilitation Program, Toronto Rehabilitation Institute-University Health Network, 550 University Avenue, Toronto, Canada. [3]Sunnybrook Health Sciences, 2075 Bayview Avenue, Toronto, Canada. [4]Department of Medicine, University of Toronto, 27 King's College Circle, Toronto, Canada. [5]Department of Exercise Sciences, Faculty of Physical Education and Health, University of Toronto, 27 King's College Circle, Toronto, Canada. [6]Music and Health Research Collaboratory, Faculty of Music, University of Toronto, 80 Queens Park, Toronto, Canada. [7]Dean's Office, Faculty of Music, University of Toronto, 80 Queens Park, Toronto, Canada. [8]Department of Health Policy, Management and Evaluation, University of Toronto, 40 St George Street, Toronto, Canada. [9]Faculty of Rehabilitation Medicine, The University of Alberta, 8205 114 Street, Alberta, Canada. [10]The University of Toronto, 27 King's College Circle, Toronto, Canada.

References

1. Woodcock J, Franco OH, Orsini N, Roberts I. Non-vigorous physical activity and all-cause mortality: systematic review and meta-analysis of cohort studies. Int J Epidemiol. 2011;40(1):121–38.
2. Nocon M, Hiemann T, Muller-Riemenschneider F, Thalau F, Roll S, Willich SN. Association of physical activity with all-cause and cardiovascular mortality: a systematic review and meta-analysis. Eur J Cardiovasc Prev Rehabil. 2008;15(3):239–46.
3. Colley RC, Garriguet D, Janssen I, Craig CL, Clarke J, Tremblay MS. Physical activity of Canadian adults: accelerometer results from the 2007 to 2009 Canadian Health Measures Survey. Health Rep. 2011;22(1):7–14.
4. Heran BS, Chen JM, Ebrahim S, Moxham T, Oldridge N, Rees K, Thompson DR, Taylor RS, Exercise-based cardiac rehabilitation for coronary heart disease. Cochrane Database Syst Rev. 2011;7:CD001800.
5. West RR, Jones DA, Henderson AH. Rehabilitation after myocardial infarction trial (RAMIT): multi-centre randomised controlled trial of comprehensive cardiac rehabilitation in patients following acute myocardial infarction. Heart. 2012;98(8):637–44.
6. Davies P, Taylor F, Beswick A, Wise F, Moxham T, Rees K, Ebrahim S, Promoting patient uptake and adherence in cardiac rehabilitation. Cochrane Database Syst Rev. 2010;7:CD007131.
7. Chase JA. Systematic review of physical activity intervention studies after cardiac rehabilitation. J Cardiovasc Nurs. 2011;26(5):351–8.
8. Yamashita S, Iwai K, Akimoto T, Sugawara J, Kono I. Effects of music during exercise on RPE, heart rate and the autonomic nervous system. J Sports Med Phys Fitness. 2006;46(3):425–30.
9. Anshel MH, Marisi D. Effect of music and rhythm on physical performance. Res Q. 1978;49(2):109–13.
10. Cervellin G, Lippi G. From music-beat to heart-beat: a journey in the complex interactions between music, brain and heart. Eur J Intern Med. 2011;22 (4):371–4.
11. Clark IN, Taylor NF, Baker F. Music interventions and physical activity in older adults: a systematic literature review and meta-analysis. J Rehabil Med. 2012;44(9):710–9.
12. Karageorghis CI, Mouzourides DA, Priest DL, Sasso TA, Morrish DJ, Walley CJ. Psychophysical and ergogenic effects of synchronous music during treadmill walking. J Sport Exerc Psychol. 2009;31(1):18–36.
13. Fritz TH, Hardikar S, Demoucron M, Niessen M, Demey M, Giot O, Li Y, Haynes JD, Villringer A, Leman M, Musical agency reduces perceived exertion during strenuous physical performance. Proc Natl Acad Sci U S A. 2013;110(44):17784–9.
14. Karageorghis C, Jones L, Stuart DP. Psychological effects of music tempi during exercise. Int J Sports Med. 2008;29(7):613–9.
15. Simpson SD, Karageorghis CI. The effects of synchronous music on 400-m sprint performance. J Sports Sci. 2006;24(10):1095–102.
16. Terry PC, Karageorghis CI, Saha AM, D'Auria S. Effects of synchronous music on treadmill running among elite triathletes. J Sci Med Sport. 2012;15(1):52–7.
17. Thaut MH, Kenyon GP, Schauer ML, McIntosh GC. The connection between rhythmicity and brain function. IEEE Eng Med Biol Mag. 1999;18(2):101–8.
18. Leman M, Moelants D, Varewyck M, Styns F, van NL Martens JP. Activating and relaxing music entrains the speed of beat synchronized walking. PLoS One. 2013;8(7):e67932.
19. Khalfa S, Roy M, Rainville P, Dalla BS, Peretz I. Role of tempo entrainment in psychophysiological differentiation of happy and sad music? Int J Psychophysiol. 2008;68(1):17–26.
20. Potteiger JA, Schroeder JM, Goff KL. Influence of music on ratings of perceived exertion during 20 minutes of moderate intensity exercise. Percept Mot Skills. 2000;91(3 Pt 1):848–54.
21. van der Vlist B, Bartneck C, Maueler S. moBeat: using interactive music to guide and motivate users during aerobic exercising. Appl Psychophysiol Biofeedback. 2011;36(2):135–45.
22. Molinari M, Leggio MG, De MM, Cerasa A, Thaut M. Neurobiology of rhythmic motor entrainment. Ann N Y Acad Sci. 2003;999:313–21.
23. Lima-Silva AE, Silva-Cavalcante MD, Pires FO, Bertuzzi R, Oliveira RS, Bishop D. Listening to music in the first, but not the last 1.5 km of a 5-km running trial alters pacing strategy and improves performance. Int J Sports Med. 2012;33(10):813–8.
24. Mendonca C, Oliveira M, Fontes L, Santos J. The effect of instruction to synchronize over step frequency while walking with auditory cues on a treadmill. Hum Mov Sci. 2014;33:33–42.
25. Sejdic E, Jeffery R, Vanden KA, Chau T. An investigation of stride interval stationarity while listening to music or viewing television. Hum Mov Sci. 2012;31(3):695–706.
26. Creel SC. Similarity-based restoration of metrical information: different listening experiences result in different perceptual inferences. Cogn Psychol. 2012;65(2):321–51.
27. Honing H. Without it no music: beat induction as a fundamental musical trait. Ann N Y Acad Sci. 2012;1252:85–91.
28. Kenyon GP, Thaut MH. Rhythm-driven optimization of motor control. In: Thaut MH, editor. Rhythm, Music, and the brain: scientific foundations and clinical applications. 1st ed. New York: Routledge; 2008. p. 85–112.
29. Will U, Berg E. Brain wave synchronization and entrainment to periodic acoustic stimuli. Neurosci Lett. 2007;424(1):55–60.
30. Nozaradan S, Peretz I, Mouraux A. Selective neuronal entrainment to the beat and meter embedded in a musical rhythm. J Neurosci. 2012;32(49):17572–81.

31. Nakamura PM, Pereira G, Papini CB, Nakamura FY, Kokubun E. Effects of preferred and nonpreferred music on continuous cycling exercise performance. Percept Mot Skills. 2010;110(1):257–64.
32. Macnay SK. The influence of preferred music on the perceived exertion, mood, and time estimation scores of patients participating in a cardiac rehabilitation exercise program. Mus Ther Perspect. 1995;13:91–6.
33. Popescu M, Otsuka A, Ioannides AA. Dynamics of brain activity in motor and frontal cortical areas during music listening: a magnetoencephalographic study. Neuroimage. 2004;21(4):1622–38.
34. Hammill BG, Curtis LH, Schulman KA, Whellan DJ. Relationship between cardiac rehabilitation and long-term risks of death and myocardial infarction among elderly Medicare beneficiaries. Circulation. 2010;121(1):63–70.
35. Alter DA, Zagorski B, Marzolini S, Forhan M, Oh PI. On-site programmatic attendance to cardiac rehabilitation and the healthy-adherer effect. Eur J Prev Cardiol. 2014. doi: 10.1177/2047487314544084.
36. Hogan T, Sundaram M. Rhythmic auditory stimulation in generalized epilepsy. Electroencephalogr Clin Neurophysiol. 1989;72(5):455–8.
37. Forhan M, Zagorski BM, Marzonlini S, Oh P, Alter DA. Predicting exercise adherence for patients with obesity and diabetes referred to a cardiac rehabilitation and secondary prevention program. Can J Diabetes. 2013;37(3):189–94.
38. Cadence software. http://www.cadenceappcom/2014.
39. Chen JL, Zatorre RJ, Penhune VB. Interactions between auditory and dorsal premotor cortex during synchronization to musical rhythms. Neuroimage. 2006;32(4):1771–81.
40. Beekman AT, Deeg DJ, Van LJ, Braam AW, De Vries MZ, Van TW. Criterion validity of the Center for Epidemiologic Studies Depression scale (CES-D): results from a community-based sample of older subjects in The Netherlands. Psychol Med. 1997;27(1):231–5.
41. Lorig KR, Sobel DS, Ritter PL, Laurent D, Hobbs M. Effect of a self-management program on patients with chronic disease. Eff Clin Pract. 2001;4(6):256–62.
42. Hedeker D, Gibbons RD, Waternaux C. Sample size estimation for longitudinal designs with attrition. J Educ Behav Stat. 1999;24:70–93.
43. Slootmaker SM, Chin A Paw JM, Schuit AJ, van Mechelen W, Koppes LL. Concurrent validity of the PAM accelerometer relative to the MTI Actigraph using oxygen consumption as a reference. Scand J Med Sci Sports. 2009;19(1):36–43.
44. Brownley KA, McMurray RG, Hackney AC. Effects of music on physiological and affective responses to graded treadmill exercise in trained and untrained runners. Int J Psychophysiol. 1995;19(3):193–201.
45. Hayakawa Y, Miki H, Takada K, Tanaka K. Effects of music on mood during bench stepping exercise. Percept Mot Skills. 2000;90(1):307–14.
46. Lim HB, Atkinson G, Karageorghis CI, Eubank MR. Effects of differentiated music on cycling time trial. Int J Sports Med. 2009;30(6):435–42.
47. Bellebaum C, Koch B, Schwarz M, Daum I. Focal basal ganglia lesions are associated with impairments in reward-based reversal learning. Brain. 2008;131(Pt 3):829–41.
48. Zatorre RJ, Salimpoor VN. From perception to pleasure: music and its neural substrates. Proc Natl Acad Sci U S A. 2013;110 Suppl 2:10430–7.
49. Karageorghis CI, Priest DL. Music in the exercise domain: a review and synthesis (Part I). Int Rev Sport Exerc Psychol. 2012;5(1):44–66.
50. Ferrier S, Blanchard CM, Vallis M, Giacomantonio N. Behavioural interventions to increase the physical activity of cardiac patients: a review. Eur J Cardiovasc Prev Rehabil. 2011;18(1):15–32.
51. Rhodes RE. Bridging the physical activity intention-behaviour gap: contemporary strategies for the clinician. Appl Physiol Nutr Metab. 2014;39(1):105–7.
52. Mangeri F, Montesi L, Forlani G, Dalle GR, Marchesini G. A standard ballroom and Latin dance program to improve fitness and adherence to physical activity in individuals with type 2 diabetes and in obesity. Diabetol Metab Syndr. 2014;6:74.
53. Cho J. The effect of music therapy on mood, perceived exertion, and exercise adherence of patients participating in a rehabilitative upper extremity exercise program. University of Kansas, Master's Thesis: Music Education & Music Therapy. 2009. https://kuscholarworks.ku.edu/bitstream/handle/1808/5529/Cho_ku_0099M_10419_DATA_1.pdf?sequence=1. Accessed April 29, 2015.
54. Edworthy J, Waring H. The effects of music tempo and loudness level on treadmill exercise. Ergonomics. 2006;49(15):1597–610.
55. Karageorghis CI, Terry PC, Lane AM, Bishop DT, Priest DL. The BASES Expert Statement on use of music in exercise. J Sports Sci. 2012;30(9):953–6.
56. Wen CP, Wai JP, Tsai MK, Yang YC, Cheng TY, Lee MC, Chan HT, Tsao CK, Tsai DS, Wu X, Minimum amount of physical activity for reduced mortality and extended life expectancy: a prospective cohort study. Lancet. 2011;378(9798):1244–53.
57. Franco OH, de Laet C, Peeters A, Jonker J, Mackenbach J, Nusselder W. Effects of physical activity on life expectancy with cardiovascular disease. Arch Intern Med. 2005;165(20):2355–60.
58. Moy ML, Teylan M, Weston NA, Gagnon DR, Garshick E. Daily step count predicts acute exacerbations in a US cohort with COPD. PLoS One. 2013;8(4):e60400.
59. LaCroix AZ, Leveille SG, Hecht JA, Grothaus LC, Wagner EH. Does walking decrease the risk of cardiovascular disease hospitalizations and death in older adults? J Am Geriatr Soc. 1996;44(2):113–20.

24

Preventive effects of regular physical exercise against cognitive decline and the risk of dementia with age advancement

Thierry Paillard

Abstract

With age advancement, cognitive function is impaired and the risk of dementia is increased under the influence of normal or pathological cortical and subcortical neuronal alterations. Significant researches has been undertaken to analyze the preventive effects of exercise against the decline of cognitive function and the risk of dementia (e.g., Alzheimer's disease), particularly during the past 10 years. The aim of this short review is to report the scientific knowledge, relating to these effects, that has been obtained during the past 10 years. Acute physical exercise raises the cardiac output in response to increased needs for oxygen and energetic substrates compared to the state of rest, which increases the cerebral blood flow. The increased cerebral blood flow triggers various neurobiological mechanisms in the brain tissue. Repeated and regular physiological modifications related to exercise facilitate the synthesis of cerebral tissue. Regular physical exercise (rPE) may thus increase angiogenesis, neurogenesis, synaptogenesis, and the synthesis of neurotransmitters in different cerebral structures involved in cognition due to an increase in the liberation of neurotrophic factors and the production of enzymatic antioxidants. There is an inversely proportional relationship between the amount of physical activity undertaken and the risk of cognitive decline and/or the development of neurodegenerative disease. The synthesis of cerebral tissue under the influence of aerobic rPE may increase the volume of the gray and white matters of the prefrontal and temporal cortical areas as well as the volume of the hippocampus. Moreover, coordination exercise stimulates cognitive function, thereby inducing positive adaptations of cerebral function when regularly practiced. The possible effects of other types of exercise that weakly stimulate the cardiovascular system or cognitive function, such as stretching and strength training, are also beneficial but their mechanistic explanations require further exploration.

Key points

- There is an inversely proportional relationship between the amount of physical activity undertaken and the risk of cognitive decline and dementia,
- Regular physical exercise may increase angiogenesis, neurogenesis, synaptogenesis in different cerebral structures involved in cognition, and
- Aerobic exercise activates and maintains the sensorimotor network while coordination exercise activates and maintains the visual-spatial network.

Correspondence: thierry.paillard@univ-pau.fr
Département STAPS, Université de Pau et des Pays de l'Adour, ZA Bastillac Sud, 11 rue Morane Saulnier, 65000 Tarbes, France

Review

Introduction

More than 50% of 85-year-old subjects present cognitive disorders ranging from simple non-pathological disorders of the memory to dementia states [1]. Cerebral alteration is inevitable as a result of age advancement even for clinically healthy subjects. The risk of dementia and the prevalence of neurodegenerative pathologies radically increase with age advancement [2,3]. Genetic and environmental factors also have an influence on the development of these pathologies [4-7]. In humans, the most frequent form of dementia is Alzheimer's disease [8].

Moreover, indirect factors can have a significant negative influence on cerebral alteration with age advancement. These include social and familial factors (e.g., persons who are socially isolated), economic factors (e.g., persons with limited financial means), and available therapeutic means (e.g., lack of effective disease-modifying treatments) [9-12]. It is difficult for individuals to overcome these unfavorable factors. However, physical exercise constitutes an ecological approach (together with food and cognitive stimulation) likely to attenuate the effects of normal cerebral aging (non-pathological) and reduce the risk of dementia [13]. The physiological adaptations resulting from chronic exercise are predicted to be favorable to cerebral health.

Indeed, acute physical exercise raises the cardiac output in response to increased needs for oxygen and energetic substrates compared to the state of rest, which increases the cerebral blood flow [14]. The increased cerebral blood flow triggers various neurobiological mechanisms in the brain tissue. Repeated and regular neurobiological modifications related to exercise facilitate the synthesis of cerebral tissue by increasing angiogenesis, neurogenesis, synaptogenesis, and the synthesis of neurotransmitters in different cerebral structures involved in cognition (e.g., memorization) [15,16]. On the basis of the above data, regular physical exercise (rPE) is likely to maintain or even improve cognitive function of healthy elderly subjects [17] and reduce the risk of dementia - e.g., Alzheimer's disease [18,19].

During the last decade, a number of observational studies as well as interventional studies have been carried out in order to determine the preventive effects of rPE against the decline of cognitive function and the risk of dementia. However, the question of the actual potential of rPE to generate neuroprotective mechanisms in healthy subjects who advance in age currently still remains open. The aim of this short review is to summarize the main scientific knowledge relating to the preventive effects of rPE against the decline of cognitive function and the risk of dementia (e.g., Alzheimer's disease) that has been published in the past 10 years. Significant results obtained by empirical studies prior to this period are also included in this review as well as the mechanistic explanations of preventive effects induced by rPE.

An electronic search strategy was carried out using the *PubMed* database on the basis of reasonable expressions of these three concepts: physical activity (exercise, physical activity, physical exercise, physical training, motor activity), cognition (cognitive function, memory, executive function, cognitive impairment, cognitive decline, dementia, Alzheimer's disease, brain), and age advancement (aging, older, elderly). A number of interventional and observational studies were identified as relevant and their methodology was in conformance with existing norms (number of subjects, protocol, etc.).

Prevention of cognitive decline with age advancement

Normal cerebral aging in healthy subjects

With age advancement, memory, and cognitive decline in healthy subjects is partly explained, at least, by the degradation of the process of synaptic plasticity [20]. At the cellular level, one can observe a loss and/or a change of dendritic arborization accompanied by a disappearance and/or a modification of the synaptic structures [21]. The neurons undergo a slowing down of their metabolic activities; their average size decreases and the cerebral blood flow as well as the glucose metabolism decline [22,23]. In mammals, with age advancement, neuronal apoptosis particularly affects cerebral areas such as the neocortex, the hippocampus, and the cerebellum [24]. The neuronal losses especially concern the neurons whose axons are myelinated [25-27]. Moreover, intense chronic psychological stress and, more particularly, the concentration in glucocorticoids that it induces, aggravate the effects of cerebral aging. Prolonged exposure to high plasmatic concentrations of cortisol damages the neurons of the hippocampus [28,29]. Finally, normal cerebral aging generally engenders an alteration of dopaminergic pathways that are essential for the activity of the executive functions [30]. In healthy subjects, age advancement results in cerebral structural modifications which induce cognitive functional decline.

Preventive effects of regular physical exercise

Normal cerebral aging (non-pathological) can induce a cognitive decline which can be slightly to moderately limited by rPE. Observational studies have shown that rPE has a prophylactic effect on cerebral health and cognitive function of elderly people. A longitudinal study carried out in Western Europe (in Finland, Italy, and Holland) over a 10-year period revealed that subjects ($n = 295$) who decreased their level of daily physical activity in amount or in intensity showed a cognitive decline that was greater than those subjects who maintained their level of physical activity in amount or in intensity [31]. Moreover, in a cohort of 347 elderly men (74.6 ± 4.3 years), the cognitive decline measured by means of the mini-mental status examination (MMSE) test was higher for individuals who practiced less than 1 h of weekly physical activity than those who were significantly more active [32]. Lytle et al. [33] reported that 30 min of aerobic activity, three times a week during a period of 2 years (929 subjects who were 76 years old completed the whole study out of 1,146 subjects who were initially recruited) reduced cognitive decline by half (MMSE test), when compared with subjects who remained physically inactive. The risk of cognitive decline appears to be inversely proportional to the amount of physical activity practiced throughout life. A longitudinal study of 5,925 subjects aged more than 65 over a 6- to 8-year period revealed that the cognitive decline was 17%, 18%, 22%, and 24%, respectively, for the highest, the third, the second, and the lowest quartiles related to the amount of physical activity daily undertaken [34]. Another study of 18,766 American women, aged between 70 and 81, over a 7-year period (between 1995 and 2001 and between 1997 and 2003) indicated that the subjects belonging to the highest quintile in terms of level of physical activity presented a risk of cognitive decline 20% lower than the subjects belonging to the lowest quintile [35]. Moreover, the preventive effects of rPE on cognitive function are also evident in the case of very old subjects aged near to 80 [36].

Prevention of the risk of dementia

Physiopathological characteristics In humans, the most frequent form of dementia is Alzheimer's disease. It seems relevant to briefly describe the cerebral disorders of this neurodegenerative disease. Alzheimer's disease is characterized by a loss of neurons and synapses in the cerebral cortex as well as in certain subcortical regions. The neuronal loss induces an atrophy of the affected regions such as the temporal lobe, the parietal lobe, and a part of the frontal cortex and the cingular gyrus [37]. Concerning the clinical aspects, the presence of amyloid plaques in the neocortex and the hippocampus reveals the existence of the disease and corresponds to the extracellular accumulation of Aβ-42 cerebral proteins which are neurotoxic. The presence of non-eliminated Tau (tubule-associated unit) proteins forming aggregates is also a sign of neurofibrillary degeneration (deterioration of the microtubules which form the cytoskeleton of axons) which prevents (blocks) the axonal transport of biological elements required for neuronal activity. Moreover, Alzheimer's disease causes Aβ deposition in the cerebral vessel wall leading to cerebral amyloid angiopathy [38]. Aβ is particularly toxic to endothelial cells and inhibits endothelial nitric oxide synthase (eNOS) in cultured endothelial cells. Hypercontractility of the affected vessels, ultimately leading to chronic impairment of cerebral blood flow (cerebral hypoperfusion), thus contributes to neurodegeneration. Furthermore, vascular risk factors (hypotension, diabetes, hyperlipidaemia, elevated homocysteine, atrial fibrillation, etc.) are highly prevalent in old subjects and closely related to cognitive impairment in later life [38]. The neurological and cardiovascular factors are closely linked to the physiopathology of dementia (e.g., Alzheimer's disease).

Preventive effects of regular physical exercise The effects of rPE are actual and beneficial against the risk of dementia. There is a relationship between the practice of physical activity and Alzheimer's disease. Larson et al. [39] have concluded through a longitudinal study that rPE delays the onset of Alzheimer's disease and dementia in very old subjects. In humans, the results of epidemiological studies have also revealed other advantages. rPE may in fact limit or even prevent the development of Alzheimer's disease, e.g., [40]. An American study of 1,740 subjects aged more than 65 showed that the incidence of dementia was 13.0 per 1,000 person-years for participants who exercised three or more times per week (≥15 min/session of walking, bicycle, swimming, aerobics, eurhythmics, aquaerobics, strength training, stretching, or other activities) compared with 19.7 per 1,000 person-years for those who exercised fewer than three times per week [39]. A meta-analysis has concluded that there is an inversely proportional relationship between the amount of rPE practiced and the risk of developing Alzheimer's disease (0.55; 95% CI 0.36 to 0.84; $p = 0.006$) [13]. Other even more recent works have confirmed this relationship [18,19,41]. Karceski [42] specified, in a comparison of active subjects and inactive subjects, that the risk of developing the disease was twice as high for the inactive subjects. Hamer and Chida [13] deduced almost the same conclusion by showing that rPE reduced the risk of developing Alzheimer's disease by 45%.

Neuroprotective mechanisms resulting from regular physical exercise The repeated and regular physiological modifications (i.e., increased cerebral blood flow) related to exercise are favorable to the synthesis of cerebral tissue, e.g., [15,17]. rPE activates the neurotrophic function and angiogenesis, thereby facilitating neurogenesis and synaptogenesis which improve the memory and the cognitive functions, e.g., [15,43-45].

In order to analyze and describe the mechanisms involved in the protective effect of rPE, studies completed with animal models have been necessary. rPE carried out between moderate and high intensities has a neuroprotective effect by increasing the production of antioxidant enzymes (particularly superoxide dismutase or SOD), endothelial nitric oxide synthases (eNOS), brain-derived neurotrophic factors (BDNF), nerve growth factors (NGF), insulin-like growth factors (IGF-1), and vascular endothelial growth factors (VEGF), and by reducing the production of free radicals (reactive oxygen species or ROS) as well as the concentration of amyloid-ß plaques (Aβ), in particular in the cerebral zones involved in cognitive function (notably the memory) such as the hippocampus [38,46,47]. In a study carried out by Van Praag et al. [48] rPE induced hippocampic neurogenesis (particularly in the dentate gyrus) which was associated with synaptogenesis and an improvement in the learning capabilities (spatial memory and long-term potentiation) of trained old mice in comparison with control mice (same model and same age), that did not have access to a running wheel. Regular and continuous training of rats (from 5 to 23 months of age) over a period of 18 months, which required them to run on a horizontal treadmill at a speed of 20 m/min for 20 min, twice a day, 5 days a week, also had a neuroprotective effect on the cerebellum [49]. Larsen et al. [49] reported that sedentary-aged rats had 11% fewer Purkinje cells and 9% smaller Purkinje cell soma volumes (both two, $p = 0.02$) than exercised aged rats, and exercised aged rats had the same number of Purkinje cells as young rats (5 months of age). Evidence suggests that, in the case of animals, rPE results in beneficial structural cerebral adaptations.

In the case of cognitively normal human subjects, rPE is likely to improve the executive function, attentional capacity, processing speed, episodic memory, and procedural memory [36,50,51]. Physical exercise of 40 min repeated four times a week (ergocycle, treadmill, and stair-climbing) for a period of 12 weeks increased the cerebral blood flow in the dentate gyrus of the hippocampus which facilitates its neurogenesis [52]. rPE engendered an increase of gray matter in the temporal and frontal lobes which improved cognitive performances [17,53]. An aerobic program (three weekly sessions of 1 h for a period of 6 months) generated a volume increase (evaluation by means of magnetic resonance imaging or MRI) of gray and white matters in certain prefrontal and temporal cortical regions (i.e., those which are substantially damaged by age advancement) for subjects aged between 60 and 79 [54]. A longitudinal study showed that there is also a relationship between the amount of physical activity practiced and the volume of the prefrontal and temporal areas as well as the volume of the hippocampus, after 9 years of monitoring of 299 subjects (178 women) aged 78 [55]. This study specified that greater gray matter volume resulting from rPE reduced the risk for cognitive impairment. One year later, the same laboratory carried out an interventional study and reported that aerobic training over 12 months (3 days/week, 40 min/session, 60% to 75% of the maximum heart rate reserve from the seventh week) generated an increase (+2%) of the hippocampal volume (and it is known that the age-related hippocampal annual volume loss is between −1% and −2% a year) which was associated with an increase in the plasmatic concentration of BDNF in old healthy subjects (120 subjects randomized into two groups, 60 × 68-year-old control subjects versus 60 × 66-year-old experimental subjects who practiced stretching exercises) [56]. Evidence also suggests that, in the case of humans, aerobic exercise generates beneficial structural and functional cerebral adaptations.

Lange-Asschenfeldt and Kojda [38] have described the molecular mechanisms of the beneficial effects of rPE on the vasculature, such as activation of the vascular NO/eNOS pathway. These authors concluded that, as well as maintaining neuronal plasticity, rPE may prevent/counteract cerebral pathophysiology by building a vascular reserve. Moreover, in the case of cognitively normal subjects, rPE is associated with Alzheimer's disease biomarkers. In a study of 61 adults aged between 55 and 88, confirmed to be cognitively normal, Liang et al. [57] recorded that individuals with elevated Pittsburgh compound-B or PIB (i.e., radiotracers were used to image amyloid-β aggregates with plaque formation, which indicated higher uptake of PIB) and cerebrospinal fluid Tau proteins and phosphorylated Tau proteins (ptau) carried out less exercise whereas active individuals had lower PIB binding. Nevertheless, the mechanical explanation is still uncertain since it has not yet been possible to attribute the causal link between the value of these biomarkers and the amount of physical activity.

rPE that focuses on motor coordination activates cerebral structures that are involved in executive control and perceptual speed, thereby improving not only the quality of motor responses (execution correctness and speed) but also the integration process of visuospatial information [58]. Voelcker-Rehage et al. [58] have shown with the use of the functional MRI technique that rPE that focuses on motor coordination enhances the activation level of the cerebral network that treats visuospatial information. These authors have specified that repeated and regular enhancements of the activation level induce structural and functional adaptations of this cerebral network thereby facilitating cognitive functioning.

For adults [17] and old adults aged between 60 and 79 [54], stretching and toning or relaxation interventions do not have any effect on the cerebral volume and cognitive function because the metabolic or cognitive demands are too low in comparison with aerobic exercise and coordination tasks. Aerobic exercise induces changes in the cardiovascular function that occur based on the energy demands, while coordination exercise induces changes in information processing that occur based on the cognitive demands. This effect of coordination exercise might be crucial for inducing molecular or cellular changes and thus might show the positive effects of physical activity on cognitive function [52,58]. Cardio-vascular training has been associated with increased activation of the sensorimotor network, whereas coordination training has been associated with increased activation of the visual-spatial network [58]. Nevertheless, other authors have reported that non-aerobic and non-visuo-motor coordination activities such as stretching and toning could improve the executive function in old subjects [59]. Tai Chi could also be beneficial for cognitive function [60-63] even if its effects need to be validated by studies of large cohorts of old subjects [64].

The contribution of each type of exercise to the cerebral structures and functions of old persons remains to be determined more precisely by future studies in this field. At this point, it is evident that aerobic exercise combined with other types of exercise (e.g., motor coordination, stretching, toning, Tai Chi) generates greater positive effects on cognitive function than aerobic exercise practiced alone [65].

Conclusions

Regular aerobic exercise can limit cognitive decline and the risk of dementia as a result of various neurobiological mechanisms that it is likely to trigger in the brain tissue especially in the temporal and prefrontal areas as well as the hippocampus. This form of exercise can activate and maintain the sensorimotor network. However, the optimal workload related to the frequency, the intensity, and the duration of sessions has still not been clearly established, and future research on this topic should particularly focus on these aspects. Regular motor coordination exercise can also generate positive adaptations of cognitive function, and this form of exercise is likely to activate and maintain the visual-spatial network. The preventive effects of other types of exercise still need to be explored.

Competing interests

Thierry Paillard declares that he has no conflict of interest. No financial support was received for the conduct of this study or preparation of this manuscript.

References

1. INSERM (2008) Activité physique - contextes et effets sur la santé. INSERM Editions: Paris; ISBN 978-2-85598-862-4
2. Bonaconsa M, Colavito V, Pifferi F, Aujard F, Schenker E, Dix S, et al. Cell clocks and neuronal networks: neuron ticking and synchronization in aging and aging - related neurodegenerative disease. Curr Alzheimer Res. 2013;10:597–608.
3. Dartigues JF, Foubert-Samier A, Helmer C. Relationship between educational level and dementia: social factor and age-related chronic disease. Rev Epidemiol Sante Publique. 2013;61 Suppl 3:195–8.
4. Paulson HL, Igo I. Genetics of dementia. Semin Neurol. 2011;31:449–60.
5. Gao HM, Hong JS. Gene-environment interactions: key to unraveling the mystery of Parkinson's disease. Prog Neurobiol. 2011;94:1–19.
6. Zawia NH, Basha MR. Environmental risk factors and the developmental basis for Alzheimer's disease. Rev Neurosci. 2005;16:325–37.
7. Logroscino G. The role of early life environmental risk factors in Parkinson disease: what is the evidence? Environ Health Perspect. 2005;113:1234–8.
8. Ibanez V. Les maladies neuro-dégénératives : problèmes cliniques. Médecine Nucléaire, Imagerie Fonctionnelle et Métabolique. 2005;29:213–9.
9. Zeki Al Hazzouri A, Haan MN, Kalbfleisch JD, Galea S, Lisabeth LD, Aiello AE. Life-course socioeconomic position and incidence of dementia and cognitive impairment without dementia in older Mexican americans: results from the Sacramento area Latino study on aging. Am J Epidemiol. 2011;173:1148–58.
10. Plassman BL, Williams Jr JW, Burke JR, Holsinger T, Benjamin S. Systematic review: factors associated with risk for and possible prevention of cognitive decline in later life. Ann Intern Med. 2010;153:182–93.
11. Osler M, Avlund K, Mortensen EL. Socio-economic position early in life, cognitive development and cognitive change from young adulthood to middle age. Eur J Public Health. 2013;23:974–80.
12. De Luca d'Alessandro E, Bonacci S, Giraldi G. Aging populations: the health and quality of life of the elderly. Clin Ter. 2011;162:e13–8.
13. Hamer M, Chida Y. Physical activity and risk of neurodegenerative disease: a systematic review of prospective evidence. Psychol Med. 2009;39:3–11.
14. Rivera-Brown AM, Frontera WR. Principles of exercise physiology: responses to acute exercise and long-term adaptations to training. PM R. 2012;4:797–804.
15. Gligoroska JP, Manchevska S. The effect of physical activity on cognition - physiological mechanisms. Mater Sociomed. 2012;24:198–202.
16. Archer T. Physical exercise alleviates debilities of normal aging and Alzheimer's disease. Acta Neurol Scand. 2011;123:221–38.
17. Voelcker-Rehage C, Niemann C. Structural and functional brain changes related to different types of physical activity across the life span. Neurosci Biobehav Rev. 2013;37:2268–95.
18. Abe K. Total daily physical activity and the risk of AD and cognitive decline in older adults. Neurology. 2012;79:1071.
19. Buchman AS, Boyle PA, Yu L, Shah RC, Wilson RS, Bennett DA. Total daily physical activity and the risk of AD and cognitive decline in older adults. Neurology. 2012;24:1323–9.
20. Bergado JA, Almaguer W. Aging and synaptic plasticity: a review. Neural Plast. 2002;9:217–32.
21. Kelly KM, Nadon NL, Morrison JH, Thibault O, Barnes CA, Blalock EM. The neurobiology of aging. Epilepsy Res. 2006;68 Suppl 1:5–20.
22. Moeller JR, Ishikawa T, Dhawan V, Spetsieris P, Mandel F, Alexander GE, et al. The metabolic topography of normal aging. J Cereb Blood Flow Metab. 1996;16:385–98.
23. Martin AJ, Friston KJ, Colebatch JG, Frackowiak RS. Decreases in regional cerebral blood flow with normal aging. J Cereb Blood Flow Metab. 1991;11:684–9.
24. Rutten BP, Korr H, Steinbusch HW, Schmitz C. The aging brain: less neurons could be better. Mech Ageing Dev. 2003;124:349–55.
25. Saver JL. Time is brain-quantified. Stroke. 2006;37:263–6.
26. Mazner L, Nyengaard JR, Tang Y, Pakkenberg B. Marked loss of myelinated nerve fibers in the human brain with age. J Comp Neurol. 2003;462:144–52.
27. Peters A. The effects of normal aging on myelin and nerve fibers: a review. J Neurocytol. 2002;31:581–93.
28. Qin S, Hermans EJ, van Marle HJ, Fernández G. Understanding low reliability of memories for neutral information encoded under stress: alterations in memory-related activation in the hippocampus and midbrain. J Neurosci. 2012;32:4032–41.
29. Hasan KM, Rahman MS, Arif KM, Sobhani ME. Psychological stress and aging: role of glucocorticoids (GCs). Age (Dordr). 2012;34:1421–33.
30. Erixon-Lindroth N, Farde L, Wahlin TB, Sovago J, Halldin C, Bäckman L. The role of the striatal dopamine transporter in cognitive aging. Psychiatry Res. 2005;138:1–12.
31. Van Gelder BM, Tijhuis MA, Kalmijn S, Giampaoli S, Nissinen A, Kromhout D. Physical activity in relation to cognitive decline in elderly men: the FINE Study. Neurology. 2004;63:2316–21.
32. Schuit AJ, Feskens EJ, Launer LJ, Kromhout D. Physical activity and cognitive decline, the role of the apolipoprotein e4 allele. Med Sci Sports Exerc. 2001;33:772–7.
33. Lytle ME, Vander Bilt J, Pandav RS, Dodge HH, Ganguli M. Exercise level and cognitive decline: the MoVIES project. Alzheimer Dis Assoc Disord. 2004;18:57–64.
34. Yaffe K, Barnes D, Nevitt M, Lui LY, Covinsky K. A prospective study of physical activity and cognitive decline in elderly women: women who walk. Arch Intern Med. 2001;161:1703–8.
35. Weuve J, Kang JH, Manson JE, Breteler MM, Ware JH, Grodstein F. Physical activity, including walking, and cognitive function in older women. JAMA. 2004;292:1454–61.
36. Colcombe S, Kramer AF. Fitness effects on the cognitive function of older adults: a meta- analytic study. Psychol Sci. 2003;14:125–30.
37. Wenk GL. Neuropathologic changes in Alzheimer's disease. J Clin Psychiatry. 2003;64 Suppl 9:7–10.
38. Lange-Asschenfeldt C, Kojda G. Alzheimer's disease, cerebrovascular dysfunction and the benefits of exercise: from vessels to neurons. Exp Gerontol. 2008;43:499–504.
39. Larson EB, Wang L, Bowen JD, McCormick WC, Teri L, Crane P, et al. Exercise is associated with reduced risk for incident dementia among persons 65 years of age and older. Ann Intern Med. 2006;144:73–81.
40. Nelson R. Exercise could prevent cerebral changes associated with AD. Lancet Neurol. 2005;4:275.
41. de Bruijn RF, Schrijvers EM, de Groot KA, Witteman JC, Hofman A, Franco OH, et al. The association between physical activity and dementia in an elderly population: the Rotterdam study. Eur J Epidemiol. 2013;28:277–83.
42. Karceski S. Preventing Alzheimer disease with exercise? Neurology. 2012;78:110–2.
43. Deslandes A, Moraes H, Ferreira C, Veiga H, Silveira H, Mouta R, et al. Exercise and mental health: many reasons to move. Neuropsychobiology. 2009;59:191–8.
44. Lista I, Sorrentino G. Biological mechanisms of physical activity in preventing cognitive decline. Cell Mol Neurobiol. 2010;30:493–503.

45. Eggermont L, Swaab D, Luiten P, Scherder E. Exercise, cognition and Alzheimer's disease: more is not necessarily better. Neurosci Biobehav Rev. 2006;30:562–75.
46. Radak Z, Hart N, Sarga L, Koltai E, Atalay M, Ohno H, et al. Exercise plays a preventive role against Alzheimer's disease. J Alzheimer's Dis. 2010;20:777–83.
47. Vaynman S, Ying Z, Gomez-Pinilla F. Hippocampal BDNF mediates the efficacy of exercise on synaptic plasticity and cognition. Eur J Neurosci. 2004;20:2580–90.
48. Van Praag H, Christie BR, Sejnowski TJ, Gage FH. Running enhances neurogenesis, learning, and long-term potentiation in mice. Proc Natl Acad Sci U S A. 1999;96:13427–31.
49. Larsen JO, Skalicky M, Viidik A. Does long-term physical exercise counteract age-related Purkinje cell loss? A stereological study of rat cerebellum. J Comp Neurol. 2000;428:213–22.
50. Angevaren M, Aufdemkampe G, Verhaar HJ, Aleman A, Vanhees L. Physical activity and enhanced fitness to improve cognitive function in older people without known cognitive impairment. Cochrane Database Syst Rev. 2008;16(2):CD005381. doi:10.1002/14651858.
51. Smith PJ, Blumenthal JA, Hoffman BM, Cooper H, Strauman TA, Welsh-Bohmer K, et al. Aerobic exercise and neurocognitive performance: a meta-analytic review of randomized controlled trials. Psychosom Med. 2010;72:239–52.
52. Pereira AC, Huddleston DE, Brickman AM, Sosunov AA, Hen R, McKhann GM, et al. An in vivo correlate of exercise-induced neurogenesis in the adult dentate gyrus. Proc Natl Acad Sci. 2007;104:5638–43.
53. Kramer AF, Colcombe S, Erickson K, Belopolsky A, McAuley E, Cohen NJ, et al. Effects of aerobic fitness training on human cortical function: a proposal. J Mol Neurosci. 2002;19:227–31.
54. Colcombe SJ, Erickson KI, Scalf PE, Kim JS, Prakash R, McAuley E, et al. Aerobic exercise training increases brain volume in aging humans. J Gerontol A Biol Sci Med Sci. 2006;61:1166–70.
55. Erickson KI, Raji CA, Lopez OL, Becker JT, Rosano C, Newman AB, et al. Physical activity predicts gray matter volume in late adulthood: the Cardiovascular Health Study. Neurology. 2010;75:1415–22.
56. Erickson KI, Voss MW, Prakash RS, Basak C, Szabo A, Chaddock L, et al. Exercise training increases size of hippocampus and improves memory. Proc Natl Acad Sci U S A. 2011;108:3017–22.
57. Liang KY, Mintun MA, Fagan AM, Goate AM, Bugg JM, Holtzman DM, et al. Exercise and Alzheimer's disease biomarkers in cognitively normal older adults. Ann Neurol. 2010;68:311–8.
58. Voelcker-Rehage C, Godde B, Staudinger UM. Cardiovascular and coordination training differentially improve cognitive performance and neural processing in older adults. Front Hum Neurosci. 2011;5:26. doi:10.3389/fnhum.2011.00026.
59. Voss MW, Prakash RS, Erickson KI, Basak C, Chaddock L, Kim JS, et al. Plasticity of brain networks in a randomized intervention trial of exercise training in older adults. Front Aging Neurosci. 2010. doi:10.3389/fnagi.2010.00032.
60. Wu Y, Wang Y, Burgess EO, Wu J. The effects of Tai Chi on cognitive function in older adults: a meta-analysis. J Sport Health Science. 2013;2:193–203.
61. Nguyen MH, Kruse A. A randomized controlled trial of Tai chi for balance, sleep quality and cognitive performance in elderly Vietnamese. Clin Interv Aging. 2012;7:185–90.
62. Chang YK, Nien YH, Tsai CL, Etnier JL. Physical activity and cognition in older adults: the potential of Tai Chi Chuan. J Aging Phys Act. 2010;18:451–72.
63. Taylor-Piliae RE, Newell KA, Cherin R, Lee MJ, King AC, Haskell WL. Effects of Tai Chi and Western exercise on physical and cognitive functioning in healthy community-dwelling older adults. J Aging Phys Act. 2010;18:261–79.
64. Blake H, Hawley H. Effects of Tai Chi exercise on physical and psychological health of older people. Curr Aging Sci. 2012;5:19–27.
65. Audiffren M, André N, Albinet C. Effets positifs de l'exercice physique chronique sur les fonctions cognitives des seniors: bilan et perspectives. Rev Neuropsychol. 2011;3:207–25.

25

Influence of Active Recovery on Cardiovascular Function During Ice Hockey

Jamie F. Burr[1,2*], Joshua T. Slysz[2], Matthew S. Boulter[2] and Darren E. R. Warburton[3]

Abstract

Background: Ice hockey is a popular sport comprised of high-intensity repeated bouts of activity. Light activity, as opposed to passive rest, has been shown to improve power output in repeated sprinting and could potentially help to offset venous pooling, poor perfusion, and the risk of an ischemic event. The objective of our study was, thus, to examine the efficacy of low-intensity lower body activity following a simulated hockey shift for altering hemodynamic function.

Methods: In a cross-over design, 15 healthy hockey players (23 ± 1 years, 54 ± 3 mL/kg/min) performed two simulated hockey shifts. In both conditions, players skated up to 85 % of age-predicted heart rate maximum, followed by either passive recovery or active recovery while hemodynamic measures were tracked for up to 180 s of rest.

Results: Light active recovery within the confines of an ice hockey bench, while wearing skates and protective gear, was effective for augmenting cardiac output (an average of 2.5 ± 0.2 L/min, $p = 0.03$) at 45, 50, and 120 s. These alterations were driven by a sustained elevation in heart rate (12 bpm, $p = 0.05$) combined with a physiological relevant but non-significant (11.6 mL, $p = 0.06$) increase in stroke volume.

Conclusions: Standing and pacing between shifts offers a realistic in-game solution to help slow the precipitous drop in cardiac output (heart rate and stroke volume) that typically occurs with passive rest. Prolonging the duration of an elevated cardiac output further into recovery may be beneficial for promoting recovery of the working skeletal muscles and also avoiding venous pooling and reduced myocardial perfusion.

Key Points:

- Evidence that light activity in the form of standing/pacing is effective for maintaining cardiac output, and thus venous return
- Increased cardiac output and venous return may help reduce the chances of poor perfusion (ischemia) and could also promote recovery for performance
- This is a simple, low-risk, intervention demonstrated for the first time to work within the confines of a player's bench while wearing hockey gear

Keywords: Impedance cardiography; Performance; Cardiac risk; Venous return; Sprint

* Correspondence: burrj@uoguelph.ca
[1]Human Performance Laboratory, University of Guelph, 50 Stone Road East, Guelph, Ontario N1G 2W1, Canada
[2]Human Performance and Health Research Laboratory, University of PEI, Charlottetown, Canada
Full list of author information is available at the end of the article

Background

The sport of ice hockey is characterized by stop and start play, with repeated high-intensity exercise interspersed with seated rest on the bench. At the highest level, on-ice shifts typically last between 30 and 60 s [1], with a work to rest ratio of 1:3. This differs somewhat from recreational "old-timer" hockey wherein the work to rest ratio is closer to 1 owing to longer less intense shifts and fewer players per team [2–4].

During competitive hockey, on-ice heart rates (HR) are often sustained as high as 85 % max and have been reported to peak >90 % [4]. Atwal et al. (2002) employed Holter monitoring to demonstrate HR ranges between 85 and 100 % of age-predicted max during recreational hockey [5], and our own lab has (unpublished) data confirming these results in recreational male hockey players (65 ± 6 years), with the average shift representing 97 ± 8 % of age predicted HRmax, and peaks of 103 ± 7 % (reflecting the variability around estimations of max HR). Goodman et al. have recently demonstrated peak on-ice HRs that actually exceeded the objectively measured maximal values observed during laboratory fitness tests (i.e., 107 % of laboratory max) [2]. Given these physical demands of ice hockey, it is logical that the level of competitive play and "success" in hockey is associated with well-developed physiological attributes [6–8]. Potentially compounding the high intensity of play is the fact that many older recreational hockey players also have poorly controlled cardiovascular risk factors [5, 9], and thus, it is perhaps not surprising that hockey is often suggested as a high-risk sport for this population. There is compelling evidence that the risk for adverse exercise-related event (such as sudden cardiac death) increases significantly in vigorous activities greater than 6 metabolic equivalents (METs) (with hockey reported to be ≥8 METs [10]), and this risk is markedly increased in previously inactive or untrained individuals [11, 12].

The intermittent nature of hockey, which requires participants to perform particularly stressful exercise followed by relative inactivity between shifts, represents an interesting cardiovascular challenge for both the competitive player and recreational "old-timer" alike. Given the evidence that higher exercise intensities lead to greater metabolite-induced vasodilation post-exercise, this is particularly salient in the sport of ice hockey [13]. For the competitive athlete, the challenge of maintaining optimal performance is paramount, whereas the avoidance of cardiac ischemia may be a primary goal for the prevention of adverse cardiac events in the aged athlete.

Given that the circulatory system can be modeled as a simple closed-circuit loop with a single pump, venous return must equal cardiac output (Q). It also follows that augmented venous return would thus ensure that Q is optimized, thus potentially augmenting both central and peripheral blood supply for either performance or health. It is for this reason that exercisers are commonly encouraged to include a "cool-down" period of light exercise following physical activity in an attempt to slow the decline in HR and stroke volume (SV), by maintaining a light cardiovascular demand and decreasing venous pooling. However, in ice hockey, it is often not possible for athletes to slowly reduce the exercise intensity through low-intensity skating following each shift, as the game play continues and the athlete is within the confines of the player's bench. Nevertheless, participants are recommended to find alternative methods of promoting recovery and venous return following the cessation of vigorous exercise to ensure adequate cerebral, musculoskeletal, and cardiac flow.

Although standing or walking in place between shifts in hockey has been suggested for those who may be at an increased risk of cardiovascular event [14], empirical evidence demonstrating the efficacy of such actions on cardiac responses for hockey players is lacking. Investigations of active versus passive recovery using cycling exercise have demonstrated active recovery to maintain Q by maintaining a higher SV and HR compared to passive recovery [15, 16] likely through alterations in systemic vascular resistance to maintain blood and perfusion pressure [17]. However, the efficacy of using the muscle pump during ice hockey could be greatly compromised considering the restrictions of the player's bench and the athlete's ability to contract the musculature of their legs. In particular, lower leg contractions involving dorsi and plantar flexion may be limited by the stiff upper boot of a hockey skate. It is also possible that related hockey-specific environmental factors (i.e., equipment, environment) might affect the ecological validity of implementing this technique for altering cardiac and hemodynamic response outside of a laboratory setting.

The objective of our study was, thus, to examine the efficacy of changing body posture (stand vs. sit) and including low-intensity lower body activity following a simulated hockey shift for altering hemodynamic function. We hypothesized that standing and pacing between shifts would assist in the maintenance of Q by augmenting venous return and SV by way of peripheral muscle pump action and through a sustained increase in HR.

Methods

We recruited 15 young (22.5 ± 0.9 years) male hockey players from the varsity men's hockey team to participate in a cross-over controlled study. Participants were of average build and fitness for competitive hockey players [7] as can be seen from the descriptive participant characteristics presented in Table 1. Player fitness was measured during a pre-season physical fitness combine, with VO_2 estimated from maximal performance on a widely used and validated field-based 20-m shuttle run, for

Table 1 Descriptive participant statistics

	$\bar{X}$	SD
Age (year)	22.5	0.9
Height (cm)	181.8	6.9
Weight (kg)	89.0	6.1
BMI (kg/m^2)	26.9	1.2
Est. VO_2max (mL/kg/min)	53.7	3
Systolic BP (mmHg)	119	2
Diastolic BP (mmHg)	77	3
Est. HRmax (bpm; 220 – age)	198	0.9
Body surface area (m^2)	2.1	0.1

which methods have been described in detail elsewhere [18]. Prior to data collection, all participants provided written informed consent, and this study was approved by the university's research ethics board (ref #6005349) for investigations involving human participants, in accordance with the Helsinki Declaration of 1975, as revised in 2008.

Cardiovascular Measurements

Cardiovascular hemodynamic measures were recorded for each player using impedance cardiography (Physioflow Enduro, Manatec Biomedical, France) with a telemetric signal relayed wirelessly to a dedicated computer, housed rink-side in the player's bench. Thoracic bio-impedance is a non-invasive and portable method of determining Q and has been shown to have good agreement with thermodilution techniques [19] at rest and also with the direct Fick method during incremental exercise to maximum exertion [20]. The Physioflow impedance cardiography (ICG) device that we employed differs from conventional ICG in that there is less reliance on the baseline thoracic impedance signal (resistance ZO) for transformation during exercise; instead, a pulsatile waveform representing the sensed impedance signal (delta Z) is processed and analyzed with its derivative over time. This signal morphology filter improves the signal to noise ratio and reduces artifact introduced by exercise, making it ideally suited for our purposes. During testing, participants wore full hockey gear, with the exception of shoulder pads so as not to interfere with the electrodes placed on the upper chest and back. Prior to testing, the participant's skin was cleaned, shaved, and abraded (Nu-prep), and surface electrodes (SkinTact FS-50) were placed according to the landmarks recommended by the manufacturer for exercise testing. On the hockey bench adjacent to the ice surface, the participant was instructed to sit quietly for 5–10 min prior to the measurement of blood pressure with a standard sphygmomanometer for calibration of the ICG device. Blood pressure was re-evaluated and corrected for ICG measures periodically during recovery.

Experimental Protocol

Baseline hemodynamic data was collected at rest on each participant prior to undertaking two skate-rest conditions. In condition 1, participants skated shuttles back and forth on the ice for 60 s, bringing their heart rate up to the typical in-game intensity [3, 4] of approximately 85 % of maximum, followed by a seated 180-s rest on the bench. In condition 2, participants again skated for 60 s at the same intensity followed by a 180-s "active" recovery on the bench. The active recovery consisted of standing and pacing on the spot or pacing within the confines of the bench that would normally be afforded to a player during a real game situation. Every participant performed both conditions consecutively in a randomized order. As such, both posture and muscular pump action were altered and compared in a cross-over design. Following baseline calibration, a short warm-up was permitted, after which time all exercise and rest was standardized to the above-noted work to rest ratio. ICG data was collected and analyzed using 15-s averages with measurements considered at 15, 30, 45, 60, 120, and 180 s post exercise.

Statistical Analysis

We employed a two-way repeated measures ANOVA comprising a 2 (recovery condition; passive or active) × 6 (time point) model. Time effects were examined using Bonferroni adjusted post hoc pairwise comparisons, and repeated measures t tests were used to compare mean differences between intervention groups at select time points, when indicated by main effects or interaction. Normality was confirmed using a Shapiro-Wilk test, and Greenhouse-Geisser correction was applied for interpretation of ANOVAs when sphericity was violated according to Mauchly's test. Exertion at peak exercise (% predicted HRmax) and hemodynamic responses were compared between conditions using paired sample t tests. All stats were performed using SPSS v21.0 and an alpha of $p < 0.05$ was selected a priori. All results are presented as mean ± SD unless otherwise noted.

Results

There was no difference in the level of exertion reached during a simulated shift between recovery conditions, with players skating up to a mean intensity of 83 ± 7 % (197 ± 1 bpm) and 84 ± 6 % (198 ± 1 bpm) of age-predicted HRmax for the passive and active trials, respectively. Similarly, no differences existed in hemodynamic variables at the end of the exercise period immediately prior to the initiation of recovery, which for the purposes of this study represent baseline values as the recovery phase was the time period of interest. As can be seen in Fig. 1, an interaction between time and recovery condition was observed for Q ($p = 0.03$), such that the difference in Q between

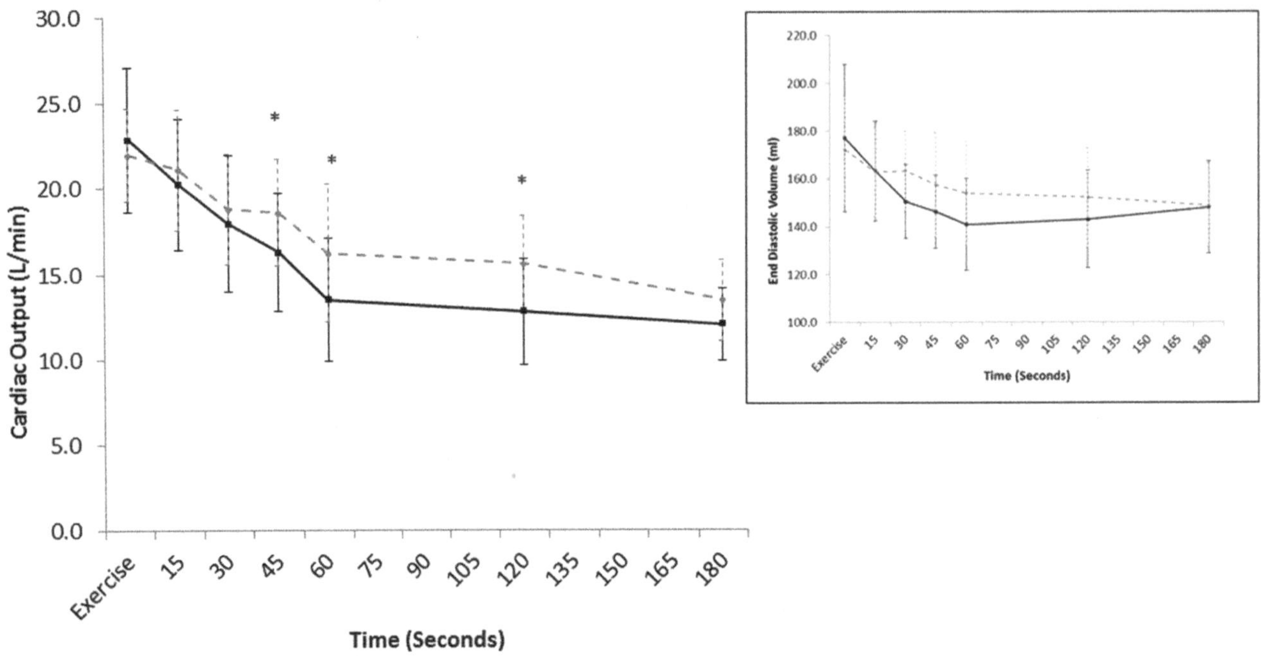

Fig. 1 A comparison of the cardiac output measured by impedance cardiography during skating exercise and following 15–180 s of recovery in hockey players who passively sat on the bench (*solid line*) or performed light activity (*dashed line*) by standing and rocking on feet. (*Inset*) End-diastolic volumes (EDV) during the same period. Statistical significance was not met for EDV which had larger variance about the mean, but the similarity in the shape of these curves is notable. * $p<0.05$

groups increased throughout rest, reaching a statistically different value of approximately 2.5 L/min at 45 s, which was maintained at 60 and 120 s post exercise before values began to converge by the final measurement at 180 s. Examination of the contributing factors to *Q* (Fig. 2) revealed alterations over time for both HR ($p < 0.001$) and SV ($p = 0.004$) as they returned toward resting levels. There was also a main effect on HR by condition ($p = 0.05$) with differences between groups presenting at 45 s of recovery and persisting until through the 120-s measurement. Although a clear trend was apparent for alterations in SV by recovery condition, this did not reach significance ($p = 0.06$). Importantly, the changes in SV would be considered to be of physiological importance [21]. Related hemodynamic variables are presented in Table 2, where it can be seen that only cardiac index (expressed relative to body size) and left heart work index differed between recovery conditions.

Discussion

Altering body posture from sitting to standing and engaging the muscle mass of the lower legs as a recovery strategy following a simulated hockey shift was found to be effective for maintaining *Q* and slowing the precipitous drop in *Q* that occurs with the abrupt cessation of exercise. This paper presents novel evidence that standing and pacing on the bench between shifts may represent an easily adopted and viable alternative to light skating to "cool down" slowly between shifts, when a player must leave the ice. This may have important implications for the high-performance athlete and aging recreational hockey player alike, both of whom face potential challenges that stem from insufficient *Q* between shifts while the body attempts to recover from a previous bout of stressful activity.

The current data supported our hypothesis regarding the overall effects on *Q*; however, the hypothesized mechanisms of this elevation were not fully supported, as elevations in SV did not reach significance. As can be observed from the graphical representation of data in Fig. 2, the elevated response of SV and HR in the active recovery condition was temporally similar; however, the larger variance around the measure of SV compared to HR almost certainly played a role in reducing the chances of reaching statistical significance ($p = 0.06$). In the current investigation, blood pressure was used to calibrate the ICG unit; however, a continuous BP signal was not recorded throughout exercise or recovery owing to the "field-based" nature of data collection, which is a limitation worth noting. Alterations in HR for time points 45–120 s, which significantly differed between active and passive recovery conditions, had a mean difference of 12 ± 3 bpm. At the matched time points, the mean alteration in SV was 12 ± 6 mL/beat, thus suggesting that the change in SV actually represented a slightly

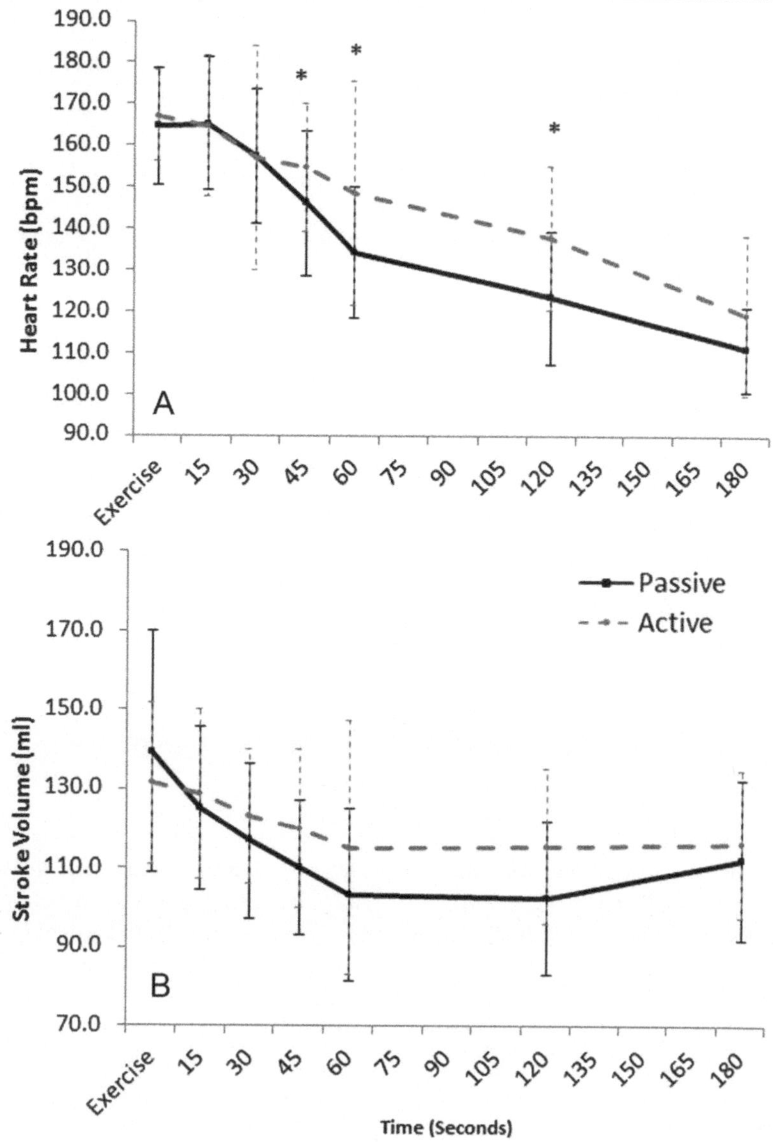

Fig. 2 Independent graphical representation of each of the components of cardiac output. These figures demonstrate the recovery response of heart rate (**a**) and stroke volume (**b**) following skating exercise in hockey players who either sat passively (*solid line*) or stood and paced (*dashed line*) at the bench. * $p<0.05$

greater relative deviation from baseline at 8.8 % compared to HR at 7.5 %. Notably, alterations did not occur within the first 30 s of recovery, which likely reflects the time necessary for the cardiovascular system to adjust to the changing exercise demands. By 180 s, difference between the active and passive conditions started to disappear, and this likely relates to the fact that the young, fit hockey players used in the current investigation were conditioned to recover in approximately 3–4 min of rest. This effect may be amplified (at both the beginning and end of the rest period) in less fit athletes, or by altering the intensity of the active recovery condition, which was intentionally light in the current investigation.

Cardiovascular Implications for Performance

There is convincing evidence from cycle ergometry models demonstrating significant decrements in repeated sprint ability when athletes recover passively between work bouts, as opposed to engaging in a light "active" recovery [22, 23]. It is suggested that this effect is primarily driven by ATP repletion and pH recovery, both of which are affected by *Q*/blood flow [22] through alterations in O_2 delivery and the maintenance of metabolite (H^+) gradients between the passing blood and local muscle tissue [24, 25]. Corresponding to the temporal demands of a hockey shift, evidence clearly demonstrates that sprints of 15–30-s duration, separated by

Table 2 Hemodynamic variables associated with cardiovascular function and recovery following a high-intensity short-duration simulated hockey shift

	Time (s)	Cardiac index (L/min/m^2)	Ejection fraction (%)	End-diastolic volume (mL)	Contractility index (no unit)	Left cardiac work index (kg.m/m^2)
Passive	Exercise	10.8 ± 1.8	78.6 ± 7.1	177 ± 30.8	372 ± 178.9	12.8 ± 2.3
	15	9.5 ± 1.7	76.2 ± 9	163.3 ± 20.9	314.9 ± 129	11.5 ± 2.2
	30	8.4 ± 1.8	74.7 ± 11.4	150.5 ± 15.4	273 ± 97.5	10 ± 2.3
	45	7.6 ± 1.6	75 ± 9.1	146.3 ± 15.2	264.1 ± 74.2	9 ± 2.1
	60	6.3 ± 1.6	70.6 ± 12.5	140.9 ± 19.2	220.6 ± 94.1	7.5 ± 2.1
	120	6 ± 1.4	71.6 ± 11.2	143 ± 20.2	229.2 ± 84.9	7.1 ± 1.7
	180	5.6 ± 0.9	72.6 ± 11.6	148.2 ± 19.2	249.1 ± 89.6	6.9 ± 0.9
Active	Exercise	10.3 ± 1.1	76.7 ± 8.5	172.1 ± 22.6	324.2 ± 147	12.3 ± 1.5
	15	9.9 ± 1.5	78.3 ± 9	162.8 ± 18.6	350.9 ± 154.7	11.5 ± 1.7
	30	8.8 ± 1.3	75.2 ± 10.6	163.4 ± 16.7	290.2 ± 116.9	10.5 ± 1.8*
	45	8.7 ± 1.3*	76.5 ± 9.6	157.5 ± 21.7	301 ± 120	10.1 ± 1.4*
	60	10.3 ± 8.5*	81.1 ± 14.9	154 ± 21.5	293.8 ± 111.3	9.8 ± 1.5*
	120	7.3 ± 1.1*	74.4 ± 10.2	152.1 ± 20.8	261.6 ± 79.5	8.9 ± 1.1
	180	6.3 ± 1	76.2 ± 7.7	148.8 ± 17.3	296.4 ± 115.2	7.7 ± 1.2
	Condition	$p = 0.01$	$p = 0.09$	$p = 0.266$	$p = 0.09$	$p = 0.003$
	Time	$p < 0.00$	$p = 0.485$	$p = 0.14$	$p = 0.07$	$p < 0.00$
	Interaction	$p = 0.03$	$p = 0.222$	$p = 0.464$	$p = 0.235$	$p = 0.02$

*Significantly different $p < 0.05$ from passive condition for select time point
p values across the bottom represent main effects and interactions across groups and time

rests of 3–4 min, show benefits to mechanical power output when light activity is substituted for passive rest, particularly in the first 10–15 s [22, 23]. As such, it would appear that competitive athletes may benefit from improved performance as a result of better recovery, but direct tests of skating speed, power, and longer term in-game adoption of this strategy are warranted.

Cardiovascular Implications for Health

By contrast, blood flow may have different, yet equally important, implications for the older recreational hockey player given the effects on central, rather than peripheral, circulation. Despite the well-accepted understanding that the risk reward of exercise greatly favors participation [11], it is undeniable that exercise can act as a trigger for a myocardial infarction or sudden cardiac death in the susceptible myocardium [12, 26]. Among the factors that might act to trigger these events in-game, or immediately after exercise, are the decrease in Q and relatively slow compensatory vasoconstriction of leg vasculature [27, 28]. This in turn can affect venous return, Q, and coronary perfusion, particularly in the vulnerable heart wherein supply and demand mismatches may be exacerbated. Prolonged intense exercise in particular (as often occurs in many recreational hockey games wherein there are suboptimal numbers of players per team to offer regular shift changes) can worsen these effects. If this type of prolonged vigorous play also leads to significant heat stress and dehydration [29], the associated reductions in blood plasma, coagulatory factors, and thermoregulatory fluid shifts have the potential to further compound the supply and demand imbalance through a reduction in stroke volume and compensatory increase in heart rate [30]. Prolonging an elevated Q further into recovery may be beneficial for promoting recovery of the working skeletal muscles and also avoiding venous pooling and reduced myocardial perfusion, particularly in persons with compromised coronary artery flow.

Mechanistic Implications

For the high-performance athlete, the mechanism for maintaining an increased Q may be of little consequence, as perfusion of the working muscles is augmented nonetheless, and improvements in blood flow-driven blood/tissue gradients (for the transfer of O_2, nutrients, and waste products) are established regardless of the underlying hemodynamic alterations. However, for the aging hockey player with a potentially susceptible myocardium, the observed mechanisms supporting an elevated Q could be further optimized for avoiding a supply and demand imbalance. This may be of greater importance for some individuals more than others given the clearly divergent responses in SV evident in the large variability in individual response, but it should be noted that the current population comprised exclusively of young ostensibly healthy men, who were of high fitness. The response of older potentially susceptible participants may be more homogenous in its response [31]. In practice, myocardial supply would be enhanced by reductions in HR, which would prolong diastolic filling time during which coronary arteries supply oxygenated blood to the cardiac tissue itself [32]. A current trend in sports performance apparel includes the wearing of compression garments to improve both performance and recovery through alterations in blood flow. If external compression devices are capable of promoting improved venous return [33], there may be a yet unexplored role for such garments in helping to bridge the gap between the benefits of activity for promoting long-term health and fitness and the acute risk posed during a given exercise session in a potentially at-risk population. External compression combined with light activity could also potentially alter the effective time-course of the observed recovery effects and should be further explored.

Conclusions

Standing and pacing on the hockey bench between shifts offers a realistic in-game solution to help slow the rapid drop in cardiac output (heart rate and stroke volume) that typically occurs with passive rest on the bench between hockey shifts. As such, adoption of an on-bench practice of standing recovery offers an easily implemented and low-cost solution with low participant risk, but a potentially high benefit.

Abbreviations

HR: heart rate; Q: cardiac output; ICG: impedance cardiography; SV: stroke volume.

Competing interests

Jamie F. Burr, Josh Slysz, Matthew Boulter, and Darren E. R. Warburton declare that they have no competing interests. J Burr and D Warburton are supported by NSERC Discovery grants. All the writing and preparation was the work of the authorship team.

Authors' contributions

JFB participated in the study design, data analysis, interpretation, and primary manuscript preparation. JS and MB were responsible for the primary data acquisition and reduction. DERW participated in the manuscript preparation, data interpretation, and critical revision. All authors read and approved the final manuscript.

Acknowledgements

We thank Aaron Rainnie for his contributions to the data acquisition with the impedance cardiography unit and general laboratory support.

Author details

[1]Human Performance Laboratory, University of Guelph, 50 Stone Road East, Guelph, Ontario N1G 2W1, Canada. [2]Human Performance and Health Research Laboratory, University of PEI, Charlottetown, Canada. [3]Cardiovascular Physiology and Rehabilitation Laboratory, University of British Columbia, Vancouver, Canada.

References

1. Cox MH, Miles DS, Verde TJ, Rhodes EC. Applied physiology of ice hockey. Sports Med. 1995;19(3):184–201.
2. Goodman Z. The cardiovascular effects of recreation hockey in middle-aged men. 2013.
3. Montgomery DL. Characteristics of "old timer" hockey play. Can J Appl Sport Sci. 1979;4(1):39–42.
4. Montgomery DL. Physiology of ice hockey. Sports Med. 1988;5(2):99–126.
5. Atwal S, Porter J, MacDonald P. Cardiovascular effects of strenuous exercise in adult recreational hockey: the Hockey Heart Study. CMAJ. 2002;166(3):303–7.
6. Quinney HA, Dewart R, Game A, Snydmiller G, Warburton D, Bell G. A 26 year physiological description of a national hockey league team. Appl Physiol Nutr Metab. 2008;33(4):753–60.
7. Burr JF, Jamnik RK, Baker J, Macpherson A, Gledhill N, McGuire EJ. Relationship of physical fitness test results and hockey playing potential in elite-level ice hockey players. J Strength Cond Res. 2008;22(5):1535–43.
8. Green MR, Pivarnik JM, Carrier DP, Womack CJ. Relationship between physiological profiles and on-ice performance of a national collegiate athletic association division I hockey team. J Strength Cond Res. 2006;20(1):43–6.
9. Mittleman MA. The double-edged blade of recreational hockey. CMAJ. 2002;166(3):331–2.
10. Warburton DE, Nicol CW, Bredin SS. Health benefits of physical activity: the evidence. CMAJ. 2006;174(6):801–9.
11. Goodman JM, Thomas SG, Burr JF. Evidence-based risk assessment and recommendations for exercise testing and physical activity clearance in apparently healthy individuals. Appl Physiol Nutr Metab. 2011;36(S1):S14–32.
12. Mittleman MA, Maclure M, Tofler GH, Sherwood JB, Goldberg RJ, Muller JE. Triggering of acute myocardial infarction by heavy physical exertion. Protection against triggering by regular exertion. Determinants of Myocardial Infarction Onset Study Investigators. N Engl J Med. 1993;329(23):1677–83.
13. Crisafulli A, Tocco F, Pittau G, Lorrai L, Porru C, Salis E, et al. Effect of differences in post-exercise lactate accumulation in athletes' haemodynamics. Appl Physiol Nutr Metab. 2006;31(4):423–31.
14. Hopkins-Rosseel DH. Cardiovascular prevention in a high risk sport, ice hockey: applications in wider sports physical therapy practice. N Am J Sports Phys Ther. 2006;1(4):187–94.
15. Crisafulli A, Orru V, Melis F, Tocco F, Concu A. Hemodynamics during active and passive recovery from a single bout of supramaximal exercise. Eur J Appl Physiol. 2003;89(2):209–16.
16. Takahashi T, Hayano J, Okada A, Saitoh T, Kamiya A. Effects of the muscle pump and body posture on cardiovascular responses during recovery from cycle exercise. Eur J Appl Physiol. 2005;94(5–6):576–83.
17. Crisafulli A, Carta C, Melis F, Tocco F, Frongia F, Santoboni UM, et al. Haemodynamic responses following intermittent supramaximal exercise in athletes. Exp Physiol. 2004;89(6):665–74.
18. Leger LA, Lambert J. A maximal multistage 20-m shuttle run test to predict VO2 max. Eur J Appl Physiol Occup Physiol. 1982;49(1):1–12.
19. Sharma V, Singh A, Kansara B, Karlekar A. Comparison of transthoracic electrical bioimpedance cardiac output measurement with thermodilution method in post coronary artery bypass graft patients. Ann Card Anaesth. 2011;14(2):104–10.
20. Richard R, Lonsdorfer-Wolf E, Charloux A, Doutreleau S, Buchheit M, Oswald-Mammosser M, et al. Non-invasive cardiac output evaluation during a maximal progressive exercise test, using a new impedance cardiograph device. Eur J Appl Physiol. 2001;85(3–4):202–7.
21. Warburton DE, Gledhill N, Jamnik VK, Krip B, Card N. Induced hypervolemia, cardiac function, VO2max, and performance of elite cyclists. Med Sci Sports Exerc. 1999;31(6):800–8.
22. Bogdanis GC, Nevill ME, Lakomy HK, Graham CM, Louis G. Effects of active recovery on power output during repeated maximal sprint cycling. Eur J Appl Physiol Occup Physiol. 1996;74(5):461–9.
23. Connolly DA, Brennan KM, Lauzon CD. Effects of active versus passive recovery on power output during repeated bouts of short term, high intensity exercise. J Sports Sci Med. 2003;2(2):47–51.

24. Gladden LB. Lactate uptake by skeletal muscle. Exerc Sport Sci Rev. 1989;17:115–55.
25. Sahlin K, Harris RC, Hultman E. Resynthesis of creatine phosphate in human muscle after exercise in relation to intramuscular pH and availability of oxygen. Scand J Clin Lab Invest. 1979;39(6):551–8.
26. Willich SN, Lewis M, Lowel H, Arntz HR, Schubert F, Schroder R. Physical exertion as a trigger of acute myocardial infarction. Triggers and Mechanisms of Myocardial Infarction Study Group. N Engl J Med. 1993;329(23):1684–90.
27. Goodman J, Thomas S, Burr JF. Physical activity series: cardiovascular risks of physical activity in apparently healthy individuals: risk evaluation for exercise clearance and prescription. Can Fam Physician. 2013;59(1):46,9. e6-e10.
28. Franklin BA. Cardiovascular events associated with exercise. The risk-protection paradox. J Cardiopulm Rehabil. 2005;25(4):189,95. quiz 196–7.
29. Logan-Sprenger HM, Palmer MS, Spriet LL. Estimated fluid and sodium balance and drink preferences in elite male junior players during an ice hockey game. Appl Physiol Nutr Metab. 2011;36(1):145–52.
30. Saltin B. Circulatory response to submaximal and maximal exercise after thermal dehydration. J Appi Physiol. 1964;19:1125.
31. Rodeheffer RJ, Gerstenblith G, Becker LC, Fleg JL, Weisfeldt ML, Lakatta EG. Exercise cardiac output is maintained with advancing age in healthy human subjects: cardiac dilatation and increased stroke volume compensate for a diminished heart rate. Circulation. 1984;69(2):203–13.
32. Merkus D, Kajiya F, Vink H, Vergroesen I, Dankelman J, Goto M, et al. Prolonged diastolic time fraction protects myocardial perfusion when coronary blood flow is reduced. Circulation. 1999;100(1):75–81.
33. Varela-Sanz A, Espana J, Carr N, Boullosa DA, Esteve-Lanao J. Effects of gradual-elastic compression stockings on running economy, kinematics, and performance in runners. J Strength Cond Res. 2011;25(10):2902–10.

26

Do Elite Athletes Live Longer? A Systematic Review of Mortality and Longevity in Elite Athletes

Srdjan Lemez* and Joseph Baker

Abstract

Background: Understanding of an athlete's lifespan is limited with a much more sophisticated knowledge of their competitive careers and little knowledge of post-career outcomes. In this review, we consider the relationship between participation at elite levels of sport and mortality risk relative to other athletes and age- and sex-matched controls from the general population. Our objective was to identify, collate, and disseminate a comprehensive list of risk factors associated with longevity and trends and causes of mortality among elite athletes.

Methods: English language articles were searched using the Web of Science database. Keywords *athletes*, *death*, *elite*, *"high performance" life expect**, *longevity*, *mortality*, *players*, *professional*, and *sport* were used to locate research articles. Seventeen additional articles were retrieved from reference lists found in these papers and a general web search. The inclusion criteria were the following: (1) publication year 1980 or later; (2) the study examined elite-level athletes; and (3) outcome data measured mortality/longevity trends and/or causes.

Results: Fifty-four peer-reviewed publications and three articles from online sources met the criteria for inclusion. Baseball, football, soccer, basketball, and cycling had the most reported data on elite athletes' lifespan longevities. A variety of mechanisms have attempted to explain mortality risk (e.g., handedness, playing position, achievement, etc.). Considerable support was found for superior longevity outcomes for elite athletes, particularly those in endurance and mixed sports.

Conclusions: Future research into the mechanisms that may affect mortality risk is important for a better understanding of life expectancies in both eminent and non-eminent populations. Participation in elite sport is generally favorable to lifespan longevity.

Key Points:

- A majority of studies included in this review reported superior lifespan longevity outcomes for elite athletes compared to age- and sex-matched controls from the general population and other athletes.
- Several mechanisms within and between sports may have powerful effects on the overall lifespan longevities of players (e.g., type of sport, playing position, race, and energy system).
- Future research on mortality in elite athletes would benefit from more comprehensive statistical measures and reliable databases to determine potential mechanisms that may influence mortality trends and causes in both athlete and non-athlete samples.

Keywords: Athletes; Death; Elite; Longevity; Mortality

* Correspondence: lemezs@yorku.ca
School of Kinesiology and Health Science, York University, 4700 Keele Street, Toronto M3J 1P3, ON, Canada

Background

Rationale

Researchers have given considerable attention to the athlete development process (e.g., positive youth development through sport) (see [1]). Interestingly, insight into post-career outcomes is significantly limited. For instance, our knowledge of how participation in elite sport affects lifespan longevity is particularly incomplete. This lack of information about later phases of athletes' lifespans may be attributable to several factors, such as the greater access to athletes during their competitive careers as well as the preponderance of participation- and performance-based theories focusing on elements related to understanding the antecedents of sporting success (e.g., [2]). Attaining a *complete* understanding of an athlete's lifespan requires knowledge of the inherent complexity of relationships that link hereditary and environmental characteristics to developmental outcomes. In this study, we focus on mortality of previously elite athletes.

An important challenge to mortality research in sport is the lack of data on the health behaviors of athletes post retirement. Much of our current understanding of trends and causes in elite athlete mortality derives from what appear to be "one-off" studies by small teams of researchers. Past work examining this issue in depth appears to be limited, although the Finnish studies that examined lifespan longevities of former elite endurance, team, and power athletes who represented Finland between the years 1920 and 1965 are exceptions (e.g., [3–6]). In addition, views on elite athlete mortality are largely shaped by popular media sources, which may downplay tenets of the lifespan and create false perceptions of early mortality in athletes (e.g., MLB's Tony Gwynn at 54 years [cancer], the NFL's Junior Seau at 43 years [suicide], boxing's Tommy Morrison at 44 years [AIDS], sailing's Andrew Simpson at 36 years [drowning] and skiing's Sarah Burke at 29 years [training fall]).

A recent meta-analysis completed by Garatachea et al. [7] indicated that elite athletes live longer than the general population, with an all-cause pooled standard mortality ratio (SMR) of 0.67 (95 % confidence interval [CI] 0.55–0.81; $P < 0.001$). Further, they found a lower risk of cardiovascular disease (CVD) and cancer in those who participated in high-performance sport, which emphasized the health benefits of exercise [7]. While their study makes an important contribution to our knowledge of longevity outcomes in elite sport, the restrictive sampling frame necessary for a meta-analysis excluded numerous studies that could inform our broader understanding of elite athlete health. For example, Garatachea et al. [7] included 10 studies of elite athlete longevity in their meta-analyses, but their inclusion criteria excluded studies that did not use SMR as a statistical measure of mortality (38 studies were excluded for this reason). As a result, studies with important information regarding longevity in elite athletes were excluded, such as greater longevity in Norwegian professional divers (hazard ratio [HR] = 0.79, 95 % CI 0.63–0.997) [8], and important mechanisms that may influence longevity, such as sex, as indicated by Olympic medal-winning females having greater longevity relative to Olympic medal-winning male athletes (HR = 0.61, 95 % CI 0.51–0.72) [9], and race, as indicated by African-American professional basketball players having a 77 % greater risk of death compared with white players (HR = 1.77, 95 % CI 1.35–2.32) [10]. Further, several studies which reported SMRs were not included in the meta-analysis (e.g., [11–15]). As such, there is an opportunity to grow our current limited understanding of longevity outcomes of elite athletes by examining a wider range of studies and sports through a systematic review.

Similarly, Teramoto and Bungum [16] completed a narrative review of mortality and longevity of elite athletes; however, a relatively small sample of 14 epidemiological studies was included. Their primary method of literature retrieval was through the PubMed (1950-) and Scopus (1960-) databases, using keywords *mortality, longevity, life expectancy, death,* and *(elite/professional) athletes* and *players*. While this literature search strategy was appropriate, a large number of studies on elite athlete mortality and longevity were published during or after their publication year of 2010 (e.g., [3, 8–10, 12, 13, 15, 17–31]). As a result, mechanisms such as race have since been validated as more consistent indicators of early mortality (e.g., [10, 19]). Currently, it may be premature to make conclusions about the long-term value of being a professional athlete considering the new evidence that has emerged from literature.

Although it appears that there are many unanswered questions concerning athletes' lifespan longevities, Teramoto and Bungum [16] presented enough empirical evidence to determine some cross-sport and energy system trends. Teramoto and Bungum [16] found a trend towards endurance (e.g., long-distance runners) and mixed-sport (e.g., soccer) athletes having more favorable survival outcomes relative to power sport (e.g., weightlifters) athletes and the general population. Similarly, a meta-analysis performed by Löllgen et al. [32] examined 38 studies that measured physical activity and all-cause mortality in samples of physically active individuals (non-elite athletes) and reported an overall significant relationship between physical activity participation and lower all-cause mortality. Light and moderate intensity levels of activity were generally associated with a reduction in mortality, whereas training at high intensities was not required for the main prevention against all-cause mortality [32]. While Löllgen and colleagues [32] provided evidence of physical activity positively influencing lifespan longevity independent of age and sex, the relationship between participation in *elite sport* and longevity can enhance our understanding of the benefits of physical activity at the highest levels of competition in unique athletic cohorts.

Teramoto and Bungum's [16] review suggested that the type and dose of elite sport participation may ultimately determine mortality risk. In addition, Teramoto and Bungum [16] highlighted the importance of considering elite athletes as a heterogeneous group with respect to mortality trends; differences between and within sports exist. In particular, the differences in health-related behaviors between and within sports may also create modifiable factors that are associated with longevity and mortality. As a result, overall mortality risk is explained by several modifiable factors, such as obesity and physical inactivity, and non-modifiable (unchangeable) factors, such as age and race, that are unique to athletes. For instance, Baron et al. [19] found an overall decrease in mortality in National Football Players (NFL) who were active between 1959 and 1988; however, defensive linemen had increased mortality from CVD and cardiomyopathy. Moreover, those with a playing time body mass index (BMI) of >30 kg/m^2 had a significantly higher risk of CVD, which was also influenced by race/ethnicity [19]. Although the effects of playing position on lifespan longevity may be more pronounced in contact sports such as football, we cannot overlook the differences and nuances in health-related behaviors between and within sports that may influence lifespan longevities.

Objectives

A subject such as death rates in professional athletes may be more susceptible to sensationalism when trends begin to emerge; therefore, it is essential that the data being disseminated are transparent and accurate. In this review, we consider the relationship between participation at elite levels of sport and mortality risk relative to other athletes and age- and sex-matched controls from the general population. Our objective was to extend the narrative review of Teramoto and Bungum [16] with a more comprehensive and up-to-date list of studies on mortality and longevity in previously elite athletes. More specifically, our aim was to advance knowledge in this area by collating athlete mortality/longevity literature that may help refine future analytic methods, form evidence-based models of athlete longevity, and determine whether elite-level participation in high-performance sport produces a lifespan longevity advantage. Similar to Teramoto and Bungum's [16] research questions, we asked the following: (1) do elite athletes have superior longevity outcomes relative to the general population, and (2) which mechanisms and risk factors are associated with longevity and are potential precursors to early mortality?

Methods

Literature Search

A systematic review of literature was performed using the Web of Science database (1 January 1980–30 September 2014; see Tables 1 and 2). Web of Science was chosen as our primary citation index as it contained over 90 million records through its 7 online databases, which would have made searches into smaller citation indexes largely redundant (e.g., EMBASE contains over 28 million records). Further, given this review's objective, Web of Science's databases appeared to be the most relevant to our study (e.g., Science Citation Index Expanded). Keywords, including *athletes, death, elite, "high performance" life expect*, longevity, mortality, players, professional*, and *sport*, were used to locate research articles. While a full electronic search strategy for at least *one* database is recommended [33], we further located research articles by searching the references of records that were identified through our database search, in addition to performing a general web search through the Google Scholar search engine.

Inclusion Criteria

The inclusion criteria were the following: (1) publication year 1980 or later; (2) the study examined elite-level athletes; and (3) outcome data measured mortality/longevity trends and/or causes. We excluded studies with no full-text availability (abstracts, conference proceedings, commentaries, and editorials), no English-text availability (a small proportion of international articles were unavailable for translation to English), other literature reviews with different inclusion criteria (e.g., non-elite samples), duplicates, case reports, studies on morbidity (i.e., CVD risk factors, etc.), psychosocial measures, collegiate athletes, and studies on the effectiveness of pre-screening strategies and prevention. For consistency, we use "elite" synonymously with any form of high-performance participation in sport (i.e., national, professional, and international competition such as the Olympics).

Data Extraction

We identified 1001 records through database searching using the aforementioned keywords. After review of title and abstract, we excluded 961 of those records (identical papers, $n = 31$; inclusion criteria not fulfilled, $n = 930$; most commonly due to studies not examining elite athletes and/or mortality/longevity trends), which left 40 eligible full-text articles from the Web of Science database search. Seventeen additional articles were retrieved from reference lists found in these papers and a general web search. In total, 57 studies filled the criteria for inclusion (Tables 1 and 2): 54 peer-reviewed publications (see Table 1), in addition to three articles from online sources included to investigate findings of mortality risk

Table 1 Peer-reviewed elite athlete mortality literature (>1980; $n = 54$)

Sport/Country	Authors	N	Key finding	LE vs. GP
MLB[a]	Abel and Kruger [35] (2004)	6038	Significant differences in longevity related to handedness ($F[2,6035] = 0.13$) (death < 2001)	–
MLB[a]	Abel and Kruger [36] (2005)	2604	LE: ~4–5 years longer ($f = 188.0$, $df = 1$, 2,555, $P < 0.001$); (1900–1950 debut)	↑
MLB[a]	Abel and Kruger [37] (2005)	3573	Median post-induction survival for HOFs was 5 years shorter than for non-inducted players, 18 years (CI 15.0–21.0) vs. 23 years (CI 22.1–23.9) for matched controls (OR = 1.37, CI 1.08–1.73); (death ≤ 2002)	–
MLB[a]	Abel and Kruger [38] (2006)	4492	LE: 4.8 years longer (SD = ±15.0); career length increased longevity ($F = 3.4$ $df = 3{,}4379$; $P < 0.02$); (1900–1939 debut)	↑
MLB[a]	Abel and Kruger [39] (2007)	3760	Earlier career debut predicted earlier death ($F[8,2898] = 7.78$, $P < 0.001$); (death < 2006; 1900–1935 debut)	–
MLB[a]	Abel and Kruger [40] (2007)	3835	Players ($n = 11$) with positive initials (e.g., A.C.E.; 80.4 ± $SE = 3.0$) lived significantly longer ($F[2904] = 3.7$, $P < 0.03$, two-tailed) by 13 years than players ($n = 30$) with negative initials (e.g., D.E.D.; 67.0 ± $SE = 3.1$) or players ($n = 864$) with neutral initials (67.1 ± $SE = 0.5$); players with positive initials lived significantly longer than their matched controls and those with negative initials ($P < 0.05$); (died before 1950)	–
MLB[a]	Boren and Erickson [41] (1998)	28	The most common toxin that lead to death by poisoning was carbon monoxide; low overall risk (death 1889–1995)	–
MLB[a]	Fudin et al. [42] (1993)	1686	*In response to Halpern and Coren's* [43] *study:* Left-handers ($n = 235$) had a *M* longevity of 64.46 years (SD = 15.34) right-handers ($n - 1451$), a difference of 38.57 days ($t[1684] - 0.09$, $P > 0.05$ for compared to 64.56 years (SD = 15.02) for years lived; Halpern and Coren [43] reported a difference of 244.72 days); (considered longevity data through 1978)	–
MLB[a]	Halpern and Coren [43] (1988)	1708	*M* age at death for right-handers was 64.64 years ($n = 1472$; SD = 15.5) and 63.97 years for left-handers ($n = 236$; SD = 15.4), a significant difference ($Z = 6.63$, $P < 0.001$)	–
MLB[a]	Hicks et al. [44] (1994)	5441	*In response to Fudin et al.'s* [42] *study:* Reliable data were confirmed for 3501 right-handers (64.3 %), 1199 mixed-handers (22.0 %) and 741 left-handers (13.6 %); the differences in *M* days of life were not significant in each group (F[2,5338] = .59, $P = 0.55$) and between just right- and left-handers ($t[4240] = -1.08$, $P = 0.28$; *M* longevity less for right-handers)	–
MLB[a]	Kalist and Peng [45] (2007)	2641	Greater longevity overall (SMR = 0.31); positive relationship between education and longevity (HR = 0.74, CI 0.56–0.977); black players had a HR 2.47 times greater than white players (1963–1996 debut)	↑
MLB[a]	Reynolds and Day [15] (2012)	14,360	Greater longevity rates throughout the last century (1900–1999 debut); (SMR = 0.87, CI 0.85–0.89; 1930–1999)	↑
MLB[a]	Saint Onge et al. [46] (2008)	6772	LE: ~5 years longer, compared to 20-year-old U.S. males; at 20 years, players from the Modern Era can expect to live 65.5 vs. 52.4 years and 58.3 years from the Early and Golden Eras, respectively (1902–2004 debut)	↑
MLB[a]	Smith [29] (2011)	–	*In response to Abel and Kruger's* [40] *study:* No relationship between name initials and longevity ($P > 0.05$)	–
MLB[a]	Smith [30] (2011)	102	*In response to Abel and Kruger's* [37] *study:* Corrected data shows that there is no statistically significant difference in the LE of HOF players ($Z = 0.06$, two-sided $P = 0.952$)	–
MLB[a]	Waterbor et al. [47] (1988)	985	Greater longevity overall (SMR = 0.94); longevity was correlated with position and in-game achievement (1911–1925 debut)	–
NBA[a]	Fafian Jr. [48] (1997)	2810	Greater longevity overall, particularly in guards (active 1946–1994)	↑
NBA[a]	Lawler and Lawler [25] (2011)	3647	Handedness was not significantly related to LE (HR = 0.92, CI 0.54–1.60; $P = 0.76$); (active 1946–2009)	–

Table 1 Peer-reviewed elite athlete mortality literature (>1980; $n = 54$) *(Continued)*

NBA[a]	Lawler et al. [10] (2012)	3366	White players lived longer (~1.5 years) than black players (HR = 1.77, CI 1.35–2.32); LE: ~4 year longer overall (active 1946–2005)	↑
NFL[a]	Abel and Kruger [49] (2006)	1512	LE: 6.1 years longer (SD = ±11.9); career length ($F = 4.7$, $df = 2{,}1504$; $P < 0.01$) and BMI ($R^2 = 0.01$, $P < 0.01$) increased longevity (debut < 1940)	↑
NFL[a]	Baron et al. [19] (2012)	3439	Greater longevity overall (SMR = 0.53, CI 0.48–0.59); BMI, race, and position were associated with longevity (active 1959–1988)	↑
NFL[a]	Lehman et al. [12] (2012)	3439	Greater longevity overall (SMR = 0.53, CI 0.48–0.59); increased overall risk of neurodegenerative MR (SMR = 2.83–3.26, CI 1.36–5.21); elevated ALS (SMR = 4.31, CI 1.73–8.87) and AD (SMR = 3.86, CI 1.55–7.95) subcategories (active 1959–1988)	↑
NFL[a]	Selden et al. [50] (2009)[b]	–	Review of recent data suggests ↑ CVD risk factors in players, particularly linemen	–
Boxing	Baird et al. [18] (2010)	339	Decline in premature MR after 1983 (rounds reduced from 15 to 12); (death 1950–2007)	–
Cricket[c]	Aggleton et al. [51] (1993)	3165	There was a significant lifespan longevity difference ($t[3163] = 2.77$, $P = 0.006$, two-tailed) between right-handers ($n = 2580$; 65.62 years) and left-handers ($n = 585$; 63.52 years); left-handers were more likely to die prematurely in accidents or in warfare (players in the British Isles from 1864–1983)	–
Cricket[c]	Aggleton et al. [52] (1994)	5960	No significant relation between mortality and handedness ($P = 0.3$); left-handers were more likely to die from unnatural causes ($P = 0.03$, log hazard 0.37, CI 0.04–0.70), particularly warfare ($P = 0.009$, log hazard 0.53, CI 0.13–0.92); (born between 1840–1960; players in the British Isles from 1864–1992)	–
Cyclists[d]	Marijon et al. [27] (2013)	786	Greater longevity overall in Tour de France participants (SMR = 0.59, CI 0.51–0.68, $P < 0.0001$); reduction in neoplasms (SMR = 0.56, CI 0.42–0.72, $P < 0.0001$) and CVD (SMR = 0.67, CI 0.50–0.88, $P = 0.004$); (1947–2012 participants)	↑
Cyclists[d]	Morcet et al. [13] (2012)	514	Greater longevity overall (SMR = 0.50, CI 0.34–0.71); although higher MR in younger cyclists (active 1960–1990)	↑
Cyclists[d,e,f]	Sanchis-Gomar et al. [28] (2011)	834	LE: ~8 years longer for Tour de France participants ($P < 0.05$); (active 1930–1964)	↑
Diving[g]	Irgens et al. [8] (2013)	3130	Greater longevity overall (HR = 0.79, CI 0.63–0.997), although increased violent deaths (born 1950–1999)	↑
Golf[a]	Coate and Schwenkenberg [21] (2012)	313	LE: 5.4 years longer (won prize money 1980–2009)	↑
Golf[h]	Farahmand et al. [11] (2009)	300,818	Greater longevity overall (SMR = 0.60, CI 0.57–0.64); greatest longevity in most skilled players (SMR = 0.53, CI 0.41–0.67); (born >1920, registered < 2001)	↑
PL[i]	Pärssinen et al. [53] (2000)	62	Increased premature MR (SMR = 4.6, CI 2.04–10.45; $P = 0.0002$), suspected from prior anabolic steroid use (placed first–fifth in Finnish championships, 1977–1982)	↓
Rugby[j]	Beaglehole and Stewart [54] (1983)	822	LE of All Blacks is the same as GP, although LE (73.0 years) for non-Māori All Blacks was ~10 years longer (CI 71.8–74.5) relative to the Māori All Blacks (1884–1981)	=
Skiing[g]	Grimsmo et al. [22] (2011)	122	Total MR was 9 % lower after a 30-year follow-up ($P = 0.04$); (study participants, 1976–1981)	↑
Soccer[e]	Belli and Vanacore [55] (2005)	350	Similar observed and expected MR, although a ten-fold increase of ALS MR (SPMR = 1158, CI 672–1998) was present (active 1960–1996)	=
Soccer[k]	Koning and Amelink [23] (2012)	371	Greater longevity overall ($P = 0.003$); (active 1970–1973)	↑
Soccer[l]	Kuss et al. [24] (2011)	812	Cumulative observed survival was smaller than cumulative expected survival; therefore, male and female players had reduced longevity (RSR ≤ 1); (active 1908–2006)	↓
Soccer[e]	Taioli [56] (2007)	5389	Greater longevity overall (SMR = 0.68, CI 0.52–0.86), although increased risk for car accident (SMR = 2.23, CI 1.46–3.27) and ALS (SMR = 18.18, CI 5.00–46.55) death (active 1975–2003)	↑

Table 1 Peer-reviewed elite athlete mortality literature (>1980; $n = 54$) *(Continued)*

SW[m]	Kanda et al. [57] (2009)	73	Deceased wrestlers had higher BMIs (OR = 1.08, CI 1.01–1.15) and winning percentages (OR = 1.29, CI 0.86–1.93); (active 1926–1989)	–
T and F[c]	Menotti et al. [58] (1990)	983	Greater longevity in males (SMR = 0.73; $n = 700$) and females (SMR = 0.48; $n = 283$); significant when analyzed together ($P = 0.0296$); (active > 1940)	↑
Mixed[a]	Abel and Kruger [17] (2010)	10,216	Decrease in longevity associated with names beginning with A–D; linear decrease for baseball and hockey players, but non-linear in football and basketball players; for each sport, A names lived longer than E–Z names, and D names had decreased longevities compared to E–Z names $F(4,10,193) = 4.16$, $P = 0.002$); football players lived the longest (72.3 ± 12.7) and baseball players lived the least years (70.8 ± 14.7); significant letter differences occurred between A and E–Z (HR = 0.80, CI 0.71–0.91, $P < 0.001$) and D and E–Z (HR = 1.16, CI 1.04–1.30, $P < 0.01$); (born 1875–1930)	–
Mixed	Bianco et al. [59] (2007)	715	Baseball (LE: 76; $n = 154$), basketball (LE: 78; $n = 58$), boxing (LE: 73; $n = 81$),football (LE: 77; $n = 81$), ice hockey (LE: 74.5; $n = 130$), swimming (LE: 74; $n = 37$), tennis (LE: 79; $n = 83$), track and field (LE: 75; $n = 59$), and wrestling (LE: 77; $n = 32$) HOFs had greater overall longevity ($P < 0.05$); ($M = 76$ years); (born 1860–1930)	↑
Mixed	Clarke et al. [20] (2012)	15,174	11,619 (76.6 %) male and 3555 (23.4 %) female Olympic Game medalists' (1896–2010) LE was 2.8 years longer (RCS = 1.08, CI 1.07–1.10); endurance (RCS = 1.13, CI 1.09–1.17) and mixed (RCS = 1.11, CI 1.09–1.13) sport athletes had a more favorable survival advantage relative to power sport athletes (RCS = 1.05, CI 1.01–1.08)	↑
Mixed[a]	Coate and Sun [9] (2013)	2690	Females ($n = 1348$; HR = 0.61, CI 0.51–0.72) had a ~6 year LE advantage over males ($n = 1342$), even though they competed in the same Olympic events (1900–2008) and tennis championships (HR = 0.65, CI 0.47–0.91; >1880); Olympic medalists' LE: 2–3 years longer if born <1920, but smaller advantage overall; tennis players' LE: 5–6 years longer if born <1920, and 2–3 years overall; *M* LE was 82 years for females and 76 years for males	↑
Mixed[n]	Gajewski and Poznańska [60] (2008)	2113	Greater longevity overall in male ($n = 1689$; SMR = 0.50, CI 0.44–0.56) and female ($n = 424$; SMR = 0.73, CI 0.48–1.05) Olympians (1924–2000)	↑
Mixed[i]	Kettunen et al. [3] (2014)	2363	LE: ~5–6 years longer overall; endurance (79.1 years; CI 76.6–80.6), team (78.8 years; CI 78.1–79.8) and power (75.6 years; CI 74.0–76.5) sport athletes who represented Finland in international competitions (active 1920–1965) had higher LE than controls (72.9 years, CI 71.8–74.3), even after adjusting for socio economic status, birth cohort, and disease-specific mortality (HR ≤ 1); boxers had increased risk of dementia mortality (HR = 4.20, CI 2.30–7.81)	↑
Mixed[i]	Kujala et al. [4] (2001)	2009	Greater longevity overall (SMR = 0.74, CI 0.69–0.79); all-cause mortality was lower for endurance (SMR = 0.57, CI 0.47–0.68), mixed (SMR = 0.68, CI 0.61–0.76), and power (SMR = 0.90, CI 0.81–1.00) sport athletes who represented Finland in international competitions (active 1920–1965); increased risk of hypertension in power sport athletes (SMR = 2.63, CI 1.06–5.42); (SMRs calculated 1971–1995)	↑
Mixed[h]	Lindqvist et al. [26] (2013)	1199	MR was not increased overall in former power sport athletes, except a slight increase at 45 years (CI 2.1–4.2); between 20 and 50 years, estimated HR = 1.44–1.46; 2.1–3.9 times increased MR from suicide between 30 and 50 years (overall, HR = 1.74, CI 1.08–2.66; $P = 0.025$); however, there was a lower malignancy MR (HR = 0.71, CI 0.50–0.98; $P = 0.036$); (active 1960–1979)	–
Mixed[n]	Poznańska and Gajewski [14] (2001)	–	Greater overall longevity (SMR = 0.42, CI 0.35–0.49), particularly between 1992 and 1998 (Olympians 1981–1998)	↑

Table 1 Peer-reviewed elite athlete mortality literature (>1980; $n = 54$) *(Continued)*

Mixed[b]	Samaras et al. [61] (2002)	1505	Modest correlation coefficients indicated that weight is only one risk factor that affected the longevities of baseball players ($n = 1278$; $r = -0.22$, $P < 0.025$) [58], football players ($n = 199$; $r = -0.33$, $P < 0.005$) [59], and Finnish elite athletes ($r = -0.51$, non-significant) [5]	–
Mixed[i]	Sarna et al. [5, 6] (1993, 1997)	2613	LE for endurance (5.7; $M = 75.6$, CI 73.6–77.5), team (4.0; $M = 73.9$, CI 72.7–75.1), and in power (1.6; $M = 71.5$, CI 70.4–72.2) sport athletes was greater than the referents (69.9); decreased CVD in endurance (OR = 0.49, CI 0.26–0.93) and team (OR = 0.61, CI 0.41–0.92) sport athletes (active 1920–1965)	↑
Mixed	Zwiers et al. [31] (2012)	9889	High-intensity sport athletes had lower longevity compared to low-intensity sport athletes (high risk of bodily collision, HR = 1.11, CI 1.06–1.15, and high levels of physical contact, HR = 1.16, CI 1.11–1.22 (Olympians 1896–1936; sex breakdown unknown)	–

Studies with no subscript analyzed multiple countries, or other sports were used as controls. Full citations provided in reference list; all LE and MR data were compared to age-matched controls from the GP and all studies were on male participants, unless stated otherwise; descriptions reflect only the key findings
AD Alzheimer's disease, *ALS* amyotrophic lateral sclerosis, *BMI* body mass index, *CI* confidence interval, *CVD* cardiovascular disease, *GP* general population, *HOF* hall of fame, *HR* hazard rate/ratio of death, *LE* life expectancy, *M* mean, *MLB* Major League Baseball, *MR* mortality rate, *NBA* National Basketball Association, *NFL* National Football League; *OR* odds ratio for mortality, *PL* powerlifting, R^2 explained variation/total variation (coefficient of determination), *RCS* relative conditional survival, *RSR* relative survival ratio, *SD* standard deviation, *SMR* standardized mortality ratio, *SPMR* standardized proportionate mortality ratio, *SW* sumo wrestling, *T and F* track and field
[a]USA
[b]Reviews met inclusion criteria
[c]United Kingdom
[d]France
[e]Italy
[f]Belgium
[g]Norway
[h]Sweden
[i]Finland
[j]New Zealand
[k]Netherlands
[l]Germany
[m]Japan
[n]Poland

in elite athletes that may be disseminated to a different cohort of the population (e.g., social media users; see Table 2). Specifically, these three additional articles were located through Google Scholar's search engine using the same keywords as used in the Web of Science database search (e.g., athletes, death, etc.). We assessed the quality of each of these records through the Newcastle-Ottawa Quality Assessment Scale for cohort studies [34]. See Fig. 1 for the PRISMA statement [33].

Measured Outcomes

This review was comprised of elite athlete mortality/longevity studies from 13 different countries: USA, France, Italy, Belgium, Norway, Sweden, Finland, New Zealand, Netherlands, Germany, Japan, Poland, and the UK. Measures of mortality included hazard rate/ratio of death (HR), life expectancy (LE), mortality rate (MR), odds ratio for mortality (OR), relative conditional survival (RCS), relative survival ratio (RSR), standardized mortality ratio (SMR), and standardized proportionate mortality ratio (SPMR). All LE and MR data were compared to age-matched controls from the general population and all studies were on male participants, unless stated otherwise in the tables.

Results

Literature Search

From 1 January 1980 to 30 September 2014, we located 54 peer-reviewed studies [3–6, 8–15, 17–31, 35–61] and three online articles [62–64] that examined mortality and longevity in elite athletes ($n = 57$). This is an addition of 43 peer-reviewed studies that were not included in Teramoto and Bungum's [16] review (11 peer-reviewed studies overlap). Three peer-reviewed studies from their review did not match our inclusion criteria (<1980).

Summary of Life Expectancy in Elite Athletes from Literature

This review included a total of 465,575 athletes: 450,295 from peer-reviewed literature (Table 1) and 15,280 from online articles (Table 2). Of those 465,575 examined, only 5610 (1.2 %) were female athletes. Although it appears that females have been grossly underrepresented in mortality and longevity studies of elite athletes, the extremely low proportion of 1.2 % is skewed by separate studies examining the same cohort of players [e.g., 12 and 19, $n = 3439$; 3–6, active Finnish athletes from 1920 to 1965), single studies that contained very large sample sizes of

Table 2 Online elite athlete mortality articles ($n = 3$)

Sport/Country	Authors	N	Key finding	LE vs. GP
NFL[a]	Baron and Rinsky [62] (*NIOSH*) (1994)	6848	NFL players had a 46 % decreased MR (SMR = 0.54); linemen had a 52 % greater risk of death from heart disease than the GP, and three times the risk compared to football players; players had a decreased risk of death from violence (79 %) and accidents (39 %); (players since 1959; death through 1991)	↑
NFL[a]	Hargrove [63] (*Scripps Howard News Service*) (2006)	3850	The heaviest NFL players were more than twice as likely to die before their 50th birthday than their teammates; players are generally not dying sooner than average, but offensive and defensive linemen had a 52 % greater risk of dying from heart disease than the GP; out of the 130 players who died before age 50, 1/69 players born since 1955 are dead, 22 % of which died of heart diseases (77 % qualified as obese) and 19 % from homicides or suicides; when compared to *2403 MLB* players who have died in the last century, NFL players are more than twice as likely to die before age 50 (born since 1905)	–
Mixed[a]	Barnwell [64] (*Grantland*) (2012)	4582	12.8 % of football players had died ($n = 3088$) compared to 15.9 % of baseball players ($n = 1494$) as of 2007 (active from 1959–1988)	–

AD Alzheimer's disease, *ALS* amyotrophic lateral sclerosis, *BMI* body mass index, *CI* confidence interval, *CVD* cardiovascular disease, *GP* general population, *HOF* hall of fame, *HR* hazard rate/ratio of death, *LE* life expectancy, *M* mean, *MLB* Major League Baseball, *MR* mortality rate, *NBA* National Basketball Association, *NFL* National Football League; *OR* odds ratio for mortality, *PL* powerlifting, R^2 explained variation/total variation (coefficient of determination), *RCS* relative conditional survival, *RSR* relative survival ratio, *SD* standard deviation, *SMR* standardized mortality ratio, *SPMR* standardized proportionate mortality ratio, *SW* sumo wrestling, *T and F* track and field

[a]USA

male athletes [e.g., 11; $n = 300{,}818$), and instances where the breakdown of sex in the sample went unreported (e.g., [31]). Nevertheless, only 6 peer-reviewed studies on elite athlete mortality and longevity that included females in their samples were identified [9, 20, 24, 31, 58, 60] and no studies that investigated females exclusively.

From the 9-point Newcastle-Ottawa Quality Assessment Scale [34], 1 study had a quality score of 6, 6 studies had a quality score of 7, 32 studies had a quality score of 8, and 15 studies had a quality score of 9 (only peer-reviewed articles were assessed). Therefore, the majority of the studies included in this review were generally of high

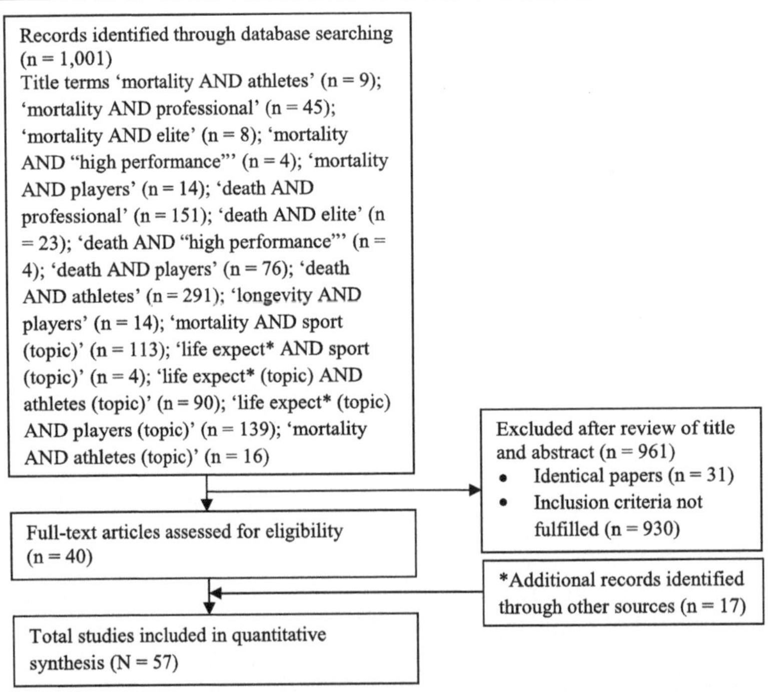

Fig. 1 Flow of information through the different phases of the systematic review, as per the PRISMA statement [33]. *Additional records were identified through searching the references of records that were identified through database searching and a general web search (i.e., Google Scholar)

quality (e.g., representative sample sizes, age- and sex-matched control groups from the general population, etc.).

Of the 54 peer-reviewed studies included, 4 were responses to the authors of different studies related to mortality and longevity of elite athletes [29, 30, 42, 44]. Aside from the studies or reviews that examined multiple sports, professional baseball players ($n = 16$), football players (4 peer-reviewed, 2 online), soccer players ($n = 4$), basketball players ($n = 3$), and cyclists ($n = 3$) were identified through our literature search as having the most reported data on elite athletes' mortality outcomes. In particular, MLB players [15, 36, 38, 45–47], NFL players [12, 19, 49, 62], cyclists [13, 27, 28], NBA players [10, 48], and golfers [11, 21] had the most robust evidence of greater longevity. These LE benefits generally ranged from 4 to 8 years [e.g., 36 and 28, respectively].

The majority of studies included in this review examined sport organizations that were primarily located in the USA and used age- and sex-matched controls that were also American (MLB, NBA, and NFL). The general finding of these studies was a greater longevity for elite athletes relative to their American controls. Notably, the majority of mixed-sport studies included in this review also found support for greater longevity for athletes who competed at elite levels of competition (e.g., Olympics). Similarly, the "one-off" studies from international researchers whose controls spanned 12 different countries also reflect a general trend towards increased survival rates for a diverse group of athletes relative to their country-specific controls from the general population. For example, elite cyclists, such as French, Italian, and Belgian Tour de France participants, had greater lifespan longevities when compared to the pooled general population from their respective countries for the appropriate age cohorts [13, 27, 28]. Further, Norwegian divers [8] and skiers [22] and Italian track and field athletes [58] had greater lifespan longevities relative to controls from their respective countries as well. Alternatively, less consistent results were found in soccer players, in which both superior survival rates in Dutch players [23] and inferior survival rates in German players [24] were reported, alongside increases in amyotrophic lateral sclerosis (ALS) prevalence in Italian players [55, 56]. In addition, elite Finnish powerlifters [53] displayed lower lifespan longevities compared to the Finnish general population.

Mechanisms of Mortality and Primary Outcomes

Considerable research attention has been given to identifying which mechanisms may be precursors to early mortality, including handedness, precocity, names and initials of players/athletes, playing position and weight, education and race, achievement, and energy system classifications. First, the relationship between handedness and mortality in elite athletes has received increased attention within the last two decades. Nevertheless, differences in longevity related to handedness appear to be non-existent in MLB [35, 42, 44] and NBA players [25]. While a relationship between longevity and handedness was identified in elite cricketers [51], the inclusion of a larger sample size appears to have washed out previous significant findings [52]. Second, the precocity-longevity hypothesis (see [65]), which investigates the relationship between precociousness (i.e., career debut) and early death, has been shown to affect MLB players' longevities [39]. Third, MLB players with positive initials in their names (e.g., A.C.E.) were found to live significantly longer than players with negative initials (e.g., D.E.D.) [40] while baseball, hockey, football and basketball players with names beginning with D had shorter lifespans than those with names beginning with E to Z [17]. It is noteworthy that there has been some criticism regarding the methodologies used in these studies, such as using selective data and the appropriateness of the statistical tests performed [29, 30]. Further, while it has been suggested that health is influenced by certain symbolic aspects of the environment [66], such as a decreased prevalence of death before birthdays (e.g., [67]), the scientific rationale behind the initials of a name affecting lifespan longevity is limited. In turn, the emergence of a hypothetical name-longevity relationship in elite athletes emphasizes the need for greater replication in this area of research.

An athlete's playing position is arguably the most obvious mechanism that influences mortality risk, largely due to perceived anthropometric differences that are determinants of health (e.g., weight). Longevity was found to be correlated with position in MLB [47] and NBA players [48]. In particular, *weight* and position significantly influenced mortality risk in NFL players [19, 49, 50, 61–63, 68]. Further, weight also influenced the lifespan longevities of baseball players [61, 69] and played a role in the longevities of Japanese sumo wrestlers, although its influence appeared to be small [OR = 1.08, CI 1.01–1.15; 57]. With regard to athlete race, this has been shown to be associated with longevity in NBA [10] and NFL players [19], as well as with education and longevity in MLB players [45]. Sixth, high achievement in sport emerged as a determinant of mortality, specifically through winning percentage in Japanese sumo wrestlers [57], handicap in Swedish golfers [11], and Hall of Fame (HOF) induction in a diverse range of sports [37, 59]. Although Abel and Kruger [37] reported differences in the life expectancies of MLB HOFs compared to non-inductees, Smith [30] did not find a statistically significant difference using corrected data from the same sample.

The last trend that developed from these studies, which served as a classification method for Teramoto and Bungum's [16] review, was the relationship between the type of sport and required energy systems for participation (i.e., aerobic/endurance, mixed, and anaerobic/power) and mortality. Similar to Teramoto and Bungum's [16] findings, the largest gains in lifespan longevities were in endurance and mixed-sport athletes. The greatest LE advantages were found in European cyclists [13, 27, 28], whereas the lowest LEs were found in Finnish powerlifters [53]. Cross-sport analyses uniformly reported LE advantages in endurance and mixed-sport athletes compared to power sport athletes [3–6, 20, 31], who had some evidence of increased premature mortality from suicide suspected from prior anabolic steroid use [26, 53]. The inconsistent mortality outcomes in power sport athletes make it difficult to generalize across all sports. Nevertheless, there was considerable support in the existing literature for superior longevity outcomes for elite athletes compared to the age- and sex-matched controls from the general population.

Discussion

The objective of our review was to advance knowledge on elite athlete mortality and longevity to ultimately determine whether elite-level participation in high-performance sport produces a lifespan longevity advantage. As a whole, the empirical evidence suggests that several mechanisms within and between sports have powerful effects on the overall lifespan longevities of players. Our first research question considered whether elite athletes had superior longevity outcomes relative to the general population. An overwhelming majority of studies included in this review reported favorable lifespan longevities for athletes compared to their age- and sex-matched controls from the general population. In fact, only two studies reported lower lifespan longevities in athletes relative to the controls: 812 male and female soccer players who participated in international matches for Germany between 1908 and 2006 ($RSR \leq 1$) [24], and 62 male Finnish powerlifters who placed first–fifth in their respective weight category in the Finnish championships between 1977 and 1982 ($SMR = 4.6$) [53]. Our second research question explored the mechanisms and risk factors associated with longevity and whether there were precursors to early mortality. Although our overall understanding of modifiable and non-modifiable factors that contribute to mortality risk in elite athletes remains limited, in part due to methodological and data source inconsistencies [29, 30], some trends emerged from our investigation. In particular, our review supports previous conclusions that aerobic and mixed-sport athletes have superior longevity outcomes relative to more anaerobic sport athletes. In addition, playing position and weight, as well as education and race, appeared to be consistent indicators of mortality risk, whereas other mechanisms such as handedness, precocity, and names and initials appeared to be less consistent and/or examined.

In their review of the relationship between body size and lifespan longevity, Samaras et al. [61] drew attention to several confounders that may positively influence longevity outcomes, such as higher socioeconomic status, smaller body size, and positive environmental and health benefits. As highlighted in this review, weight is an important predictor of mortality risk. Likewise, significant empirical evidence suggests that obesity is one of the major risk factors for premature death (e.g., [70]). While it is premature to undervalue the relationship between weight and mortality in athletes, particularly post-retirement, research has also highlighted the importance of accounting for body composition. For example, it has been suggested that a measure of BMI is likely to overestimate adiposity in muscular athletes (e.g., [71]), particularly in NFL players [19]. In addition, Koning and Amelink [23] highlighted that self-selecting to participate in an occupation where health is important may predispose athletes to favorable survival outcomes relative to population comparisons. Factors such as these, in addition to a bevy of other confounders such as access to high-quality medical care [23], are what make LE a difficult outcome to accurately predict.

As a variety of confounders may impact longevity, the reasons for the differences in lifespans between elite athletes and the general population are likely to be multifactorial. Teramoto and Bungum [16] provided possible explanations of increased survival in the elite athlete cohort; namely, participation in higher volumes of exercise training leading to higher physical fitness levels, the likelihood that elite athletes are comprised of the healthiest and fittest individuals, and the maintenance of active and healthy lifestyles later in life. The extents to which these confounders contribute to mortality risk are still largely unknown however, as survival statistics may undermine the interplay of complex socioeconomic factors [72]. For example, medical care accessibility made available by higher income may improve the LE of athletes when compared to other groups. Further, plenty of corroborating evidence suggests health-care services alone do not result in improved health outcomes, but a variety of social factors such as education and employment produce these widespread biases in health (e.g., [73]). As a result, the historical investigations of elite athletes and longevity outcomes need to be cautiously interpreted and discussed in the contexts of a variety of possible influential factors of mortality.

Abel and Kruger [17] discussed two advantages to studying elite athletes with regards to longevity. First, they represent a relatively homogenous occupational population, similar to Teramoto and Bungum's [16] classification of a distinct physically fit and healthy group, and, perhaps more importantly, many sports contain detailed statistical and historical databases that track a variety of variables that can influence longevity (e.g., anthropometrics, performance-based indicators such as induction into the HOF, etc.). These advantages help contribute to the growing body of research on elite athlete mortality trends, which in turn can advance research by forming evidence-based models of athlete longevity through investigations into a variety of variables. In contrast, a caveat to this tendency of measuring the effects of sport-specific variables on mortality is that the amount of data available varies from sport to sport and may be somewhat arbitrary. For example, handedness is unlikely to be measured in soccer players, and the influence of position in non-contact sports may be more relevant in life quality research rather than life longevity. In addition, each sport will have a different inaugural season, which limits the amount of deceased players in the relatively newer sports (e.g., mixed martial arts). Therefore, each sport will have unique statistical variables that may make it more difficult for researchers to draw cross-sport comparisons.

Limitations

The main finding of this systematic review indicates favorable lifespan longevity advantages for elite athletes relative to age- and sex-matched controls from the general population; however, limitations in reviewing literature on mortality and longevity in elite athletes exist. We will first examine the possible biases in epidemiological research in historical samples of athletes.

Databases

The use of accurate and up-to-date databases is extremely important when analyzing a sample longitudinally; however, some statistical databases for past players have been found to be incomplete. For example, Smith [30] discovered a substantial portion of missing death date data (e.g., unknown death dates) in former MLB players in the Sean Lahman Baseball Archive [74]. Unfortunately, Smith's [30] critique of Abel and Kruger's [37] conclusion (cases without death date data were treated as living players) that HOF non-inductees had a 5-year lifespan longevity advantage was not the only study on MLB player longevity that used the same database (e.g., [17, 35, 36, 38–40, 45]). Although it may be premature to conclude that other databases have similar fallibility (e.g., missing death date data), we must be cautious of the possible incongruency between reported and unreported/unknown death date data in other studies that bias lifespan longevity results.

Holistic Health

As a variety of socioeconomic, demographic, and epidemiologic factors dynamically interact to shape population change [72], so do factors that influence holistic health. Arguably, the most objective measurement of elite athlete health is rate of mortality. Using mortality statistics of elite athletes who played in the earlier decades to make inferences regarding holistic health in present-day athletes may be deceptive. The information age has made information on elite athletes easy to access, whereas information on elite athletes from the earlier eras often fails to depict the mental and social wellbeing characteristics that encompass holistic health. Sorenson et al.'s [75] investigation of lifespan exercise among elite intercollegiate athletes is one of few studies that have presented empirical evidence of lifetime health and wellbeing in modern competitive athletes relative to age- and sex-matched controls. They found that current student athletes reported higher volumes of weekly exercise, perceived exercise importance, and likelihood of compliance with American College of Sports Medicine (ACSM) exercise guidelines relative to non-athletes [75]. Interestingly, Sorenson et al. [75] found no significant differences between alumni student athletes and non-athletes, suggesting that former athletes failed to maintain higher exercise levels later in life. Further, in their follow-up study on the same sample, Sorenson et al. [76] found that relatively older former student athletes (age 43+ years) had a greater risk for joint health concerns later in life compared to a non-athlete control group. These findings seem counterintuitive since physical activity is often associated with a substantial reduction of chronic disease risk and being important to overall health and wellbeing (e.g., [77]).

To broaden our knowledge on holistic health outcomes and behavior in former athletes, it is important to consider the totality of data that have been collected and analyzed to date, particularly as research pertaining to the "whole person" (e.g., physical and psychosocial measures) in modern competitive athletes gains momentum. It is equally important to make the distinction between "quality of life" and "longevity," as physical health likely moderates psychosocial health. For example, evidence suggests that physical activity plays an important role in managing mental health diseases, such as anxiety and depression (e.g., [78]). Thus, factors such as being physically capable to participate in physical activity are important to consider when determining an individual's quality of life. As such, our current understanding of elite athletes' quality of life during and after sport is limited relative to their lifespan longevity trends.

Statistical Measures

Another criticism of the athlete-mortality literature is on methodological grounds; more specifically, cross-study discrepancies in the statistical tests and/or measures used. Although the relative paucity of lifespan longevity studies of elite athletes may serve as a temporary explanation for why different measures and control variables are used to analyze mortality, we cannot ignore the impact of possible statistical bias risk. Risk of bias can affect the cumulative evidence of a review of literature [33], such as selective reporting within studies, whereby researchers may under-report variables that were found to have less statistical impact on longevity outcomes in the course of reporting results that support the direction of their findings. As a result, the extent of our knowledge about the influence of certain variables on longevity may be restricted. Future work in this area of research would benefit from replication of control variables when analyzing the same or similar athletic populations to better establish important predictors of longevity. Further, meta-analyses on the longevity of elite athletes, such as the review completed by Garatachea and colleagues [7], can provide more evidence-based data on the benefits of participating in physical activity. Moreover, it is notable that the sports examined have examined periods of different length. Ideally, comparisons would be best when comparing timespans of similar length; however, the timespans investigated have ranged from players being born from as early as 1840 [52] to being active as recently as 2012 [27]. These differences could affect the proportion of those living or dead in a sample, which may affect measures such as SMR. The implication of these biases on the cumulative evidence of this review is unclear, and as a result, it is important to consider how publication bias can under- and overestimate certain predictors of longevity.

Longitudinal Lifestyle Factors

Given that empirical evidence is necessary for coherent explanations of longevity outcomes of elite athletes, do mechanisms that influence mortality become ineffective and/or less powerful if maintenance of physical activity ceases? Although there has been some evidence that former intercollegiate student athletes fail to maintain higher exercise levels later in life [75], our understanding of the impact of different longitudinal lifestyle factors influencing lifespan longevity remains incomplete. For example, former male Finnish world class athletes were found to be more active than their non-competitive controls [79], and participation in physical activity at a young age predicted later life involvement, which reduced the prevalence of coronary heart disease [80]. In addition, former athletes have been found to partake in fewer negative health habits, such as smoking and drinking alcohol [79].

Another issue that is emerging from more recent research relates to the possible detrimental effects of high levels of training. In particular, O'Keefe (e.g., [81, 82]) has advocated that "excessive" aerobic training can result in cardiovascular damage (e.g., atrial fibrillation, coronary artery disease, and malignant ventricular arrhythmias). These effects may have particular relevance for studies of mortality in previously elite athletes. It is important for future research to determine which factors are more robust predictors of longevity and if they continue to be relevant in later life. In turn, these findings will have implications on the generalizability of factors found to predict mortality and longevity in elite athletes that were measured at one point in time (i.e., active athletic career).

Future Directions

The relationship between sport and health has evolved considerably over the past 100 years. The context in which the historical data are transferable is important to consider, particularly when discussing the social determinants of health [73]. Despite its limitations, historical analyses of sport and health shape our present understanding of its relationship and influence.

Reliable Databases, Repetition, Causes of Mortality, and Follow-up Studies

Continued contributions to the growing body of research on longevity outcomes of elite athletes should utilize appropriate statistical testing with reliable and complete databases. Although there are a variety ways to statistically measure and report mortality, research must be substantiated through repetition. An important first step is locating or comprising a reliable and comprehensive database that embodies all accessible and applicable data. To this end, future research of athlete lifespan outcomes can arguably have the greatest impact by determining the *causes* of mortality. Current empirical evidence on the rates of mortality in athletes is far superior to our knowledge on the causes of mortality. Epidemiological studies with long-term follow-ups are also rare [55]. For example, available evidence suggests a possible connection between dietary supplements and/or drug use and the high prevalence of amyotrophic lateral sclerosis (ALS) in former soccer players [55, 56]. This potential association emphasizes negative long-term neurological outcomes of performance demands that are not reflected in MR occurrence.

Cross-sport Comparisons and Generalizability

Several sports were noticeably absent from the elite athlete mortality literature (e.g., ice hockey, field hockey, handball, snowboarding, table tennis, volleyball, and motorsports). In addition, sex-related differences in lifespan longevity remain largely unknown due to the paucity of studies on elite female athletes. This raises an important concern about the cross-sport generalizability disseminated in this review. Perhaps more importantly, the applicability of these results to the general population (i.e., non-elite-athletes) can likely be best explained by mechanisms of mortality that have not been extensively examined to date in the athlete cohort. Some examples include smoking and diet/nutrition (as stated by Teramoto and Bungum) [16], lifespan health (psychosocial and physical, such as the influence of morbidity on life quality, etc.), and the interplay of nature (hereditary, such as superior genotypes for physical fitness) (e.g., [83]) and nurture (environmental influences). Presumably, elite athletes possess advantageous genetic traits. Research on the heritability of physical fitness (e.g., [84]) suggests that we cannot discount the influence of advantageous genetic inheritance coupled with high levels of participation and competition in sport.

Conclusions

Mechanisms such as type of sport, playing position, weight, education, and race can inform our understanding of lifespan longevity, which places increased responsibility on future research to demystify and contextualize mortality risk in both eminent and non-eminent populations. In conclusion, while additional research studies are needed to address quality of life and wellness outcomes, this review highlights mortality trends among elite athletes and concludes that participation in elite sport is generally favorable to lifespan longevity.

Ethical Standards

This manuscript does not contain clinical studies or patient data.

Competing Interests

Both authors declare that they have no competing interests.

Authors' contribution

SL and JB designed the study, developed the methodology, interpreted the data, and drafted the manuscript. SL collected the data. All authors read and approved the final manuscript.

Acknowledgements

This project was not funded.

References

1. Holt NL. Positive youth development through sport. UK: Routledge; 2008.
2. Baker J, Horton S. A review of primary and secondary influences on sport expertise. High Abil Stud. 2004;15:211–28.
3. Kettunen JA, Kujala UM, Kaprio J, Bäckmand H, Peltonen M, Eriksson JG, et al. All-cause and disease-specific mortality among male, former elite athletes: an average 50-year follow-up. Br J Sports Med. Published Online First: [2 Sept 2014]. doi:10.1136/bjsports-2013-093347
4. Kujala UM, Tikkanen HO, Sarna S, Pukkala E, Kaprio J, Koskenvuo M. Disease-specific mortality among elite athletes. The J of the Am Med Assoc. 2001;285:43–4.
5. Sarna S, Sahi T, Koskenvuo M, Kaprio J. Increased life expectancy of world class male athletes. Med and Sci in Sports and Exerc. 1993;2:237–44.
6. Sarna S, Kaprio J, Kujala UM, Koskenvuo M. Health status of former elite athletes. The Finnish experience. Aging Clin Exp Res. 1997;9:35–41.
7. Garatachea N, Santos-Lozano A, Sanchis-Gomar F, Fiuza-Luces C, Pareja-Galeano H, Emanuele E, et al. Elite athletes live longer than the general population: A meta-analysis. Mayo Clin Proc. 2014 Sep;89:1195–200. doi:10.1016/h.mayocp.2014.06.004. Epub 2014 Aug 12.
8. Irgens Å, Troland K, Thorsen E, Grønning M. Mortality among professional divers in Norway. Occup Med. 2013;63:537–43.
9. Coate D, Sun R. Survival estimates for elite male and female Olympic athletes and tennis championship competitors. Scand J of Med and Sci in Sports. 2013;23:722–7.
10. Lawler TP, Lawler FH, Gibson J, Murray R. Does the African-American-white mortality gap persist after playing professional basketball? A 59-year historical cohort study. Ann of Epidemiol. 2012;22:406–12.
11. Farahmand B, Broman G, de Faire U, Vågerö D, Ahlbom A. Golf: a game of life and death—reduced mortality in Swedish golf players. Scand J of Med and Sci in Sports. 2009;19:419–24.
12. Lehman EJ, Hein MJ, Baron SL, Gersic CM. Neurodegenerative causes of death among retired National Football League players. Neurol. 2012;79:1970–4.
13. Morcet J, Perrin M, Trégaro M, Carré F, Deugnier Y. Mortality in a cohort of 514 elite road cyclists. Sci and Sports. 2012;27:9–15.
14. Poznańska A, Gajewski AK. Mortality of male members of the Polish Olympic teams in 1981–1998. Przeglad Epidemiologiczny. 2001;55:305–12.
15. Reynolds R, Day S. Life expectancy and comparative mortality of Major League Baseball players, 1900–1999. Webmed Central Sports Medicine. 2012;3(5):WMC003380. doi:10.9754/journal.wmc.2012.003380.
16. Teramoto M, Bungum TJ. Mortality and longevity of elite athletes. J of Sci and Med in Sport. 2010;13:410–6.
17. Abel EL, Kruger ML. Athletes, doctors, and lawyers with first names beginning with "D" die sooner. Death Stud. 2010;34:71–81.
18. Baird LC, Newman CB, Volk H, Svinth JR, Conklin J, Levy ML. Mortality resulting from head injury in professional boxing. Neurosurg. 2010;67:1444–50.
19. Baron SL, Hein MJ, Lehman E, Gersic CM. Body mass index, playing position, race, and the cardiovascular mortality of retired professional football players. The Am J of Cardiol. 2012;109:889–96.
20. Clarke PM, Walter SJ, Hayen A, Mallon WJ, Heijmans J, Studdert DM. Survival of the fittest: retrospective cohort study of the longevity of Olympic medallists in the modern era. Br Med J. 2012. doi:10.1136/bmj.e8308.
21. Coate D, Schwenkenberg J. Survival function estimates for champions tour golfers. J of Sports Econ. 2012;14:656–63.
22. Grimsmo J, Maehlum S, Moelstad P, Arnesen H. Mortality and cardiovascular morbidity among long-term endurance male cross country skiers followed for 28–30 years. Scand J of Med and Sci in Sports. 2011;21:351–8. doi:10.1055/s-0028-1128150.
23. Koning RH, Amelink R. Medium-term mortality of Dutch professional soccer players. The Econ and Labour Relations Rev. 2012;23:55–68.
24. Kuss O, Kluttig A, Greiser KH. Longevity of soccer players: an investigation of all German internationals from 1908 to 2006. Scand J of Med and Sci in Sports. 2011;21:260–5.
25. Lawler TP, Lawler FH. Left-handedness in professional basketball: prevalence, performance, and survival. Percept and Mot Skills. 2011;113:815–24.
26. Lindqvist AS, Moberg T, Ehrnborg C, et al. Increased mortality rate and suicide in Swedish former elite male athletes in power sports. Scand J of Med and Sci in Sports. 2013. doi:10.1111/sms.12122.
27. Marijon E, Tafflet M, Antero-Jacquemin J, El Helou N, Berthelot G, Celermajer DS, et al. Mortality of French participants in the Tour de France (1947–2012). Eur Heart J. 2013;34:3145–50.
28. Sanchis-Gomar F, Olaso-Gonzalez G, Corella D, Gomez-Cabrera MC, Vina J. Increased average longevity among the "Tour de France" cyclists. Int J of Sports Med. 2011;32:644–7.
29. Smith G. Another look at baseball player initials and longevity. Percept and Mot Skills. 2011;112:211–6.
30. Smith G. The baseball hall of fame is not the kiss of death. Death Stud. 2011;35:949–55.
31. Zwiers R, Zantvoord FWA, Engelaer FM, van Bodegom D, van der Ouderaa FJG, Westendorp RGJ. Mortality in former Olympic athletes: retrospective cohort analysis. Br Med J. 2012;345:19–27.
32. Löllgen H, Böckenhoff A, Knapp G. Int J Sports Med. 2009 Mar;30:213–24. doi:10.1055/s-0028-1128150. Epub 2009 Feb 6.
33. Moher D, Liberati A, Tetzlaff J, Altman DG; PRISMA Group. Preferred reporting items for systematic reviews and meta-analyses: the PRISMA statement. PLoS Med. 2009;e1000097. doi:10.1371/journal.pmed1000097
34. Wells GA, Shea B, O'Connell D, Peterson J, Welch V, Losos M, et al. Newcastle-Ottawa Scale for assessing the quality of non-randomized studies in meta-analysis. Ottawa Hospital Research Institute website. http://www.ohri.ca/programs/clinical_epidemiology/oxford.asp. Accessed March 14, 2015.
35. Abel EL, Kruger ML. Left-handed major-league baseball players and longevity re-examined. Percept and Mot Skills. 2004;99:990–2.
36. Abel EL, Kruger ML. Longevity of Major League Baseball players. Res in Sports Med. 2005;13:1–5.

37. Abel EL, Kruger ML. The longevity of baseball hall of famers compared to other players. Death Stud. 2005;29:959–63.
38. Abel EL, Kruger ML. The healthy worker effect in Major League Baseball revisited. Res in Sports Med. 2006;14:83–7.
39. Abel EL, Kruger ML. Precocity predicts shorter life for major league baseball players: confirmation of McCann's precocity-longevity hypothesis. Death Stud. 2007;31:933–40.
40. Abel EL, Kruger ML. Symbolic significance of initials on longevity. Percept and Mot Skills. 2007;104:179–82.
41. Boren S, Erickson TB. Toxicological deaths of Major League Baseball players. J of Toxicol: Clin Toxicol. 1998;36:737–42.
42. Fudin R, Renninger L, Lembessis E, Hirshon J. Sinistrality and reduced longevity: Reichler's 1979 data on baseball players do not indicate a relationship. Percept Mot Skills. 1993;76:171–82.
43. Halpern DF, Coren S. Do right-handers live longer? Nature. 1988;333:213.
44. Hicks RA, Johnson C, Cuevas T, Deharo D, Bautista J. Do right handers live longer? An updated assessment of baseball player data. Percept and Mot Skills. 1994;78:1243–7.
45. Kalist DE, Peng Y. Does education matter? Major League Baseball players and longevity. Death Stud. 2007;31:653–70.
46. Saint Onge JM, Rogers RG, Krueger PM. Major League Baseball players' life expectancies. Soc Sci Q. 2008;89:817–30.
47. Waterbor J, Cloe P, Delzell E, Andjelkovich D. The mortality experience of Major League Baseball players. New Engl J of Med. 1988;318:1278–80.
48. Fafian Jr J. Mortality experience of National Basketball Association players. North Am Actuar J. 1997;1:45–8.
49. Abel EL, Kruger ML. The healthy worker effect in professional football. Res in Sports Med: An Int J. 2006;14:239–43.
50. Selden MA, Helzberg JH, Waeckerle JF. Early cardiovascular mortality in professional football players: fact or fiction? The Am J of Med. 2009;122:811–4.
51. Aggleton JP, Kentridge RW, Neave NJ. Evidence for longevity differences between left handed and right handed men: an archival study of cricketers. J Epidemiol Community Health. 1993;47:206–9.
52. Aggleton JP, Bland JM, Kentridge RW, Neave NJ. Handedness and longevity: archival study of cricketers. Br Med J. 1994;309:24–31.
53. Pärssinen M, Kujala U, Vartiainen E, Sarna S, Seppälä T. Increased premature mortality of competitive powerlifters suspected to have used anabolic agents. Int J of Sports Med. 2000;21:225–7.
54. Beaglehole R, Stewart A. The longevity of international rugby players. The NZ Med J. 1983;96:513–5.
55. Belli S, Vanacore N. Proportionate mortality of Italian soccer players: is amyotrophic lateral sclerosis an occupational disease? Euro J of Epidemiol. 2005;20:237–42.
56. Taioli E. All causes of mortality in male professional soccer players. Euro J of Public Heal. 2007;17:600–4.
57. Kanda H, Hayakawa T, Tsuboi S, Mori Y, Takahashi T, Fukushima T. Higher body mass index is a predictor of death among professional sumo wrestlers. J of Sports Sci and Med. 2009;8:711–2.
58. Menotti A, Amici E, Gambelli GC, Milazzotto F, Bellotti P, Capocaccia R, et al. Life expectancy in Italian track and field athletes. Euro J of Epidemiol. 1990;6:257–60.
59. Bianco M, Fabbricatore C, Sanna N, Fabiano C, Palmieri V, Zeppilli P. Elite athletes: is survival shortened in boxers? Int J of Sports Med. 2007;28:697–702.
60. Gajewski AK, Poznańska A. Mortality of top athletes, actors and clergy in Poland: 1924–2000 follow-up study of the longer term effect of physical activity. Euro J of Epidemiol. 2008;23:335–40.
61. Samaras TT, Storms LH, Elrick H. Longevity, mortality and body weight. Ageing Res Rev. 2002;1:673–91.
62. Baron S, Rinsky R. Health hazard evaluation report, National Football League players mortality study. Report No. HETA 88–085. Atlanta, GA: Centers for Disease Control and Prevention, National Institute for Occupational Safety and Health, 1994. http://www.cdc.gov/niosh/pdfs/nflfactsheet.pdf. Accessed 15 Sept 2014.
63. Hargrove T. Supersized in the NFL: many ex-players dying young. Scripps Howard News Service Online. 31 Jan 2006. http://sports.espn.go.com/nfl/news/story?id=2313476. Accessed 15 Sept 2014.
64. Barnwell B. Mere mortals: what we learned by comparing the mortality rates of baseball players and their NFL counterparts. Grantland. 17 Aug 2012.
65. McCann SJH. The precocity-longevity hypothesis: earlier peaks in career achievement predict shorter lives. Per Soc Psych Bull. 2001;27:1429–39.
66. Christenfeld N, Phillips DP, Glynn LM. What's in a name: mortality and the power of symbols. J of Psychosom Res. 1999;47:241–54.
67. Phillips DP, Van Voorhees CA, Ruth TE. The birthday: lifeline or deadline? Psychosom Med. 1992;54:532–42.
68. Maher T, Gill B. Pro Football Encyclopedia. Macmillan, New York; 1997. http://grantland.com/features/comparing-mortality-rates-football-baseball/. Accessed 12 Sept 2014.
69. Samaras TT, Storms LH. Impact of height and weight on life span. Bull of the World Health Organ. 1992;70:259–67.
70. Bahrami H, Bluemke DA, Kronmal R, Bertoni AG, Lloyd-Jones DM, Shahar E, et al. Novel metabolic risk factors for incident heart failure and their relationship with obesity: the MESA (Multi-Ethnic Study of Atherosclerosis) study. J Am Coll Cardiol. 2008;51:1775–83.
71. Okorodudu DO, Jumean MF, Montori VM, Romero-Corral A, Somers VK, Erwin PJ, et al. Diagnostic performance of body mass index to identify obesity as defined by body adiposity: a systematic review and meta- analysis. Int J Obes (Lond). 2010;34:791–9.
72. Omran AR. The epidemiologic transition: a theory of the epidemiology of population change. The Milbank Quart. 2005;83:731–57.
73. Kelly MP, Morgan A, Bonnefoy J, Butt J, Bergman V. The social determinants of health: developing an evidence base for political action. Final Report to World Health Organization Commission on the Social Determinants of Health. National Institute for Health and Clinical Excellence. 2007;1–165.
74. Sean Lahman's Baseball Archive. 2010. http://www.baseball1.com.
75. Sorenson SC, Romano R, Azen SP, Schroeder T, Salem GJ. Life span exercise among elite intercollegiate student athletes. Sports Helath. 2014. doi:10.1177/1941738114534813.
76. Sorenson SC, Romano R, Scholefield RM, Martin BE, Gordon JE, Azen SP, et al. Holistic life-span health outcomes among elite intercollegiate student-athletes. J of Athl Train. 2014. doi:http://dx.doi.org/10.4085/1062-6050-49.3.18
77. Miles L. Physical activity and health. Nutr Bull. 2007;32:314–63.
78. Paluska SA, Schwenk TL. Physical activity and mental health. Sports Med. 2000;29:167–80.
79. Fogelholm M, Kaprio J, Sarna S. Healthy lifestyles of former Finnish world class athletes. Med Sci Sports Exerc. 1994;26:224–9.
80. Kujala UM, Sarna S, Kaprio J, Tikkanen HO, Koskenvuo M. Natural selection to sports, later physical activity habits, and coronary heart disease. Br J Sports Med. 2000;34:445–9.
81. Lavie CJ, O'Keefe JH, Sallis RE. Exercise and the heart—the harm of too little and too much. Curr Sports Med Rep. 2015;14:104–9.
82. O'Keefe JH, Patil HR, Lavie CJ, Magalski A, Vogel RA, McCullough PA. Potential adverse cardiovascular effects from excessive endurance exercise. Mayo Clin Proc. 2012;87:587–95.
83. Montgomery H, Safari L. Genetic basis of physical fitness. Annu Rev Anthropol. 2007;36:391–405.
84. Garatachea N, Lucia A. Genes, physical fitness and ageing. Ageing Res Rev. 2013;12:90–102.

27

Bra strap orientations and designs to minimise bra strap discomfort and pressure during sport and exercise in women with large breasts

Celeste E Coltman*, Deirdre E McGhee and Julie R Steele

Abstract

Background: Bra straps are a primary source of discomfort during sport and exercise, particularly for women with large breasts. This study aimed to investigate the effects of altering bra strap orientation and design on bra strap comfort, pressure and breast support in women with large breasts. This is a descriptive laboratory study.

Methods: Bra strap discomfort (visual analogue scale, 0 to 10), pressure (custom-designed 10 mm^2 calibrated pressure sensor, 0.5 to 24 kPa range, 50 Hz, S2011, Novel GmbH, Munich, Germany, placed under the right bra strap at the crest of each participant's shoulder), preference ranking and vertical breast displacement (VBD; Optotrak Certus® motion capture system, 200 Hz, Northern Digital, Ontario, Canada) data during dynamic treadmill running and static upright standing (pressure only) were collected for 23 active women with large breasts (D+ cup size) while they wore an encapsulation sports bra with six different bra strap conditions (two bra strap orientations: vertical and cross-back; three bra strap designs: standard width, wide and gel).

Results: Bra strap discomfort was significantly less ($p \leq 0.001$) in the vertical compared to the cross-back strap orientation, which was the most preferred orientation despite no significant difference in strap pressure. The wide strap design had the lowest discomfort scores, significantly lower strap pressure compared to the standard width and gel strap designs ($p < 0.001$), and was equally the most preferred design with the gel straps. There was no significant difference in VBD among the six strap conditions.

Conclusions: Bra straps that are vertically orientated and wide (approximately 4.5 cm in width) are preferable for women with large breasts during sport and exercise to minimise bra strap pressure and discomfort. The addition of gel pads under bra straps may also decrease discomfort and prevent straps slipping off the shoulders, although this notion warrants further investigation.

Key points

- This study provides evidence upon which sports medicine practitioners can offer advice regarding bra strap orientations and designs most suitable to minimise bra strap discomfort and pressure in active women with large breasts.
- Encapsulation sports bras with bra straps that are vertically orientated and wide (approximately 4.5 cm in width) are preferable for women with large breasts to wear during sport and exercise in order to minimise bra strap pressure and discomfort.
- The addition of gel pads under bra straps may also decrease discomfort and potentially prevent straps slipping off the shoulders.

Background

Women with large breasts suffer from musculoskeletal pains secondary to their breasts, including head, neck, back and shoulder pain [1,2,3]. Although bras provide external support to the breasts, they also contribute to these musculoskeletal pains experienced by women with large breasts [4]. One bra component that contributes to these pains is the bra straps. Providing secondary breast support to the band of the bra, straps have been rated as the most disliked features of current bra design [5]. The weight of large breasts, which is exerted through the bra straps onto

* Correspondence: cc721@uowmail.edu.au
Biomechanics Research Laboratory, University of Wollongong, Northfields Avenue, Wollongong, New South Wales 2522, Australia

the superior aspect of the shoulders, often over prolonged durations of bra wear, can create deep furrows and soft tissue damage at the bra strap-shoulder interface [6]. In extreme cases, the prolonged pressure and tissue deformation caused by excessive bra strap loading can lead to neurological symptoms in the upper limbs [6]. Reducing this loading through reduction mammoplasty surgery has been found to be effective in relieving bra strap discomfort and neurological symptoms [7]. Breast reduction surgery, however, is not always feasible due to the high financial and personal costs of surgery and the risks of post-surgery complications in women with a body mass index (BMI) greater than 26 [8-11].

One treatment strategy that has been found to decrease the local discomfort and tissue tenderness at the bra strap-shoulder interface is bra removal [4]. Removing the external breast support provided by a bra, however, is likely to have a negative impact on the posture of women with large breasts [1,12]. Research has shown an increased flexion torque on the thoracic spine among women with large breasts, with this torque thought to contribute to the greater thoracic kyphosis found in women with large breasts compared to women with small breasts [1,12]. It is acknowledged that breast mass is also affected by breast density, which varies widely among women [8,13]. Furthermore, bra removal may also have a negative effect on the physical activity level of women with large breasts because breast discomfort and embarrassment related to excessive breast movement are barriers to women participating in sport and exercise [14-16]. Promoting physical activity in women with large breasts is particularly important as breast mass and BMI are positively correlated [17], and it is imperative that all women, irrespective of breast mass, are able to enjoy the health benefits associated with an active lifestyle. Therefore, improving sports bra design is a more sensible treatment strategy to reduce local discomfort and tissue tenderness at the bra strap-shoulder interface compared to bra removal [4].

Currently, sports bras have several different strap orientations, with some bras being able to convert from one strap orientation to another. The common strap orientations are a vertical orientation, where the straps run vertically over the shoulders, lying on the acromion process and lateral clavicle at the apex of the shoulder, and a cross-back orientation, where the straps cross the back and lie on the upper trapezius muscles at the apex of each shoulder (Figure 1). In terms of design, bra straps also vary in width and the materials the straps are made of. The standard commercially available sports bra strap width at the apex of the shoulder is approximately 2.5 cm (e.g. High Performance Non-Padded Sports Bra, Berlei, Wentworthville, NSW, Australia), although this width can vary. Indeed, the bra strap width of fashion bras can be as narrow as 0.8 cm (Wind Chime Balconette bra, Elle Macpherson Intimates, Sydney, NSW, Australia). Different materials, such as gel pads, are also incorporated into some commercially available sports bra straps (e.g. Triaction Sports bra, Triumph, Bad Zurzach, Switzerland).

Only one previous study has investigated the effect of altering bra strap orientation and design on both bra strap discomfort and pressure [5]. Vertical and cross-back bra strap orientations were compared with and without the addition of a small cushioned pad placed under the strap at the apex of the shoulder. Bra strap discomfort was not significantly different in any condition and bra strap pressure was only reduced with the addition of the cushioned pad in the cross-back orientation, which had higher pressures than in the vertical strap orientation, both with and without the cushioned pad. Although the results of this previous study suggest that bra strap discomfort and pressure cannot be reduced by altering bra strap orientation and design, the study had several limitations. For example, the authors reported that the cushioned pad was not effective in increasing strap width or, in turn, surface area of contact at the shoulder-strap interface as it was found to curl under the strap in the vertical condition [5]. The higher strap pressures in the cross-back orientation may also have been due to tighter straps in this orientation because the bra straps used in the study were commercially available convertible straps, which do not always allow for the greater distance required between the attachment sites of the bra in the cross-back orientation compared to the vertical orientation. It is also conflicting that the cross-back orientation was the most preferred by the 14 participants when it had the same level of discomfort as the vertical orientation and higher strap pressures. The participant number was also low, and the bra sizes, and in turn breast sizes, were at the small end of the spectrum for women with large breast [17-20]. It is also recognised that a range of reasons can affect bra strap preference, such as aesthetics and personal preference, which may have resulted in the cross-back orientation being the preferred orientation in the study cohort.

Due to the limitations listed above, further research is required to determine whether alterations in bra strap orientation and design can decrease bra strap discomfort and pressure in women with large breasts. Such research could provide sports medicine practitioners with evidence regarding which bra strap orientations and designs are most suitable for their female patients with large breasts to wear during sport and exercise to minimise breast movement and discomfort considering age, breast size and level of physical activity [21]. The aim of this study was therefore to investigate the effects of altering bra strap orientation and design on bra strap comfort, pressure and breast support for active women with large breasts. It was hypothesised that both strap orientation and design would affect the pressures exerted at the bra strap-

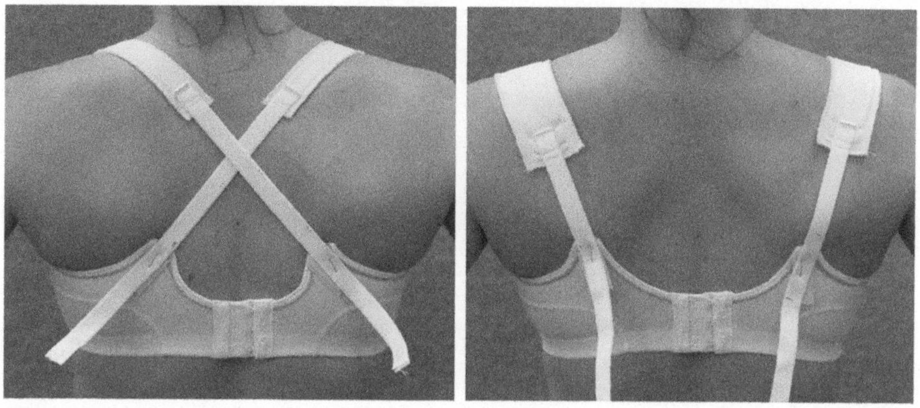

Figure 1 Strap design. The standard width strap design in the cross-back orientation (left) and the wide strap design in the vertical strap orientation (right). All bra straps were constructed using the same industrial grade bra wadding (outer layer: 100% polyester; inner layer: 65% polyprople, 35% polyester), cotton spandex (95% cotton, 5% spandex) and satin power mesh (88% nylon, 12% spandex), as typically used in the straps of commercially available encapsulation bras.

shoulder interface and, in turn, ratings of self-reported bra strap discomfort and preference, without compromising breast support.

Methods

Participants

Twenty-three women (22.3 ± 2.6 years of age, 168.5 ± 5.0 cm height, 66.3 ± 6.5 kg body mass) who were professionally fitted [22] to wear a D+ cup bra size (average cup size DD, range D to E; average band size 10, range 10 to 16) were recruited as representative of women with large breasts. The cohort was deliberately homogenous in age range, mass and physical activity levels (all reported to exercise in a sports bra approximately 5 h per week) [23] to eliminate differences due to these variables and to ensure that sports bras were commonly used by the participants. Exclusion criteria included previous breast surgery, currently experiencing menopause, being pregnant or breastfeeding, or suffering from any musculoskeletal disorder or pain that prevented treadmill running. Based on a power analysis using G*power 3.1.3 and that a difference of ±2 on a visual analogue scale (VAS; rated 0 to 10) measuring discomfort was deemed significant [19], it was estimated that a minimum sample size of 22 participants was required to achieve statistical power of at least 80% (with a significance level of $p < 0.05$). To account for potential participant drop out, 23 participants were recruited for the present study. Participants were not tested if they were experiencing any breast tenderness associated with their menstrual cycle. Each participant completed a short questionnaire about their current sports bra usage and provided written informed consent before participating in the study. The University of Wollongong Human Research Ethics Committee (HE12/118) approved recruitment and testing procedures, and all testing was conducted in accordance with the National Statement on Ethical Conduct in Human Research [24].

Experimental design

A within-subject design was used, where participants ran in a standardised manner and speed (average speed: 9.1 ± 0.3 kph) on a treadmill (PowerJog, GX-100; Expert Fitness UK, Glamorgan, UK) while wearing the same style of encapsulation sports bra (New Legend Underwire sports bra, Berlei, Wentworthville, NSW, Australia), which provided a high level of support and is recommended for women with large breasts to wear during high-impact physical activity [22]. Six randomly [25] allocated bra strap conditions were trialled, including two bra strap orientations (vertical and cross-back) and three different bra strap designs (standard width, wide and gel). All of the straps were made and sewn by the primary investigator [CEC] to ensure a standardised bra strap structure across the three strap designs and a standardised length of the two strap orientations per participant, which were longer in the cross-back orientation compared to the vertical orientation. Professional bra fitting criteria [5,22] were used to ensure the bras fitted the participants correctly and that each strap was the correct length for each participant, in each strap condition (strap length was adjusted once the gel pad was added), as both incorrect bra fit and insufficient strap length could bias both bra strap discomfort and pressure measurements. Following adequate familiarisation, the participants ran in each bra strap condition for 3 min, with data collected while the participants stood motionless (static condition) prior to running and then between the first and third minute of running (dynamic condition). A three-minute duration was chosen as the baseline duration for each condition to minimise participant burden and to facilitate comparison of the strap conditions by limiting the time between them, although it is acknowledged that women commonly exercise and wear sports bras for much longer durations. All the running trials were closely supervised to standardise both the mode of running and the speed, and at least 5 min of rest was allowed between conditions. Participants wore their own running shorts and shoes, which were checked to ensure that they were appropriate for the running task.

Experimental bra strap conditions

The standard width and wide strap designs were made of the same material, consistent with commercially available encapsulation sports bra straps (see Figure 1). The gel strap design consisted of the standard width strap, with the addition of a 2.5-cm-wide gel pad (Dermis Plus Polymer gel; MacMed Health Care, Mudgeeraba, Queensland, Australia) placed under the bra strap (see Figure 2). Each strap was secured to the test bra in the same manner, anteriorly with bikini hooks (15 mm × 2 mm white plastic hooks; Birch Haberdashery & Craft, Heidelberg, Victoria, Australia) and posteriorly with hook and loop tape (Birch Haberdashery & Craft, Heidelberg, Victoria, Australia), staples and strapping tape. Each participant was provided with a new test bra, two new sets of bra straps (standard width (2.5 cm) and wide (4.5 cm)) and two unused gel strips for hygiene purposes and to eliminate potential effects of wear or washing on the bra straps.

Bra strap discomfort and strap preference

Bra strap discomfort was measured immediately after the running trials using a VAS (rated 0 to 10), whereby 0 represented 'no discomfort' and 10 represented 'worst possible discomfort'. The perceived reason for any bra strap discomfort was also reported, and at the end of the test session, participants selected their most and least preferred bra strap orientation and design.

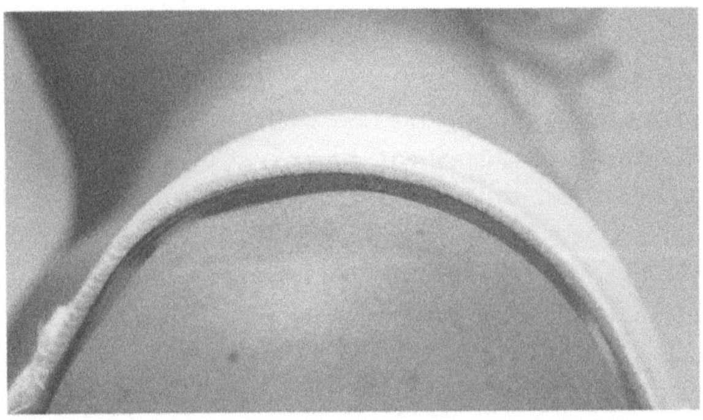

Figure 2 The Dermis Plus Polymer gel pads. These were cut into strips and placed under the standard width bra strap design to create the gel strap design. Each gel pad was cut into four equal 10 cm × 2.5 cm strips, which were positioned end to end and then placed under the standard width bra straps, so that the gel material was flush with the bra strap and in direct contact with the participant's skin.

Bra strap pressure

Strap pressure exerted on the shoulders (bra strap-shoulder interface) was measured while the participants stood stationary and upright prior to running (static condition) and then while they ran on the treadmill (dynamic condition) during each strap condition. Pressure was measured using a custom-designed 10 mm^2 calibrated pressure sensor (0.5 to 24 kPa range, 50 Hz, S2011, Novel GmbH, Munich, Germany) placed under the right bra strap at the crest of each participant's shoulder, where the bra strap traversed the shoulder and exerted a downward force on the sensor. The sensors were secured with micropore surgical tape (3M™ Australia, Sydney, NSW, Australia) and zeroed prior to the 10-s of static pressure data collection, the six 10-s samples during the steady state treadmill running and the 10-s static pressure recording once the running was completed. Pliance-x Expert Online software (Version 10.3, Novel GmbH, Munich, Germany) was used to calculate the average static pressure (kPa), and the average dynamic peak pressure (kPa), which was taken as the average of the six 10-s periods per bra strap condition.

Vertical breast displacement

Vertical breast displacement (VBD; cm) relative to the torso was measured using an Optotrak Certus® motion capture system (200 Hz, Northern Digital, Ontario, Canada) during dynamic treadmill running to determine whether breast motion was consistent among the different strap conditions. Two infrared-emitting diodes (2 mm diameter) were placed on each nipple using double-sided toupee tape (Creative Hair Products, Melbourne, Victoria, Australia), which was placed over micropore surgical tape (3M™ Australia, NSW). A third diode was placed on the sternal notch as a reference point to characterise trunk motion in the vertical plane. Three-dimensional motion of the three markers was recorded during each running trial for six 10-s periods using First Principles software (Version 1.2.2, Northern Digital Inc., Ontario, Canada). The average VBD (minimum from maximum during dynamic treadmill running) relative to the trunk was calculated from a representative 8-s epoch (equivalent to 15 to 20 consecutive breast cycles) for each of the six 10-s data recordings per condition.

Statistical analysis

Frequencies of the questionnaire responses and the bra strap preference data for each bra strap condition were calculated. After confirming the data were normally distributed, means and standard deviations were calculated for, these data, as well as, bra strap pressure and VBD data for each strap condition. A two-way ANOVA design with two within factors (strap orientation and strap design) was then used to determine whether there were any significant main effects or interactions of strap orientation (vertical, cross-back) or strap design (standard width, wide, gel) on the outcome variables, with Tukey *post hoc* analyses used to determine where any significant difference lay. All statistical procedures were conducted using the Statistical Package for the Social Sciences (Version 15.0; SPSS Inc., Chicago, IL, USA).

Results

Bra strap orientation

The bra strap discomfort scores ($p \le 0.001$; Table 1) were significantly less in the vertical strap orientation (0.9 ± 1.2 VAS score) compared to the cross-back strap orientation (1.9 ± 2.1 VAS score). Participants reported greater strap tightness, pressure and 'digging in' in the cross-back strap orientation, despite the correct bra fit and bra strap length (vertical mean length 28.9 cm, range 24.0 to 33.5 cm; cross-back length 35.5 cm, range 28.0 to 41.0 cm). The vertical strap orientation was the most preferred orientation by 70% of participants with reports of 'feelings of less pressure on the trapezius muscle', 'straps did not pull on their shoulder blades' and 'feelings of superior comfort' compared to the cross-back orientation. This was despite no significant difference in the mean or peak strap pressure between the two strap orientations ($p = 0.398$; Table 2).

Bra strap design

There was no significant difference in the bra strap discomfort scores among the three strap designs, although the wide design had the lowest VAS scores (Table 1). Strap preference was similar for the gel and wide designs (gel $n = 11$, 48%; wide $n = 10$, 43%), and the standard width strap was the least preferred design ($n = 13$, 57%; Table 1). When the data were pooled across designs, both the mean static and the dynamic mean peak bra strap pressures were significantly lower in the wide strap design compared to both the standard width and the gel designs ($p < 0.001$). There was no difference in dynamic mean peak pressure between the standard and gel designs ($p > 0.05$; Table 2), although there was a significantly greater mean static pressure in the gel design compared to the standard width design ($p < 0.001$; Table 2). There was no significant difference in VBD among any of the six bra strap conditions (Table 3). Participants' responses to the questionnaire are provided in Table 4.

Table 1 Mean ± standard deviations for strap discomfort and frequency of most and least preferred conditions ($n = 23$)

Strap condition	Bra strap discomfort	Most preferred *n* (%)	Least preferred *n* (%)
Vertical orientation			
Standard	1.4 ± 1.6	1 (4)	5 (22)
Wide	0.5 ± 0.9	8 (35)	0 (0)
Gel	0.7 ± 1.0	7 (31)	2 (9)
Cross-back orientation			
Standard	2.1 ± 2.1*	1 (4)	8 (35)
Wide	1.8 ± 2.3*	2 (9)	7 (30)
Gel	1.9 ± 1.8*	4 (17)	1 (4)

*Indicates a significant main effect of bra strap orientation ($p < 0.05$).

Discussion

Sports medicine practitioners should routinely include breast support assessment and education as an integral part of treating active women, particularly those who experience high frequencies and long durations of breast bounce, or to alleviate the musculoskeletal pains suffered by women with large breasts so they can exercise in comfort [12,26,27]. This study provides evidence for sports medicine practitioners upon which to base recommendations on the bra strap orientation and designs most suitable for their female patients, particularly those with large breasts. As breast support should not be compromised for the sake of greater bra strap comfort, the current study ensured the level of breast support was standardised among the six strap conditions, with no significant between-strap condition difference found in VBD (Table 3).

Bra strap orientation

A vertical bra strap orientation appears to be more suitable for women with large breasts due to the significantly lower strap discomfort and the preference for this orientation compared to the cross-back strap orientation. Although the mean static and dynamic mean peak pressure data were not significantly lower in the vertical bra strap orientation compared to the cross-back orientation, participants consistently reported that the vertical orientation did not 'dig in' or 'create pressure or tension on the trapezius muscle' compared to the cross-back orientation. It is possible that this between-strap orientation difference in perception of pressure, despite the lack of any quantitative difference in strap pressure, may be due to variations in the anatomical structures at the strap/pressure sensor interface. That is, in the vertical orientation, the strap lays across the bone, which is better designed to tolerate compressive forces relative to the muscle tissue at the cross-back orientation strap/pressure sensor interface (upper trapezius muscle) [28]. As the effect of different tissue interfaces on pressure measurements is unknown, this is a recommended topic for future research.

The lack of difference in strap pressure in the two strap orientation conditions was in contrast to the previous study

Table 2 Mean ± standard deviation and confidence interval (CI) values for the mean and peak bra strap pressures (kPa) recorded at the bra strap-shoulder interface for each of the six bra strap conditions ($n = 15$)[a]

	Mean static pressure			Mean peak pressure		
	Mean ± SD	95% CI		Mean ± SD	95% CI	
		Lower bound	Upper bound		Lower bound	Upper bound
Vertical orientation						
Standard	4.3 ± 1.2*	3.7	4.9	9.1 ± 3.6	7.7	10.5
Wide	3.5 ± 1.2*	2.8	4.1	6.2 ± 2.3*	4.8	7.6
Gel	5.6 ± 1.1*	4.9	6.2	10.6 ± 2.4	9.2	12.0
Cross-back orientation						
Standard	4.9 ± 1.5*	4.3	5.5	9.0 ± 2.5	7.6	10.4
Wide	3.2 ± 1.0*	2.5	3.8	5.7 ± 1.5*	4.3	7.1
Gel	5.8 ± 1.2*	5.2	6.4	9.8 ± 3.4	8.4	11.2

*Indicates a significant main effect of bra strap design ($p < 0.05$). [a]Due to technical issues, pressure data were available for only 15 of the 23 participants. This reduced the statistical power of the pressure data to 68%.

of Bowles and Steele [5] that reported higher strap pressures in cross-back orientated straps compared to vertical straps [5]. The mean peak pressures were of a lower range in the current study compared to those reported by Bowles and Steele [5] (current study 5.7 to 10.6 versus 11.7 to 14.9 kPa) [5], which is likely to be attributed to differences in the measurement devices (current study: one 10 mm^2 sensor versus ten 1 cm^2 sensors positioned in parallel) [5]. Ideally, it would be preferable to have the pressure sensors the same width as the bra strap. However, it is also possible that pressures in the cross-back orientation measured by Bowles and Steele [5] were falsely high due to overly tight straps. That is, the straps used by Bowles and Steele [5] were commercially available convertible bra straps of a fixed length, which did not allow for the additional length required to traverse the torso in the cross-back orientation. Tighter straps will cause higher strap pressures and more strap discomfort. An objective measure of strap tension would provide further insight into the strap pressure/discomfort relationship and is a suggested area of study for future research. Irrespective of differences in strap tension, it is imperative that both bra manufacturers and consumers ensure that the strap length is sufficient for bras with a cross-back strap orientation, taking into consideration the wide range of women's torso morphology.

The significantly lower strap discomfort and the strap preference of the vertical orientation compared to the cross-back orientation were also in contrast to previous research [5]. It should be noted, however, that the bra strap discomfort VAS scores for both studies were low, confirming that 3 to 5 min of treadmill running is insufficient to assess the long-term impact of bra strap discomfort; as for this cohort, 63% reported discomfort and problems with the bra straps of their own bras (Tables 1 and 4). Future research should therefore ensure that the duration over which bra strap discomfort and pressure are measured are longer to truly represent times that women wear sports bras while they participate in sport and exercise. Other factors may have also contributed to strap preference, such as the clothing to be worn on top of the

Table 3 Mean ± standard deviation values for right vertical breast displacement (cm) during treadmill running ($n = 23$)

Strap condition	Vertical breast displacement (cm)
Vertical orientation	
Standard	3.3 ± 1.0
Wide	3.2 ± 1.1
Gel	3.3 ± 1.1
Cross-back orientation	
Standard	3.1 ± 1.1
Wide	3.1 ± 1.0
Gel	3.2 ± 1.1

Table 4 Questionnaire responses for the participants ($n = 23$)

Questionnaire response	Number	Percentage (%)
Bra strap orientation of own sports bra		
Vertical	12	52
Cross-back	11	48
Report problems specifically associated with bra straps	15	65
Change bra strap orientation based on clothing worn over bra	8	35
Sacrifice comfort for this change in bra strap orientation	14	61
Report difficulty finding a good sports bra	20	87
Commonly wear more than one bra during exercise	12	52
Have never been professionally fitted for a sports bra	20	87

bra, whether it was acceptable for the bra straps to be visible or not, as well as personal preference. We attempted to control these factors in the current study by assessing personal preference and by recruiting an equal percentage of the participants who reported to commonly wear either strap orientation. Interestingly, 80% of the participants stated that they sacrificed comfort for appearance when changing their bra strap orientation to suit the clothing to be worn over the bra (Table 4).

Bra strap design

A wide strap design, approximately 4.5 cm in width, is more suitable for women with large breasts compared to the standard width (2.5 cm) or a gel strap design for sports bras, as evidenced by the strap preference and the bra strap pressure data. Participants consistently perceived that the wide straps better cushioned the load borne by the straps, which is logical considering the greater surface area over which to distribute the load generated at the bra strap-shoulder interface. This was also evident in the significantly lower mean static and dynamic mean peak pressure recordings in the wider bra strap conditions compared to the other strap conditions [29]. However, although the wide strap design had the lowest VAS scores, no significant difference was found in strap discomfort among the three strap designs, which may also be attributed to the short durations over which the straps were worn.

The gel strap design had some interesting results that warrant further investigation in future research, in particular combining the gel and the wide strap design. The gel design had equivalent strap discomfort and preference compared to the wide strap design, with participants consistently reporting that they 'liked' the feeling of the gel material on their shoulders and felt it 'cushioned' the load borne by the straps. This was despite the gel design having the highest mean bra strap pressure. This apparently conflicting result might have been due to limitations in the pressure measurement device used in the current study. That is, only one sensor was placed at the apex of the shoulder, which in the gel condition may have masked the true effect of the gel pad by limiting the surface area that the gel covered, as the gel pad was placed under the standard width bra strap. Furthermore, pressure data were only extracted for 15 of the 23 participants. Future research should measure bra strap pressure using several pressure sensors placed along the entire length of the bra strap or incorporate the gel within the bra strap. The tacky nature of the gel may also have the potential to decrease strap slippage, a problem reported by 57% of women [30], and which also warrants further investigation.

It is common for women with large breasts to experience tissue deformation at the bra strap-shoulder interface, with deep grooves and tissue tenderness caused by their bra straps. The magnitude of bra strap pressures that may cause this deformation, over the long durations (12 to 14 h/day, for up to 60 or 70 years) that women wear bras for, is unknown. Back-pack strap studies have reported pressures as low as 9 kPa caused by carrying 20-kg back-packs for 2 h can produce skin and subcutaneous soft tissue damage in animal studies [31], as well as cause restrictions in circulation within the upper trapezius muscle [32-34]. The bra strap pressures in the current study were mostly below this magnitude (mean static: 3.2 to 5.8 kPa; mean peak dynamic: 5.7 to 10.6 kPa). When considered, however, from an accumulation perspective, the static bra strap pressures are typically sustained for 12 to 14 h a day over many years with the higher dynamic pressures experienced every time a woman participates in sport and exercise. The magnitude of the mean peak bra strap pressures during the running trials also suggest that the frequency of breast bounce should be considered when advising active women on breast support, regardless of their breast size. That is, the breasts bounce with each heel strike. Therefore, if active women are involved in hours per week of impact activity, which could equate to tens of thousands of breast bounces per week, they should ensure that the bras they wear have straps that are designed to minimise strap pressure in order to reduce development of tissue tenderness and deformation at the bra strap-shoulder interface. Further research is required to investigate the effects of longer durations and higher frequencies of dynamic bra strap pressures on tissue loading and circulation within the upper trapezius muscles in women with a range of breast sizes [31,32].

Conclusions

The current study provides evidence upon which sports medicine practitioners can offer advice regarding bra strap orientations and designs most suitable to minimise bra strap discomfort and pressure in active women, particularly those women with large breasts. Encapsulation sports bras with bra straps that are vertically orientated and wide (approximately 4.5 cm in width) are preferable for women with large breasts to wear during sport and exercise in order to minimise bra strap pressure and discomfort. The addition of gel pads under the bra strap may also decrease discomfort and potentially prevent the strap slipping off the shoulders, although this notion warrants further investigation.

Competing interests
The authors declare that they have no competing interests.

Authors' contributions
CC was the primary investigator. She was responsible for the study design; recruiting the participants; collecting, analysing and interpreting the data, writing the first full draft of the manuscript and approving the final version of the manuscript. DM was a co-supervisor of CC. She was responsible for helping to develop the study design, assisting to interpret the data, providing substantial feedback on versions of the manuscript and approving the final version of the manuscript. JS was a primary supervisor of CC. She

was responsible for helping to develop the study design, assisting to interpret the data, providing substantial feedback on versions of the manuscript, assisting with the figures and approving the final version of the manuscript. All authors read and approved the final manuscript.

Acknowledgements
Funding for this study was provided by the University of Wollongong.

References

1. Findikcioglu K, Findikcioglu F, Ozmen S, Guclu T. The impact of breast size on the vertebral column: a radiologic study. Aesthet Plas Surg. 2007;31:23–7.
2. Greenbaum AR, Heslop T, Morris J, Dunn KW. An investigation of the suitability of bra fit in women referred for reduction mammaplasty. Brit J Plast Surg. 2003;56:230–6.
3. Letterman G, Schurter M. The effects of mammary hypertrophy on the skeletal system. Ann Plas Surg. 1980;5:425–30.
4. Ryan EL. Pectoral girdle myalgia in women: a new function for pectoralis major? Clin J Pain. 2009;25:734–6.
5. Bowles KA, Steele JR. Effects of strap cushions and strap orientation on comfort and sports bra performance. Med Sci Sport Exer. 2013;45:1113–9.
6. Kaye BL. Neurologic changes with excessively large breasts. South Med J. 1972;65:177–80.
7. Goulart Jr R, Detanico D, Vasconcellos RP, Schütz GR, Santos SGD. Reduction mammoplasty improves body posture and decreases the perception of pain. Can J Plast Surg. 2013;21:29–32.
8. Boyd N, Martin L, Charez S, Gunasekara A, Salleh A, Melnichouk O, et al. Breast-tissue composition and other risk factors for breast cancer in young women: a cross-sectional study. Lancet Oncology. 2009;10:569–80.
9. Chun YS, Schwartz MA, Gu X, Lipsitz SR, Carty MJ. Body mass index as a predictor of postoperative complications in reduction mammaplasty. Plast Reconstr Surg. 2012;129:228e–33.
10. Fischer JP, Cleveland EC, Shang EK, Nelson JA, Serletti JM. Complications following reduction mammaplasty: a review of 3538 cases from the 2005–2010 NSQIP data sets. Aesthet Surg J. 2014;34:66–73.
11. Shah R, Al-Ajam Y, Stott D, Kang N. Obesity in mammaplasty: a study of complications following breast reduction. J Plast Reconstr Aes. 2011;64:508–14.
12. Coltman KA, McGhee DE, Harland DL, Steele JR. Does breast size affect posture? Conference Proceedings of the 24th Congress of the International Society of Biomechanics. Natal, Brazil. 2013.
13. Haahr M. List Randomizer. 2012. http://www.random.org/lists/. Accessed April 2012.
14. Lorentzen D, Lawson L. Selected sports bras: a biomechanical analysis of breast motion while jogging. Physician Sportsmed. 1987;15:128–39.
15. McGhee DE, Steele JR. Optimising breast support in female patients through correct bra fit. A cross-sectional study. J Sci Med Sport. 2010;13:568–72.
16. Starr C, Branson D, Shehab R, Farr C, Ownbey S, Swinney J. Biomechanical analysis of a prototype sports bra. JTATM. 2005;4:1-14.
17. Spencer L, Briffa K. Breast size, thoracic kyphosis & thoracic spine pain - association & relevance of bra fitting in post-menopausal women: a correlational study. Chiropr Man Therap. 2013;21:20-4.
18. Dundas KL, Atyeo J, Cox J. What is a large breast? Measuring and categorizing breast size for tangential breast radiation therapy. Australas Radiol. 2007;51:589–93.
19. McGhee DE, Steele JR. Breast elevation and compression decrease exercise-induced breast discomfort. Med Sci Sport Exer. 2010;42:1333–8.
20. McGhee DE, Steele JR, Zealey WJ, Takacs GJ. Bra-breast forces generated in women with large breasts while standing and during treadmill running: implications for sports bra design. App Ergon. 2013;44:112–8.
21. McGhee DE, Steele JR. Exercise and breast support. Breast Research Australia (BRA) with Sports Medicine Australia Wollongong (NSW). Albert Park, Australia: Sports Medicine Australia; 2012.
22. McGhee DE, Steele JR, Sports MB, Fitness B. Sports bra fitness. Wollongong (NSW): Breast Research Australia (BRA); 2008.
23. ACSM. 2008 Physical Activity Guidelines for Americans: U.S. Department of Health and Human Services; 2008. http://www.health.gov/paguidelines/pdf/paguide.pdf Accessed April 2012.
24. National Health and Medical Research Council, Australian Research Council, Australian Vice-Chancellors' Committee. National Statement on Ethical Conduct in Human Research. Australian Government. 2007. http://www.nhmrc.gov.au/health-ethics/human-research-ethics-committees-hrecs/human-research-ethics-committees-hrecs/national. Accessed April 2012.
25. Lee NA, Rusinek H, Weinreb J, Chandra R, Toth H, Singer C, et al. Fatty and fibroglandular tissue volumes in the breasts of women 20-83 years old: comparison of X-ray mammography and computer-assisted MR imaging. Am J Roentgenol. 1997;168:501–6.16.
26. BeLieu RM. Mastodynia. Obstet Gyn Clin N AM. 1994;21:461–77.
27. Ryan EL. Pectoral girdle myalgia in women: a 5-year study in a clinical setting. Clin J Pain. 2000;16:298–303.
28. Oatis CA. Kinesiology: the mechanics and pathomechanics of human movement. 2nd ed. Philadelphia: Lippincott Williams & Wilkins; 2009.
29. Zhou J. New methods of evaluating breast motion in braless and sports bra conditions. Hong Kong (China): Institute of Textiles and Clothing, The Hong Kong Polytechnic University; 2011.
30. Bowles KA, Steele JR, Munro BJ. Features of sports bras that deter their use by Australian women. J Sci Med Sport. 2012;15:195–200.
31. Linder-Ganz E, Engelberg S, Scheinowitz M, Gefen A. Pressure-time cell death threshold for albino rat skeletal muscles as related to pressure sore biomechanics. J Biomech. 2006;39:2725–32.
32. Hadid A, Epstein Y, Shabshin N, Gefen A. Modeling mechanical strains and stresses in soft tissues of the shoulder during load carriage based on load-bearing open MRI. Appl Physiol. 2012;112:597–606.
33. Mackie HW, Stevenson JM, Reid SA, Legg SJ. The effect of simulated school load carriage configurations on shoulder strap tension forces and shoulder interface pressure. Appl Ergon. 2005;36:199–206.
34. Vacheron JJ, Poumarat G, Chandezon R, Vanneuville G. The effect of loads carried on the shoulders. Mil Med. 1999;164:597–9.

Permissions

All chapters in this book were first published in SMO, by Springer; hereby published with permission under the Creative Commons Attribution License or equivalent. Every chapter published in this book has been scrutinized by our experts. Their significance has been extensively debated. The topics covered herein carry significant findings which will fuel the growth of the discipline. They may even be implemented as practical applications or may be referred to as a beginning point for another development.

The contributors of this book come from diverse backgrounds, making this book a truly international effort. This book will bring forth new frontiers with its revolutionizing research information and detailed analysis of the nascent developments around the world.

We would like to thank all the contributing authors for lending their expertise to make the book truly unique. They have played a crucial role in the development of this book. Without their invaluable contributions this book wouldn't have been possible. They have made vital efforts to compile up to date information on the varied aspects of this subject to make this book a valuable addition to the collection of many professionals and students.

This book was conceptualized with the vision of imparting up-to-date information and advanced data in this field. To ensure the same, a matchless editorial board was set up. Every individual on the board went through rigorous rounds of assessment to prove their worth. After which they invested a large part of their time researching and compiling the most relevant data for our readers.

The editorial board has been involved in producing this book since its inception. They have spent rigorous hours researching and exploring the diverse topics which have resulted in the successful publishing of this book. They have passed on their knowledge of decades through this book. To expedite this challenging task, the publisher supported the team at every step. A small team of assistant editors was also appointed to further simplify the editing procedure and attain best results for the readers.

Apart from the editorial board, the designing team has also invested a significant amount of their time in understanding the subject and creating the most relevant covers. They scrutinized every image to scout for the most suitable representation of the subject and create an appropriate cover for the book.

The publishing team has been an ardent support to the editorial, designing and production team. Their endless efforts to recruit the best for this project, has resulted in the accomplishment of this book. They are a veteran in the field of academics and their pool of knowledge is as vast as their experience in printing. Their expertise and guidance has proved useful at every step. Their uncompromising quality standards have made this book an exceptional effort. Their encouragement from time to time has been an inspiration for everyone.

The publisher and the editorial board hope that this book will prove to be a valuable piece of knowledge for researchers, students, practitioners and scholars across the globe.

List of Contributors

Paolo T. Pianosi
Department of Pediatric and Adolescent Medicine, Mayo Clinic, 200 First St. SW, Rochester, MN 55905, USA

Zhen Zhang
Department of Statistics, University of Chicago, Eckhart 7 #5. 5734 S. University Avenue, Chicago, IL 60637, USA

Marianne Huebner
Department of Statistics and Probability, Michigan State University, 619 Red Cedar Rd, Rm C422 Wells Hall, East Lansing, MI 48824, USA

Paul Hernandez
Department of Medicine, Queen Elizabeth II Health Sciences Centre and Dalhousie University, 1796 Summer Street Halifax, Halifax B3H 4G2 NS, Canada

Tom Porter and Alison Rushton
School of Sport, Exercise and Rehabilitation Sciences, College of Life and Environmental Sciences, University of Birmingham, Edgbaston, Birmingham B15 2TT, UK

Hailee L Wingfield, Abbie E Smith-Ryan, Malia N Melvin, Erica J Roelofs, Eric T Trexler, Anthony C Hackney and Eric D Ryan
Department of Exercise and Sport Science, University of North Carolina, 209 Fetzer Hall, CB #8700, Chapel Hill, NC 27599-8700, USA

Anthony C Hackney
Department of Nutrition - Gillings School of Global Public Health, University of North Carolina, Chapel Hill, NC, USA

Mark A Weaver
Departments of Medicine and Biostatistics, University of North Carolina, Chapel Hill, NC, USA

Robert Buresh
Department of Exercise Science and Sport Management, Kennesaw State University, 520 Parliament Garden Way NW, Kennesaw, GA 30144, USA

Kris Berg
School of Health, Physical Education, and Recreation, University of Nebraska at Omaha, Omaha, NE, USA

François Potdevin
Univ. Lille, EA 7369 - URePSSS - Unité de Recherche Pluridisciplinaire Sport Santé Société, F-59000 Lille, France

Gilles Vanlerberghe
Univ. Littoral Côte d'Opale, Département STAPS, F- 62100 Calais, France

Gautier Zunquin, Thierry Pezé and Denis Theunynck
Univ. Littoral Côte d'Opale, EA 7369 - URePSSS - Unité de Recherche Pluridisciplinaire Sport Santé Société, F-59144 Dunkerque, France

Martin D Hoffman
Department of Physical Medicine & Rehabilitation, Department of Veterans Affairs, Northern California Health Care System, and University of California Davis Medical Center, 10535 Hospital Way, Sacramento, CA, USA

Kristin J Stuempfle
Health Sciences Department, Gettysburg College, Gettysburg, PA, USA

Viola C Altmann
Rehabilitation Centre, Sint Maartenskliniek, P.O. Box 90116500 GM Nijmegen, The Netherlands

Anne L Hart
Department of Physical Therapy and Athlete Training, Northern Arizona University, Flagstaff, Arizona, USA

Yves C Vanlandewijck
Department of Rehabilitation sciences, Katholieke Universiteit Leuven, Leuven, Belgium

Jacques van Limbeek
Achmea Health Insurance Company, Amersfoort, The Netherlands

Miranda L van Hooff
Sint Maartenskliniek, Research, Nijmegen, The Netherlands

Karim Chamari
Athlete Health and Performance Research Centre, ASPETAR, Qatar Orthopaedic and Sports Medicine Hospital, Doha, Qatar

Johnny Padulo
University e-Campus, Via Isimbardi, 10-22060 Novedrate, CO, Italy
Tunisian Research Laboratory "Sports Performance Optimization", National Center of Medicine and Science in Sports, Tunis, Tunisia

Ruben Tobias Goebel
Sport Science Program, Qatar University, P.O. Box 2713, Doha, Qatar

Heinz Kleinöder and Joachim Mester
Institute of Training Science and Sport Informatics, German Sport University Cologne, Cologne, Germany

Zengyuan Yue
The German Research Center, Center of Elite Sport, German Sport University Cologne, Cologne, Germany

Ranajay Gosh
Department of Mechanical and Industrial Engineering, Northeastern University, Boston, MA, USA

John Singhammer
Department of Physiotherapy, VIA University College, Hedeager 2, DK8200 Aarhus, Denmark

Mathias Ried-Larsen, Niels Christian Møller, Peter Lund-Kristensen, Karsten Froberg and Lars Bo Andersen
Institute of Sports Science and Clinical Biomechanics, Centre of Research in Childhood Health, University of Southern Denmark, Odense, Denmark

Sebastian Bohm, Falk Mersmann and Adamantios Arampatzis
Department of Training and Movement Sciences, Humboldt-Universität zu Berlin, Philippstr 13, Haus 11, 10115 Berlin, Germany

Ricardo J. S. Costa, Rhiannon Snipe and Vera Camões-Costa
Department of Nutrition & Dietetics, Monash University, Notting Hill, Victoria, Australia

Volker Scheer
British Forces Germany Health Services, Paderborn, Germany

Andrew Murray
Centre of Sports & Exercise, Edinburgh University, Edinburgh, UK

Terry K. Morgan and Emilie Jensen
Department of Pathology, Oregon Health & Science University, 3181 SW Sam Jackson, Mail Code L-471, Portland, OR 97239, USA

Jeong Lim
Department of Public Health & Preventative Medicine, Oregon Health & Science University, Portland, OR, USA

Russell Riggs
Reflex Clinic, Portland, OR, USA

Lindy-Lee Folscher, Catharina C Grant and Dina Christina Janse van Rensberg
Section Sports Medicine, Faculty of Health Sciences, University of Pretoria, Hatfield, Pretoria 0002, South Africa

Lizelle Fletcher
Department of Statistics, University of Pretoria, Hatfield, Pretoria 0002, South Africa

Chun-Jung Huang, Aaron L. Slusher and J. Thomas Mock
Exercise Biochemistry Laboratory, Department of Exercise Science and Health Promotion, Florida Atlantic University, 777 Glades Road, FH11A-126B, Boca Raton, FL 33431, USA

Matthew J. McAllister
Department of Kinesiology, Mississippi State University, Starkville, MS, USA

Edmund O. Acevedo and Aaron L. Slusher
Department of Kinesiology and Health Sciences, Virginia Commonwealth University, Richmond, VA, USA

Heather E. Webb
Department of Kinesiology, Texas A&M University-Corpus Christi, Corpus
Christi, TX, USA

K L Morgan
Department of Musculoskeletal Biology, Institute of Ageing and Chronic Disease, University of Liverpool, Leahurst Campus, Neston CH64 7TE, UK

C M Inness and K L Morgan
School of Veterinary Sciences, University of Liverpool, Leahurst Campus, Neston CH64 7TE, UK

Mark D Griffiths
Nottingham Trent University, Nottingham, UK

Attila Szabo
Institute of Health Promotion and Sport Sciences, Faculty of Education and Psychology, Eötvös
Loránd University, Budapest, Hungary

Mia B Lichtenstein
University of Southern Denmark, Odense, Denmark

Ricardo de la Vega and Roberto Ruiz-Barquín
Autonomous University of Madrid, Madrid, Spain

Jason Youngman
University of Miami, Coral Gables, FL, USA

Robert Urbán, Zsolt Demetrovics and Bernadette Kun
Institute of Psychology, Faculty of Education and Psychology, Eötvös Loránd University, Budapest, Hungary

Myosotis Massidda, Valeria Bachis, Laura Corrias, Claudia Culigioni and Carla M Calò
Department of Life and Environmental Sciences, University of Cagliari, SS 554, km 4.500, Monserrato 09042, Italy

Francesco Piras and Marco Scorcu
FMSI CR Sardegna and Cagliari Calcio SpA, Viale Tiziano, Cagliari 70-00196, Italy

Daniele Masala
University of Cassino, Viale dell'Università, Cassino 03043, Italy

Rich D Johnston and Tim J Gabbett
School of Exercise Science, Australian Catholic University, Brisbane, Queensland 4014, Australia

Tim J Gabbett and David G Jenkins
School of Human Movement Studies, University of Queensland, Brisbane, Queensland 4072, Australia

George P Nassis and João R Silva
National Sports Medicine Programme Excellence in Football Project, Aspetar-Qatar Orthopaedic and Sports Medicine Hospital, P.O BOX 29222, Doha, Qatar

João R Silva and Antonio Rebelo
Center of Research, Education, Innovation and Intervention in Sport (CIFI2D), Porto, Portugal

Edith Van Dyck, Bart Moens, Jeska Buhmann, Michiel Demey, Esther Coorevits, and Marc Leman
IPEM, Department of Arts, Music and Theatre Sciences, Ghent University, Technicum Blok 2, Sint-Pietersnieuwstraat 41, Ghent, Belgium

Simone Dalla Bella
EuroMov, Movement 2 Health Laboratory (M2H), University of Montpellier, 700 Avenue du Pic Saint Loup, Montpellier, France

Sigal Ben-Zaken, Moran Rabinovich and Yoav Meckel
Genetics and Molecular Biology Laboratory, The Zinman College of Physical Education and Sports Sciences at the Wingate Institute, Netanya 42902, Israel

Alon Eliakim and Dan Nemet
Child Health and Sports Center, Pediatric Department, Meir Medical Center, Sackler School of Medicine, Tel-Aviv University, Tel-Aviv, Israel

Eias Kassem
Pediatric Department, Hillel-Yafe Medical Center, Hadera, Israel

Donald A Redelmeier and David A Alter
Institute for Clinical Evaluative Sciences, 2075 Bayview Avenue, Toronto, ON M4N 3M5, Canada

David A Alter, Mary O'Sullivan, Susan Marzolini, Paul I Oh, Richard Liu, Mary Forhan, Michael Silver and Jack M Goodman
University Health Network Cardiovascular Prevention and Rehabilitation Program, Toronto Rehabilitation Institute-University Health Network, 550 University Avenue, Toronto, Canada

Donald A Redelmeier
Sunnybrook Health Sciences, 2075 Bayview Avenue, Toronto, Canada

Paul I Oh, Donald A Redelmeier and David A Alter
Department of Medicine, University of Toronto, 27 King's College Circle, Toronto, Canada

Jack M Goodman
Department of Exercise Sciences, Faculty of Physical Education and Health, University of Toronto, 27 King's College Circle, Toronto, Canada

Lee R Bartel
Music and Health Research Collaboratory, Faculty of Music, University of Toronto, 80 Queens Park, Toronto, Canada
Dean's Office, Faculty of Music, University of Toronto, 80 Queens Park, Toronto, Canada

David A Alter and Redelmeier
Department of Health Policy, Management and Evaluation, University of Toronto, 40 St George Street, Toronto, Canada

Mary Forhan
Faculty of Rehabilitation Medicine, The University of Alberta, 8205 114 Street, Alberta, Canada

David A Alter, Mary O'Sullivan, Paul I Oh, Donald A Redelmeier, Susan Marzolini, Richard Liu, Mary Forhan, Michael Silver, Jack M Goodman and Lee R Bartel
The University of Toronto, 27 King's College Circle, Toronto, Canada

Thierry Paillard
Département STAPS, Université de Pau et des Pays de l'Adour, ZA Bastillac Sud, 11 rue Morane Saulnier, 65000 Tarbes, France

Jamie F. Burr
Human Performance Laboratory, University of Guelph, 50 Stone Road East, Guelph, Ontario N1G 2W1, Canada

Jamie F. Burr, Joshua T. Slysz and Matthew S. Boulter
Human Performance and Health Research Laboratory, University of PEI, Charlottetown, Canada

Darren E. R. Warburton
Cardiovascular Physiology and Rehabilitation Laboratory, University of British Columbia, Vancouver, Canada

Srdjan Lemez and Joseph Baker
School of Kinesiology and Health Science, York University, 4700 Keele Street, Toronto M3J 1P3, ON, Canada

Celeste E Coltman, Deirdre E McGhee and Julie R Steele
Biomechanics Research Laboratory, University of Wollongong, Northfields Avenue, Wollongong, New South Wales 2522, Australia